D1072389

Children's Nutrition

The Jones and Bartlett Series in Nursing

Basic Steps in Planning Nursing Research,
Third Edition
Brink/Wood

Bone Marrow Transplantation
Whedon

Cancer Chemotherapy: A Nursing Process Approach
Burke et al.

Cancer Nursing: Principles and Practice,
Second Edition
Groenwald et al.

Chronic Illness: Impact and Intervention,
Second Edition
Lubkin

Clinical Nursing Procedures
Belland/Wells

Comprehensive Maternity Nursing, Second Edition
Auvenshine/Enriquez

Critical Elements for Nursing Preoperative Practice
Fairchild

Emergency Care of Children
Thompson

Fundamentals of Nursing with Clinical Procedures, Second Edition
Sundberg

1991-1992 Handbook of Intravenous Medications
Nentwich

Health Assessment in Nursing Practice,
Second Edition
Grimes/Burns

Healthy People 2000
U.S. Department of Health & Human Services

Human Development: A Life-Span Approach,
Third Edition
Frieberg

Intravenous Therapy
Nentwich

Introduction to the Health Professions
Stanfield

Management and Leadership for Nurse Managers
Swansburg

Management of Spinal Cord Injury,
Second Edition
Zejdlik

Medical Terminology: Principles and Practices
Stanfield

Mental Health and Psychiatric Nursing
Davies/Janosik

The Nation's Health, Third Edition
Lee/Estes

Nursing Assessment, A Multidimensional Approach, Second Edition
Bellack/Bamford

Nursing Diagnosis Care Plans for Diagnosis-Related Groups
Neal/Paquette/Mirch

Nursing Management of Children
Servonsky/Opas

Nursing Research: A Quantitative and Qualitative Approach
Roberts/Burke

Nutrition and Diet Therapy: Self-Instructional Modules
Stanfield

Psychiatric Mental Health Nursing,
Second Edition
Janosik/Davies

Writing a Succesful Grant Application,
Second Edition
Reif-Lehrer

Children's Nutrition

Fima Lifshitz, M.D., F.A.C.N.
Nancy Moses Finch, M.N.S., R.D.
Jere Ziffer Lifshitz, B.S.N., R.N.

Department of Pediatrics
North Shore University Hospital—
Cornell University Medical College
Manhasset, New York

JONES AND BARTLETT PUBLISHERS
BOSTON

Editorial, Sales, and Customer Service Offices
Jones and Bartlett Publishers
20 Park Plaza
Boston, MA 02116

Library of Congress Cataloging-in-Publication Data

Lifshitz, Fima, 1938-
Children's nutrition / by Fima Lifshitz, Nancy Moses Finch, Jere Ziffer Lifshitz.
p. cm.
Includes bibliographical references and index.
ISBN 0-86720-186-X
1. Children—Nutrition. 2. Diet therapy for children. 3. Pregnancy—Nutritional aspects. I. Finch, Nancy Moses. II. Lifshitz, Jere Ziffer. III. Title.
[DNLM: 1. Child Nutrition. 2. Diet Therapy—in infancy & childhood. 3. Infant Nutrition. 4. Nutrition—in adolescence. 5. Nutrition—in pregnancy. WS 115 L722c]
RJ206.L515 1991
613.2'083—dc20
DLC
for Library of Congress 91-7011
CIP

Cover design: Hannus Design Associates
Interior design: Rafael Millán

Cover art: *Breakfast in Bed* by Mary Cassatt. From the Virginia Steel Scott Collection, Huntington Library and Art Gallery.
Photo credits: Page xiv, courtesy of Rafael Millan; pages 82 and 494, courtesy of Tufts Health Sciences Center, Tufts University, Boston; page 250, courtesy of New England Medical Center, Boston.

Printed in the United States of America
95 94 93 92 91 10 9 8 7 6 5 4 3 2 1

To those who nourish and nurture us

Table of Contents

Part III: Nutrition for Special Needs

Part IV: High-Tech Nutrition

Preface

Lori is 15 pounds overweight. She has decided not to gain much weight during her pregnancy "to keep in shape." Lori read that she can "get away with little weight gain during pregnancy without adversely affecting the baby."

Robert's baby is one month old and is spitting up. He calls his mother-in-law, who advises him to "put some cereal in the baby's bottle; it will make the formula heavier and more likely to stay down."

On a television commercial, a very thin model with bulging eyes says that her pharmacist has recommended diet pills to lose weight.

A woman about 7 months pregnant on a television commercial is working out in a gym with a can of diet soda in one hand. . . .

A kind old country storekeeper is the object of a little girl's admiration. "You sure know a lot 'bout 'trition, Mr. Green," she says after he informs her in this commercial that canned vegetables have as many vitamins and minerals as fresh ones.

These are some real examples that represent the fact that the public often receives its nutrition information from advertisements and self-proclaimed nutrition experts. Many health care professionals may even advise their patients on nutritional practices without giving much thought to the individual's medical status and with little knowledge of the complex subject of nutrition. At best, the person receiving the misinformation will simply not receive optimal nutrition. At worst, a life, or a potential life, will be jeopardized.

The goal of this book is to provide the reader with accurate facts about current concepts in children's nutrition in an easily understood style. The book, written with the health care professionals in mind, procures the theories of nutrition to practice better health care of children from conception through adolescence, in health and in disease. The nutrition knowledge to date is reviewed in simple terms and presented in a manner that may facilitate physicians to impart nutrition concepts to their patients and may encourage lay persons to read this book. All the chapters systematically expose the process of nutritional analysis, leading to pertinent conclusions and practical information needed for appropriate counseling. It was written by a pediatrician, a nutritionist, and a nurse, whose objectives are to present accurate information in a straightforward manner to distinguish between the myths and realities of the many nutrition issues that often worry parents and affect children's health and well being.

Fima Lifshitz, M.D.

Foreword

This book is both current and complete and covers in detail the most important areas in children's nutrition from pregnancy through early childhood and adolescence. The book is designed for health care professionals. It is extremely comprehensive not only in the material it covers but also in the references cited. Equally impressive is the simple, straightforward, and easily understandable style of the authors. This makes it a useful book for reading by anyone interested in nutrition and health including the general public. Thus, this book should be an important resource for your personal reference library. Anyone needing to look up an important fact relating to nutrition in pregnancy and childhood should be able to find it easily. The authors not only tell the reader *what* is important but also *why* it is important; and then, perhaps more importantly, what foods in what quantities are most appropriate in a given situation. This book will make good reading both for persons with a serious interest in nutrition and those with only a casual interest.

Myron Winick, M.D.
President
Distinguished Professor of Pediatrics and Nutrition
University of Health Sciences/The Chicago Medical School

Acknowledgments

The expertise and dedication of Amy Karr made writing this book so much easier, and we are very grateful to her. We also acknowledge the secretarial assistance of Carol Meisner and the contribution of Marie Fasano on Chapter 18, and of Pat Larsen on Chapter 14, and the comments on the book by Melanie Smith. In addition, we recognize and salute the support of all our associates and personnel of the Division of Pediatric Endocrinology, Metabolism and Nutrition of North Shore University Hospital–Cornell University Medical College.

This book came about while on a fellowship at Bellagio Study Center, the Rockefeller Foundation, Villa Serbelloni, Bellagio, Italy. There the book was seeded and drafted . . . but the long evenings after dusk and the mornings before dawn in New York and Great Barrington brought about the polished final version.

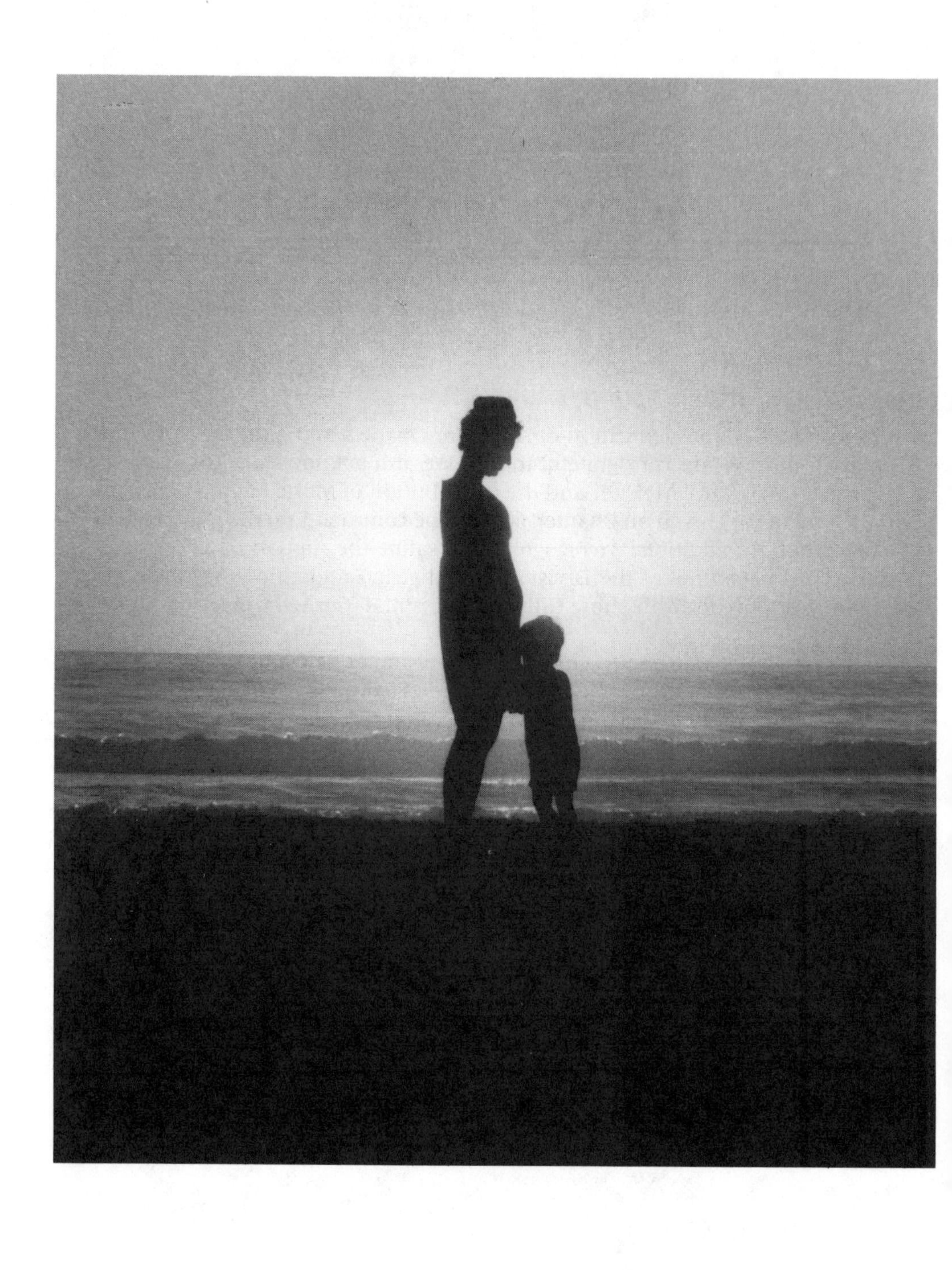

PART I

Nutrition Before the Baby Is Born

1

Mother's and Baby's Weight Gain During Pregnancy

Nutrition myths during pregnancy seem to haunt us from one generation to the next. It has long been the fashion in some circles that a pregnant woman who is overweight should gain no weight during pregnancy, and that weight gain should be restricted during pregnancy for all women. For centuries, it has been known that this practice of dietary restriction may lead to tragic results. In 1817, obstetrician Sir Richard Croft regularly bled his patient, Princess Charlotte, and prescribed a "low diet" during pregnancy. The princess died soon after the delivery of her stillborn son. In the early 1900s, obstetrician Ludwig Prochownick recommended semistarvation of the mother because "curtailment of food would produce a small, light-weight baby easier to deliver." Even in these modern times, mothers are often admonished by their doctors not to gain much weight.

Pregnancy is no time to diet!

MATERNAL WEIGHT GAIN

Most authorities currently recommend that pregnant women receive ample nutrients to achieve optimal anabolism during pregnancy (Brown 1988). The mother-to-be who has an appropriate weight gain during pregnancy can be assured that both she and her baby are adequately nourished. The National Research Council Committee on Maternal Nutrition and the Committee on Nutrition of the American College of Obstetrics and Gynecology recommend a gain of about 24.2 pounds (11 kg) for women who start pregnancy at a normal weight. A recently published investigation showed that in a sample of almost 3000 women, the mean weight gain during pregnancy was somewhat greater, at 33.6 pounds (15.3 kg) (Abrams & Laros 1986).

During the first trimester, total gain should be about 4 pounds (1.8 kg). During the second and third trimesters, weight gain is greater, usually 9 and 10 pounds, respectively (4.1 and 4.3 kg). The best reproductive performance is associated with a weight gain of a little less than 20 pounds (9 kg) in the last half of pregnancy—that is, a weight gain of 1.0 pound (0.45 kg) per week. Women who have had several pregnancies gain about 2 pounds (0.9 kg) less than women during their first pregnancy. The distribution of 30 pounds (13.6 kg) of weight gain is shown in Figure 1–1 (Hytten & Leitch 1971).

These rates of weight gain are meant for women who start pregnancy with a normal body weight. To monitor weight gain during pregnancy, a standard graph has typically been used (Fig. 1–2). However, this chart may underestimate necessary weight gain for the underweight woman and overestimate weight gain for an overweight or obese mother-to-be. Women with a below-normal prepregnancy weight should gain more weight during pregnancy to ensure delivery of a healthy baby. In contrast, overweight or obese mothers-to-be should gain less during pregnancy, but must gain weight nonetheless (Fig. 1–3).

According to Naeye (1979), the optimal weight gain associated with the lowest perinatal mortality rates is 30 pounds (13.6 kg) for very thin mothers, 20 pounds (9.1 kg) for normally proportioned mothers, and 16 pounds (7.3 kg) for overweight mothers. The perinatal mortality rates increase when mothers gain more than 32 pounds (14.5 kg) at term, regardless of their weight prior to pregnancy. Thus, very high or very low pregnancy weight gains are usually associated with mortality rates that are increased several-fold.

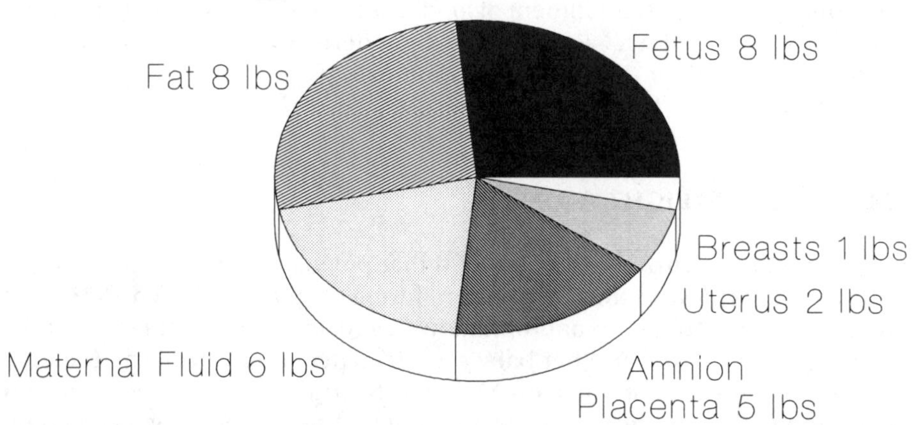

Figure 1–1. Distribution of weight gain during pregnancy (30 pounds [13.6 kg]).

Data derived from Hytten FE, Leitch I. The physiology of human pregnancy. 2nd ed. London: Blackwell, 1971:265–387.

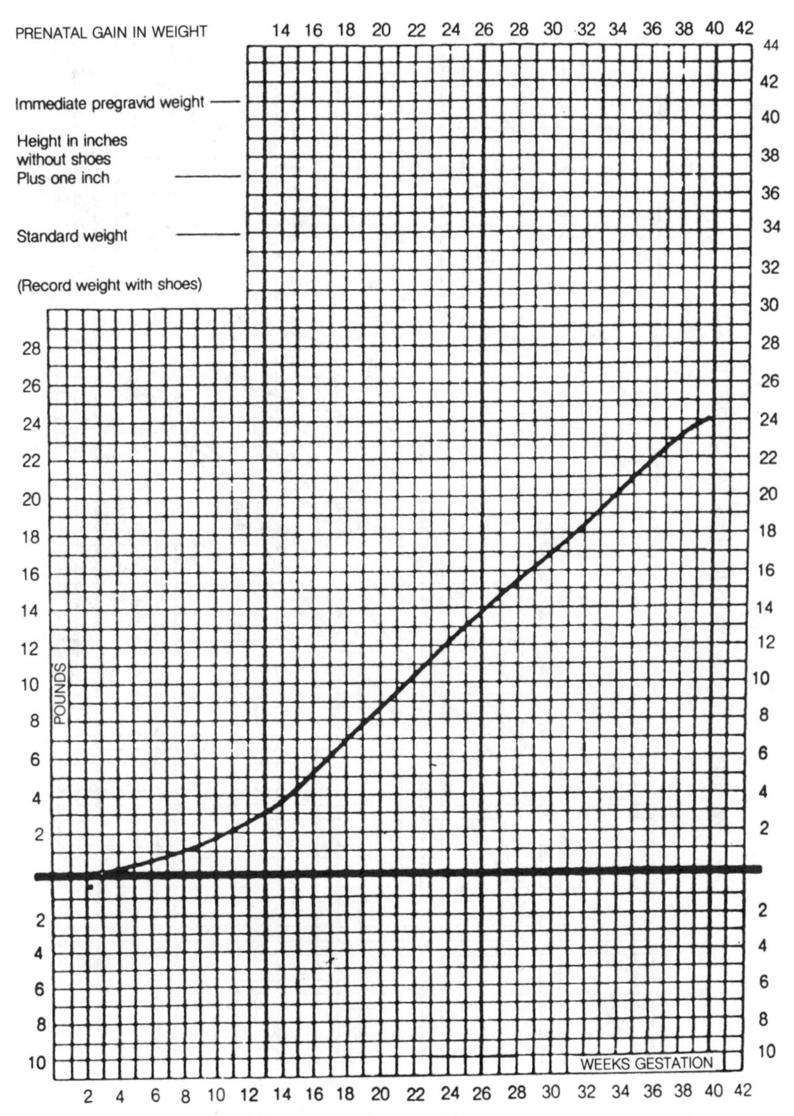

Figure 1–2. Chart to monitor weight gain during pregnancy for women at their appropriate weight for height prior to pregnancy.

Reprinted with permission from Clinical Obstetrics, eds. Clifford B. Lull & Robert A. Timbrough, 1953, J.B. Lippincott and Co., Philadelphia, Pa.

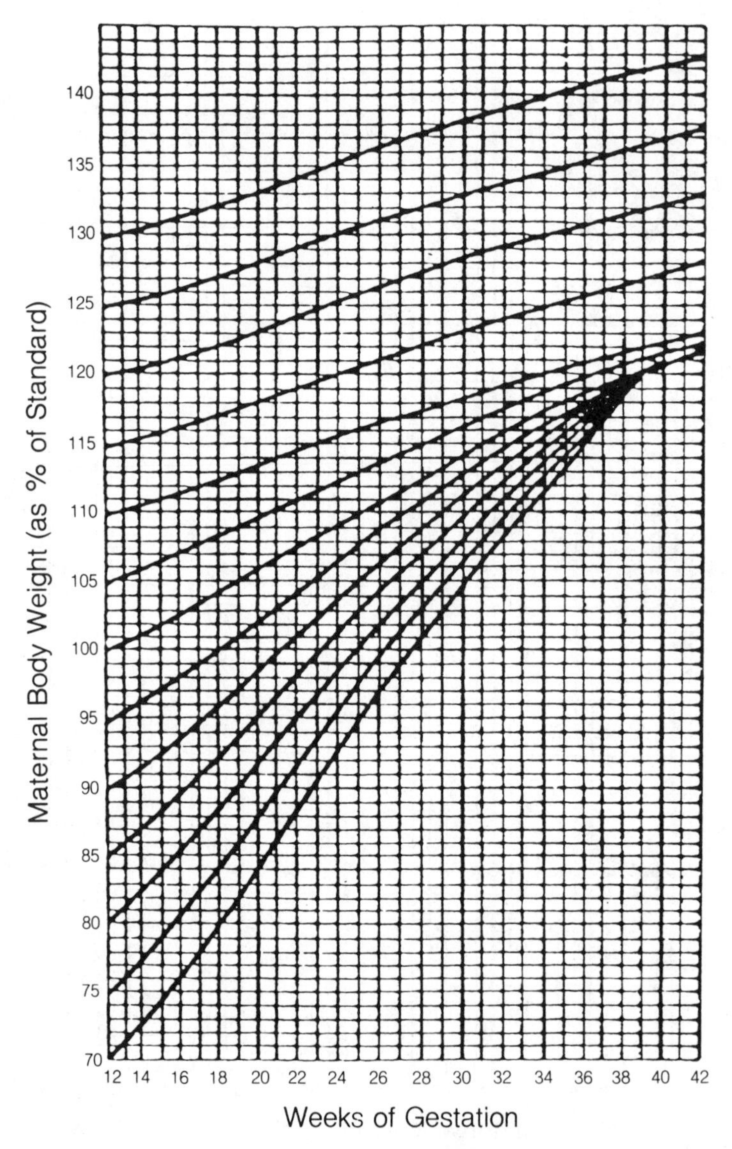

Figure 1–3. Chart to monitor weight gain during pregnancy considering pre-pregnancy weight and height. Maternal body weight as a percent of standard is calculated as follows: Actual Body Weight/Ideal Body Weight × 100.

Reprinted with permission from Rosso P. A new chart to monitor weight gain during pregnancy. Am J Clin Nutr 1985; 41:644–652. © Am J Clin Nutr American Society for Clinical Nutrition.

The amount of weight gain necessary for optimum outcome of twin gestations has not been determined. In general, maternal weight gain in twin pregnancies mimics that of singleton pregnancies during the first trimester but increases in the subsequent trimesters, with total weight gains ranging from 32 to 80 pounds (14.5 to 36.4 kg) (Leonard 1982, Campbell 1986, Worthington-Roberts 1988). In healthy women who were pregnant with twins, mean maternal weight gain of 44 pounds (20 kg) was associated with optimal outcomes, whereas mothers who gained 37 pounds (16.8 kg) had less than optimum outcomes. Limited information is available on ideal maternal weight gain with triplet gestations.

Whereas most of the overall weight gain occurs during the latter half of pregnancy, maternal fat stores are deposited by midpregnancy. The so-called centripetal fat deposits are noticeable early during the first half of pregnancy and may account for up to 9 pounds (4.1 kg). This fat is capable of supplying approximately 35,000 calories, which is sufficient to sustain fetal growth in the last trimester of pregnancy. At that time the fetus more than doubles its weight, from an average of 3.3 pounds (1.5 kg) at 30 weeks' gestation to over 6 pounds (3.3 kg) at 40 weeks' gestation. Thus, more than 40 percent of the maximum energy required to support the routine pregnancy can be found in the fat deposited as maternal stores in early pregnancy.

In addition to prepregnancy weight and multiple-birth pregnancies, other factors need to be considered to interpret the data on maternal weight gain and pregnancy outcome (Lederman 1985). The health of the woman and her age, parity, and nutritional history are important. It is also necessary to distinguish between overweight due to obesity and overweight related to a large, lean body mass, as would be seen in some very muscular women. Increased body fluid is a third possible cause for excessive weight gain.

RISKS OF DIETING

The risks of dieting during pregnancy associated with inadequate weight gain have been generally underemphasized. Mothers-to-be who diet may be subject to deficiencies of essential nutrients in addition to insufficient energy intake and thereby have an increased risk of delivering a low-birth-weight infant. However, they may have other complications, such as toxemia, characterized by hypertension and fluid retention (edema) (preeclampsia) (see Chapter 6). This complication may develop in women who are markedly underweight at conception and who fail to gain weight normally during the antenatal period (Belizan & Villar 1980, Schulman 1982). Pregnant women who diet and gain small amounts of weight during pregnancy have twice the perinatal mortality rates of overweight mothers who have somewhat larger weight gains.

Dieting during pregnancy adversely affects infant mortality (Chez 1979, Coetzee, Jackson & Berman 1980, Naeye & Chez 1981) by creating a metabolic derangement that results in catabolism of fat stores. This leads to ketosis (accumulation of fat breakdown products) and other metabolic abnormalities, including hypoglycemia and hypoinsulinemia, which develop sooner and are more severe in fasting pregnant women than in fasting nonpregnant women. Changes in the maternal blood glucose and ketone levels are mirrored in the amniotic fluid, creating an abnormal environment for the fetus. The presence of maternal ketosis may impair fetal neurologic development (Dobbing 1985). Children born to such mothers have been found to have lower I.Q. scores at 4 years of age even without any alterations in the birth weight (Chez 1979, Coetzee, Jackson & Berman 1980), but others did not confirm these observations (Naeye & Chez 1981). Women with ketosis also have been reported to have a significant increase in the perinatal mortality rate. Ketosis is often seen in pregnant women who lost weight or whose weight gain was less than 25 percent of the recommended level.

There is a consensus among experts that there is no advantage in prescribing weight-reduction regimens for obese patients during pregnancy; weight reduction should be undertaken only after delivery. A much greater emphasis should be placed on the value of a good diet during pregnancy, particularly for women entering pregnancy with poor nutritional status and poor dietary habits.

Women need not worry about not returning to their prepregnancy body weight. Most studies demonstrate that the average maternal weight after pregnancy is higher than the prepregnancy weight even when normal weight gain occurs during pregnancy. However, in most instances, the mother's body weight slowly readjusts following delivery.

INFANTS' BIRTH WEIGHT

Women need to be well nourished and to have about 22 percent of their body weight as fat to maintain normal menstrual cycles and hence conceive (Frisch & McArthur 1974, Frisch 1988). Women also need to gain appropriate amounts of weight during pregnancy to deliver a baby with a normal birth weight (Gormican, Valentine & Satter 1980, Abrams & Laros 1986). Many years ago it was recognized that those women who manage to get pregnant despite poor dietary intake may have a baby with a reduced birth weight. For example, during the winter of 1944 to 1945, a 28-week famine occurred in the Netherlands as a result of German occupation (Stein et al 1975). The average dietary consumption by most of the population was about 1200 calories per day. Thus, many pregnant women were undernourished. They gained less weight, their placentas were smaller, and their babies were born with reduced body weights (Fig. 1–4). An intake of 1500 calories per day appeared to be the nutritional breakpoint, as maternal caloric intakes below this amount during the last trimester produced small babies. When the famine was over and food became available to the Dutch people, maternal postpartum weight increased approximately 4 weeks prior to an improvement in fetal growth. This suggests that adequate nutrition of the mother must be achieved before birth weight is enhanced (see Fig. 1–4).

The Collaborative Perinatal Project of the National Institute of Neurologic and Communicative Disorders and Stroke (1959–1966) supported the observation that poor maternal weight gain is associated with a decreased infant birth weight. Additional studies also concluded that there is a linear relationship between the mother's weight at the beginning of pregnancy, the weight gain during pregnancy, and the birth weight of the offspring. It was further noted that the association of weight gain of the mother and birth weight of the infant varied with the mother's prepregnancy weight. As the prepregnancy weight increased, the influence of the maternal weight gain during the pregnancy was reduced (Naeye 1979, Susser 1981, Falkner 1981, Rosso 1985).

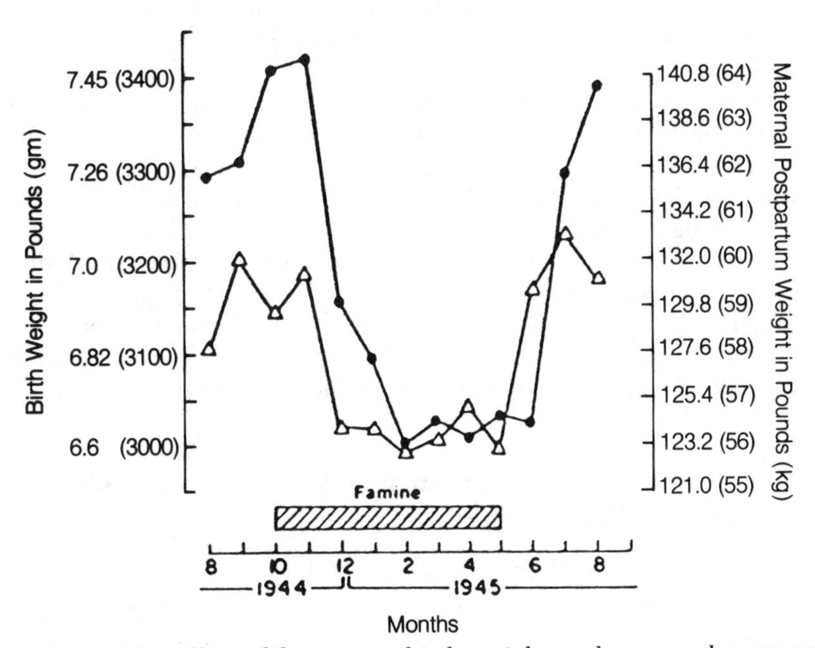

Figure 1–4. The effect of famine on birth weight and maternal postpartum weight in a Dutch population. (Δ = maternal weight; ● = birth weight.)

Adapted from Stein Z, Susser M, Saenger G, Marolla F. Famine and human development, the Dutch Hunger Winter of 1944–45. New York: Oxford University Press, 1975.

Field studies in different parts of the world also showed that in malnourished populations, nutritional supplementation during pregnancy increased the birth weight of the newborn child (Adams, Barr & Huenemann 1978, Rush, Stein & Susser 1980, Viegas et al 1982). In Guatemala, women who were given high-calorie, high-protein supplementation while breastfeeding their first offspring (245 kcal/d) and during the second pregnancy (180 kcal/d and 20 g protein/d) had babies with birth weights approaching those of industrialized populations (Villar & Rivera 1988). However, further increases in nutritional supplementation did not yield better birth weights, and when 470 calories and 40 grams of protein were given daily there were more premature births and neonatal deaths. A complete balanced nutrient supplement (170 kcal/d) improved the pregnancy outcome and the baby's weight (Mardones-Santander et al 1988).

A myriad of animal studies also show that when food is restricted during pregnancy, the mother and fetus compete for the available nutrients. The fetus, unlike a true parasite, *does not* always "win" under these circumstances. For example, Table 1–1 shows that when pregnant animals are subjected to food restriction, the growth of the fetus is impaired. The effect of malnutrition on growth is more marked in the fetus than in the mother. A review of other available experimental data has verified that the mother protects her own body stores from her fetus during precarious dietary conditions (Rosso 1981).

Excess weight gain before or during pregnancy will also have an impact on infants' birth weight. Obese women whose prepregnancy weights are greater than 135 percent of ideal weight for height may have large infants (Harrison, Udall & Morrow 1980). Maternal weight gains in excess of 45 pounds have been associated with large-sized babies and, as a result, with increased cesarean section rates and prolonged labor (Shepard, Hellenbrand & Bracken 1986). Big babies, greater than 10 pounds (>4500 g), certainly can be problematic to deliver (Sack 1969). Large babies born to mothers who were healthy but gained excess weight during pregnancy usually do not have serious health problems. However, large babies born to mothers who have

Table 1–1. Maternal Body Weight and Birth-Weight Changes Caused by Food Restriction in Animals.

SPECIES	TYPE OF RESTRICTION	PERCENTAGE CHANGE IN BODY WEIGHT (%)	
		Mother	Fetus
Rat	50% of food intake	−10	−12
	75% of food intake	−32	−51
Guinea pig	60% of food intake	−12	−22

Adapted from Rosso P. Nutrition and maternal-fetal exchange. Am J Clin Nutr 1981; 34:744–755.

diabetes or are a postterm delivery can have many medical complications, such as respiratory distress or hypoglycemia (Garbaciak et al 1985, Kleigman et al 1984, Spellacy et al 1985).

THE LOW-BIRTH-WEIGHT INFANT

The toll of having a low-birth-weight baby is a heavy one. These babies often spend considerable time in newborn nurseries and require intensive medical care and costly hospitalizations. Their mortality and morbidity rates are high, and few of these babies manage to survive with intact neurologic development. The causes of low birth weight vary greatly; malnutrition during pregnancy is only one of the many causes (Gormican, Valentine & Satter 1980, Susser 1981, Oh & Coustan 1989), although it is one of the most prominent preventable causes (Worthington, Vermeersch & Williams 1977).

There are two types of low-birth-weight infants: (1) premature babies—that is, babies who are born before 37 weeks' gestation with normal intrauterine growth (the body weight of these babies at birth is above the 10th percentile for gestational age); and (2) "small for dates" babies—that is, babies who, regardless of gestational age, have had intrauterine growth retardation (IUGR). The body weight of these babies at birth is always below the 10th percentile for gestational age. When the incidence of low-birth-weight babies is increased in a given population, the proportion of IUGR infants or "small for dates" babies becomes greater compared with the number of premature infants.

Low-birth-weight infants may be born with alterations in length as well as in weight (proportionate IUGR), or may be born with an appropriate body length but a reduced body weight (disproportionate IUGR) (Pitkin 1981). The type of IUGR may reflect the time during pregnancy when the nutritional insult takes place. Since linear growth peaks during the second trimester, proportionate IUGR infants have probably suffered an insult, such as inadequate dietary intake, early in the pregnancy; the effects are sustained until delivery. Since weight gain is predominantly a phenomenon of the third trimester, disproportionate IUGR babies were probably exposed to caloric deprivation only during the latter part of the pregnancy.

Another type of nutritional problem in low-birth-weight infants can occur during the last 2 to 3 weeks of gestation, after both length and weight growth are almost completed. In the absence of adequate nutrition during the last part of pregnancy, these fetuses may have to use their own fat stores and thus lose weight before they are born. The fetus exposed to inadequate nutrition for only the last few weeks in utero has very low fat but relatively normal muscle mass, whereas the disproportionate IUGR baby who did not gain adequate weight throughout the last trimester of pregnancy shows reductions in both muscle and fat. Thus, skinfold measurements taken at birth may differentiate these two types of IUGR babies (see Chapter 10).

Clearly, the burden of compromised fetal growth during nutritional deprivation is not shared equally by all organ systems at the time of the nutritional insult (Paige & Villar 1982). Even within each organ, a distinct histologic region may have its own intrinsic time for maximum growth and therefore show different effects after a nutritional insult. For example, within the brain, the timing and rate of growth of the cerebrum and cerebellum are distinct. In animals, maternal dietary deficiencies from gestation through weaning cause a 40 percent decline in brain cells and a lesser decline in cerebellum cells. Although the experimental animal data are indicative of the potential damage of poor maternal nutrition on brain development of the offspring, data in human beings are less apparent (Winick 1989).

THE PLACENTA

Maternal malnutrition also affects fetal growth by its detrimental effect on placental growth and development (Laga, Driscoll & Munro 1972a & b, Munro et al 1983). Poor women in developing countries have placental weights 14 to 50% less than those of well-nourished mothers. This effect appears to be more severe among malnourished mothers who were in precarious dietary condition even before pregnancy than among the women who were acutely deprived at some point in gestation. These data support the hypothesis that improving nutritional status prior to pregnancy may lessen the negative impact produced by low nutrient intake during pregnancy (Villar & Rivera 1988).

It is important to note that in undernourished women, placental weight is proportionately more affected than fetal weight. In contrast, IUGR owing to nonnutritional factors such as smoking or high altitude results in relatively larger placentas compared to fetal weight. This suggests that malnutrition may affect fetal growth through a reduction in placental size, whereas nonnutritional insults such as tobacco affect the fetus directly and stimulate a partial placental functional compensation. The placentas of malnourished mothers show many other alterations besides weight, including decreased DNA (reduced cell number), villous mass, and steroid hormones such as pregnanediol, progesterone, and peptide hormones like lactogen. These data suggest that the major effect of an inadequate diet may be the inhibition of protein synthesis in the placenta.

Also, in conditions of maternal malnutrition the blood flow through the placenta may be diminished, thereby minimizing transport of nutrients to the fetus. It should also be noted that dietary deficits of specific nutrients (e.g., calcium or essential fatty acids) may reduce placental circulation in otherwise well-nourished pregnant women. For example, a low fat intake may provide insufficient dietary linoleic acid, and a diet low in calcium or vitamin D may lead to a decreased calcium availability. Either of these deficits may reduce prostaglandin levels, which control the volume of blood flowing through the vessels in the placenta. Whenever the placenta is affected, the nutritional status of the unborn baby is at stake.

CLINICAL INTERVENTION

Expectant mothers need to be aware of the importance of proper nutrition and weight gain to optimize their fetus' growth and development (Paige & Villar 1982). One of the most important goals of nutrition counseling for these women is to stress the importance of eating a wholesome, varied, and mixed diet (see Chapter 2). The specific quantity of weight gain ideal for each woman is based upon her percent of ideal body weight (IBW) prior to conception. Women who begin pregnancy thin, average, and overweight have different nutritional requirements, which will affect their baby.

An easy rule of thumb to determine IBW for nonpregnant women is 100 pounds for the first 5 feet of height plus 5 pounds for each additional inch (±10 percent for small- or large-frame women). That means that a 5′4″ woman of average build will have a prepregnancy IBW of 120 pounds. If she started her pregnancy at 100 pounds she is underweight and must gain 30 pounds during the course of pregnancy (see Fig. 1–3). If this same woman started pregnancy at 115 pounds she is close to her IBW for height (±5 percent) and should be expected to gain about 24 pounds. A woman who starts pregnancy more than 20 percent above her IBW should only gain 16 pounds.

Under no circumstances should a woman diet to lose weight while pregnant (Lederman 1985). The frequent habit of omitting breakfast and/or skipping meals should be avoided, as it may have serious consequences. It is very important for all pregnant women to eat at least three meals a day to avoid the risks of ketosis. Furthermore, some women will eat sufficient calories while pregnant but engage in compulsive and excessive exercising to avoid "losing their tone and gaining too much weight." This behavior can be equally troublesome to the fetus, as insufficient nutrients are delivered to the fetus as they are used for meeting the demands of the increased activity of the pregnant woman.

Women who have trouble gaining weight (3 to 4 pounds during the first 10 weeks, and 1 pound per week for the remainder of their pregnancy) should have nutritional counseling to help them ingest the necessary calories. This problem may be common during the first trimester of pregnancy when nausea and vomiting are often present (see Chapter 5). Small, frequent meals, low in bulk and high in energy (such as peanut butter sandwiches, milk shakes, orange juice, or hamburgers) are helpful.

If a woman is gaining excessive weight (more than 1 pound per week during the last 20 weeks), she should closely monitor her caloric intake and restrict it to 2500 calories per day. If she is hungry and desires a greater quantity of food, she should decrease the caloric density of her foods and increase the volume of low-calorie foods. For example, snacks of fresh raw vegetables instead of cookies can increase the volume and quantity of a diet while decreasing the calories without interfering with nutrition quality (see Chapter 2).

In addition, the pregnant woman may find it helpful to increase the bulk and fiber content of her diet in order to quench appetite as well as diminish the common problems of constipation and hemorrhoids. Meals that are more frequent and smaller, or between-meal snacks, may help the woman avoid overeating. This eating pattern may diminish between-meal hunger and decrease gastric reflux, which is also a frequent occurrence during the latter months of pregnancy. Whatever the woman chooses as her diet, it is important to reemphasize the necessity of a mixed and varied diet (see Chapter 2).

If the woman continues to gain an excess amount of weight with a 2500-calorie diet, her calories may need to be further restricted. This is especially necessary for sedentary women. The diet restriction should be monitored; it should not fall below 2000 calories per day and should include foods from all food groups.

Calorie control during pregnancy can be particularly problematic given the increased vitamin and mineral requirements (see Chapter 3). Therefore, special guidance is warranted to help the pregnant woman maintain adequate caloric intake to promote appropriate gain without jeopardizing the nutrient quality of her diet. Remember, one can eat 2000 calories of ice cream, and demonstrate weight gain, but fail miserably at achieving the goal of good nutrition.

REFERENCES

Abrams BF, Laros RK. Prepregnancy weight, weight gain, and birth weight. Am J Obstet Gynecol 1986; 154:503–509.

Adams SO, Barr GD, Huenemann RL. Effect of nutritional supplementation during pregnancy. J Am Diet Assoc 1978; 72:144–147.

Belizan JM, Villar J. The relationship between calcium intake and edema-proteinuria and hypertension gestasis. Am J Clin Nutr 1980; 33:2202–2210.

Brown JE. Weight gain during pregnancy: What is "optimal"? Clin Nutr 1988; 7:181–190.

Campbell DM. Maternal adaptation in twin pregnancy. Semin Perinatol 1986; 10:14–18.

Chez RA. Pregnancy: Metabolism, diabetes and the fetus. Ciba Foundation Symposium (new series). New York: Excerpta Medica, 1979.

Coetzee EJ, Jackson WPO, Berman PA. Ketonuria in pregnancy with special references to calorie restricted food intake in obese diabetics. Diabetes 1980; 29:177–181.

Dobbing J. Maternal nutrition in pregnancy and later achievement of offspring: A personal interpretation. Early Human Dev 1985; 12:1–8.

Falkner F. Maternal nutrition and fetal growth. Am J Clin Nutr 1981; 34:769–774.

Frisch RE, McArthur JN. Menstrual cycles: Fatness as a determinant of minimum weight for height necessary for their maintenance or onset. Science 1974; 185:949–951.

Frisch RE. Fatness and fertility. Sci Am 1988; 258:88–95.

Garbaciak JA Jr, Richter M, Miller S, Barton JJ. Maternal weight and pregnancy complications. Am J Obstet Gynecol 1985; 152:238–245.

Gormican A Valentine J, Satter E. Relationships of maternal weight gain, prepregnancy weight, and infant birth weight. J Am Diet Assoc 1980; 77:662–667.

Harrison GG, Udall JN, Morrow G. Maternal obesity, weight gain in pregnancy, and infant birth weight. Am J Obstet Gynecol 1980; 136:411–412.

Hytten FE, Leitch I. The physiology of human pregnancy. 2nd ed. London: Blackwell, 1971:265–387.

Kleigman R, Gross T, Morton S, Dunnington R. Intrauterine growth and postnatal fasting metabolism in infants of obese mothers. J Pediatr 1984; 404:601–607.

Laga EM, Driscoll SG, Munro HN. Comparison of placentas from two socioeconomic groups. I. Morphometry. Pediatrics 1972a; 50:24–32.

Laga EM, Driscoll SG, Munro HN. Comparison of placentas from two socioeconomic groups. II. Biochemical characteristics. Pediatrics 1972b; 50:33–39.

Lederman SA. Physiological changes of pregnancy and their relation to nutrient needs. In Winick M, ed. Feeding the mother and infant. New York: John Wiley and Sons, 1985:13–43.

Leonard LG. Twin pregnancy. Maternal-fetal nutrition. J Obstet Gynecol-Neonatal Nurs 1982; 11:139–145.

Mardones-Santander F, Rosso P, Stekel A, et al. Effect of milk-based food supplement on maternal nutritional status and fetal growth in underweight Chilean women. Am J Clin Nutr 1988; 47:413–419.

Munro HN, Pilistine SJ, Fant ME. The placenta in nutrition. Annu Rev Nutr 1983; 3:97–124.

Naeye RL. Weight gain and the outcome of pregnancy. Am J Obstet Gynecol 1979; 135:3–9.

Naeye RL, Chez RA. Effects of maternal acetonuria and low pregnancy weight gain on children's psychomotor development. Am J Obstet Gynecol 1981; 139:189–193.

Oh W, Coustan DR. Intrauterine growth retardation. In Lebenthal E, ed. Textbook of gastroenterology and nutrition in infancy. New York, Raven Press, 1989:35–44.

Paige DM, Villar J. Maternal and fetal nutrition. In Lifshitz F, ed. Pediatric nutrition: Infant feedings, deficiencies, diseases. New York: Marcel Dekker, 1982:3–34.

Pitkin RM. Assessment of nutritional status of mother, fetus, and newborn. Am J Clin Nutr 1981; 34:658–668.

Rosso P. Nutrition and fetal maternal exchange. Am J Clin Nutr 1981; 34:744–755.

Rosso P. A new chart to monitor weight gain during pregnancy. Am J Clin Nutr 1985; 41:644–652.

Rush D, Stein Z, Susser M. Diet in pregnancy: A randomized controlled trial of nutritional supplements. March of Dimes Birth Defects Foundation. New York: Alan R. Liss, 1980.

Sack RA. The large infant. Am J Obstet Gynecol 1969; 104:195-202.

Schulman PK. Hyperemesis gravidarium: An approach to the nutritional aspects of care. J Am Diet Assoc 1982; 80:577–578.

Shepard MJ, Hellenbrand KG, Bracken MB. Proportional weight gain and complications of pregnancy, labor, and delivery in healthy women of normal prepregnant stature. Am J Obstet Gynecol 1987; 155:947–954.

Spellacy WN, Muler S. Winegar A, Peterson PQ. Macrosomia—maternal characteristics and infant complications. Obstet Gynecol 1985; 66:158–161.

Stein Z, Susser M, Saenger G, Marolla F. Famine and human development, the Dutch Hunger Winter of 1944–45. New York: Oxford University Press, 1975.

Susser M. Prenatal nutrition, birthweight, and psychological development: An overview of experiments, quasi-experiments, and natural experiments in the past decade. Am J Clin Nutr 1981; 34:784–803.

Viegas OA, Scott PH, Cole TJ, et al. Dietary protein energy supplementation of pregnant Asian mothers at Sorrento, Birmingham. II. Selective during third trimester only. Br Med J 1982; 285:592–595.

Villar J, Rivera J. Nutritional supplementation during two consecutive pregnancies and the interim period: Effect on birth weight. Pediatrics 1988; 81:51–57.

Winick M. Early nutrition and brain development. In Lebenthal E, ed. Textbook of gastroenterology and nutrition in infancy. New York: Raven Press, 1989:45–50.

Worthington BS, Vermeersch J, Williams SR. In Nutrition in pregnancy and lactation. St. Louis: C.V. Mosby Co., 1977:31–54.

Worthington-Roberts B. Weight gain pattern in twin pregnancies with desirable outcomes. Clin Nutr 1988; 7:191–196.

2

Nutrient Requirements and Meal Planning During Pregnancy

Lori, who is 15 pounds overweight, decided not to gain any weight during her pregnancy. She did not want to get any heavier and she certainly did not want to be fat after the baby was born. She was not concerned that dieting during pregnancy would cause her and her unborn baby to receive inadequate amounts of protein, vitamins, and minerals. She held to the obsolete view that the unborn baby is like a parasite that can take whatever nutrition it requires from the mother's own stores, regardless of the mother's diet.

We now know, however, that if the mother is inadequately nourished during pregnancy, her body does not adapt itself to provide optimal fetal growth. On the contrary, the mother will maintain her own nutritional status and the baby will not grow appropriately.

PRENATAL NUTRITIONAL REQUIREMENTS

A woman's nutritional needs during pregnancy are increased for all nutrients as compared with other times (Table 2–1). In addition, nutrient requirements vary depending on the age of the woman; younger women tend to have greater needs than older women (Nichols & Nichols 1983). Changes in body composition, with increased fat and reduced metabolically active tissue, combined with a reduction in physical activity contributes to the lower nutrient needs associated with aging. Most of the recommended dietary allowances (RDAs) for a pregnant woman can easily be met by eating ordinary, readily available food (Worthington, Vermeersch & Williams 1982), although iron and folic acid often must be supplemented (see Chapter 3).

Table 2–1. Recommended Dietary Allowances for Nonpregnant and Pregnant Women.

	RECOMMENDED DAILY REQUIREMENTS FOR NONPREGNANT WOMEN		MAXIMUM INCREASE IN NUTRIENT REQUIREMENTS FOR PREGNANCY
NUTRIENT	19 to 24 Years	25–50 Years	
Energy (kcal/kg)	38	36	+300 kcal/d
Protein (g/kg)	0.8	0.8	+10–14 g/d
Vitamin A (μg RE*)	800	800	0
Vitamin D (μg)†	10	5.0	+ 5
Vitamin E (mg)‡	8	8	+ 2
Vitamin C (mg)	60	60	+ 10
Vitamin K (μg)	60	65	+ 5
Folic acid (μg)	180	180	+220
Niacin (mg)	15	15	+ 2
Riboflavin (mg)	1.3	1.3	+ 0.3
Thiamin (mg)	1.1	1.1	+ 0.4
Vitamin B_6 (mg)	1.6	1.6	+ 0.6
Vitamin B_{12} (μg)	2.0	2.0	+ 0.2
Calcium (mg)	1200	800	+400
Phosphorus (mg)	1200	800	+400
Iron (mg)	15	15	+ 15
Magnesium (mg)	280	280	+ 40
Zinc (mg)	12	12	+ 3
Iodine (μg)	150	150	+ 25
Selenium (μg)	55	55	+ 10

*Retinol Equivalents; 1 RE equals 3.33 International Units (IU).
†1 μg equals 40 IU.
‡1 mg equals 1.49 IU.

Adapted from the Committee on Dietary Allowances, Food and Nutrition Board, National Research Council. Recommended daily allowances. 10th ed. Washington, D.C.: National Academy Press, 1989.

Energy

Energy requirements are increased during pregnancy for three major reasons: (1) new fetal and maternal tissue is being produced; (2) the new tissues require additional metabolism; and (3) increased energy is needed to move the increased body mass of the pregnant woman during physical activity (Paige & Villar 1982). It has been calculated that pregnancy requires an additional 65,000 to 85,000 calories, which represents an average increment of 275 to 300 calories per day throughout the duration of pregnancy (280 days). However, the demand for energy is not equally distributed throughout the pregnancy. The greatest energy is needed during the second and third trimesters of pregnancy, when fat deposition takes place and the demands for fetal growth are greatest. Additional energy requirements during pregnancy are distributed as shown in Figure 2–1.

The additional energy allowance does not take into account variation in

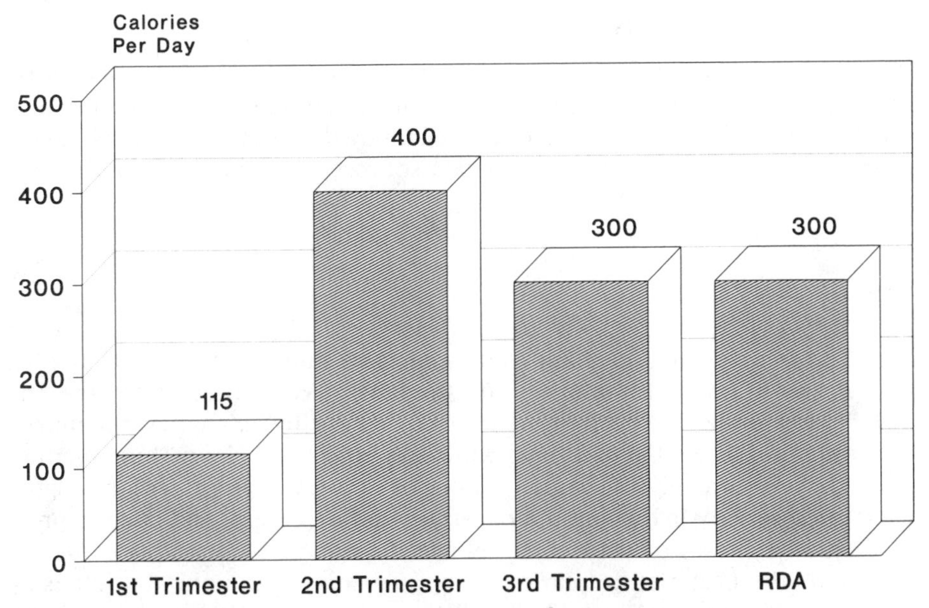

Figure 2–1. Additional energy requirements during pregnancy.
From Paige DM, Villar J. Maternal and fetal nutrition. In Lifshitz F, ed. Pediatric nutrition: Infant feedings, deficiencies, diseases. New York: Marcel Dekker, 1982:167–196.

physical activity during pregnancy (Nagy & King 1983). Physically active pregnant women require more than 300 extra calories per day to maintain maternal and fetal tissue weight gains, and even sedentary women require a minimum daily intake of 2000 to 2100 calories during pregnancy.

Protein

During pregnancy new tissue is synthesized at a faster rate than at any other time in a woman's life (Nutrition Reviews 1984). A total of 925 grams of protein is stored in fetal and maternal tissues. An increase in protein deposition is noted throughout pregnancy, from 0.6 gram per day in the first quarter of pregnancy to 6.1 grams per day in the last months.

The National Research Council RDAs advise the liberal daily addition of 10 grams of high-quality protein to the usual diet of a healthy pregnant woman. This estimation fails to take into consideration the energy-protein interaction, which suggests that an increased energy intake may compensate for a low protein intake in pregnancy. However, epidemiologic observations suggest that pregnancy outcome is better when additional protein is consumed (see Chapter 1). The daily protein requirements during pregnancy can be met from a variety of plentiful food sources, such as fish, meat, and milk.

Vitamins and Minerals

The adequacy of a diet during pregnancy goes beyond the provision of appropriate amounts of calories and protein. The needs for other essential nutrients must also be met (Table 2–1). During pregnancy the needs for iron and folic acid may be difficult to meet from dietary sources alone, even when the diet is ''ideal'' (see Chapter 3).

DIETARY INTAKE

The dietary intake of a pregnant woman must be sufficient to provide all the energy and nutrients the mother and the fetus need during pregnancy. In order to emphasize the need to eat a varied diet during pregnancy, the nutrient content of three different meal choices is analyzed below. These menus contain approximately the same number of calories appropriate for weight gain, but they vary in the amount of carbohydrate, protein, and fat, and provide either excesses or deficiencies of specific minerals, vitamins, or both. Therefore, the best diet to follow during pregnancy is the one that offers a *variety* of all foods, with specific supplementation as needed.

The selection of foods in the first menu described below represents one that aims for a ''wholesome'' diet, with adequate calories, protein, and calcium and avoidance of so-called ''junk food'' and other processed items. It also limits fat and cholesterol by eliminating red meats and eggs. High-fiber foods, including whole grains, breads, and fresh fruits and vegetables, are emphasized.

MENU 1

Breakfast
2 ounces unsweetened cereal
1 ounce raisins
1 banana
½ cup whole milk
1 cup orange juice

Lunch
½ cup tuna salad
2 slices whole wheat bread
2 cups lettuce, tomato, red pepper salad with 1 tablespoon dressing
½ cup cranberry juice
½ cup frozen yogurt

Dinner
4 ounces roast chicken
½ cup brown rice

¾ cup stringbeans with mushrooms
¼ cantaloupe
1 piece carrot cake
1 cup apple-grape juice

Snacks
½ cup cottage cheese with ¼ cup sliced peaches
2 tablespoons unsalted peanut butter on whole wheat crackers
1 cup vanilla yogurt with ¼ cup granola

Although this menu provides adequate calories for maternal weight gain and may appear wholesome and nutritious, it does not meet all the RDAs of pregnancy (Fig. 2–2). The mother-to-be who selected this meal plan was overzealous in her effort to consume a "healthy" diet; as a consequence, by eliminating items such as red meat, this diet does not provide the recommended requirements for iron, zinc and vitamin D. It is, therefore, not a meal plan that is ideal for pregnant women.

In contrast to the first meal plan, Menu 2 depicts a more well-balanced approach to nutrition during pregnancy. An effort has been made to eat three meals and snacks to assure adequate calories while including milk for calcium and eggs and red meat as good iron and zinc sources.

MENU 2

Breakfast
2 scrambled eggs
2 slices whole wheat toast with 2 teaspoons margarine
8 ounces orange juice

Lunch
1 cup vegetable soup
3 ounces roast beef sandwich with lettuce, tomato, mayonnaise (2 teaspoons)
1 cup 2 percent milk
½ cup grapes

Snack
½ cup raisins with ¼ cup peanuts mixture
peach

Dinner
1 cup salad with dressing
1 average serving lasagna
½ cup broccoli
1 piece garlic bread
1 cup fresh-fruit cocktail

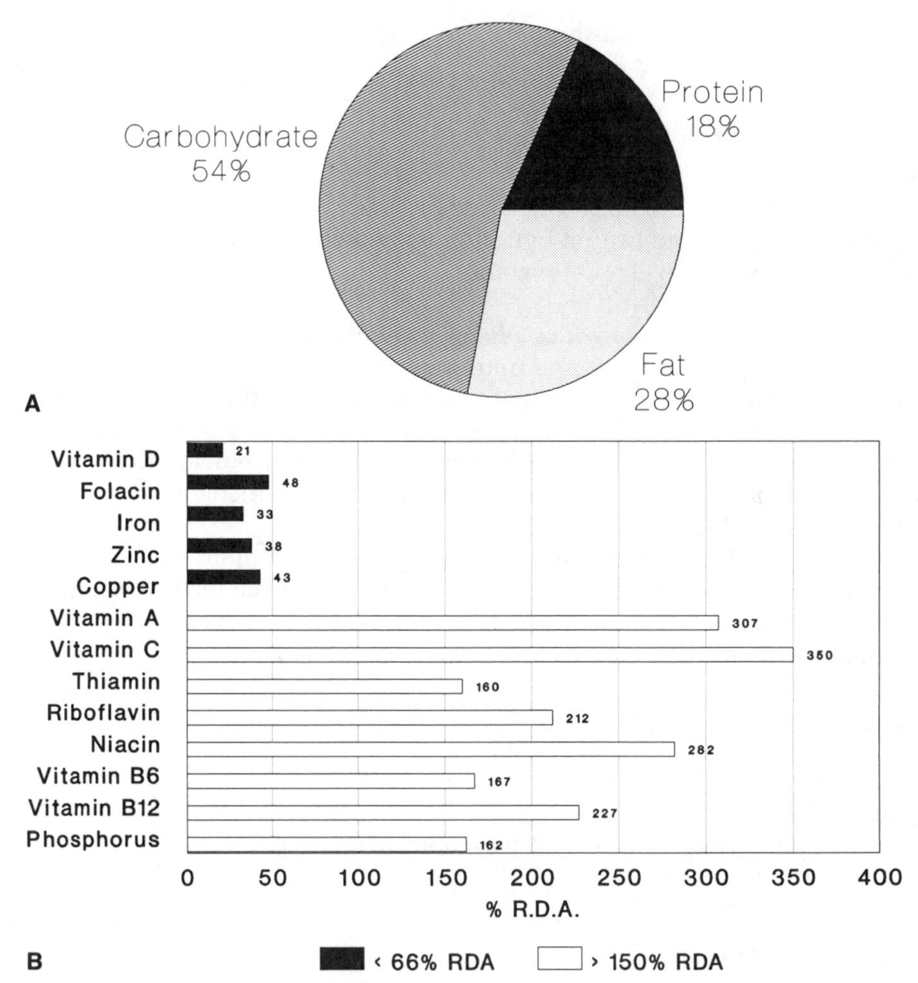

Figure 2–2. **A.** Caloric distribution of Menu 1. **B.** Inappropriate nutrient intakes.

Snack
1 cup 2 percent milk
2 sandwich-type cookies

As with the previous meal plan, Menu 2 provides adequate calories for gestation. This typical American-style diet contains more than enough protein to meet the increased requirements of pregnancy. The distribution of calories is close to the recommended ideal diet for healthy women (Fig. 2–3). All nutrient requirements are now met in this meal pattern except for folacin and

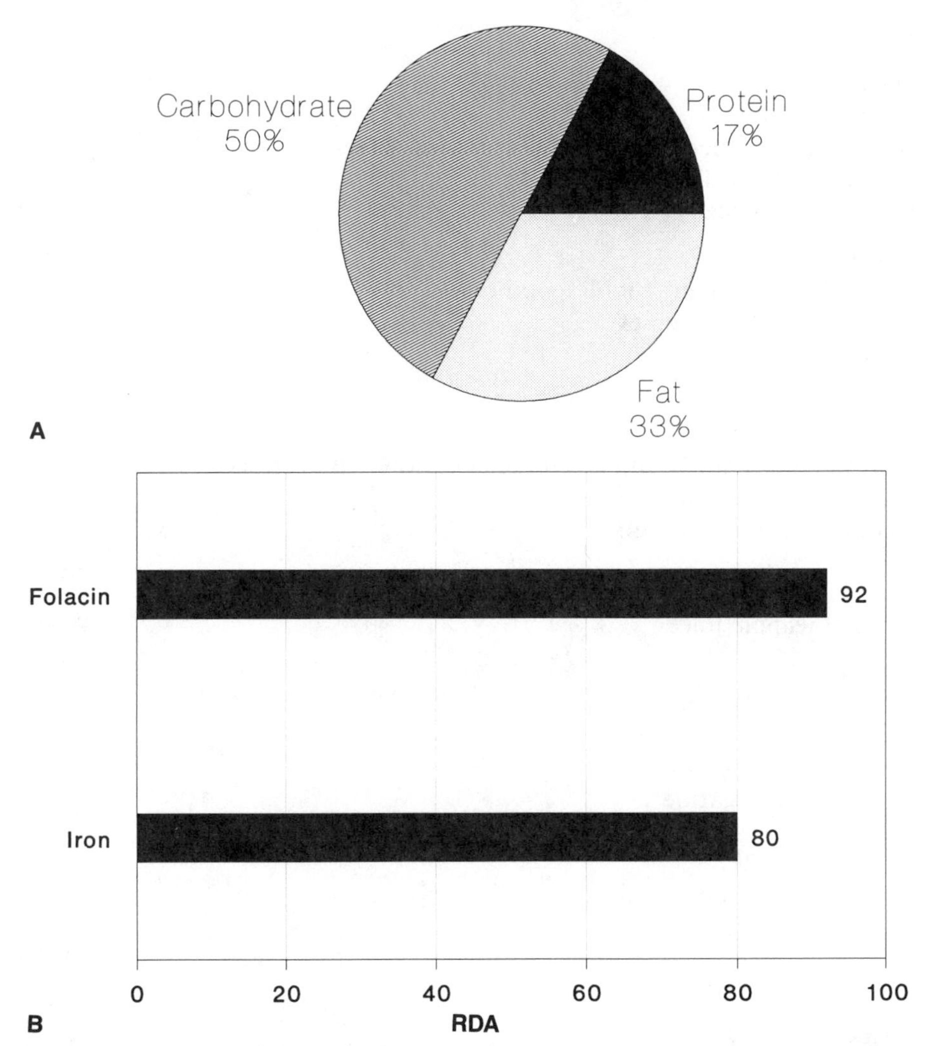

Figure 2–3. **A.** Caloric distribution of Menu 2. **B.** Inappropriate nutrient intakes.

iron. Therefore, even a diet that contains rich sources of protein and other essential minerals may not fully supply these two important elements during pregnancy.

The third menu provides a low-fat choice for the pregnant woman, offering low-fat dairy products and lean meats. Many women now believe that by ingesting foods low in fat they may avoid the long-term problems of atherosclerosis and obesity. This diet may also be selected by the mother-to-be who is troubled by the nausea and vomiting of pregnancy (see Chapter 5).

MENU 3

Breakfast
1 cup skim milk
¾ cup unsweetened cereal and ½ cup bran flakes
2 tablespoons raisins
1 cup orange juice

Snack
1 English muffin with 1 tablespoon margarine
1 teaspoon jelly preserves
1 cup skim milk

Lunch
2 ounces feta cheese
2 cups lettuce with ¼ cup green pepper and ¼ cup carrots
1 tablespoon oil and vinegar
6 rye-whole wheat wafers
1 peach
1 corn muffin
1 cup pineapple juice

Dinner
3 ounces turkey breast
1 cup peas
1 cup mashed potatoes
1 teaspoon margarine
1 cup salad tossed—no dressing
1 cup skim milk
1 slice pound cake
½ cup blueberries

Snack
1 banana
2 pretzels
1 cup apple juice

Menu 3 is a meal plan that provides adequate calories and protein but is relatively low in fat and high in carbohydrate (Fig. 2–4). Also, note that with this diet a large volume of food must be consumed in order to meet calorie requirements during pregnancy. Many women may find this to be unacceptable and may inadvertently not consume sufficient calories for maternal weight gain. The amount of vitamin C in this diet is in excess of requirements while intakes of iron, zinc, and folacin are still below recommended requirements.

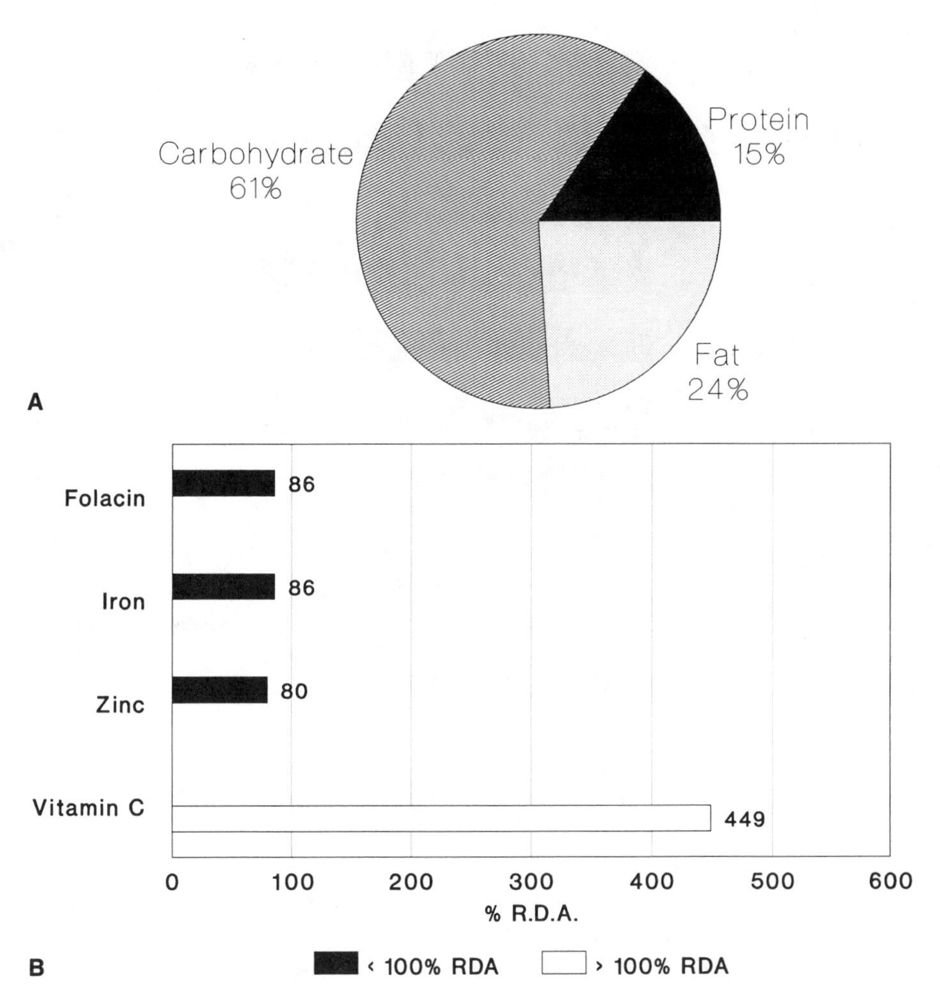

Figure 2–4. **A.** Caloric distribution of Menu 3. **B.** Inappropriate nutrient intakes.

CLINICAL INTERVENTION

During pregnancy, many factors affect a woman's diet, and all medical professionals who care for pregnant women should inform their patients of the necessity of proper nutrition and prenatal care (Truswell 1985) (Fig. 2–5). Women who have poor nutritional intake during prepregnancy and gestation are least likely to seek and receive prenatal care. However, they may receive health care and advice from other professionals such as social workers, pharmacists, dentists, community health nurses, and so on. Often, pregnant

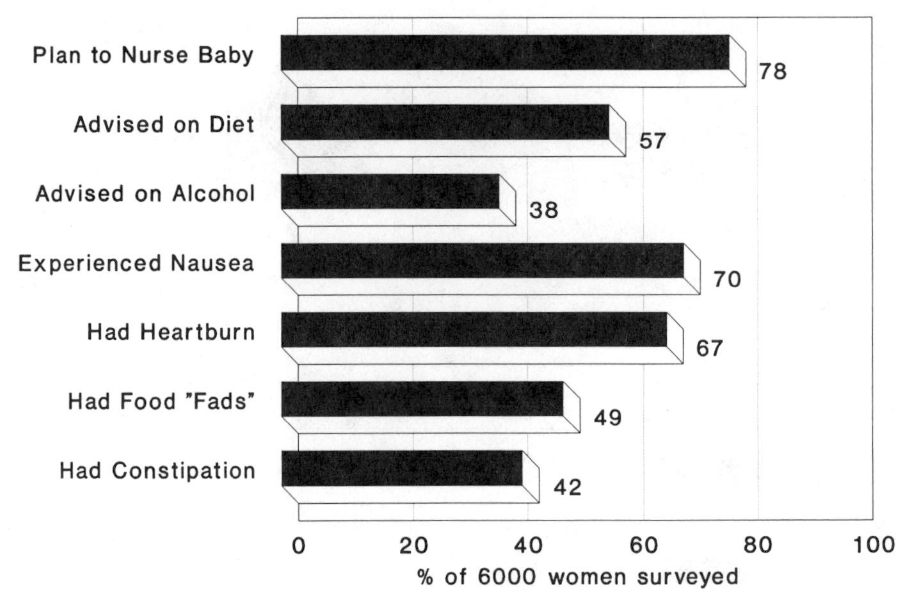

Figure 2–5. Factors that may alter a woman's diet during pregnancy. Modified from data obtained via a BBC TV survey of 6000 women.

Modified from Truswell AS. ABC of nutrition: Nutrition for pregnancy. Br Med J 1985; 291:263–266.

women do not seek or expect nutrition advice from their obstetrician but instead rely on family, friends, and media sources for their nutrition information. Thus, health professionals who provide appropriate nutrition information to the expectant mother set a precedent for pregnant women to rely on knowledgeable sources for their care (King 1986). Appropriate nutrition before and during pregnancy may reduce the risk of having low-birth-weight infants (see Chapter 1).

Health care professionals must provide nutrition education to women prior to conception and continue with further teaching and monitoring throughout the course of pregnancy. Most women are not aware of the magnitude or significance of their diet during pregnancy, and most of them do not receive supervised guidance in this aspect of their prenatal care. With optimal instruction and learning, an appropriate diet suitable for each individual can easily be achieved. A guide for good eating during pregnancy is shown in Table 2–2.

Nutrition education and monitoring is needed for all pregnant women regardless of their preconception weight (underweight to obese), nutritional status, educational level, or economic situation. If the woman has had a poor nutritional intake prior to conception, she must be taught appropriate nutri-

Table 2–2. A Guide for Good Eating During Pregnancy*

FOOD GROUP	RECOMMENDED NUMBER OF SERVINGS PER DAY
MILK/CHEESE	
1 serving is:	
1 cup milk or yogurt	3–4
1 1/3 ounces cheddar or Swiss cheese	
2 ounces processed cheese food	
1 1/2 cups ice cream or ice milk	
2 cups cottage cheese	
MEAT/POULTRY/FISH/BEANS	
1 serving is:	
2 ounces cooked meat, fish, or poultry	2–3
2 eggs	
2 ounces cheddar cheese	
1/2 cup cottage cheese	
4 tablespoons peanut butter	
1 1/2 cups cooked dry beans, peas, lentils, or soy beans	
1/2 to 1 cup nuts, sesame, or sunflower seeds	
VEGETABLE	
1 serving is:	
1/2 cup juice	2–3
1/2 cup cooked vegetables	
1 cup raw vegetables	
FRUIT	
1 serving is:	
1/2 cup juice	3–6
1/2 grapefruit	
portion commonly served, i.e., medium apple, banana, etc.	
BREAD/CEREAL	
1 serving is:	
2 slices bread	2–6
1 cup cooked cereal or pasta	
2 cups ready-to-eat cereal	
FAT	
1 serving is:	
2 teaspoons margarine, butter, or oil	3–4
2 tablespoons salad dressing	
2 teaspoons mayonnaise	

*The number of servings may vary depending on the calorie needs of the pregnant woman. A diet containing 3 servings of meat or equivalent, 3 servings of vegetables, 6 servings of fruit, 6 servings of bread, and 4 servings of fat will provide a pregnant woman with 2500 calories and sufficient protein intake. Selecting a variety of foods within each food group will assure adequate vitamin and mineral intake, with the possible exception of iron and folic acid.

tion practices (Villar & Rivera 1988). She may need information on the updated six basic food groups and direction on what type of food to consume during pregnancy (see Table 2–2). It is essential to obtain a dietary history. This will help determine the prepregnant nutritional status, food preferences, and eating habits. Also, inquiries must be made regarding presence of food sensitivities or allergies; presence of any eating disorders; and if there is an excessive consumption of any particular foods, alcohol, vitamins, or minerals. Additionally, ethnic, religious, and economic considerations should also be obtained to help plan an acceptable diet for the mother-to-be. If the woman is concerned about obesity or is preoccupied with dieting, careful reassurance and monitoring of nutritional intake and body weight will be necessary to avoid excess worries or deviations from the recommended diet. Some guidelines to modify caloric intake during pregnancy are shown in Table 2–3.

Suggestions for alterations in dietary intake necessary during pregnancy must (1) fit within the framework of the woman's tastes and preferences; (2) include written material (or pictures for the illiterate patient) as well as verbal instructions; and (3) provide for monitoring of nutritional status. When instructing women in a proper gestational diet, the rationale for the recommended diet should be included (e.g., appropriate dietary intake is necessary

Table 2–3. How to Modify Caloric Intake During Pregnancy Without Jeopardizing Nutrition.

	HIGHER CALORIE FOODS	LOWER CALORIE FOODS
Dairy	Whole milk; hard and processed cheeses; yogurt made from whole milk; ice cream; puddings	Low-fat, skim milk; low-fat cheeses; frozen yogurt; ice milk
Meat, poultry, fish	Fatty cuts of beef, lamb, pork; cold cuts; sausage; hot dogs; duck; organ meats; fried meat, chicken, or fish; canned fish in oil; nuts; nut butters	Lean meat; poultry without skin; fish; fish canned in water; dried beans
Fruits and vegetables	Fruits/vegetables with added butter, margarine, creams, and sauces; dried fruits; canned fruits in heavy syrup; avocados; olives	Fresh, frozen fruits and vegetables without added sauces or syrups
Breads and cereals	Baked goods (pies, muffins, cakes, cookies); grains/pastas with cream sauces, cheese, butter, margarine; sweetened cereals; potato chips; corn chips	Whole grains; unsweetened cereals; pasta with no added sauces; plain crackers; pretzels; popcorn; ginger-snap cookies; graham crackers
Fats	Butter; margarine; oils; mayonnaise; dressings; cream; shortening; chocolate; dips	Try to decrease total amount

for optimal fetal growth and development) and the potential problems that may occur (e.g., dieting may lead to ketosis and fetal damage).

Most women will be able to meet most of their nutritional needs if they ingest a varied, balanced diet. However, iron, folic acid, and perhaps other minerals may require supplementation (see Chapter 3). It is necessary to keep in mind that an appropriate diet for a pregnant woman can be achieved only if the selection of food is varied (Jacobson 1987). No single diet with a limited number of food choices can suffice to meet all the requirements of the mother and her baby (Munro 1981). If the mother needs to limit her intake because of excess weight gain during pregnancy, it should be done with supervision to avoid intake of an inappropriate, unbalanced diet.

REFERENCES

Jacobson HN. Maternal nutrition in the 1980's. J Am Diet Assoc 1987; 80:216–219.

King JC. Nutrition during pregnancy. In Kretchmer N, ed. Frontiers in clinical nutrition. Rockville: Aspen Systems Corporation, 1986:3–13.

Munro HN. Nutrient requirements during pregnancy II. Am J Clin Nutr 1981; 34:679–684.

Nagy LE, King JC. Energy expenditure of pregnant women at rest or walking self-paced. Am J Clin Nutr 1983; 38:369–376.

Nichols BL, Nichols VN. Nutritional physiology in pregnancy and lactation. In Barness LA, ed. Advances in pediatrics. Chicago: Year Book Medical Publishers, 1983:473–515.

Nutrition Reviews. Present knowledge in nutrition. 5th ed. Washington, D.C.: The Nutrition Foundation Inc., 1984.

Paige DM, Villar J. Maternal and fetal nutrition. In Lifshitz F, ed. Pediatric nutrition: Infant feedings, deficiencies, diseases. New York: Marcel Dekker, 1982:167–196.

Truswell AS. ABC of nutrition: Nutrition for pregnancy. Br Med J 1985; 291:263–266.

Villar J, Rivera J. Nutritional supplementation during two consecutive pregnancies and the interim lactation period: Effect on birth weight. Pediatrics 1988; 81:51–57.

Worthington B, Vermeersch J, Williams S. Nutrition in pregnancy and lactation. St Louis: C.V. Mosby Co., 1982.

3

Vitamins and Minerals for the Pregnant Woman

"The first vitamins your body will accept as food." That is what the advertisement stated and that is what Ricki believed. She read the advertisement and regularly took her daily pills while dieting during her pregnancy. After all, the brand she bought cost $40 per month, contained every vitamin and mineral she would need, and "did not have to be taken with meals. . . ."

Vitamin and mineral supplementation during pregnancy is a ritual in our population, but it is not a substitute for a healthy wholesome diet. Indeed, vitamins may not be needed or may lead to problems if taken in excess. Supplementation of iron and folic acid may be the only exceptions, since it may be difficult to meet the RDAs of these two nutrients by consuming an ordinary diet (see Chapter 2).

FAT-SOLUBLE VITAMINS

During pregnancy the fetal requirements for fat-soluble vitamins are increased (see Chapter 1), but intake of an ordinary, well-balanced diet by the mother-to-be will provide all the fat-soluble vitamins she and her baby need.

Vitamin A is needed for a series of special metabolic processes during pregnancy. These include fetal development and liver storage, maternal formation of colostrum and lactation, and possibly hormone synthesis. The adult RDA for vitamin A is set at 800 microgram retinol equivalents (RE) (2640 IU) for both nonpregnant and pregnant females. During pregnancy, two or three extra servings of fresh vegetables can assure adequate intake of vitamin A. However, it should be kept in mind that there is evidence that either an excess or a deficit of vitamin A may produce congenital anomalies.

Large doses of vitamin A given to animals during pregnancy has resulted in offspring with cleft palate, urinary tract anomalies, and other malformations. Vitamin A deficiency in lower animals has been shown to cause eye defects as well as congenital abnormalities of the skeleton and other organs (Robens 1970). In humans, there are reported cases of birth defects (teratogenesis) with findings similar to those of animals associated with vitamin A supplementation during pregnancy of greater than 25,000 IU per day (Lammer et al 1985, Rosa, Wilk & Kesley 1986). Also, young women with high vitamin A intake due to retinol treatment for acne had babies with small heads, deformed ears, cleft palate, heart defects, and hypoplastic kidneys.

Vitamin D has a role in promoting a positive calcium balance in pregnant women. Furthermore, one of the metabolites of vitamin D, 25-hydroxyvitamin D, is capable of crossing the placenta and may therefore play a part in promoting fetal calcium balance. Plasma levels of the active form of the vitamin, 1, 25-dihydroxyvitamin D (the hormone responsible for the regulation of calcium absorption), are increased in plasma during pregnancy (Reddy et al 1983). This is an unusual finding since plasma levels of most other vitamins are decreased during gestation. The rise of the active metabolite of vitamin D during pregnancy may be due to an increased rate of synthesis by the kidney or by the placenta itself as a compensatory mechanism to meet the fetal demands of calcium. The RDA for vitamin D in adult females varies from 5 to 10 micrograms (200–400 IU) daily; doubling the requirement is recommended during pregnancy. Consumption of milk and milk products assures the supply of this essential nutrient, but sunlight exposure may also provide the necessary vitamin D for the pregnant woman. Vitamin D deficiency is unlikely, as fortification of milk and other products is a common practice in our country. Excess vitamin D intake may lead to toxicity in the mother and perhaps in the unborn baby. There have been claims that infantile hypercalcemia is the result of intake of large doses of vitamin D during pregnancy (Hurley 1980).

The role of *vitamin E* is not yet clearly understood, even 50 years after its discovery. During pregnancy the fetus accumulates vitamin E (alpha tocopherol). The content of this metabolite in the fetal liver increases progressively from about 1.8 milligrams per gram of liver at 3 months of gestational age to 4.4 milligrams per gram at 6 months of age. These levels continue to increase until adulthood. The RDA of vitamin E in adult women is 8 milligrams (11.9 IU), but during pregnancy a total of 10 milligrams (14.9 IU) per day is recommended. Consumption of vegetable oils and cereals will usually satisfy the need for this essential nutrient. Vitamin E in high doses was thought to be useful for the treatment and prevention of spontaneous abortion, but this effect has never been well established (Pitkin 1975).

Vitamin K is a fat-soluble vitamin derived from bacterial metabolism in the intestine (K_2 form) and from the intake of vegetables rich in vitamin K (K_1 form). In general, the usual dietary intake is enough for pregnant women to cover all their needs for this vitamin. There is no evidence of the effectiveness of the use of vitamin K supplementation during pregnancy as a preventive measure of hemorrhagic disease in newborns.

WATER-SOLUBLE VITAMINS

The requirements of the *B-complex vitamins* are generally increased during pregnancy. The blood levels of these vitamins usually decline in the mother, the urinary excretion increases, and the fetal blood level exceeds those of the mother as a consequence of the active transport of these vitamins across the placenta. Low biochemical blood levels of the B-complex vitamins during pregnancy should be interpreted as normal physiologic adjustments of the mother's system, and are not indicative of a nutrient deficiency. Consumption of an ordinary varied diet by the mother will assure the intake of all the needed B-complex vitamins for her and her baby. Nonetheless, vitamin B deficiency during pregnancy can occur, as there is limited storage of these vitamins in the body, particularly among women whose diets contain few vegetables, a good source of most B-complex vitamins.

The effects of deficiencies of B vitamins is not clear, but they could play an important role in the neurologic development of the fetus. The growth of the central nervous system requires vitamin B_6; a deficiency of this vitamin could have important adverse consequences. Furthermore, immunologic alterations in the presence of pantothenic acid deficiency have been reported in animals. Although none of these results have been confirmed in human beings, it is prudent for mothers to increase their intake of these vitamins during pregnancy by eating a varied diet.

FOLACIN

Folacin is the term used to describe compounds with biologic folic acid activity. The minimum daily requirements of these substances during pregnancy have been estimated at 400 micrograms, which is greater than twofold the usual dose for nonpregnant women. This amount will suffice only if adequate folacin stores are present at the onset of pregnancy; higher amounts are needed if that is not the case. For diets to be adequate in folacin, not only must there be sufficient amounts in the diet, but folacin must be available for absorption. The bioavailability of this substance in food varies; it is usually only about 50 percent but may be as low as 25 percent. Since the typical

Western diet only contains about 200 micrograms of folacin per daily portion, a woman may easily become deficient in this vitamin (see Chapter 2). In addition, ingestion of alcohol further inhibits folacin absorption, and anticonvulsant drug therapy enhances folacin metabolism.

A high prevalence of folic acid deficiency has been reported during gestation. About 25 percent of healthy pregnant women in the United States have marginal-to-low serum folate levels, and in less developed countries this problem is even more prevalent. In the United States, low serum folacin levels are reported in the majority of low-income pregnant adolescents (Bailey, Mahan & Dimperio 1980). A deficiency of this vitamin was shown several years ago to lead to infertility and sterility (Jackson, Daig & McDonald 1967). When pregnancy does occur in the presence of folacin deficiency, it may lead to fetal and placental malformations, particularly neural-tube defects. Since the folacin content of the diet is usually insufficient to provide for all needs, supplementation with folic acid is routinely recommended for pregnant women. Moreover, in patients with histories of inadequate dietary intake, faulty absorption, multiple pregnancies, and anticonvulsant drug therapy, a higher folic acid supplementation is necessary even before pregnancy.

VITAMIN C

The RDA for ascorbic acid is increased during pregnancy from 60 to 70 milligrams per day. The increased need during pregnancy is often entirely met by diet, since the content of vitamin C in food is plentiful. However, pregnant women should be more concerned about ingesting too much of this vitamin rather than consuming insufficient amounts. A condition called vitamin C dependency, which resembles scurvy, was recognized many years ago in human infants whose mothers had ingested an excess of 400 milligrams per day of ascorbic acid during pregnancy (Cochrane 1965). When the fetus is exposed to large amounts of vitamin C in utero, the excess vitamin C begins to be rapidly excreted. This process may continue after the baby is born even though the large supply of vitamin C is no longer given.

MINERALS

Unlike iron and calcium, which are generally accepted as needing supplementation during pregnancy, deficiencies of magnesium, zinc, and chromium receive little attention by most obstetricians and pediatricians. The extent to which these deficiencies during pregnancy contribute to gestational complications and failures, and to neonatal and infantile morbidity and mortality, requires more study. The prevalence of mineral deficiencies at birth, as well as the immediate and longer-term sequelae in the baby and in the mother, also need further investigation.

IRON

During pregnancy, iron is needed to cover the basal needs of the mother (±240 mg), the increase in her red cell mass (±500 mg), and the requirements of the fetus and placenta (±300 mg). The total iron requirements during the entire course of pregnancy can be estimated at 1000 milligrams. However, the increased iron needs are not uniformly required throughout pregnancy. The needs are distributed as follows: 0.8 milligrams per day during the first trimester; 4.4 milligrams per day during the second trimester; and 8.4 milligrams per day during the last part of gestation. After delivery, much of the iron used to increase the red cell mass is returned to the iron stores of the mother. However, about 200 milligrams are lost as hemorrhage during delivery. Therefore, the net total requirement of iron during pregnancy is 800 milligrams.

The demand for iron may be met either by mobilizing the maternal iron stores or by increasing iron absorption from the diet. If a woman begins pregnancy with optimal iron reserves (750 mg) and maintains an ideal diet, she may be capable of carrying the gestation to term without becoming iron-deficient. However, this situation does not generally prevail in either developed or developing countries. Data from Canada, the United States, and Sweden show that about 30 percent of women between the ages of 15 and 45 do not have appropriate iron deposits. In women who have never been pregnant, iron stores have been found to be 300 milligrams at best, and almost 33 percent of women have no stores at all.

The amount of iron absorbed from the diet varies tremendously. The bioavailability of iron in Western diets varies about tenfold depending on a number of factors, including the type of iron ingested (heme vs. nonheme), as well as the overall composition of the diet. For example, increased acidity of the meal enhances iron absorption, while the presence of phytate in cereals or ingestion of tea interferes with iron absorption.

Due to the great variation in iron bioavailability from different meals, neither the total iron content of food nor the content of iron per 1000 calories (nutrient density) is a useful measure of the adequacy of the iron supplied by the diet. The ideal nutrient density of iron (average, 1.1 mg/1000 kcal) is not usually achieved in Western diets, and during the last part of gestation, when the iron requirements are enormous, it is highly unlikely that diet alone will meet these needs despite increased intestinal absorption. Whereas the nonpregnant menstruating woman may absorb 32 percent of iron ingested, a woman in her sixth month of pregnancy has an increased absorptive capacity of 84 percent.

Daily supplementation of elemental iron may preserve iron stores in the mother and positively influence her hemoglobin, hematocrit, and erythrocyte counts, with a general improvement in the health of the mother. However, it should be noted that improving the blood count or the maternal iron stores does not necessarily induce beneficial effects on the length of gestation, birth weight, or infant and maternal morbidity and mortality (Hemminki & Starfield 1978). For this reason some experts believe that routine supplements may not be warranted. However, as discussed in Chapter 2, no matter what menu choices the mother makes during pregnancy, the dietary iron content is usually low. Thus, iron supplementation is recommended.

Iron supplied as a component of a prenatal multivitamin supplement has been shown to be poorly absorbed (Seligman et al 1983). The calcium carbonate and magnesium oxide present in supplements appear to interfere with iron absorption. Therefore, if iron supplementation is deemed necessary, specific oral iron preparations may be advised (Table 3–1). A supplement with a dose of 15 to 30 milligrams per day is generally recommended for pregnant women. If anemia is present, a therapeutic dose is necessary.

Calcium

The fetus requires a 120 to 150 milligrams per kilogram of body weight per day of calcium for accretion of bone (Tsang 1985). Most of this calcium is

Table 3–1. Oral iron preparations.*

NAME	ELEMENTAL IRON (%)	TABLET SIZE (mg)	ELEMENTAL IRON PER TABLET
Ferrous fumarate	33	150	50 mg
Ferrous sulfate	20	325	65 mg
Ferrocholinate	12	333	40 mg
Ferrous gluconate	11.5	325	38 mg
		435	50 mg
Iron-FA (ferrous fumarate)	33	—	82 mg iron
			1 mg folic acid
Fero-Folic 500	20	—	105 mg iron
			0.8 mg folic acid
			500 mg vitamin C
Pronemia (ferrous fumarate)	33	—	115 mg iron
			0.1 mg folic acid
			150 mg vitamin C
			0.15 μg vitamin B_{12}

*Ferrous iron is much better absorbed than the ferric form. All combinations of ferrous iron available for supplementation are equally effective for oral iron therapy. Additionally, there are no differences among these iron preparations in terms of side effects and intolerances. Change in stool consistency, whether it be diarrhea or constipation, are non–dose-related side effects that may occur with all iron preparations. Nausea and epigastric distress are usually not a concern with doses less than 200 mg of elemental iron daily. Although delayed-release and enteric-coated iron preparations are marketed as causing fewer gastrointestinal problems, they are more poorly absorbed and, therefore, are not recommended. Since ferrous sulfate is 3 to 20 times less expensive than the other iron preparations, this is usually the supplement of choice.

deposited during the third trimester of pregnancy. This increased need for calcium occurs at the same time that other hormonal changes in pregnancy are working against the homeostasis of this ion. For example, calcium reabsorbed from the bone (parathormone effect) is inhibited by estrogens released during pregnancy, and renal excretion of calcium is increased during gestation. Fortunately, calcium absorption from the intestine is nearly doubled during pregnancy.

The usual RDA for calcium is 1200 milligrams per day during gestation, compared with 800 to 1200 milligrams for nonpregnant women. However, older studies suggest that pregnant women cannot achieve a positive calcium balance until 2000 milligrams per day are consumed (Duggin et al 1974). The amount of calcium needed by pregnant women can be met by appropriate dietary intake, but women who are unable to tolerate milk may have problems. For women who do not ingest dairy products because of lactose intolerance, a predigested lactose-containing milk may be an alternative (see Chapter 19). Calcium supplements may be another option to assure adequate intake of this mineral (Table 3–2).

Appropriate calcium intake is important not only for fetal bone accretion, it also decreases calcium losses from the mother's bone, which could lead to maternal osteoporosis. Calcium intake may also be important to prevent other complications of pregnancy, such as preeclampsia. However, since there is no relationship between the incidence of osteoporosis and parity, the rationale for calcium supplementation during pregnancy has been questioned. Moreover, increased urinary excretion of calcium during pregnancy

Table 3–2. Oral calcium supplements.*

NAME	CALCIUM (%)	TABLET SIZE (mg)	ELEMENTAL CALCIUM PER TABLET (mg)
Calcium carbonate	40	625	250
		1500	600
Calcium lactate	13	325	42
		650	85
Calcium gluconate	9.4	500	47
		650	61
		1000	94
Calcium glubionate (Neo-Calglucon)	6	1 teaspoon* (5 mL) syrup	115*

*Calcium, by itself, cannot be absorbed and is, therefore, always available in combination with other chemicals. However, each of the above calcium supplements is absorbed equally well. The differences among these supplements are their concentration of calcium, cost, and contamination with other metals. The more concentrated calcium supplements are often preferable to minimize the number of pills needed to meet an individual's requirement. "Natural" calcium supplements made from bone meal, oyster shell, and dolomite may contain toxic levels of lead or mercury. These natural calcium supplements may be particularly unsafe for pregnant and lactating women as well as for children.

may be a consequence of increased calcium absorption secondary to elevated vitamin D levels (Gertner et al 1986), and this may pose a potential risk for nephrolithiasis (kidney stones).

Phosphorus

Phosphorus is the second most abundant mineral in the body. About 85 percent of this element is found in bone as calcium phosphate and hydroxyapatite salts. The fetal accretion of phosphorus is about 70 to 85 milligrams per kilogram per day. Phosphorus is important in the formation of the crystalline structure of the skeleton as well as being a constituent of nucleic acid and cell membranes and an essential factor in all energy-producing reactions of the cells. However, little attention is paid to phosphorus because it is abundantly available in a wide variety of foodstuffs. Therefore, nutritional deficiencies of phosphorus are rare except under unusual circumstances, such as in the small prematurely born infant and in patients being treated with total parenteral nutrition.

Magnesium

Until recently, there has been little cognizance taken of possible magnesium deficiencies during gestation, even though a large body of knowledge of its metabolic importance and risks have already accumulated. An average of 2.6 to 3.75 milligrams per kilogram per day of magnesium is needed for fetal accretion, and the RDA for magnesium during pregnancy is 320 milligrams per day. However, the average daily intake of magnesium is usually much lower, and the diet may contain nutrients and substances that decrease magnesium bioavailability. Two studies that evaluated the diets of middle-class pregnant women reported their daily magnesium intakes to be only 103 to 333 milligrams, with an average net magnesium loss of 40 milligrams (Ashe, Schofield & Gram 1979, Johnson & Phillips 1980).

The decreased dietary intake and the increased needs of magnesium by pregnant women explain the lower serum levels seen in pregnant women. Magnesium deficits have been found even after correction for hemodilution. The possible contribution of magnesium deficiency to the pathogenesis of preeclampsia and eclampsia has been widely discussed, though no definite proof is yet available. Similarly, the possible effects of magnesium deficiency on the baby are not clear, but experimental evidence suggests that in deprived animals the mother retains magnesium at fetal expense, resulting in an increased mortality and morbidity of the offspring.

Zinc

Zinc requirements are also increased during pregnancy. It is estimated that the pregnant woman must retain 750 micrograms of zinc daily during the last two trimesters of pregnancy for optimal fetal growth and development. The intake of dietary zinc required to achieve all the needs of a pregnant woman is 15 milligrams per day, as compared with 12 milligrams for a nonpregnant woman. A high dietary zinc intake is needed because only a small portion (20 percent) of this mineral is absorbed from dietary sources. The amount absorbed varies; two important modulators of zinc absorption are dietary nitrogen and phosphorus. The higher the level of nitrogen and phosphorus in the diet, the lower the zinc absorption. To ensure an appropriate dietary intake of this element, a mixed, varied diet must be ingested throughout gestation. However, it has been suggested that zinc intake during pregnancy may be suboptimal, and mild zinc deficiency among pregnant women may not be a rare phenomenon in the United States and in other industrialized Western countries.

It has long been known that in animals marginal-to-low intake of zinc during gestation, even for short periods, can cause fetal abnormalities, particularly neural-tube defects (Warkany & Petering 1972). This indicates that even when zinc deficits are severe enough to cause fetal abnormalities the mother does not mobilize sufficient zinc from her own stores (e.g., bone) to meet the fetal requirements (Hurley 1980). The teratogenic effects of low zinc intake in rats predominantly involve the development of bone, brain, eyes, and lungs.

Human studies also point toward an important role of zinc deficiency as a teratogenic agent with a high incidence of anencephaly (Sever & Emanuel 1973). In the United States, an epidemiologic association has also been made between maternal zinc deficiency and fetal central nervous system malformations. Additionally, women with acrodermatitis enteropathica, malabsorption of zinc, have increased spontaneous abortions or deliver babies with major congenital malformations such as multiple skeletal abnormalities and anencephaly. After institution of appropriate zinc therapy, one of these mothers had three normal infants (Brenton, Jackson & Young 1981). However, routine zinc supplementation to pregnant women has not been shown to improve pregnancy outcome (Hambidge et al 1983, Swanson & King 1987).

Chromium

Fetal chromium levels are maintained at the cost of maternal supplies. In human fetal tissue, chromium concentrations increase from the second through the seventh month of gestation and fall after birth. There is a close correlation between the serum chromium concentration of mothers at delivery and the hair chromium content of their newborn infants. However, the mean value of maternal hair chromium is less than half that of the newborn infant. Transfer of chromium across the placenta might lead to maternal chromium deficiency, which prevents the normal maternal response to a glucose load and therefore causes an impaired glucose tolerance. These data suggest that gestational chromium deficiency may play a role in the genesis of gestational diabetes mellitus (Seelig 1982).

Therefore, an appropriate chromium intake during pregnancy should be ensured. This element is contained in meat, particularly liver and other organ meats, brewer's yeast, whole grains, nuts, cheeses, and black pepper. The chromium content of American diets ranges from 5 to 150 micrograms per day. Other countries, such as Japan, consume more than 200 micrograms per day. The recommended dietary intake of chromium is 50 to 200 milligrams per day as per the National Research Council. The amount of chromium available from food for metabolic use is dependent on its bioavailability. Organically bound chromium, as is present in food, is much better absorbed in the gut than the inorganic form of chromium.

The precise quantitation of the role of chromium during pregnancy remains to be established. Supplementation with this mineral is not recommended as we do not yet know the possible toxic effects on the fetus.

SUPPLEMENTAL VITAMINS AND MINERALS

Although it is customary to prescribe vitamin and mineral supplements to pregnant women, an appropriate well-balanced diet will be sufficient, in most instances, to meet the increased vitamin requirements of the mother-to-be and the unborn baby. Folic acid and iron are the exceptions, and supplementation is recommended. Attention should also be paid to ensure adequate intake of magnesium, zinc, and chromium, which could easily be insufficient in the usual diet. When that is the case, supplements may be necessary.

It should be kept in mind that there are reports that suggest a positive effect of multivitamin supplementation during pregnancy, reducing neural-tube defects in babies (Smithells et al 1980 & 1981). The use of multivitamins for the 3 months before conception and through the first 3 months of pregnancy has also been shown to have an overall protective effect against neural-tube defects (Mulinare et al 1988). However, other studies have shown that overall malnutrition was an important factor. Women with nutritionally poor diets had a higher recurrence rate of neural-tube defects than that observed among those who were eating more appropriate diets (Lawrence et al 1980). Despite the limitation of these studies, the results should be considered carefully, and malnutrition of any type before and during pregnancy should be avoided.

During pregnancy women should rely on a wholesome, varied diet to ingest all the necessary nutrients, including vitamins and minerals. Supplemental vitamins and minerals are no substitute for a healthy diet, and the general use of multivitamin or mineral supplements provided on a routine basis to well nourished individuals does not improve pregnancy outcome. Megadoses of vitamins are clearly contraindicated during pregnancy. The reports already discussed on congenital malformations associated with vitamins A, C, and D support this conclusion. The only supplements that are routinely recommended are iron and folacin.

CLINICAL INTERVENTION

Pregnant women should be instructed that it is more beneficial to eat a well-balanced diet rich in necessary vitamins and minerals than to take pharmaceutical supplements. The practice of using medications could even be dangerous if inappropriate meals are ingested because of the belief that vitamin and mineral capsules or tablets would compensate for the dietary deficits. For example, a woman may receive iron from a vitamin and mineral tablet, but it may not be sufficient or it may be inadequately absorbed.

Prenatal vitamins are available as both nonprescription and prescription items. Although these are marketed directly for the pregnant woman, they differ very little from routine over-the-counter vitamins assigned for use by the general public (although they tend to be much more expensive).

Most vitamin formulations offer advantages and disadvantages that need to be weighed individually in relation to the woman's diet and needs. Careful attention should be taken to note the composition of the prenatal vitamins. For example, Filibum (Lederle) contains 100 percent of the folate but it provides a little more than half the minimum iron requirement. Another over-the-counter prenatal vitamin, Natabec (Parke Davis) does not contain any folic acid, a nutrient that is usually deficient in a pregnant woman's diet. It is an incomplete supplement for other vitamins and minerals but provides 100 percent of the needed iron. Another vitamin marketed for pregnant women, Niferex Elixir (Central Pharmaceuticals), contains alcohol, and although it is a small quantity, alcohol is a substance that should be avoided during pregnancy (see Chapter 7).

Vitamins are advertised as being ideal for the pregnant woman, boasting about providing more than 100 percent of the vitamins and minerals required by the mother-to-be. However, such vitamins may introduce potential dangers. For example, Mission Prenatal (Mission), which contains 343 percent of the RDA for vitamin C (240 mg), and 300 percent of the RDA for vitamin A (8000 IU), may lead to an excessive intake of these vitamins, with potentially serious side effects. A pregnant woman who receives this supplement and eats a normal diet (see Menu 2, Chapter 2) would consume 21,637 IU of vitamin A and 546 milligrams of vitamin C. These quantities provide the woman with over 812 percent of the RDA for vitamin A and 780 percent of

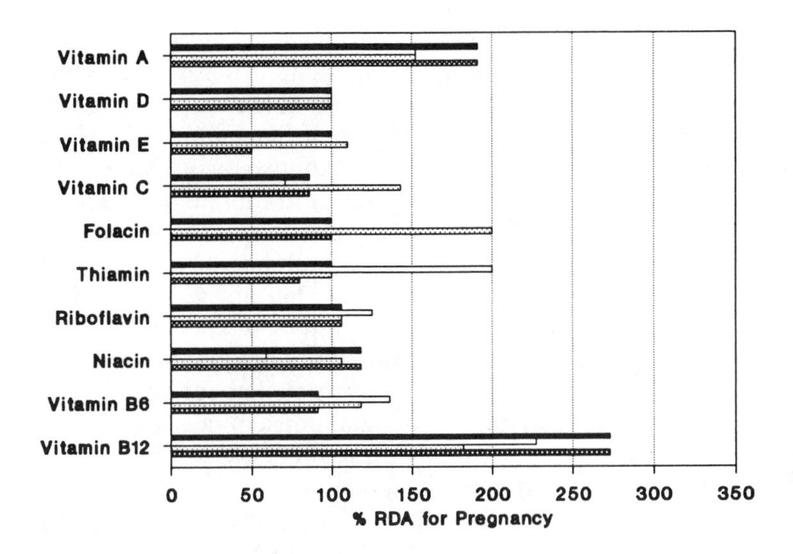

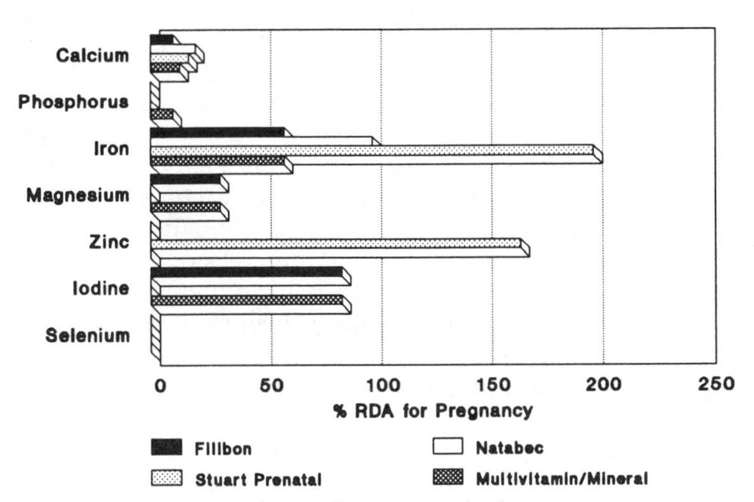

Figure 3–1. Comparison of prenatal supplements.

From Physician's desk reference for nonprescription drugs. 11th ed. Oradell, NJ: Medical Economics Co., Inc., 1990.

the RDA for vitamin C; levels that are potentially toxic for the mother and fetus. Therefore, any vitamins and minerals ordered for pregnant women must be carefully evaluated for inadequacy and excess in the context of each woman's dietary intake. If a well-balanced diet is eaten, most supplemental vitamins and minerals are not needed!

However, it is difficult to consume enough bioavailable folic acid and iron by diet alone. One example of an available supplement is Iron-FA, which contains 1 milligram of folic acid and 250 milligrams of ferrous gluconate (82 mg elemental iron) (see Table 3–1). This is an appropriate amount to be administered to most pregnant women and is inexpensive compared with other, more complicated, supplements, which may also contain other unnecessary additions such as "intrinsic factor concentrate" and other B vitamins.

The pregnant woman should be instructed about the dangers to the fetus of excessive consumption of vitamins, particularly vitamins C, A, and D. If these are being taken in large quantities, they should be discontinued. If the dietary intake demonstrates that insufficient quantities of vitamins and minerals are ingested, then the woman should be instructed about an adequate diet. If she is unable to meet the maternal and fetal nutrient needs by dietary means, then specific supplements should be prescribed. Often, zinc, magnesium, and calcium intake may require supplementation. Only women who are unable to consume dairy products and therefore do not take in enough calcium may need calcium supplements. It is important to note that calcium supplements may cause constipation and gas. Women may find that taking calcium in more frequent, smaller quantities (i.e., 250 mg four times a day) causes fewer gastrointestinal problems and is better absorbed.

A review of all the available prescription and nonprescription vitamin and mineral supplements listed in the *Physicians' Desk Reference* (1989) indicates that none of them is ideal (Fig. 3–1). They either provide excessive nutrient supplementation or insufficient quantities of essential elements, further stressing the necessity for eating a well-balanced diet with specific supplementation when required. Moreover, the bioavailability of all the nutrients may be changed by adding vitamin and mineral supplementation. The excessive nutrient intakes from supplements may interfere with absorption of other vitamins and minerals. For example, calcium will interfere with zinc absorption, and zinc will compete with copper absorption. This is an example of when some might be good, but more is not necessarily better.

REFERENCES

Ashe JR, Schofield FA, Gram MR. The retention of calcium, iron, phosphorus, and magnesium during pregnancy: The adequacy of prenatal diets with and without supplementation. Am J Clin Nutr 1979; 32:286–291.

Bailey LB, Mahan CS, Dimperio D. Folacin and iron status in low income pregnant adolescents and mature women. Am J Clin Nutr 1980; 33:1997–2001.

Brenton DP, Jackson MJ, Young A. Two pregnancies in a patient with acrodermatitis enteropathica treated with zinc sulphate. Lancet 1981; 2:500–502.

Cochrane WA. Overnutrition in prenatal and neonatal life: A problem? Can Med Assoc J 1965; 93:893–899.

Duggin GG, Lyneham RC, Date WE, Evans RA, Tiller DJ. Calcium balance in pregnancy. Lancet 1974; 2:926–927.

Gertner JM, Coustan DR, Kliger AS, et al. Pregnancy as state of physiologic absorptive hypercalciuria. Am J Med 1986; 81:451–456.

Hambidge KM, Krebs NF, Jacobs MA, et al. Zinc nutritional status during pregnancy: A longitudinal study. Am J Clin Nutr 1983; 37:429–442.

Hemminki E, Starfield B. Routine administration of iron and vitamins during pregnancy: Review of controlled clinical trials. Br J Obstet Gynaecol 1978; 85:404–410.

Hurley LS. Developmental nutrition. Englewood Cliffs, NJ: Prentice-Hall, Inc., 1980.

Jackson I, Doig WB, McDonald G. Pernicious anemia as a cause of infertility. Lancet 1967; 2:1159–1160.

Johnson NE, Phillips C. Magnesium content of diets of pregnant women. In Cantin M, Seelig MS, eds. Magnesium in health and disease. Jamaica, NY: SP Medical and Scientific Books, 1980:827–831.

Lawrence KM, James N, Miller M, Campbell H. Increased risk of recurrence of pregnancies complicated by fetal neural tube defects in mother receiving poor diets and possible benefit of dietary counseling. Br Med J 1980; 281:1592–1594.

Lammer EJ, Chen DT, Haar RM, et al. Retinoic acid embryopathy. New Engl J Med 1985; 313:835–841.

Mulinare J, Cordero JF, Erickson JO, Berry RJ. Periconceptional use of multivitamins and the occurrence of neural tube defects. JAMA 1988; 260:3141–3145.

Pitkin RM. Vitamins and minerals in pregnancy. Clin Perinatal 1975; 2:221–232.

Physicians' desk reference. Oradell, NJ: Medical Economics Co., Inc., 1989.

Reddy GS, Norman AW, Willis DM, et al. Regulation of vitamin D metabolism in normal human pregnancy. J Clin Endocrinol Metab 1983; 56:363–370.

Robens JF. Teratogenic effects of hypervitaminosis A in the hamster and guinea pig. Toxicol Appl Pharm 1970; 16:88–99.

Rosa FW, Wilk AL, Kesley FO. Teratogen update: Vitamin A congener. Teratology 1986; 33:355–364.

Seelig MS. Prenatal and neonatal mineral deficiencies: Magnesium, zinc, and chromium. In Lifshitz F, ed. Pediatric nutrition: Infant feedings, deficiencies, diseases. New York: Marcel Dekker, 1982:167–196.

Seligman PA, Caskey JH, Frazier JL, et al. Measurements of iron absorption from prenatal multivitamin-mineral supplements. Obstet Gynecol 1983; 61:356–362.

Sever LE, Emanuel I. Is there a connection between maternal zinc deficiency and congenital malformations of the central nervous system in man? Teratology 1973; 7:117–118.

Smithells RW, Sheppard S, Schorch CJ, et al. Possible prevention of neural tube defects by periconceptual vitamin supplementation. Lancet 1980; 1:339–340.

Smithells RW, Sheppard S, Schorch CJ, et al. Apparent prevention of neural tube defects by periconceptual vitamin supplementation. Arch Dis Child 1981; 56:911–918.

Swanson CA, King JC. Zinc and pregnancy outcome. Am J Clin Nutr 1987; 46:763–771.

Tsang RC, ed. Vitamin and mineral requirements in preterm infants. New York: Marcel Dekker, 1985.

Warkany J, Petering HG. Congenital malformations of the central nervous system in rats produced by maternal zinc deficiency. Teratology 1972; 5:319–334.

4

Teenage Pregnancy

Sue was looking forward to celebrating her "sweet 16" birthday party. Not so long ago she had such a good time at her best friend's sixteenth birthday party where she met her boyfriend, Joe. But today, she woke up feeling sick. She vomited all morning and had an upset stomach throughout the day. The party was no fun and her friends asked her what was wrong and Joe remarked that she was "no fun to be with." After many more days of the same "puking feeling," she found out that she was pregnant. When the doctor told her, she couldn't even believe it; after all, she had only "been" with Joe that one day!

THE PROBLEM

Sue's story is not unusual; indeed there are approximately 1 million teenagers who become pregnant annually in the United States. Approximately 40 percent of them elect to terminate their pregnancies (Maciak et al 1987). Adolescent pregnancies have profound health, social, psychologic, and vocational implications (Naeye 1981a, b, & 1983, Zuckerman et al 1983, Frisancho et al, 1983 & 1985). The obstetric and medical problems are related to biologic maturation of the adolescent. Those at the highest risk are obviously the youngest ones. Nearly all of these young women have had their first period 3 to 5 years before becoming pregnant, with menarche in the United States today occurring at an average age of 12.5 years. This high-risk group of very young adolescent pregnancies accounts for about 13,000 births a year. While they are small in number, these pregnancies are associated with a poor outcome and a high cost to society. An intermediate-risk group accounts for more than a quarter of a million pregnant adolescents 15 to 17 years old. Those at lowest risk are 18- and 19-year-olds, whose risks associated with pregnancy are similar to those of women in their twenties.

There are many social consequences of childbearing during adolescence. These include the potential for discontinuation of secondary education, unstable peer group relations, and altered relationship with the parents of the teenager, as well as economic and financial difficulties. Young mothers are also at a high nutritional risk. If they conceived shortly after menarche, their own growth may still be incomplete. Often, these young women enter prenatal care late, in poor nutritional status, with low prepregnancy weights and with low weight gains during pregnancy. Alcohol, tobacco, and drug abuse may also complicate the picture (see Chapter 7). Therefore, teenage pregnancy is associated with a higher proportion of low-birth-weight infants, greater neonatal mortality rates, and higher rates of premature delivery.

NUTRITION NEEDS

Teenagers who are pregnant have higher nutrient requirements than other pregnant women (Frisancho, Matos & Bollettino 1984) (Table 4–1). The energy needs of adolescent girls, especially those under 15, are higher than those of mature women because of their need for further growth and their increased physical energy expenditure (Blackburn & Calloway 1974, Dwyer 1987). Pregnant adolescents require an average of 400 to 500 calories per day in addition to the normal energy requirements of a growing teenager. Age and level of physical activity will affect these recommendations and should be taken into consideration when determining individual guidelines.

The protein needs of pregnant adolescents are nearly double those of nonpregnant adults (see Table 4–1). The RDA for protein from the second month of pregnancy until term is 74 to 76 grams per day for adolescent girls. It has been suggested that pregnant adolescents under 15 years of age receive 1.7 grams of protein per kilogram of pregnant body weight per day. For girls 15 to 18 years of age, an intake of 1.5 grams of protein per kilogram of pregnant body weight is necessary.

The mineral and vitamin needs of pregnant adolescents are also increased beyond the needs of mature pregnant women (see Table 4–1). The requirements of teenage pregnant girls for iron, calcium, phosphorus, vitamin D, and folacin are increased 200 percent or more over the RDA for nonpregnant adult women. At least a 120 percent increase is needed for vitamin E, magnesium, zinc, thiamin, and the other B vitamins.

The dietary intakes of adolescents have generally been found to be deficient in many nutrients other than calories. The nutrients most often found to be inadequate are calcium; iron; zinc; vitamins A, B_6, and C; and folacin.

Table 4–1. Recommended Dietary Allowances for Nonpregnant and Pregnant Teenagers.

	RECOMMENDED DAILY REQUIREMENTS FOR NONPREGNANT TEENAGERS		DAILY NUTRIENT REQUIREMENTS FOR PREGNANT TEENAGERS	
NUTRIENT	**11 to 14 Years**	**15 to 18 Years**	**11 to 14 Years**	**15 to 18 Years**
Energy (kcal/kg)	48	38	+500 kcal/d	+400 kcal/d
Protein (g/kg)	1.0	0.8	1.7	1.5
Vitamin A (μg RE)*	800	800	800	800
Vitamin D (μg)†	10	10	15	15
Vitamin E (mg)‡	8	8	10	10
Vitamin K (μg)	45	55	50	60
Vitamin C (mg)	50	60	60	70
Folacin (μg)	150	180	370	400
Niacin (mg)	15	15	17	17
Riboflavin (mg)	1.3	1.3	1.6	1.6
Thiamin (mg)	1.1	1.1	1.5	1.5
Vitamin B_6 (mg)	1.4	1.5	2.0	2.1
Vitamin B_{12} (μg)	2.0	2.0	2.2	2.2
Calcium (mg)	1200	1200	1600	1600
Phosphorus (mg)	1200	1200	1600	1600
Iron (mg)	15	15	30§	30§
Magnesium (mg)	280	300	320	340
Zinc (mg)	12	12	15	15
Iodine (μg)	150	150	175	175
Selenium (μg)	45	50	55	60

*Retinol Equivalents: 1 RE = 3.33 International Units (IU)
†1 μg equals 40 IU.
‡1 mg equals 1.49 IU.
§If teenager has underlying iron deficiency and anemia, iron supplementation is necessary.

Adapted from the Committee on Dietary Allowances, Food and Nutrition Board, National Research Council. Recommended daily allowances. 10th ed. Washington, D.C.: National Academy Press, 1989.

Consequently, pregnant adolescents often demonstrate multiple nutritional deficiencies, especially iron and folacin deficiency (Baily, Mahon & Dimperio 1980). Thus, they may need additional nutritional supplementation during pregnancy above that recommended for nonpregnant adolescents and for adult pregnant women (Loris, Dewey & Poirier-Brode 1985).

SPECIAL CONSIDERATIONS

Many of the risk factors that determine the outcome of a pregnancy are stacked against the teenager who is pregnant. Childbearing during this period of life is usually associated with an unstable lifestyle, emotional immaturity, and an insecure economic base. Moreover, other problems such as smoking, drugs, and alcohol may add to the fetus' undernutrition owing to their association with placental insufficiency. Frequently, these teenagers have infections and lack access to medical care. Often, they report insufficient food intake, poor food selection, and poor eating habits, with inadequate distribution of food throughout the day (Marino & King 1980, Frisancho et al 1985). They also may report pica (Anonymous 1976), which is consumption of nonfood objects such as clay, dirt, or paint. The reason for this behavior is not clear but according to folklore these cravings are caused by the increased need for minerals.

Many adolescents who become pregnant may start their pregnancy with inappropriate body weights, often being either 15 percent or more below their ideal body weight or 20 percent or more over it (Rosso & Lederman 1982). They may also have inappropriate weight gain during pregnancy due to common adolescent concerns regarding body image and appearance. Marked weight losses are also encountered more frequently among pregnant adolescents, particularly during the initial stages of pregnancy. Even if a pregnant adolescent gains the same amount of weight during pregnancy as a mature woman, her fetus faces increased competition for nutrients since she has greater nutrient requirements. Another explanation for the reduced birth weights of babies born to adolescents is a deficiency in placental functioning associated with the immature endocrine functioning of teenagers. Younger adolescents, those aged 13 to 16 years, need to gain approximately 35 pounds (16 kg) during pregnancy to produce an infant with an average birth weight (Fig. 4–1), whereas adolescent mothers older than 16 years of age may require about 24 pounds (10.9 kg) gestational weight gain for a similar outcome.

Another special consideration for the teenage mother is lactation. In one study, 19 to 27 percent of young mothers elected to breastfeed their babies (Lipsman, Dewey & Lonnerdal 1985). Lactation may be beneficial to the teenager and to her infant (Shotland & Peterson 1985), but it may also add a number of concerns, including the variability in the quality of the breast milk and the calcium losses incurred by the young mother (Chan et al 1982a, b). Additionally, the added social disruption of nursing for the adolescent mother could impede her own personal development. However, all things considered it appears that it is inappropriate to discourage breastfeeding among adolescents, although one must recognize the enormous commitment required on the part of the adolescent mother if breastfeeding is to be successful.

CLINICAL INTERVENTION

Most teenagers behave in quite unpredictable ways, a condition that may be exaggerated in the pregnant adolescent. They do whatever they want, do not often listen to adults, and at times seem as if they are from another world. The

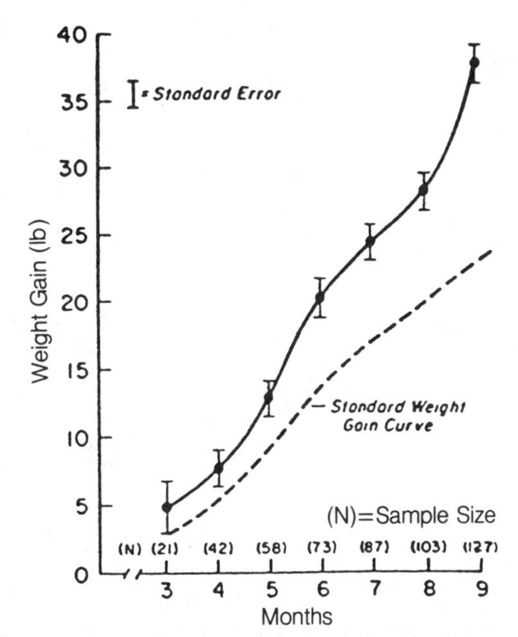

Figure 4–1. Weight gain of adolescent girls (13–19 years) delivering at term.
Reprinted with permission from Loris P, Dewey KG, Poirier-Brode K. Weight gain and dietary intake of pregnant teenagers. J Am Diet Assoc 1985; 85:1296–1305.

young pregnant woman may also be struggling with her parents and the father of the baby over continuing the pregnancy, abortion, adoption, and marriage. At the same time she may be attempting to deal with typical teenage rebellion, "raging hormones," confusion over her role, coping with dropping out of school, and feelings of rejection by her peers. Usually she is in turmoil and does not know where to turn for help.

It is difficult and often challenging to establish a good rapport with these young women. It takes time and patience to develop the type of relationship required for appropriate counseling. Teenagers need help to understand the nutritional needs of the baby as well as their own. Patience is required to assist the pregnant teenager develop a diet that will fit with her lifestyle and food preferences. For example, if a teenage mother-to-be prefers fast food, a diet that includes hamburgers, milkshakes, pizza, and so on (such as the following sample menu) will increase her compliance.

MENU 1

Breakfast
1 cup ready-to-eat cereal
8 ounces whole milk
8 ounces apple juice

Snack
Banana

Lunch
Cheeseburger
1 serving french fries
Salad with dressing
8 ounces milkshake

Snack
1 cup orange sherbet

Dinner
2 cups spaghetti with meat sauce
8 ounces grape juice
½ cup fruit cocktail

Snack
1 cup whole milk
6 ginger snap cookies

This meal selection is not unusual among our adolescent population (see Chapter 15). It provides the necessary food choices and the calories required by an average pregnant adolescent. This diet is high in energy and is relatively low in fat, with good quality and quantity of protein (Fig. 4–2). Pregnancy may not be the time to worry about so called "junk food." If this is what the adolescent will eat, let it be; after all, fast food can be part of a well-balanced diet.

However, the vitamin and mineral requirements of the pregnant teenager may not be met by this diet alone. This sample menu does not meet the following nutrient needs: vitamin D, vitamin E, folacin, iron, zinc and copper. Intake of thiamin is also slightly above the RDA for a pregnant teenager (see Fig. 4–2). The nutrients that are not ingested in sufficient quantities must be supplemented to meet the RDAs.

Given the difficulties in consuming a diet that meets all the nutrient requirements of pregnancy during adolescence, a vitamin and mineral supplement may be routinely advised. For example, a prenatal vitamin preparation such as Precare (Russ) would supplement all the needs of a pregnant adolescent for iron, zinc, folacin, magnesium, and calcium. However, it contains no vitamin E and, more importantly, would provide excessive amounts of some nutrients (e.g., 8000 IU of vitamin A and 90 mg of vitamin C). Added to the dietary intake, the RDAs are exceeded by 488 percent for vitamin A and 289 percent for vitamin C. For these reasons, supplementation is recommended only for those elements that may be deficient in the diet.

Teenage pregnancy and childbearing are serious problems (Pratt et al

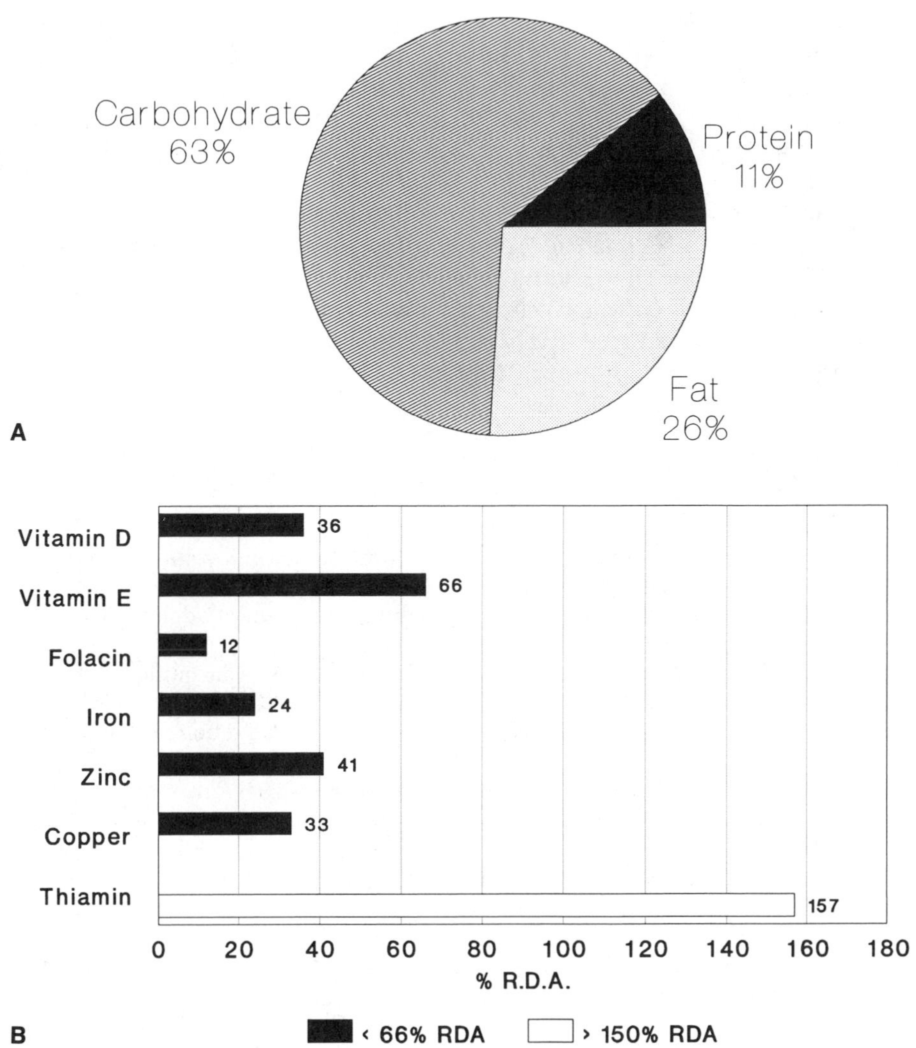

Figure 4–2. **A.** Caloric distribution of Menu 1. **B.** Inappropriate nutrient intakes.

1984), and the rates in this country are higher than in other developed countries. Approximately 8 percent of all teens, and 18 percent of sexually active adolescents, become pregnant each year (Westoff, Calot & Foster 1983). Blacks have a higher rate of teenage pregnancy than whites in America. Efforts must be aimed at delaying early sexual activity among teens and encouraging and promoting the use of contraception. For those who become pregnant and decide to carry the pregnancy to term, intense nutritional and prenatal counseling is necessary. Some of the risks of teenage pregnancy can be altered with appropriate medical, social, and nutritional intervention (Leppert, Namerow & Barker 1986). In fact, comprehensive prenatal care has been shown to be a more important factor in relation to pregnancy outcome than is maternal age.

Young adolescents who are pregnant often qualify for federal supplementary food programs such as the Women, Infant, and Children (WIC) Program and/or food stamps. They should be encouraged to participate in these programs and nutrition education classes. However, the risks of adolescent pregnancy can only be reduced by appropriate maternal behaviors and a will to take on a challenging task during and after pregnancy.

REFERENCES

Anonymous. Pica: A full report. JAMA 1976; 235:2765.

Baily LB, Mahon CS, Dimperio D. Folacin and iron studies in low income pregnant adolescents and mature women. Am J Clin Nutr 1980; 33:1997–2001.

Blackburn ML, Calloway DH. Energy expenditure of pregnant adolescents. J Am Diet Assoc 1974; 65:24–30.

Chan GM, Slater P, Ronald N, et al. Bone mineral status of lactating mothers of different ages. Am J Obstet Gynecol 1982a; 144:438–441.

Chan GM, Ronald N, Slater P, Hollis J, Thomas MR. Decreased bone mineral status in lactating adolescent mothers. J Pediatr 1982b; 101:718–719.

Dwyer J. Maternal nutrition in pregnancy with emphasis on adolescence. In Grand RJ, Stephen JL, Dietz WH, eds. Pediatric nutrition. Boston: Butterworths, 1987:205–220.

Frisancho AR, Matos J, Bollettino LA. Influence of growth status and placental function on birth weight of infants born to young still-growing teenagers. Am J Clin Nutr 1984; 40:801–807.

Frisancho AR, Matos J, Flegel P. Maternal nutritional status and adolescent pregnancy outcome. Am J Clin Nutr 1983; 38:739–746.

Frisancho AR, Matos J, Leonard WR, Yaroch LA. Developmental and nutritional determinants of pregnancy outcome among teenagers. Am J Phys Anthr 1985; 66:247–261.

Leppert PC, Namerow PB, Barker D. Pregnancy outcome among adolescent and older women receiving comprehensive prenatal care. J Adolesc Health Care 1986; 7:112–117.

Lipsman S, Dewey KG, Lonnerdal B. Breast-feeding among teenage mothers: Milk composition, infant growth and maternal dietary intake. J Pediatr Gastroenterol Nutr 1985; 4:1–9.

Loris P, Dewey KG, Poirier-Brode K. Weight gain and dietary intake of pregnant teenagers. J Am Diet Assoc 1985; 85:1296–1305.

Maciak BJ, Spitz AM, Strauss LT, Morris L, Warren CW, Marks JS. Pregnancy and

birth rates among sexually experienced US teenagers—1974, 1980, and 1983. JAMA 1987; 258:2069–2071.
Marino DD, King JC. Nutritional concerns during adolescence. Pediatric Clin North Am 1980; 27:125–138.
Naeye RL. Nutritional/nonnutritional interactions that affect the outcome of pregnancy. Am J Clin Nutr 1981a; 34:727–731.
Naeye RL. Teenaged and pre-teenaged pregnancies: Consequences of the fetal-maternal competition for nutrients. Pediatrics 1981b; 67:146–150.
Naeye RL. Maternal age, obstetric complications, and the outcome of pregnancy. Obstet Gynecol 1983; 61:210–216.
Pratt WF, Mosher WD, Bachrach CA, et al. Understanding US fertility: findings from the National Survey of Family Growth, cycle III. Popul Bull 1984; 39:1–42.
Rosso P, Lederman SA. Nutrition in the pregnant adolescent. In Winick M, ed. Adolescent nutrition, current conepts in nutrition. Vol 11. New York: John Wiley & Sons, 1982:47.
Shotland NL, Peterson C. A modest proposal: Breastfeeding for the infants of adolescent mothers. Adv Psychosom Med 1985; 12:81–90.
Westoff CF, Calot G, Foster AD. Teenage fertility in developed nations. Fam Plann Perspect 1983; 15:105–110.
Zuckerman B, Alpert JJ, Dooling E, et al. Neonatal outcome: Is adolescent pregnancy a risk factor? Pediatrics 1983; 71:489–493.

5

Nausea and Vomiting During Pregnancy

In the second month of pregnancy, Margie experienced "morning sickness," "afternoon sickness," and "evening sickness." Because she was unable to eat without feeling nauseated or vomiting, Margie began to lose weight. She tried every bit of advice to help her cope with sickness. She ate smaller, more frequent meals, kept crackers and dry toast at her bedside to eat before getting up, avoided greasy foods and foods with strong odors, . . . Finally, after losing 10 pounds, Margie had to be hospitalized.

MILD NAUSEA AND VOMITING

Approximately 50 percent of all pregnant women experience some nausea and vomiting during the first trimester of pregnancy (Fairweather 1968, Jarnfelt-Samsoe, Samsoe & Velindar 1983, Dilorio 1985). Indeed, this was first recognized 3000 years ago and is commonly accepted as one of the "discomforts" of a mother-to-be. At times, morning sickness is the first clue that a woman may be pregnant. In most cases, these symptoms are mild, occur most severely in the morning, and alter the appetite. However, these problems usually do not produce any disturbance in nutritional status or electrolyte balance. The symptoms usually disappear by the end of the first trimester without any severe consequence (Beaton 1983). The occurrence of vomiting in the latter part of pregnancy is a different type of problem, perhaps due to other alterations such as so-called hiatus hernia, and will not be addressed here.

The cause of pregnancy-induced nausea and vomiting has not been determined (Pritchard, MacDonald & Garit 1985). Changes in hormone concentrations, including increased chorionic gonadotropin and progesterone levels, have been implicated. Other causal factors that have been identified are so-called allergic factors to the pregnancy and gastric hypotonicity, hyposecretion, and hypoperistalsis. Nausea and vomiting during pregnancy have also been considered to be a manifestation of emotional or psychological influences. Furthermore, nutritional and metabolic disturbances have been implicated in the etiology of nausea and vomiting, including carbohydrate or glycogen deficiency, vitamin B deficiency, and electrolyte deficits.

Treatment of nausea and vomiting is as varied as the theories to explain the reason for this common problem of pregnancy (Biggs 1975, Beaton 1983). Clinicians often attempt nutritional rehabilitation and advise small frequent meals high in carbohydrate and replacement of electrolyte losses. Additional recommendations include the avoidance of fatty foods or any food or activity which appears to aggravate the symptoms, the limitation of liquids, and selection of dry foods like crackers, or to lying down in a dark, quiet room during an episode. The pregnant woman, through trial and error, usually finds the foods and food combinations that "stay down." One of the few reported studies on the measures used to control nausea and vomiting during pregnancy and their effectiveness was performed on 44 pregnant teenagers ages 14 to 19 years. A variety of nonpharmacological methods were used to control nausea and vomiting (Dilorio 1985) (Fig. 5–1). Often these common measures are not very helpful and further studies are needed to identify other practices which may be more effective in minimizing the nausea and vomiting of pregnancy.

In addition to a nutritional and behavioral approach to treating nausea and vomiting of pregnancy, many pharmacological treatments have been employed, none being greatly effective and some having potentially adverse side effects (Biggs 1975). An example is Bendectin, which was possibly associated with fetal malformations and discontinued because of liability, though no clear scientific evidence of its teratogenicity existed. Drug therapies have ranged from the bizarre use of intravenously administered honey to the use of antiemetic-antimotion sickness medications or vitamin B_6. There is really no effective remedy for nausea and vomiting of pregnancy. The only cure is time. Usually by the end of the fourth month, morning sickness is no longer a problem.

HYPEREMESIS GRAVIDARUM

Hyperemesis gravidarum, or pernicious vomiting of pregnancy, is a syndrome of severe nausea and vomiting which results in serious metabolic derangements in the mother and fetus (Pritchard et al 1985). Dehydration, electrolyte and acid-base imbalances, ketosis, ketonuria, and weight loss may

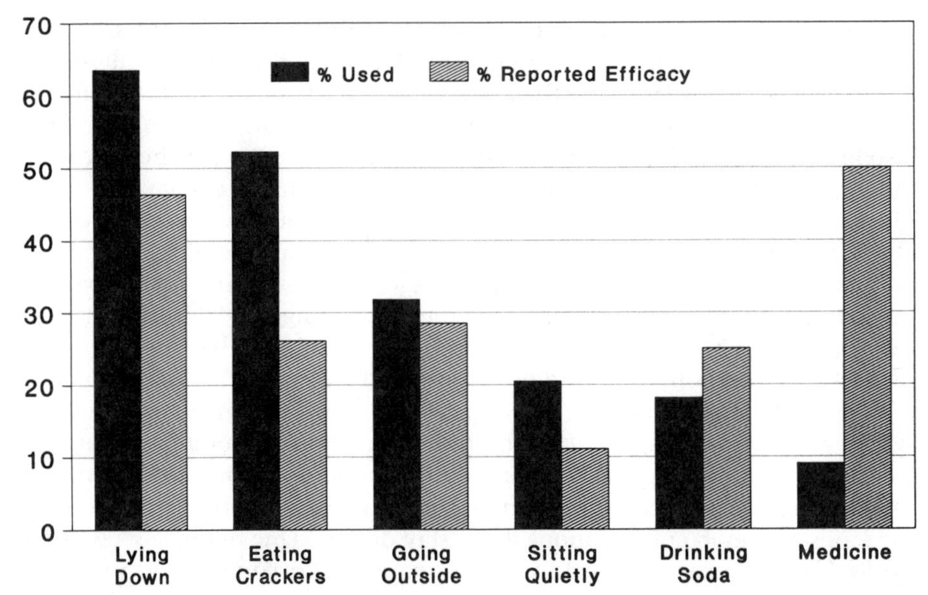

Figure 5–1. Frequency and effectiveness of methods used to control nausea and vomiting among pregnant teenagers (n = 44).

Modified from Dilorio C. First trimester nausea in pregnant teenagers: Incidence, characteristics, intervention. Nurs Res 1985; 34:372–374.

occur. The incidence of this severe complication of pregnancy in the United States and Britain is 3–4 per thousand, but in Oriental countries it is less than 2 per thousand. During war, when food was scarce and rationed, the incidence in Western countries was also reduced, probably due to the increased consumption of carbohydrates as well as to psychological factors. Hyperemesis gravidarum occurs more frequently in multiple pregnancies, and it recurs in up to 25 percent of subsequent pregnancies. However, the highest group at risk are women who have had previous unsuccessful pregnancies. The cause of this severe problem, like the cause of simple nausea and vomiting during pregnancy, is not known.

The outcome of pregnancy when this complication occurs may be associated with increased incidence of spontaneous abortions. Women often have nausea and vomiting before cramps, vaginal bleeding, and abortion. Women with hyperemesis gravidarum often deliver babies without apparent detrimental effects on the birth weight, but this condition has been associated with an increased incidence of birth defects when antiemetic drugs are used. In pregnant women who abstain from antiemetic and other drugs, hyperemesis gravidarum per se does not appear to cause an increased risk of having a deformed child. However, the pregnant woman herself is at high risk due to gross disturbances of fluid and electrolyte, particularly potassium. Reduced maternal mortality in hyperemesis gravidarum is due to the early and more efficient treatment in correcting the fluid and electrolyte imbalances.

In all instances, water and electrolyte imbalances produced by frequent vomiting must be corrected immediately. When the vomiting is mild, a liquid diet with supplementary small sips of water and juices may be sufficient. In more severe vomiting, when no food is tolerated, fluids should be provided by intravenous glucose solutions, supplemented with intravenous vitamins and minerals as needed. The patient with hyperemesis gravidarum should not even be given plain water to drink, though she may be given ice chips. Complete bed rest and a quiet, dark room often help. Once the vomiting has stopped, the patient may progress to a liquid diet. Once these diets are tolerated, the IV fluid may be discontinued. The patient may then receive her calorie requirements in the form of a liquid supplemental food such as Sustacal®, Meritene®, or Carnation Instant Breakfast® (Chapter 27).

When the woman can finally return to "regular" foods, then foods should be of a bland nature, and contain no strong odors. Her personal likes and dislikes, even idiosyncrasies, should be taken into account. When at home, she should avoid cooking foods for others, as even the smell of an offending food may set off a bout of vomiting. Setbacks may occur during the early months, and hospital readmissions for hyperemesis gravidarum are common.

In some cases the severe nausea and vomiting may persist throughout pregnancy, resulting in an inadequate maternal diet to support fetal growth. Parenteral nutrition during pregnancy has been employed successfully in a limited number of pregnant women (Chapter 28).

CLINICAL INTERVENTION

The main concern for controlling nausea and vomiting is to avoid dehydration and to provide sufficient nutrients to allow the pregnancy to proceed normally. To prevent dehydration, the mother-to-be will need to drink at least one glass (8 ounces; 240 ml) of fluid each time she vomits. Carbonated beverages or mineral water which are often selected by the pregnant woman will only replace the fluid losses; they will not replace the sodium and potassium losses secondary to vomiting (Table 5–1). It is evident that the sodium content of some beverages varies from minimal to insignificant amounts and the potassium content is negligible. Thus, even if dehydration may be prevented by drinking these types of fluids there may be electrolyte imbalances, particularly potassium deficits. A better choice of fluid intake if tolerated is to drink juices, beef and chicken bouillon which contain larger quantities of electrolytes and additional calories. Note that Gatorade®, which is often given

Table 5–1. Sodium and Potassium Content of Selected Beverages.

BEVERAGE	Sodium Per 8 Ounces		Potassium Per 8 Ounces	
	mg	mEq	mg	mEq
Mineral water, Perrier	5.0	0.2	0.0	0.0
Club soda, Canada Dry	50.4	2.2	0.0	0.0
Club soda, No Cal	< 10.0	<0.4	NA*	NA*
Seltzer, dietetic	< 10.0	<0.4	NA*	NA*
Tonic water	4.0	0.2	2.0	0.05
Coca-Cola	9.3	0.4	0.0	0.0
Pepsi-Cola	6.0	0.3	8.7	0.2
Ginger ale	20.0	0.9	3.3	0.08
7-Up	2.7	0.1	0.0	0.0
Sprite	31.3	1.4	0.0	0.0
Root beer	32.7	1.4	2.7	0.07
Diet Coke	22.0	1.0	0.0	0.0
Diet Pepsi	42.0	1.8	8.0	0.2
Diet Ginger Ale, Canada Dry	15.0	0.7	NA*	NA*
Diet Sprite	30.0	1.3	0.0	0.0
Diet root beer	39.3	1.7	0.0	0.0
Tea, brewed	19.0	0.8	58.0	1.5
Tea, instant (1 tsp.)	0.0	0.0	50.0	1.3
Coffee, brewed	2.7	0.1	156.0	4.0
Coffee, instant (2 tsp.)	0.0	0.0	72.0	1.8
Apple juice, canned	7.0	0.3	296.0	7.6
Grape juice, canned	7.0	0.3	334.0	8.6
Orange juice, canned	6.0	0.3	436.0	11.2
Tomato juice, canned	676.0	29.4	598.0	15.3
Gatorade	123.0	5.3	23.0	0.6
Beef broth, bouillon	782.0	34.0	130.0	3.3
Chicken broth	776.0	33.7	210.0	5.4

*Information not available.

Modified from Pennington JAT, Church HN. Bowes and Church's food values of portions commonly used. 14th ed. Philadelphia: JB Lippincott Co., 1985.

to replace water and electrolyte losses, does not contain as much electrolytes as some of the other liquid foods.

If the woman continues to vomit, a physician will have to determine whether there is dehydration and electrolyte imbalances which may need to be treated. This can be done with oral rehydration solutions (Chapter 18). Electrolyte replacement tablets are also available as supplements (Table 5–2). Whenever a pregnant woman vomits, the following parameters should be monitored: weight, skin turgor, oral intake, emesis output, urine volume, and specific gravity. If she loses weight, cannot tolerate any fluids, or her urine output markedly decreases, she may be dehydrated and should be examined by a physician.

If the woman continues to vomit and does not tolerate oral rehydrating solutions, she may require intravenous fluids. Electrolytes, especially potas-

Table 5–2. Electrolyte Preparations.

PREPARATION	DOSE	POTASSIUM mg	POTASSIUM mEq	SODIUM mg	SODIUM mEq
Potassium gluconate					
Kaon tablet	1 tablet	195	5	—	—
Potassium bicarbonate					
Klorvess effervescent granules	1 packet	780	20	—	—
K-lyte	1 tablet	975	25	—	—
Potassium chloride					
K-lyte Ce	1 tablet	978	25	—	—
K-lyte Cl50	1 tablet	1955	50	—	—
Micro-K Extencaps	1 capsule	312	8	—	—
Potassium phosphate					
Neutra-Phos	1 capsule	278	7	164	7
Neutra-Phos K	1 capsule	556	14	0	0
Sodium chloride (Salt)	1 teaspoon (6 g)	—	—	2300	100

From Physician's Desk Reference. 41st ed. Oradell, NJ; Medical Economics Co., Inc., 1987.

sium, should be added to the intravenous fluid. If necessary, vitamins and minerals may also be added to the intravenous fluid. Intravenous fluids can be administered either in the home, physician's office, or hospital, depending on the woman's condition. If vomiting persists and the mother-to-be does not gain weight appropriately, dietary supplements may be necessary. Nutritional supplements should be bland. If the woman finds one particular supplement unpalatable, she should try another type until she finds one she can tolerate.

Extreme cases of vomiting—hyperemesis gravidarum—require total parenteral nutrition (TPN) for several weeks, a few months, or even for the duration of the pregnancy (Martin et al 1985). Because TPN has become easier to provide in the home setting, more women are benefiting from this treatment without hospitalization and go on to complete their pregnancies and deliver healthy babies.

REFERENCES

Beaton JG. Nausea of pregnancy: A "natural" remedy. Postgrad Med 1983; 74:50.

Biggs JSG. Vomiting in pregnancy: Causes and management. Drugs 1975; 9:299–306.

DiIorio C. First trimester nausea in pregnant teenagers: Incidence, characteristics, intervention. Nurs Res 1985; 34:372–374.

Fairweather DVI. Nausea and vomiting in pregnancy. Am J Obstet Gynecol 1968; 102:135–175.

Jarnfelt-Samsoe A, Samsoe G, Velindar G. Nausea and vomiting in pregnancy—a contribution to its epidemiology. Gynecol Obstet Invest 1983; 16:221–229.
Martin R, Trubow M, Bistrian BR, Benotti P, Blackburn GL. Hyperalimentation during pregnancy: A case report. JPEN 1985; 9:212–215.
Pritchard JA, MacDonald PC, Garit NF. William's obstetrics. 17th ed. Norwalk, CT: Appleton-Century-Crofts, 1985.

6

Water Retention

In the 1970s, a newsletter from SPUN (Society for the Protection of the Unborn Through Nutrition) told the horror tale of a young mother-to-be who was admonished by her doctor not to gain much weight, and who was prescribed diuretics by the same doctor. Her baby was stillborn. . . .

Recently, Diane, who worked in a drugstore, complained to the pharmacy assistant that she was "retaining water" during her pregnancy. He handed her a package of over-the-counter "water pills."

EDEMA, HIGH BLOOD PRESSURE, PREECLAMPSIA, AND ECLAMPSIA

The presence of edema, high blood pressure, preeclampsia, and eclampsia in pregnancy has been generally referred to as toxemia when at least two of these conditions occur. However, it is now more accepted to refer to the precise problem rather than to use the vague term of toxemia (Pritchard, Macdonald & Gant 1985).

During pregnancy, women normally gain a total of 6 to 9 liters of body water and store 900 mEq (20.7 g) of sodium in maternal and fetal tissues (Robertson 1971). The water and sodium retention starts in the first trimester, but is most marked during the second and is sustained to term. Fetal storage of sodium is greatest during the final trimester of pregnancy. Fluid retention with dependent edema, especially of the lower extremities, is an uncomfortable phenomenon that occurs in up to 80 percent of pregnant women. The veins of the legs appear to be particularly susceptible because of the pressure exerted by the enlarging uterus.

Hypertension during pregnancy, defined as elevated blood pressure (higher than 140/90) without proteinuria or significant edema, occurs in 6 percent of pregnancies (Belizan & Villar 1980). Simple hypertension is not associated with adverse maternal or fetal outcomes. In contrast, preeclampsia, which occurs in 6 to 9 percent of pregnant women, is primarily seen during the first pregnancy after 20 weeks of gestation and is characterized by elevated blood pressure, proteinuria, generalized edema, and blood coagulation abnormalities. In its severe form, eclampsia is a life-threatening disease for both mother and infant. Preexisting chronic hypertension that is worsened by pregnancy occurs in 1 to 2 percent of pregnant women. It is also associated with elevated blood pressure, proteinuria, and edema and may also create significant fetal or maternal problems.

NUTRITIONAL ASPECTS OF PREECLAMPSIA–ECLAMPSIA

For many years, nutrition during pregnancy has been thought to have a significant role in the etiology of preeclampsia–eclampsia (Quilligan 1986). Although the observations concerning the relationship of diet to disease tend often to be contradictory and unclear, a significant amount of literature does implicate nutritional causes in pregnancy-induced edema, hypertension, and preeclampsia–eclampsia (Belizan & Villar 1980). No specific single nutrient is the clear culprit; rather, a complex combination of nutritional factors and deficiencies may be involved in development of the disease.

Several studies have implied that calcium, iron, and vitamin A are consistently low in the diets of most young women who are at a greater risk of complications of pregnancy, especially preeclampsia–eclampsia (Belizan & Villar 1980). Magnesium and folate deficiency have also been found to be factors that increase the incidence of this disease. Other vitamin deficiencies associated with these complications of pregnancy include thiamin, riboflavin, vitamin B_6, and niacin. The placentas of pregnant women with eclampsia have decreased contents of vitamin B_6 and thiamin.

The role of protein deprivation in the etiology of pregnancy-induced hypertension and preeclampsia–eclampsia is very controversial (Gibbs & Seitchik 1980). Some studies indicate that reduced protein intake or a suboptimal protein quality plays a part in the incidence of pregnancy-induced hypertension and that ingestion of adequate protein during pregnancy may eliminate the disease and/or reduce its frequency. However, other studies cast doubt on the role of protein deficiency. Some studies have found a greater intake of essential amino acids and protein in toxemia patients. Moreover, studies of nitrogen balance in carefully controlled pregnant women revealed no difference between those who developed toxemia and those who did not.

An increased intake of total fat and total fatty acids has also been considered in the etiology of preeclampsia–eclampsia. Fatty acids may be involved through their action on prostaglandins and uterine vascular reactivity (see Chapter 1). It may be reasonable to assume that a diet deficient in essential fatty acids may lead to deficient prostaglandin function and thus to hypertension. However, this hypothesis remains to be confirmed.

SODIUM

The theory that excess sodium intake during pregnancy causes preeclampsia or worsens preeclampsia stems from work performed over 30 years ago (Robinson 1958). At that time, it was believed that diets high in salt led to a higher incidence of eclampsia and that patients placed on a low-salt diet had improvement of the edema. However, when some preeclamptic patients were given huge amounts of sodium they gained more weight but did not have any difference in blood pressure or proteinuria. Despite the lack of evidence, salt restriction during pregnancy was the rule until the 1960s.

Pregnancy results in salt loss and requires increased sodium as compared with the nonpregnant condition. For a long time it has been known that during gestation there is an increased need for sodium, up to 74 milligrams per day or 20.7 grams (900 mEq) for the total pregnancy (Lindheimer & Katz 1973). This would be equivalent to about 50 grams of extra salt for the whole pregnancy. Since diets in the United States provide 2300 to 6900 milligrams of sodium per day—that is, about 6 to 14 grams of salt per day—there is no reason to increase sodium intake to meet the increased requirements of pregnancy. However, be aware that sodium restrictions are seldom necessary during pregnancy. The Food and Nutrition Board of the National Academy of Sciences has called the use of salt-free diets and diuretics during pregnancy potentially dangerous and stated: "It is difficult to justify dietary sodium limitation in healthy women during pregnancy on the basis of either animal or clinical evidence."

In general, patients can be advised not to limit their usual salt intake. Even severe sodium restriction (e.g., 1000 mg/d of salt) will not improve the fluid retention and the hypertensive disorders of pregnancy. On the other hand, since sodium is essential for the growth of the fetus, sodium restriction may adversely affect the fetus. Neonatal hyponatremia (low blood sodium) has been found in babies born to women who were on sodium-restricted diets.

The pregnant woman can easily get the additional 90 milligrams of sodium per day to cover the sodium needs of the fetus and the mother. One level teaspoon (5 g) of salt contains 2.5 grams of sodium, so an extra one-twentieth of a teaspoon would be necessary. However, excessive sodium intake during pregnancy should be avoided. Moderation of sodium intake can easily be achieved by avoiding foods high in sodium (Table 6–1). Only in the rare instance when pregnancy is complicated by congestive heart failure or chronic renal disease does sodium restriction become necessary.

DIURETICS IN PREGNANCY

Diuretics have long been prescribed during pregnancy to prevent or to treat preeclampsia and to alleviate excessive weight gain or edema (Robertson 1971). Prophylactic use of diuretics has been said to reduce the incidence of preeclampsia in certain susceptible populations, but these results have not been confirmed. Although diuretics will successfully decrease edema, it is

Table 6–1. Foods to Recommend or Avoid Because of Their Sodium Content.*

	RECOMMEND	AVOID
Milk/dairy	Milk: whole, low-fat, skim, unsalted buttermilk Cheese: gruyere, mozzarella, neufchatel, ricotta, Swiss, unsalted cottage cheese	Commercial foods made with milk: chocolate milk, cocoa, ice cream, sherbet; buttermilk Cheese: American, cheddar, cottage, provolone, brie, blue, roquefort, cheese spreads and dips
Meat, poultry, fish, legumes	Fresh or frozen meat and poultry; fresh fish; eggs	Organ meats; luncheon meats; canned, salted, or smoked meat or fish; shellfish; salted peanut butter; canned beans and peas
Fruits and vegetables	Fresh fruits and vegetables; fruit juices	Canned vegetables; vegetable juices; some frozen peas and lima beans processed with salt; sauerkraut; pickles; olives
Grains	Breads; most cereals; pasta; unsalted crackers; potatoes	Salted crackers and other bread products; salty snack foods: chips, pretzels; bread mixes for stuffing or casseroles
Fats	Most oils	Salt pork; bacon fat; commercial dressings; salted nuts
Other	Spices; seasonings; herbs; vinegar	Bouillon cubes; catsup; barbecue sauce; celery, onion, garlic salts; meat extracts and tenderizers; soy sauce; canned or dry soup mixes

*For further details of food salt content, the reader is referred to more complete tables (see Manual of clinical nutrition. D.M. Paige, ed. Pleasantville, NJ, Nutrition Publications, Inc., 1983:111–112).

unclear whether such an effect will favorably influence the course of the disease; and real risks have been associated with diuretic use (Pritchard, Macdonald & Gant 1985). Maternal complications of diuretics include volume constriction and electrolyte disturbances, alkalosis, decreased carbohydrate tolerance, low potassium or sodium, and high uric acid. The electrolyte imbalances per se may produce fetal malformations. Pancreatitis has also been reported to result from use of these agents. Moreover, the infant of the mother who uses diuretics is at risk for developing bleeding problems (petechiae) and may be low-birth-weight.

Since proof of benefit from diuretic agents during pregnancy is lacking, and because risks associated with its use are many, their use should be limited to specific patients who have cardiac or renal disease; they should not be used for patients with hypertension or edema of pregnancy.

CLINICAL INTERVENTION

Some pregnant women, in their desire to have a perfect, healthy baby, restrict foods that they consider harmful. Salt may fall into this category since people are accustomed to hearing "salt is bad" from the media, advertising, and physicians. Thus, salt may unjustly be considered a culprit during gestation. Pregnant women should continue to consume a normal amount of salt (Dwyer 1982). However, salt need not be taken in excessive quantities during pregnancy. Most pregnant women moderate their intake of salt by decreasing the amount of salt they add to their food. However, salt may be present in many foods, often in high quantity (e.g., processed or cured foods). It is not advisable to use salt substitutes. The use of spices and seasonings are excellent ways to enhance the taste of food without salt. The use of catsup or mustard on various foods will also eliminate the desire for added salt, but these condiments have a high sodium content themselves! The use of other salts, such as onion salt, garlic salt, lemon salt, and seasoned salt, should be moderate; they are all salts.

Each prenatal visit, which includes monitoring for high blood pressure, checking for the presence of proteinuria, and a physical assessment for edema, will reassure the mother that there is no reason to restrict salt. Even when one of these factors is abnormal, salt restriction may not be indicated. If hypertension, proteinuria, or edema are present the physician should determine the course of therapy (Pritchard, Macdonald & Gant 1985).

Over-the-counter "water pills" should not be taken during pregnancy, and diuretics are rarely needed and should be prescribed only when indicated by a physician. There are often other alternatives to a "water pill"; if the woman complains of swollen feet, she should elevate them on a stool when sitting or on a pillow when sleeping. This will improve the pedal edema and increase her comfort.

REFERENCES

Belizan JM, Villar J. The relationship between calcium intake and edema—proteinuria and hypertension gestasis. Am J Clin Nutr 1980; 33:2202–2210.

Dwyer J. Nutritional support during pregnancy and lactation. Primary Care 1982; 9:475–496.

Gibbs CE, Seitchik J. Nutrition in pregnancy. In Goodhart RS, Shils ME, eds. Modern nutrition in health and disease. 6th ed. Philadelphia: Lea & Febiger, 1980:743–752.

Lindheimer MD, Katz AI. Sodium and diuretics in pregnancy. N Engl J Med 1973; 288:891–894.

Pritchard JA, Macdonald PC, Gant NF, eds. William's obstetrics. 17th ed. Norwalk, CT: Appleton-Century-Crofts, 1985.

Quilligan EJ. Nutritional aspects of pregnancy-induced hypertension. In Kretchmer N, ed. Frontiers in clinical nutrition. Rockville: Aspen Systems Corp., 1986:49–56.

Robertson EG. The natural history of oedema during pregnancy. J Obstet Gynaecol Br Commonw 1971; 78:520–529.

Robinson M. Salt in pregnancy. Lancet 1958; 1:178–181.

7

What About a Drink?

"Behold, thou shalt conceive and bear a son and now drink no wine or strong drink." (Old Testament, Judges 13:7.)

"Drunken women bring forth children likened unto themselves." (Aristotle, 322 BC.)

Samantha was a cute baby with a delicate appearance. However, something was not quite right. She was born full-term but with a low birth weight, below-average length, and a small head. Although her caloric intake was adequate during her first year of life, she did not gain weight or grow properly. Samantha also was slow in reaching developmental milestones such as sitting up and responding to stimuli. She was admitted to the hospital for evaluation of "failure to thrive."

The hospital's social worker learned that Samantha's mother liked to drink a couple of beers with dinner and occasionally a martini. Even during pregnancy, she had continued to engage in these drinking practices. She had stopped drinking shortly before Samantha was born but unfortunately, not soon enough for her daughter to escape being a victim of FAS—fetal alcohol syndrome.

FETAL ALCOHOL SYNDROME

Fetal alcohol syndrome was first described in this country in 1973 (Jones et al 1973, Jones & Smith 1973). Moderate to heavy alcohol ingestion during pregnancy is detrimental to embryonic and fetal development (AMA 1983). It may result in FAS, characterized by small head circumference, mental retardation, decreased fat stores, reduction in birth weight and length, failure to thrive, facial abnormalities, hypotonia (poor muscle tone), poor coordination, and irritability/hyperactivity. These clinical manifestations may be sufficiently pronounced to allow for their recognition in the newborn period. More often, however, the physical features are extremely subtle, necessitating careful observations and measurements by an astute clinician (Sokol & Miller 1980).

The facial features of the affected offspring include short palpebral fissures, giving the appearance of small eyes (Fig. 7–1). A short, upturned nose and hypoplastic philtrum (the vertical groove over the center of the upper lip beneath the nose), are also part of the features. These patients also show a hypoplastic maxilla, thinned upper vermilion border of the lip, and retrognathia,

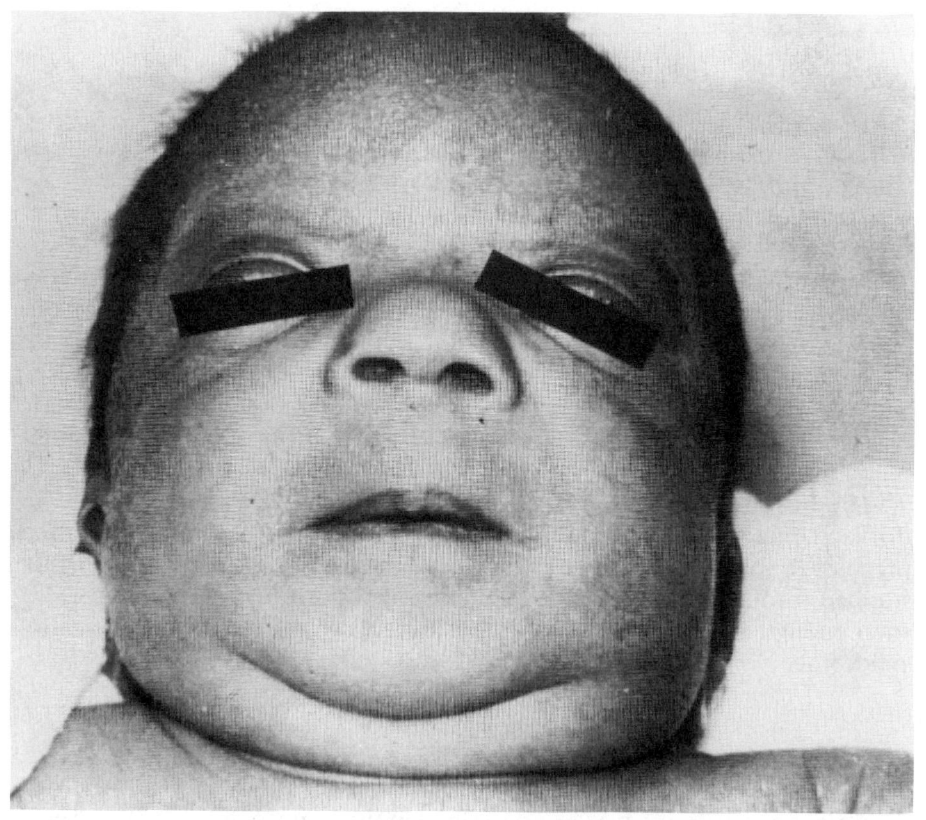

Figure 7–1. A Newborn with FAS.
Note the broad upper lip, hypoplastic philtrum, thin vermilion border, and short, upturned nose.

Reprinted with permission of the publisher from Fisher S. Fetal alcohol syndrome. In Lifshitz F, ed. Pediatric endocrinology. New York: Marcel Dekker, 1985:134.

altogether suggesting a smaller upper mouth as compared with the jaw and lower part of the mouth. Joint and limb abnormalities, cardiac defects, and mental retardation are also common (Little 1977, Beagle 1981).

EFFECT OF MATERNAL DRINKING PATTERN ON FETAL OUTCOME

The severity of morphologic alterations seen in FAS depends on the extent of alcohol abuse (Ouellete et al 1977, Tennes & Blackard 1980, Mills & Graubard 1987). Moderate prenatal alcohol exposure results in craniofacial abnormalities and genitourinary malformations, whereas higher alcohol consumption during pregnancy induces other anomalies (Table 7–1). It has been suggested that the equivalent of two drinks per day has a mild effect on fetal growth and sex organ and genitourinary malformations; three or more drinks per day increases the risk of full FAS. It is often incorrectly believed that certain alcoholic beverages may be safer than others (Table 7–2). However, the nutritional status of the mother-to-be, as well as the use of other drugs and cigarettes, may magnify the damaging potential of drinking during pregnancy (Harlap & Shimo 1980, Hingson et al 1982).

Alcohol intake *prior to conception* may also be of concern. Eleven percent of women consuming the equivalent of 1 to 2 ounces of absolute alcohol (see Table 7–2) per day in the month preceding recognition of pregnancy delivered children with features suggestive of FAS, even though they stopped

Table 7–1. Effects of Maternal Drinking Pattern on Fetal Outcome.

	MATERNAL DRINKING PATTERN (%)*		
RESULTS OF NEWBORN EXAM	**Rare**	**Moderate**	**Heavy**
Abnormal	35	36	71
Small for gestational age	8	7	27
Congenital anomalies	9	14	32
Minor anomalies	5	12	15
Small head circumference	0.4†	0.4†	12
Postmature	8	9	20
Premature	5	3	17
Hypotonia	9	12	17
Jitteriness	10	11	29
Poor suck	2	6	12

*Data are percentages of patients in each group found to have abnormalities. Rare = less than one drink per month; moderate = intermediate drinking between rare and heavy; heavy = one drink per day: 5 or more drinks on occasion, or a consistent daily average intake of more than 45 mL absolute alcohol.
†For both groups combined.

Modified from Ouellette EM, Rosett HL, Rosman NP, Weiner L. Adverse effects on offspring of maternal alcohol abuse during pregnancy. N Engl J Med 1977; 297:528–530 and Fisher S. Fetal alcohol syndrome. In Lifshitz F, ed. Pediatric endocrinology. New York: Marcel Dekker, 1985:129–139.

Table 7–2. Alcohol Content in Beverages.

	AMOUNT PER SERVING (oz)	PERCENT OF ALCOHOL (by vol)	ABSOLUTE ALCOHOL CONTENT PER SERVING (oz)
Beers/ales			
Light lager	12	4.5	0.54
Bock, porter, stout	12	6–7	0.72–0.84
Wines			
French/German	6	8.5–10	0.51–0.68
American	6	12–14	0.72–0.84
Japanese (sake)	4	17	0.68
Sherry/port	3	18–21	0.54–0.63
Distilled spirits (Scotch, Gin, Whiskey, Rum, Vodka, Brandy, Cognac)			
80 proof	1½*	38.9	0.58
86 proof	1½	41.9	0.63
90 proof	1½	44.2	0.66
94 proof	1½	46.4	0.70
100 proof	1½	49.7	0.75

*1½ oz = 1 jigger.

Modified from Brody J. Jane Brody's nutrition book. New York: W.W. Norton and Co., 1981:264–265.

drinking once they knew they were pregnant (Little et al 1980). Abstinence during pregnancy improves the birth weight of the offspring, although pregnancy outcome is not improved in women with no past history of alcohol abuse.

The critical period for alcohol to produce congenital defects (teratogenicity) is around the time of conception; a time when many women might not know they are pregnant! Thus, the risk for alcohol-related dysmorphology is greatest while the baby is just being formed (embryogenesis). Similar teratogenic effects of alcohol have been demonstrated in mice even when other factors such as intake of calories, protein, and vitamins were controlled. A dose-dependent effect of alcohol on growth and morphogenesis was demonstrated (Chernoff 1977).

The molecular basis of FAS is not known. The metabolic effects of alcohol intake, such as hypoglycemia, ketosis, and increased levels of lactic acid, may be the cause of some of the congenital defects. Also, the protein–calorie malnutrition that is common in alcoholics, particularly those with liver disease, may play a role and contribute to teratogenic and growth effects on the unborn baby (Fisher 1985).

However, the American Council on Science and Health (ACSH) as late as 1981 declared: Moderate drinking may even be good for the expectant mother's mental health. ASCH concluded that it is acceptable for pregnant women to drink socially as long as "they limit their daily intake to two drinks or less of beer, wine, or liquor. . . ."

In contrast, others have said that there is no known safe level of alcohol consumption during pregnancy (Blume 1985). Thus, it would be prudent for women who are pregnant or planning pregnancy to cease alcohol consumption altogether, or reduce such consumption "to a minimum level," in order to avoid alcohol-related abnormalities in their offspring. Any real or imagined psychologic benefit of drinking a glass or two of wine with dinner has to be weighed against the possible risk of alcohol-induced damage to the offspring. However, it is unlikely that all women will give up alcohol because of the medical adverse effects associated with moderately heavy drinking during pregnancy.

CLINICAL INTERVENTION

In answer to the question, "What about a drink during pregnancy?" it should be stated that an occasional drink can be taken without fear of consequences (Hatfield 1985). Dogmatic pronouncements to eliminate alcohol altogether are not based on firm scientific data and may frustrate women and decrease the likelihood of compliance. However, it should be stressed that only a small amount taken occasionally during pregnancy might be tolerated without consequences to the baby. A small amount does not mean "two beers per day"; this is considered moderate drinking, as the amount of alcohol in beer is high (see Table 7–2). Everybody agrees that binge drinking and alcohol intoxication must be avoided by mothers-to-be at all times to avoid FAS and to decrease the danger of spontaneous abortion.

It is often difficult to determine how much someone drinks. When obtaining the initial history, a vague answer on how much the person drinks might be elicited. Thus, querying the woman in a nonjudgmental way might yield more accurate information regarding alcohol consumption. For example, asking whether someone drinks may lead to a negative answer, whereas asking how much she drinks may elicit a different response. A woman may consider she drinks a "small" amount, this being two or three beers a day! Only after eliciting how much the woman drinks can appropriate education and counseling on the hazards associated with drinking be done.

Pregnant women can omit alcohol and still drink. Nonalcoholic wine and beer substitutes may be a good alternative for the woman who is accustomed to having a beer or wine with dinner and does not want to give up this ritual. If these are not available at cocktail parties, sodas, juices, or drinks such as "virgin" daiquiris and marys are good options.

It should be emphasized to pregnant women that a drink is a drink, be it one beer, one glass of wine or champagne, or a shot of liquor in a mixed drink (see Table 7–2). Light beer and light wine or wine coolers still contain alcohol and are also considered drinks. These so-called light drinks may contain less alcohol, often about two thirds their nonlight counterparts, but they are still alcoholic.

REFERENCES

AMA Council on Scientific Affairs. Fetal effects of maternal alcohol use. JAMA 1983; 249:2517–2521.

Beagle WS. Fetal alcohol syndrome: A review. J Am Diet Assoc 1981; 79:274–276.

Blume SB. Is social drinking during pregnancy harmless? There is reason to think not. Adv Alcohol Subst Abuse 1985; 5:209–219.

Chernoff GF. The fetal alcohol syndrome in mice: An animal model. Teratology 1977; 15:223–229.

Fisher S. Fetal alcohol syndrome. In Lifshitz F, ed. Pediatric endocrinology. New York: Marcel Dekker, 1985:129–139.

Harlap D, Shimo PH. Alcohol, smoking, and incidence of spontaneous abortions in the first and second trimester. Lancet 1980; 2:176–180.

Hatfield D. Is social drinking during pregnancy harmless? Adv Alcohol Subst Abuse 1985; 5:221–226.

Hingson R, Alpert JJ, Day N, et al. Effects of maternal drinking and marijuana use on fetal growth and development. Pediatrics 1982; 70:539–546.

Jones KS, Smith DW, Ulleland CN, Streissguth AP. Pattern of malformation in offspring of chronic alcoholic women. Lancet 1973; 1:1267–1273.

Jones KS, Smith DW. Recognition of the fetal alcohol syndrome in early infancy. Lancet 1973; 2:999–1001.

Little RE. Moderate alcohol use during pregnancy and decreased infant birth weight. Am J Public Health 1977; 67:1154–1156.

Little RE, Streissguth AP, Barr HM, Herman CS. Decreased birth weight in infants of alcoholic women who abstained during pregnancy. J Pediatr 1980; 96:974–977.

Mills JL, Graubard BI. Is moderate drinking during pregnancy associated with an increased risk for malformations? Pediatrics 1987; 80:309–314.

Ouellette EM, Rosett HL, Rosman NP, Weiner L. Adverse effects on offspring of maternal alcohol abuse during pregnancy. N Engl J Med 1977; 297:528–530.

Sokol RJ, Miller SI, Reed G. Alcohol abuse during pregnancy: An epidemiologic study. Alcoholism 1980; 4:135–145.

Tennes K, Blackard C. Maternal alcohol consumption, birth weight and minor physical anomalies. Am J Obstet Gynecol 1980; 138:774–780.

8

Caffeine, Dietetic Foods, and Sweeteners

CAFFEINE

It was ten o'clock in the morning. All of Joan's friends abandoned their typewriters in midsentence to participate in the all-American ritual called the coffee break. Joan did not do so; she was pregnant and wanted to "play it safe" by avoiding caffeine-containing beverages. However, she really missed her coffee!

Caffeine's Effects on the Unborn Baby

In 1980, the Food and Drug Administration issued a statement warning pregnant women to avoid caffeine-containing foods and drugs, if possible, or consume them only sparingly (Goyan 1980). Studies had shown that pregnant rats fed caffeine gave birth to offspring with birth defects. In the animal model, caffeine not only produced a higher incidence of congenital anomalies but was also associated with higher rates of reproductive losses.

Caffeine causes an increase in catecholamines, which may result in vasoconstriction and fetus hypoxia (Hill 1979). It has also been theorized that since caffeine is chemically similar in structure to molecules found in genetic material, it may have the potential to affect cell multiplication and cause chromosome aberrations. Caffeine crosses the placenta readily, with rapid penetration into fetal circulation. However, the fetus lacks the necessary enzymes to metabolize caffeine.

The effects of caffeine on the unborn baby are controversial. Rats process caffeine differently than human beings do, and no definitive detrimental effect of caffeine has been demonstrated in human fetuses. It has been suggested that caffeine is a culprit in prematurity and low birth weight in human beings (Rosenberg et al 1982, Linn et al 1982), but this link between coffee drinking and prematurity appears now to be due mainly to the effects of cigarette smoking among the pregnant women studied, not coffee drinking. Women who ingest large quantities of caffeine often tend to smoke a lot and may also ingest alcohol during pregnancy. The role of caffeine in the etiology of congenital anomalies and spontaneous abortions has not been clearly documented in human subjects (Srisuphan & Bracken 1986).

However, caffeine has other effects that may affect the overall health of the pregnant woman. Coffee intake has been associated with nutritional problems, including alterations in calcium metabolism (Hollingberg & Massey 1986) and lowered thiamin status (Vimokesant et al 1982). In addition, zinc and iron absorption have been shown to be negatively influenced by coffee intake (Pecoud, Donzel & Schelling 1975, Morck, Lynch & Cook 1983). Coffee consumption (> 1.8 cups a day) among third-trimester pregnant, low-income Costa Rican women was associated with lower maternal iron status, lower infant birth weight, and lower breast-milk iron concentration as compared with those pregnant women who did not drink coffee (Munoz et al 1988).

Caffeine is a potent stimulator, and consumption of large amounts of caffeine may produce rapid heart beat (tachycardia) and increase blood pressure levels. It may also result in gastric reflux and increased gastric acid secretion associated with heartburn (Cohen & Booth 1975). As in nonpregnant women, it may interfere with normal sleep patterns (Greden 1974). Therefore, it would be prudent for pregnant women to limit their intake of coffee and other caffeine-containing beverages.

To achieve a moderate intake of caffeine during pregnancy, an awareness of the caffeine content of foods is necessary (Gilbert et al 1976). Varying amounts of caffeine are contained in different blends of coffee; the method of preparation (i.e., freshly brewed versus instant) also affects its caffeine content. In addition to coffee, there are many other frequently consumed beverages that contain caffeine (Table 8–1). Also, over 2000 nonprescription drugs contain caffeine, which is an additional reason pregnant women should not take any drug without a precise knowledge of its contents and a prescription by a physician.

DIETETIC FOODS AND NONNUTRITIVE SWEETENERS

In 1902, Harvey Washington Wiley, chief chemist of the Department of Agriculture, formed a "poison squad" of 12 volunteers to test numerous substances. After the testing of saccharin, Wiley reported to President Theodore Roosevelt that saccharin should be banned as "highly injurious to health." President Roosevelt, himself a saccharin user, replied angrily, "You say sac-

Table 8–1. Caffeine Content of Selected Foods and Drugs.

	AVERAGE CAFFEINE CONTENT (mg/serving)
Coffee	
Brewed, ground	85/c
Percolated	110/c
Dripolated	146/c
Instant	66/c
Instant, decaffeinated	3/c
Tea	
Regular, bagged (brewed 5 min)	46/c
Green, bagged (brewed 5 min)	31/c
Regular, instant dry powder	32/1 tsp
Carbonated beverages	
Coca-Cola	65/12 oz
Pepsi-Cola	43/12 oz
Diet-Rite Cola	33/12 oz
Tab	45/12 oz
Dr Pepper	61/12 oz
Mountain Dew	55/12 oz
Chocolate beverages	
Cocoa, dry	10/T
Cocoa, instant	10/T
Cocoa/hot chocolate beverage	13/c
Chocolate-containing foods	
Milk chocolate	6/1 oz
Semi-sweet chocolate	17/1 oz
Sweet (dark) chocolate	20/1 oz
Chocolate powder for milk	10/T
Chocolate ice cream	8/c
Nonprescription drugs	
Anacin Analgesic	32/tablet
Dristan	16/tablet
Excedrin	65/tablet
Triaminicin	30/tablet

From Pennington JAT, Church HN. Bower and Church's food values of portions commonly used. 14th ed. New York: Harper and Row, 1985.

charine is injurious to health? Why, my doctor gives it to me every day. Anybody who says saccarin is injurious to health is an idiot!"

Dietetic Foods

Special dietetic foods are not necessary during pregnancy and do not offer any advantage to the pregnant woman. At present, there are no known specific therapeutic properties in dietetic food products; consumers may be misled since they appear to permit consumption without regard to energy content or nutrient composition.

Many individuals use dietetic products, and physicians and other health care professionals often recommend them in the hope of achieving better weight control. In most instances the consumer receives little or no nutritional benefit from costly dietetic products. Often, these special foods constitute only a fraction of the day's food intake and have little or no effect on the total caloric intake. The nutritional value of many of these products does not always differ from regular items (Table 8–2), but the cost is usually higher. In addition, there is the danger that the use of dietary products may replace foods containing important nutrients, particularly in the case of a low-calorie food plan with restricted overall intake. For the pregnant woman, the most beneficial diet is one derived from a wide variety of ordinary foods without dietetic substitutes.

Nonnutritive Sweeteners

The use of artificial sweeteners has been controversial for many years, but people continue to consume these products at an unabated rate. Consumption studies today show that the highest users of artificial and nonnutritive sweeteners and dietetic foods are teenagers and women of childbearing years. In our culture, there is a need for noncaloric sweeteners to replace sugar, which is a significant part of our diet. As long as the demand for sugar-flavored foods is high, there will be a demand for artificial and nonnutritive sweeteners, and pregnant women will ingest them. This is occurring even though there is no scientific evidence that saccharin or other nonnutritive sweeteners have greatly improved the care or eased the management of obesity or diabetes (Kalkhoff & Levin 1978, Brunzell 1978, Talbot & Fisher 1978). However, limiting caloric intake by using foods with nonnutritive sweeteners should always be done with caution during pregnancy (Pitkin 1984, Sturtevant 1985).

When the Federal Drug Administration banned the artificial sweetener cyclamate in 1969, saccharin was used in its place. Controversy regarding this noncaloric sweetener began in 1977, when a study showed that rats fed saccharine developed bladder cancer. The dose administered was equivalent to 10 to 20 times the level that would result if human beings ate it constantly for many years. Subsequent mutogenicity studies and animal-feeding experiments have raised questions regarding whether saccharin posed a serious risk for human beings, particularly unborn babies who may be vulnerable to its negative effects because it readily crosses the placenta. However, there have been no reports to date linking the use of saccharin or other sweeteners during pregnancy to defects in the fetus or cancer in babies. Although we cannot define the risks of these sweeteners with 100 percent certainty, one can place the use of saccharine in some perspective. In pregnant women, the use of saccharine appears to be lowest on a continuum of risk factors. Smoking,

Table 8–2. Comparison of Dietetic and Regular Foods.*

FOOD ITEM	AMOUNT (oz)	CALORIES (kcal)	CARBOHYDRATE (g)	FAT (g)	COST PER AMOUNT ($)
Flavor drops, dietetic	1	14	2.9	0.0	0.35
Hard candy, regular	1	108	27.2	0.8	0.08
Chocolate, dietetic	2	168	14.0	14.0	1.19
Chocolate, regular	2	150	16.0	9.0	0.22
Ice cream, dietetic	4	87	15.6	0.9	2.25
Ice cream, regular	4	130	16.0	7.0	1.50
Pancake syrup, lite	1	60	15.0	0.0	0.13
Pancake syrup, regular	1	100	26.0	0.0	0.13
Fudge cookie, dietetic	1	120	16.0	4.0	0.21
Fudge cookie, regular	1	124	20.0	4.0	0.03
Apple sauce, dietetic	4	50	12.0	0.0	0.40
Apple sauce, unsweetened regular	4	46	11.0	0.1	0.19

*Note that the calorie content of some dietetic foods differs very slightly from the nondietetic products. At times it may even be higher, as shown for chocolate, where the dietetic product yields higher calories due to the high fat content. The cost of dietetic products also is usually higher.

which is a proven etiologic factor in the growth retardation of unborn babies, poses a far greater risk.

Over 80 percent of people report that if saccharine were banned, they would revert to using other nonnutritive sweeteners to satisfy their desire for sweet foods and beverages. In addition to saccharin, other sweeteners available include fructose or sugar alcohols such as sorbitol, xylitol, mannitol, maltitol (Brunzell 1978) and the now very popular aspartame (Nutrasweet). Aspartame is a newcomer to the artificial sweetener arena (Mazur 1984). It is a synthetic compound comprising two amino acids, L-aspartic acid and the methyl ester of L-phenylalanine. Aspartame has the same calorie value as regular table sugar—4 calories per gram—but is 180 times sweeter than ordinary table sugar and has no bitter aftertaste.

This popular nonnutritive sweetener may turn out to be the most thoroughly studied and scrutinized food additive ever approved by the Food and Drug Administration (FDA) (Hayes 1981, Hile 1981). The FDA approved aspartame in 1974 for use in certain foods and for certain technologic purposes. But, as late as 1984, the American Academy of Pediatrics was still concerned about its use during pregnancy because of concerns regarding the potential toxicity of each of its three components: aspartate, phenylalanine, and methanol. Aspartate is toxic in rodents and nonhuman primates; when given in large doses it produces hypothalamic neuronal necrosis (Applebaum et al 1984). The phenylalanine content of aspartame could potentially increase plasma phenylalanine levels, which are associated with mental retardation. The ingestion of methanol could lead to high blood methanol and formate concentrations, leading to metabolic acidosis and blindness.

However, data available to date indicate little risk associated with aspartame ingestion at projected intake levels (Council on Scientific Affairs 1985). Blood formate concentrations as well as plasma aspartate and phenylalanine concentrations remain at levels far below concentrations associated with adverse effects. Moreover, primate studies report that aspartate and glutamate do not cross the placenta and the amount of methanol ingested from an aspartame-sweetened beverage is less than that from ordinary fruit juice. Thus, the FDA recently approved the use of this sweetener during pregnancy. The allowable daily intake of aspartame established by the FDA is 50 milligrams per kilogram of body weight. For a 50-kilogram individual, the allowable daily intake equals a dozen 12-ounce cans of 100 percent sweetened soda or 71 packets of Equal.

CLINICAL INTERVENTION

Caffeine

Women should be told that caffeine need not be eliminated during pregnancy. However, it is recommended that if caffeine is consumed, it should be done so in moderation. The pregnant woman may need to be instructed in the caffeine content of various foods (see Table 8–1) so that she may moderate her intake of caffeine on her own.

There is no precise quantity of caffeine that would be considered too high. Caffeine intake should be decreased in women who develop symptoms from this stimulant. Heartburn is one of the more common effects of caffeine consumption during pregnancy; this is particularly true if taken prior to sleeping. Women who cannot sleep, those who are jittery or have tachycardia might be drinking too much caffeine. They should try to reduce the amount of caffeine taken, or better yet eliminate it all together. A glass of milk would be a great substitute; they should try hot milk if they want something nutritious and warm.

Coffee is often eliminated by substituting herb tea. Herb teas are available that taste similar to coffee and are caffeine-free. However, it should be kept in mind that not all herb teas and natural teas are safe (see Chapter 15). Some, such as comfrey tea, have been implicated as the cause of liver disease. Hot water with lemon juice, often called white tea, is popular among those who want to decrease coffee consumption. Women who consume excessive quantities of caffeine in carbonated beverages may substitute caffeine-free sodas or seltzers.

Dietetic Foods and Artificial Sweeteners

There is no use for artificial sweeteners and dietetic foods during pregnancy. Although the risks associated with their use are nebulous, their potential benefit in reducing total caloric intake is doubtful. Additionally, the cost of these products is generally high. Therefore, when decreased caloric intake is desired, consumption of low-calorie, high-bulk foods may be more "dietetic" and filling than artificial sweeteners. However, if women desire sweets without the calories, artificial sweeteners may be ingested in moderation without risk to their babies.

The use of artificial sweeteners and special dietetic products may give the individual or family a false perception of benefit when, in fact, the most beneficial diet is one derived from a variety of ordinary foods. Awareness of the relationship between food consumption and weight control is the key; avoidance of sugar per se is not a panacea.

REFERENCES

CAFFEINE

Cohen S, Booth GH. Gastric acid secretion and lower-esophageal sphincter pressure in response to coffee and caffeine. N Engl J Med 1975; 293:897–899.

Gilbert RM, Marshman JA, Schwieder M, Berg R. Caffeine content of beverages as consumed. Can Med Assoc J 1976; 114:205–208.

Goyan JE. Statement by the Commissioner of Food and Drugs, FDA press release. Washington, D.C., Sept. 4, 1980 (p 80–36), p 3.
Greden JF. Anxiety or caffeinism: A diagnostic dilemna. Am J Psychiatr 1974; 131:1089–1092.
Hill RM. Perinatal pharmacology: Maternal drug ingestion, and fetal effect. Evansville, IN: Mead-Johnson, Inc., 1979.
Hollingberg P, Massey LK. Effect of dietary caffeine and sucrose on urinary calcium excretion in adolescents. Fed Proc 1986; 45:375 (abstract).
Linn S, Schoenbaum SC, Monson RR, et al. No association between coffee consumption and adverse outcomes of pregnancy. N Engl J Med 1982; 306:141–145.
Morck TA, Lynch SR, Cook J. Inhibition of food iron by coffee. Am J Clin Nutr 1983; 37:416–420.
Munoz LM, Lonnerdal B, Keen CL, Dewey KG. Coffee consumption as a factor in iron-deficiency anemia among pregnant women and their infants in Costa Rica. Am J Clin Nutr 1988; 48:645–651.
Pecoud A, Donzel P, Schelling JL. Effect of foodstuffs on the absorption of zinc sulfate. Clin Pharmacol Ther 1975; 17:469–474.
Rosenberg L, Mitchell AA, Shapiro S, Slone D. Selected birth defects in relation to caffeine-containing beverages. JAMA 1982; 247:1429–1432.
Srisuphan W, Bracken MB. Caffeine consumption during pregnancy and association with late spontaneous abortion. Am J Obstet Gynecol 1986; 154:14–20.
Vimokesant SL, Kunjara S, Rungruangsak K, Nahornehai S, Panijpan B. Beriberi caused by antithiamin factors in food and its prevention. Ann NY Acad Sci 1982; 378:123–136.

DIETETIC FOODS AND SWEETENERS

Applebaum AE, Daabees TT, Stegink LD, Finkelstein MW. Aspartate-induced neurotoxicity in infant mice. In Stegink LD, Filer LJ Jr, eds. Aspartame physiology and biochemistry. New York: Marcel Dekker, 1984:349–362.
Brunzell JD. Use of fructose, xylitol or sorbitol as a sweetener in diabetes mellitus. Diabetes Care 1978; 1:223–230.
Council on Scientific Affairs. Aspartame: Review of safety issues. JAMA 1985; 253:400–402.
Hayes AH. Aspartame: Commissioner's final decision. Fed Reg 1981; 46:(July 24):38283–38308.
Hile JP. Aspartame: Commissioner's final decision, correction. Fed Reg 1981; 46:46394.
Kalkhoff RK, Levin MF. The saccharine controversy. Diabetes Care 1978; 1:211–222.
Mazur RH. Discovery of aspartame. In Stegnik LD, Filer LJ Jr, eds. Aspartame physiology and biochemistry. New York: Marcel Dekker, 1984:3–9.
Pitkin RN. Aspartame ingestion during pregnancy. In Stegnik LD, Filer LJ Jr, eds. Aspartame physiology and biochemistry. New York: Marcel Dekker, 1984:555–563.
Sturtevant FM. Use of aspartame in pregnancy. Int J Fertil 1985; 30:85–87.
Talbot JM, Fisher KD. The need for special foods and sugar substitutes by individuals with diabetes mellitus. Diabetes Care 1978; 1:231–240.

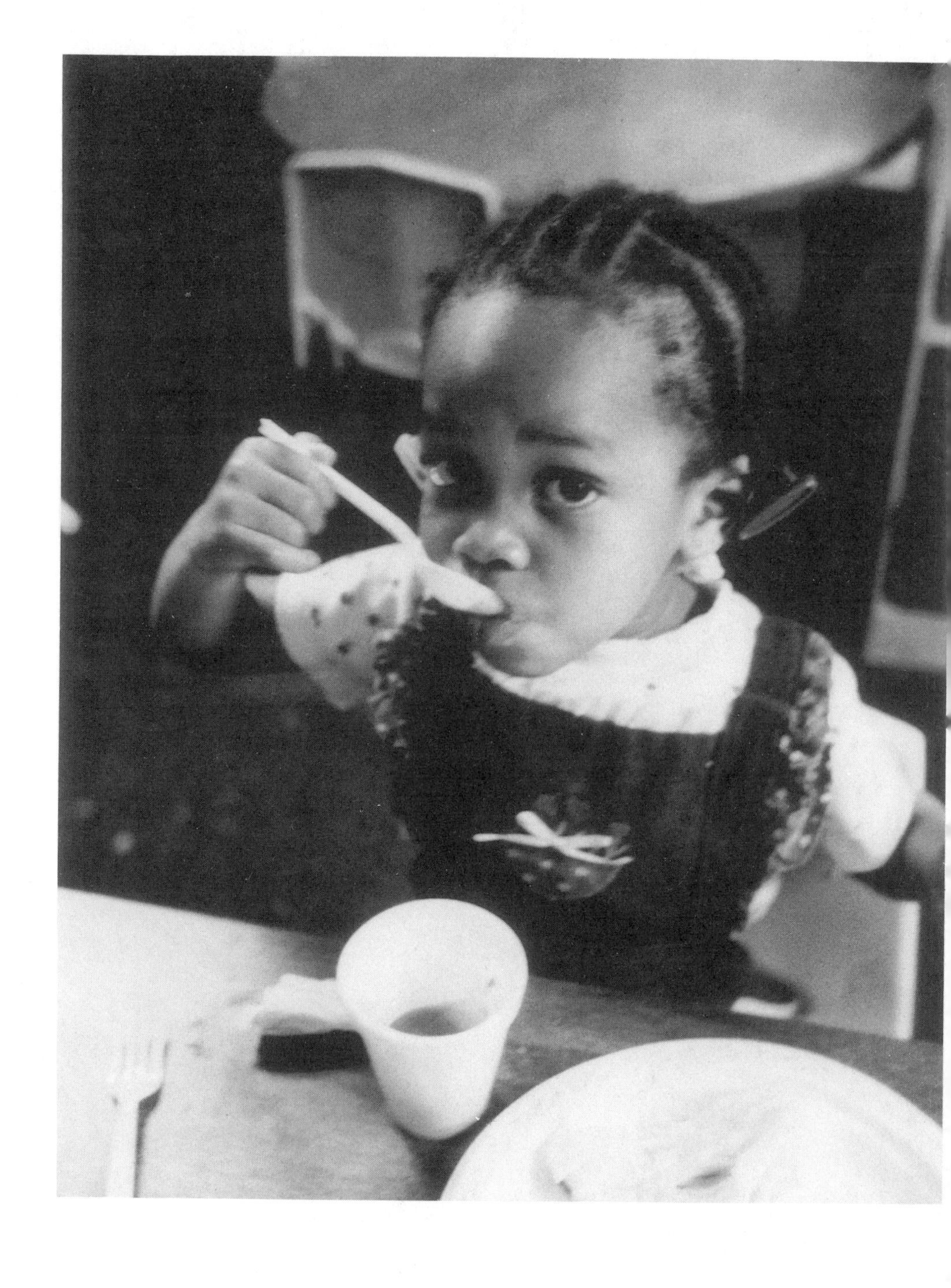

PART II

Nutrition for Infants, Children, and Adolescents

9

Nutrition Needs of Normal Babies, Children, and Adolescents

In the beginning, 40,000 years ago, the first human beings roamed the fruited plains of this earth and subsisted on roots, berries, fruits, and whatever meat rumbled by. Even after the domestication of plants and animals 30,000 years later, people did not indulge in fatty dairy products or fried foods. They consumed no butter, no sugar, and practically no salt. In those days, children's diets were much like their parents'; they consumed whatever was available, but did not even dream of eating "junk food." It was a tough life, of course, but according to a new book, *The Paleolithic Prescription* (Eaton, Shostak & Konner 1988) this diet was in many ways healthier than ours. The authors claimed that such a diet protected our ancestors against heart disease, certain cancers, strokes, and other "diseases of civilization." Everything man ate those days was "100 percent natural," yet their life span was only 31 years!

NUTRITION GOALS

It has been repeatedly noted that five of the 10 leading causes of death in the United States—coronary heart disease, certain types of cancers, stroke, diabetes mellitus, and atherosclerosis—are diseases in which diet has a role (Byrne 1988). Since these diseases may have their roots in childhood, an early start for disease prevention through diet modification has been widely recommended. Most nutrition experts agree on the human nutrition goals for the population, though there may be a lack of consensus about the recommended dietary allowances for specific nutrients (Norton & Gillespie 1988). The recommendations for desirable dietary intakes issued by the U.S. Department of Agriculture (1985) for adults are shown in Table 9–1. Most of the human nutrition goals are aimed at avoiding obesity and reducing the possible dietary factors implicated in the development of the above-mentioned conditions. The American Cancer Society (1984) and the American Heart Association (1986) also echo these recommendations for a health-promoting diet to be achieved by all people.

In accordance with the above goals, a clear-cut change in dietary habits has already occurred in America over the past two decades (Wolinsky 1980, National Research Council 1988). The per capita consumption of fluid milk and cream declined about 20 percent from 1963 to 1985. During this period, butter intake dropped over 30 percent, and intake of animal fats and oils fell 12 percent. There was also a decline of 12 percent in egg consumption since the peak intake, which occurred in 1950. Assuming the cholesterol content of a single egg to be 212 milligrams, the intake of egg cholesterol alone declined 70 milligrams per day per person in the United States! The overall mean animal fat intake (saturated fat) has also decreased slightly (4 percent), and vegetable oil intake (polyunsaturated fat) has increased greatly (about 55 percent). It appears that persons in the upper socioeconomic groups and those with a higher education level are those most likely to redirect their nutritional habits.

Attention has also been paid to other common health problems that are nutritional in nature and prevalent in the general population: namely, spe-

Table 9–1. Human Nutritional Needs.*

1. Eat a variety of foods. (Build to a variety of foods.)
2. Avoid obesity and maintain normal weight and growth. (Listen to your child's appetite to avoid over- or underfeeding.)
3. Increase consumption of unrefined complex sugars to 48 percent of total energy intake.
4. Decrease consumption of refined sugars to 10 percent of total energy intake. (Sugar is OK, but in moderation.)
5. Decrease fat intake to 30 to 33 percent of total energy intake. (Do not restrict fat in children less than 2 years of age.)
6. Decrease intake of saturated fats maximum 10 percent of total energy intake.
7. Reduce cholesterol intake not to exceed 150 mg per 1000 kcal or 300 mg per day. (Do not restrict fat or cholesterol too much.)
8. Increase dietary fiber. (Do not over-do high-fiber foods.)
9. Moderate salt intake to 5 g per day. (Salt is OK, but in moderation.)
10. Increase iron and calcium intake, fluoridate water, and limit alcohol consumption. (Children need more iron, pound for pound, than adults.)

*These needs are ideal for adults. However, children's needs differ, as indicated in parentheses. The needs of children less than 2 years of age are particularly different from those recommended for adults.

From the Committee on Dietary Allowances, Food and Nutrition Board, National Research Council. Recommended dietary allowances. 10th ed. Washington D.C.: National Academy of Sciences, 1989; the Dairy Council. A national nutrition policy: Current and emerging issues. Dairy Council Digest, 1977; 48:31–36; the U.S. Department of Agriculture, U.S. Department of Health and Human Services. Nutrition and your health: Dietary guidelines for Americans. Washington D.C.: U.S. Government Printing Office, 1985; and Pediatric Basics, Gerber Products Company, 1989.

cific nutrient deficiencies such as iron and calcium, and excess alcohol and sodium consumption. Therefore, it has been recommended that dietary iron and calcium intakes be increased, water be fluoridated, sodium intake limited, and alcohol avoided altogether.

Although the human nutrition goals are well-intended, the dietary recommendations to attain these goals for adults may not always be ideal for children. Families who attempt to zealously meet these goals may be faced with children who do not grow well (Pugliese et al 1987, Lifshitz & Moses 1988, Lifshitz, Moses, Cervantes et al 1987). The American Academy of Pediatrics has long recognized this problem and has advised that these recommendations be followed in moderation and with caution in children (American Academy of Pediatrics 1986). Children, especially those less than 2 years old, have a different set of nutrition goals, as discussed below (see Table 9–1). However, it should be kept in mind that the general health of the population may be improved even without changes in food consumption (American Medical Association 1977). Changes in lifestyle such as increased physical activity and reduced smoking have resulted in a decline in major risk factors associated with atherosclerotic disease even without dietary modifications (Wolinsky 1980).

WHAT IS GOOD TO EAT?

To achieve the nutritional goals discussed above, the following changes in food selection have been recommended. First, efforts should be made to eat a variety of all types of foods and to balance food intake (energy consumption) and physical activity (energy expenditure) to avoid obesity. In children, food intake must promote normal growth and development. If overweight, energy intake should be decreased and exercise should be encouraged to increase energy expenditure. However, in children, weight loss efforts need to be avoided in most instances (see Chapter 18).

Energy needs of schoolaged children vary according to their sex, age, body size (height and weight), onset of puberty, and physical activity (Committee on Dietary Allowances 1989). Consequently, it is difficult to determine the exact energy requirements for an individual child. The recommended energy requirements established by the Food and Nutrition Board are based on estimates of energy intake related to average body weights and represent estimated energy needs (RDAs) for children involved in light activity (Fig. 9–1). Therefore, additional energy intake may be needed in children who are more physically active (see Chapter 14). To ensure that energy requirements are met, growth should be monitored in all schoolaged children. In those who consume appropriate calories, weight and height will progress along consistent growth channels or percentiles (see Chapter 10). Let the child's appetite

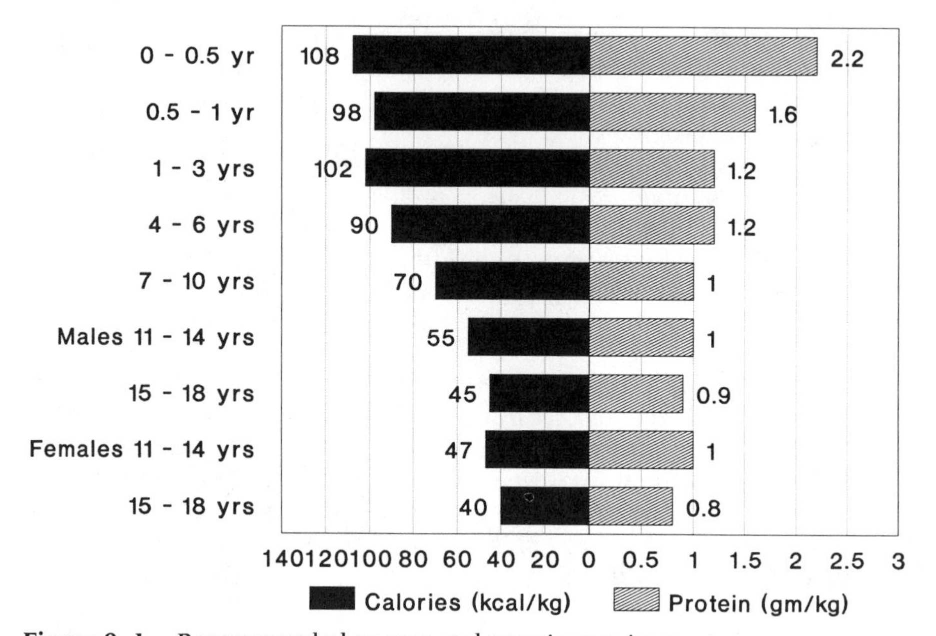

Figure 9–1. Recommended energy and protein requirements.
Adapted from the Committee on Dietary Allowances, Food and Nutrition Board, National Research Council. Recommended dietary allowances. 10th ed. Washington, D.C.: National Academy of Sciences, 1989.

be the guide for food intake as long as he or she maintains appropriate growth.

Most health experts recommend increasing starches (complex carbohydrates) in the diet. Eating more complex carbohydrates will automatically decrease total fat intake; cereal, grains, and other plant products replace food derived from animal products, which contain cholesterol and are generally higher in saturated fat. Protein quality from individual grains and vegetables is often less desirable than protein from animal products (see Chapter 15), but a varied selection of vegetables, legumes, meat, and dairy products usually suffices to meet all human protein needs.

Perhaps one of the most difficult nutrition goals to achieve among children and adolescents is the reduction of refined sugar intake. It has been estimated that the ingestion of table sugar (sucrose) in the United States exceeds 110 pounds (50 kg) per person per year (Dairy Council 1977). Sucrose is present in sweets, pastries, sodas, and candies and is used as an additive in many foods that children eat. Attempts are being made to reduce the amount of refined sugar in the diet through the use of artificial and nonnutritive sweeteners. However, despite the increased use of these sweeteners, they have not made a dent in the rates of obesity or sugar consumption in our population (USDA 1985, Gortmaker et al 1987). Moreover, elimination of sugar-containing foods from a child's or adolescent's diet without appropriate substitution of other energy-rich foods may lead to dietary intakes that do not provide sufficient calories and thus result in poor growth (Lifshitz et al 1987, Lifshitz & Moses 1988). Children need a ready source of energy; thus, carbohydrate intake is appropriate if ingested in moderation. Children have a preference for sweets from birth, since sugar is naturally found in children's diets. Breast milk contains 7 to 8 percent milk sugar (lactose) (see Chapters 12 and 13), and one third of the calories from an apple come from a fruit sugar (fructose).

To reduce the total amount of fat in our diet and to decrease animal fat and cholesterol intake, the following dietary recommendations have been made: (1) decrease consumption of foods high in fat, and partially replace saturated fats with vegetable oils; (2) decrease consumption of red meats and substitute poultry and fish, which contain less saturated fat; (3) use low-fat milk and dairy products; and (4) decrease consumption of butterfat, eggs, and other high-cholesterol foods (see Chapter 24). However, these recommendations are not meant for children, particularly those less than 2 years of age. In children less than 2 years of age the recommendation to reduce fat and cholesterol intake is a *big* no. Breast milk, which is the ideal baby food designed by nature, is neither low in fat nor low in cholesterol. It should be used as the norm in recommending ideal feedings for infants (see Chapters 11 and 12). Fat provides twice as many calories as any other food and is the source of essential fatty acids. Any restriction in total fat intake may lead to an inadequate energy consumption even in children older than 2 years, or an essential fatty acid deficiency in the young infant.

Insufficient mineral intake to support growth in the schoolaged child is another concern that may arise from the recommendations to reduce consumption of animal products. Red meat and eggs are excellent sources of essential minerals for growth, such as zinc and iron, that are not easily obtained when pasta and cereals are substituted. For example, one would have to eat a large amount of enriched pasta to get the same nourishment as is in a piece of small lean meat. The nutritional equivalency of 1 cup of enriched macaroni and sauce is comparable to 3 ounces of flank steak for calories, but 3½ and 7 cups of macaroni would be required to provide the protein and zinc, respectively, of 3 ounces of flank steak.

Fake fat is now trying to make its way onto our supermarket shelves. Olestra, a sucrose polyester made by Proctor and Gamble, is an undigestable, noncaloric replacement for fat in baking and cooking, and Simplesse is an "all natural" fat substitute produced by Nutrasweet that can be used in products that are not baked or fried. These products were just approved by the FDA and will most likely be widely available in the future. Although these fat substitutes were developed in an effort to reduce obesity and lower heart disease risks by replacing dietary fat, their effectiveness is questionable. Just as artificial sweeteners have not reduced sugar consumption in the United States, fake fats will most likely face the same fate. Moreover, the use of these fat substitutes may replace foods in the diet that contribute important nutrients. For example, fake-fat ice cream for dessert instead of an apple will not improve the nutritional quality of the diet.

Increased consumption of fiber derived from complex carbohydrates is another human nutrition goal that has received attention. A high fiber intake has been recommended to reduce the chances of getting diseases of the colon, cancer, diabetes, and cardiovascular problems related to atherosclerosis (Eastwood 1984). In general, increased consumption of whole wheat and other whole grain cereals, fruits, and vegetables will increase dietary fiber. However, there may also be some negative nutritional consequences of high fiber intake, particularly for the young child and adolescent. Adding too much fiber too quickly to a child's diet may lead to gastrointestinal problems such as abdominal pain, gas, and bowel-movement irregularities. Additionally, complex carbohydrates such as whole grains, fruit and vegetables may cause the child to become full very rapidly because they are not accustomed to eating large amounts of "bulky" foods. This could lead to inadequate energy intake. Moreover, the long-term use of high-fiber diets have been shown to interfere with absorption of vitamins and minerals (Kelsay 1978).

Avoidance of salt is widely regarded as an ideal recommendation for all human beings. However, efforts to reduce the salt intake of children's diets may lead to insufficient sodium intake. The estimated minimum daily needs of sodium range from 120 to 500 milligrams depending on the age of the child (Table 9–2). These needs must be met in all instances to allow for normal growth and avoid electrolyte imbalances. Only under medical supervision for the treatment of specific diseases may the sodium intake be curtailed below these limits.

Although there is little evidence to suggest that American children have vitamin and mineral deficiencies, there is widespread use of vitamin and mineral supplements in our health-conscious society. In a nationally representative survey (Kovar 1985), 36 percent of children less than 18 years of age

Table 9–2. Estimated Minimum Requirements (EMRs) for Sodium, Chloride, and Potassium for Healthy Persons.

	INFANTS		CHILDREN			
	0–5 mo	6–11 mo	1 yr	2–5 yr	6–9 yr	10–18 yr
Sodium (mg)	120	200	225	300	400	500
Chloride (mg)	180	300	350	500	600	750
Potassium (mg)	500	700	1000	1400	1600	2000

Adapted from the Committee on Dietary Allowances, Food and Nutrition Board, National Research Council. Recommended dietary allowances. 10th ed. Washington, D.C.: National Academy of Sciences, 1989.

reported daily use of vitamin and mineral preparations. The NHANES IV data revealed that there is greater use of vitamin and mineral supplements among young children than older children, with usages decreasing from 39 percent for 2-year-olds to slightly more than 10 percent of teenagers (Fig. 9–2). However, all healthy children should meet their vitamin and mineral needs from food, not from medication and other supplements (Tables 9–3 to 9–9).

Iron deficiency is frequently cited as the most common single nutritional deficiency in the world, and is the most common nutritional deficiency in the United States (Dallman, Yip & Johnson 1984). The RDA for iron increases from 10 milligrams for 1- to 10-year-olds to 12 milligrams for boys 11 to 18 years of age and to 15 milligrams for girls 11 to 18 years of age (Committee on Dietary Allowances 1989). Children need more iron for their weight than adults! The usual American diet provides approximately 6 milligrams of iron per 1000 calories (Hallberg 1984). However, this level of dietary intake may be even lower in children whose diets are restricted in iron-containing foods such as meat and eggs. Other minerals and vitamins that are important for the growing child may also be deficient in diets restricting animal products.

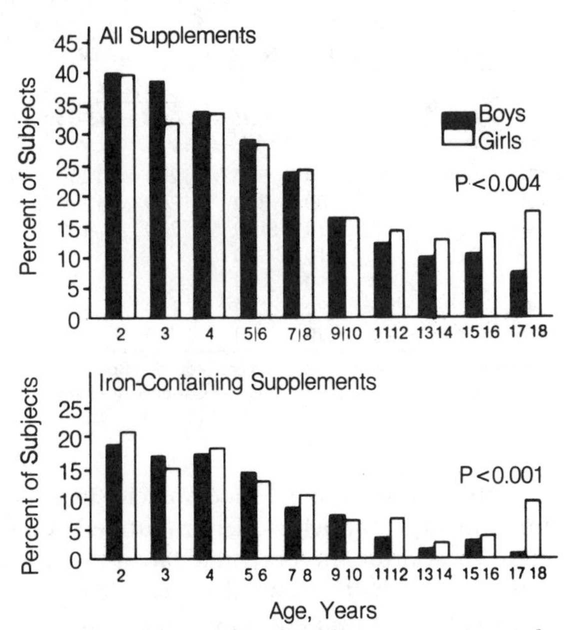

Figure 9–2. Percentage of boys and girls receiving supplements at different ages.

From Bowering J, Clancy KL. Nutritional status of children and teenagers in relation to vitamin and mineral use. J Am Dietetic Assoc 1986; 86:1033–1038.

Table 9–3. Estimated Safe and Adequate Daily Dietary Intakes of Selected Vitamins and Minerals.

	INFANTS		CHILDREN		ADOLESCENTS	
	0–6 mo	6–12 mo	1–3 yr	4–6 yr	7–10 yr	11+ yr
Biotin (μg)	10	15	20	25	30	30–100
Pantothenic acid (mg)	2	3	3	3–4	4–5	4–7
Copper (mg)	0.4–0.6	0.6–0.7	0.7–1.0	1.0–1.5	1.0–2.0	1.5–2.5
Manganese (mg)	0.3–0.6	0.6–1.0	1.0–1.5	1.5–2.0	2.0–3.0	2.5–5.0
Fluoride (mg)	0.1–0.5	0.2–1.0	0.5–1.5	1.0–2.5	1.5–2.5	1.5–2.5
Chromium (μg)	10–40	20–60	20–80	30–120	50–200	50–200
Molybdenum (μg)	15–30	20–40	25–50	30–75	50–150	75–250

Adapted from the Committee on Dietary Allowances, Food and Nutrition Board, National Research Council. Recommended dietary allowances. 10th ed. Washington, D.C.: National Academy of Sciences, 1989.

Table 9–4. Recommended Dietary Allowances of Minerals for Babies, Children, and Adolescents.

MINERALS	INFANTS		CHILDREN			ADOLESCENTS			
						Males		Females	
	0–6 mo	*6–12 mo*	*1–3 yr*	*4–6 yr*	*7–10 yr*	*11–14 yr*	*15–18 yr*	*11–14 yr*	*15–18 yr*
Calcium (mg)	400	600	800	800	800	1200	1200	1200	1200
Phosphorus (mg)	300	500	800	800	800	1200	1200	1200	1200
Magnesium (mg)	40	60	80	120	170	270	400	280	300
Iron (mg)	6	10	10	10	10	12	12	15	15
Zinc (mg)	5	5	10	10	10	15	15	12	12
Iodine (μg)	40	50	70	90	120	150	150	150	150
Selenium (μg)	10	15	20	20	30	40	50	45	50

Adapted from the Committee on Dietary Allowances, Food and Nutrition Board, National Research Council. Recommended dietary allowances. 10th ed. Washington, D.C.: National Academy of Sciences, 1989.

The most frequently seen nutritional inadequacies in children's diets include zinc, calcium, iron, and folic acid. Calcium-fortified orange juice is now available in an effort to address the potential calcium inadequacy in children's diets. Although studies have shown that the calcium in orange juice is available to the body for absorption and that it does not interfere with iron absorption, orange juice is not a substitute for milk (Mehansho et al 1989). Orange juice does not contribute the same total nutrition as milk, as it has no protein.

Table 9–5. Recommended Dietary Allowances of Vitamins for Babies, Children and Adolescents.

VITAMIN	INFANTS		CHILDREN			ADOLESCENTS			
						Males		Females	
	0–6 mo	*6–12 mo*	*1–3 yr*	*4–6 yr*	*7–10 yr*	*11–14 yr*	*15–18 yr*	*11–14 yr*	*15–18 yr*
Vitamin A (IU)	1875	1875	2000	2500	3500	5000	5000	4000	4000
[μg]*	[375]	[375]	[400]	[500]	[700]	[1000]	[1000]	[800]	[800]
Vitamin D (IU)	300	400	400	400	400	400	400	400	400
[μg]†	[7.5]	[10]	[10]	[10]	[10]	[10]	[10]	[10]	[10]
Vitamin E (IU)	4.5	6.0	8.9	10.4	10.4	14.9	14.9	11.9	11.9
[mg TE]‡	[3]	[4]	[6]	[7]	[7]	[10]	[10]	[8]	[8]
Vitamin K (μg)	5	10	<15	<20	<30	<45	65	45	55
Vitamin C (mg)	30	35	40	45	45	50	60	50	60
Thiamin (mg)	0.3	0.4	0.7	0.9	1.0	1.3	1.5	1.1	1.1
Riboflavin (mg)	0.4	0.5	0.8	1.1	1.2	1.5	1.8	1.3	1.3
Niacin (mg)	5	6	9	12	13	17	20	15	15
Vitamin B_6 (mg)	0.3	0.6	1.0	1.1	1.4	1.7	2.0	1.4	1.5
Folacin (μg)	25	35	50	75	100	150	200	150	180
Vitamin B_{12} (μg)	0.3	0.5	0.7	1.0	1.4	2.0	2.0	2.0	2.0

Adapted from the Committee on Dietary Allowances, Food and Nutrition Board, National Research Council. Recommended dietary allowances. 10th ed. Washington, D.C.: National Academy of Sciences, 1989.

*1 Retinol Equivalent (RE) = 1 μg retinol = 3.33 IU Vitamin Activity from retinol or 10 IU Vitamin A activity from B-carotene.
†10 μg cholecalciferol = 400 IU vitamin D.
‡1 mg tocopherol equivalent = 1.49 in vitamin E activity.

Table 9–6. Role of Selected Vitamins and Minerals and Their Food Sources.

	MAJOR FUNCTIONS	FOOD SOURCES*
Vitamin K	Blood coagulation	Green leafy vegetables; pork; liver; tomatoes; cheese; egg yolk
Biotin	Fat and carbohydrate metabolism	Liver; kidney; egg yolk
Pantothenic acid	Energy production from fat and carbohydrate	Meat; fish; poultry; whole grain; legumes
Copper	Bone formation and structures within the nervous system; necessary for hemoglobin	Oysters; nuts; beef and pork livers; legumes; corn oil
Manganese	Bone formation; excretion of nitrogenous wastes	Nuts; whole grains; fruits and vegetables; tea; instant coffee; cocoa powder
Fluoride	Structure of bones and teeth; prevents dental caries	Fish; tea; most animal products; fluoridated water
Chromium	Cofactor for insulin; maintains fat metabolism; DNA/RNA synthesis	Meat; cheese; whole grains; legumes; peanuts; brewer's yeast
Selenium	Vitamin E metabolism	Whole grains; seafood; meat
Molybdenum	Component of enzyme systems	Legumes; grain and cereals; organ meats
Sodium	Acid-base balance in the extracellular fluid; maintains osmotic pressure	Salt; dairy products; seafood; whole grains; legumes
Potassium	Acid-base balance in the intracellular fluid; maintains osmotic pressure	Veal; chicken; beef; dried fruits; citrus fruits
Chloride	Water balance; acid–base balance	Salt; meat; milk; eggs

*Specific amounts of nutrients not clearly known.

Fluoride is an important element in the nutrition of children and adolescents because of its beneficial effect in dental health. For many years we have known that water fluoridation significantly decreases the prevalence of dental caries. Whereas the majority of children suffered from cavities and dental caries just two decades ago, this problem has been reduced by more than 60 percent by the addition of fluoride to drinking water. However, to avoid fluoride toxicity in situations where the municipal water supply is fluoridated, fluoride supplementation by other means such as vitamin prescriptions or fluoride-containing mouthwashes should not be provided (Hennon, Stookey & Beiswanger 1977).

Although alcohol use and abuse among children and adolescents is a significant public health problem, its effect on children's nutritional status and growth has not been fully studied (Semlitz & Gold 1987, Farrow, Rees & Worthington-Roberts 1987). In general, folate deficiency, thiamin deficiency,

Table 9–7. Role of Vitamins and Food Sources.

VITAMIN	MAJOR FUNCTIONS	FOOD SOURCES	AMOUNT
Vitamin A	Vision in dim light (rhodopsin and iodopsin formation); bone and teeth development; maintains skin and other epithelial structures	1 cup fortified milk	340 IU
		4½-ounce jar strained squash	1692 IU
		small sweet potato	8100 IU
		⅔ cup cooked carrots	10500 IU
Vitamin D	Calcium and phosphorus absorption and maintains serum levels; bone calcification	1 medium egg yolk	27 IU
		1 cup fortified cow's milk	100 IU
Vitamin E	Protect breakdown of fat; regulates prostaglandin synthesis and breakdown	1 tablespoon corn oil	6.4 IU (4.3 mg)
		1 tablespoon safflower oil	7.2 IU (4.8 mg)
Vitamin C	Maintains structure of cartilage, bone, and teeth; involved in the formation of adrenal steroids	5 whole strawberries	30 mg
		1 medium orange	80 mg
		⅔ cup cooked broccoli	90 mg
		1 cup orange juice	105 mg
Thiamin (vitamin B_1)	Carbohydrate metabolism	1 tablespoon peanut butter	0.02 mg
		1 slice whole wheat bread	0.04 mg
		1 cup ready-to-eat cereal	0.3–0.7 mg
		1 lean pork chop (2½ oz)	0.80 mg
Riboflavin (vitamin B_2)	Energy metabolism	1 ounce American cheese	0.11 mg
		1 cup whole milk	0.42 mg
		1 cup ready-to-eat cereal	0.25–0.80 mg
Niacin	Energy metabolism	1 tablespoon peanut butter	2.4 mg
		1 cup ready-to-eat cereal	5–15 mg
		1 chicken drumstick (3½ oz)	5.6 mg
		1 lean hamburger patty (3 oz)	7.1 mg

Table 9–7. Role of Vitamins and Food Sources. *(cont.)*

VITAMIN	MAJOR FUNCTIONS	FOOD SOURCES	AMOUNT
Vitamin B_6	Protein metabolism	1 slice whole wheat bread	0.03 mg
		3½ ounces peanuts	0.30 mg
		3 ounces beef fillet	0.42 mg
Folacin	Protein synthesis	1 small banana	20 μg
		1 medium orange	38 μg
		½ cup cooked spinach	70 μg
Vitamin B_{12}	Development of nerve tissue; maturation of red blood cells	1 ounce veal	0.3 μg
		1 ounce cheddar cheese	0.3 μg
		1 medium egg yolk	0.4 μg
		1 cup whole milk	1.02 μg

Table 9–8. Role of Minerals and Food Sources.

MINERAL	MAJOR FUNCTIONS	FOOD SOURCES	AMOUNT
Calcium	Formation of bones and teeth; neuromuscular contractions; blood coagulation	1 medium orange	62 mg
		1 cup whole milk	293 mg
		½ cup spinach	106 mg
Phosphorus	Energy metabolism; protein and fat synthesis	1 medium orange	30 mg
		1 egg	110 mg
		1 cup whole milk	225 mg
		1 ounce beef	58 mg
Magnesium	Energy metabolism; nerve impulse and muscle contraction	½ cup cashews	134 mg
		½ cup spinach	56 mg
		1 slice whole wheat bread	18 mg
Iron	Component in red blood cells; important for many enzyme functions; energy metabolism	1 medium egg yolk	0.9 mg
		1 ounce beef	0.9 mg
		3 tablespoons raisins	1.2 mg
Zinc	Important for many enzyme systems; necessary for vitamin A utilization	1 whole egg	0.9 mg
		1 cup whole milk	0.9 mg
		1 ounce beef	1.2 mg
Iodine	Synthesis of thyroid hormones	Iodized salt	—

and vitamin B_6 deficiency are frequent consequences of excessive alcohol drinking in adults. Recent studies in adolescent drug and alcohol abusers did not demonstrate any nutritional deficiencies (Farrow et al 1987). However, regardless of the lack of nutritional effects reported, it is obvious that children should not drink alcohol.

WHAT TO FEED CHILDREN

The ability to provide optimal nutrition for children is often beyond the control of parents. Public health officials have already introduced changes into our foods that enrich their quality and safety and therefore lead to better diets for our children. For example, the development of iodized salt and vitamin D–enriched milk came from the need to compensate for inadequacies in these vital nutrients. The elimination of iodine-deficiency goiter and rickets are only a few of the successes of these dietary modifications. Clean, uncontaminated water and food and pasteurized products have further improved the nutrition and health of our population. To date, the Western diet is rich and generally contains adequate amounts of essential nutrients for children, adolescents, and adults. A recent report by the Surgeon General noted that "the health of the American people has never been better" (Byrne 1988).

Table 9–9. Potential Vitamin Toxicities.

NUTRIENT	TOXIC LEVELS	SYMPTOMS
Vitamin A (retinol)*	Acute: ≥330,000 IU Chronic: 14,000–20,000 IU	Nausea, vomiting, headache, dizziness, blurred (double) vision, muscular uncoordination. *Infants:* bulging of the forehead (fontanelle) due to increased pressure
Vitamin D	Acute: 200,000 IU/day taken for 2 weeks Chronic: 10,000 IU/day taken for 4 months	Elevated calcium levels in blood, nausea, weight loss, frequent urination, diarrhea; may cause brain and kidney damage
Vitamin E	Adults: >1200 IU/day Low-birth-weight infants (intravenous): 25–50 mg/day tocopherol acetate	Nausea, blurred vision, gas, diarrhea; interferes with vitamin K absorption; necrotizing enterocolitis in infants
Vitamin C	>1000 mg/day	Gastrointestinal disturbances, kidney stones, low blood sugar, reduced immune functioning, rebound scurvy, enhanced iron absorption and reduced copper absorption with anemia, interference with blood clotting
Niacin	>2 g/day	Flushing of the neck, face, and chest; abnormal heart rhythms, fast heart beat; dry skin with itching; liver damage; aggravates peptic ulcer; headache; cramps, nausea, vomiting, and diarrhea; low blood pressure; high blood sugar
Vitamin B_6	>500 mg/day	Neurologic problems such as numbness, difficulty walking, loss of reflexes

*Accutane, a synthetic derivative of vitamin A used for the treatment of cystic acne, may result in malformation patterns including craniofacial, cardiac, thymic, and CNS structures in offspring of mothers who use this agent early in pregnancy. This may be of concern for the sexually active teenager who may be vulnerable to pregnancy.

Yet parents have options for food choices and diet selection that will allow their children to eat a healthier diet that meets most of the human nutrition goals discussed above. We will review two typical diets that are well-liked by children as examples of what to feed a child and how to improve the quality of the menu without losing the battle between tastes and preferences of children and health choices.

A typical menu of a 1½ year old toddler weighing 24 pounds (11 kg) might include the following choices:

MENU 1

Breakfast

¾ cup juice

½ slice toast with ½ tsp. margarine

½ scrambled egg
½ cup milk

Snack
½ banana
½ cup Cheerios

Lunch
½ grilled cheese sandwich
½ cup green beans
1 cup apple juice

Snack
½ cup juice
1 cookie

Dinner
½ cup macaroni with meat sauce
½ cup peaches
½ cup milk

Snack
1 cup apple juice

This menu is very well liked by toddlers who enjoy juices. Parents encourage the selection of juices, as these are considered healthy and natural. However, the large quantities of juice in the diet of this toddler replaced many important foods necessary for a well-balanced diet, not withstanding that even water intake might be inadequate because the child gets filled up by juice. The 1100 calories provided by the above menu are sufficient for the 24 pound (11 kg) toddler. However, the amount of protein and fat that the diet provides are inappropriate, with carbohydrate intake being excessive (Fig. 9–3). Moreover, the quality of protein is less than ideal, since 40 percent of the total protein supplied by the diet is from nonanimal sources (see Chapter 15). The low amount of fat in this menu has not been recommended for children under 2 years of age (AAP 1985 & 1986), and such severe fat restriction is not even generally recommended for children requiring dietary treatment for treatment of high blood cholesterol! Additionally, this diet does not provide sufficient quantities of various minerals and vitamins (Fig. 9–4). The intakes of vitamin D, niacin, calcium, phosphorus, zinc, and copper fall below the RDAs established for an 18-month-old toddler, and the intake of iron is 85 percent of the RDA. Ingestion of such a diet could lead to failure to thrive and to nutrient deficiencies (Chapter 17).

This menu could easily be improved by simple dietary substitutions. Juices can be replaced with healthy, wholesome milk, which the child may

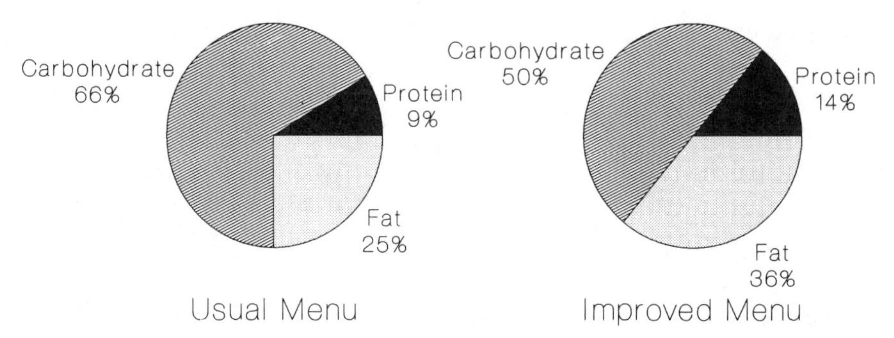

Figure 9–3. Caloric distribution of menus for an 18-month-old toddler. Usual menu-menu 1; improved menu-menu 2.

also like. For those who do not like milk, added chocolate flavoring might facilitate the change from excess juices. Iron-fortified cereal can also be added to this child's diet who, like many toddlers, may not like meat.

MENU 2

Breakfast
¼ cup apple juice
½ cup fortified baby cereal
1 cup whole milk

Snack
½ banana
½ cup Cheerios
¼ cup apple juice

Lunch
½ grilled cheese sandwich
½ cup green beans
½ cup whole milk

Snack
½ cup cranberry juice
1 chocolate cookie

Dinner
½ cup macaroni and cheese
¼ cup broccoli with ½ tsp. margarine
½ cup peaches
½ cup apple juice

Snack
½ cup whole milk

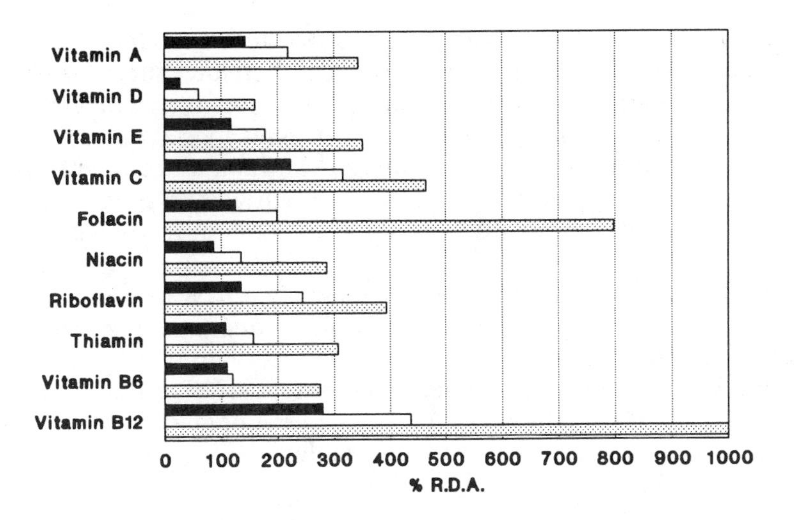

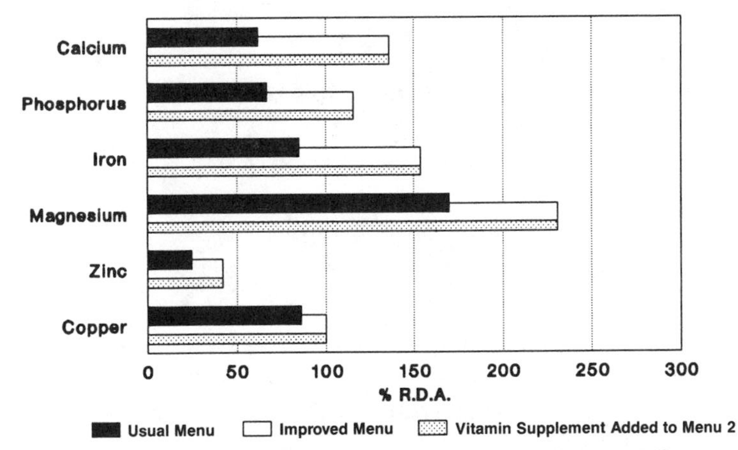

Figure 9–4. Nutrient analysis of menus for an 18-month-old toddler.
Please note that adding a vitamin supplement may not improve mineral intake since most vitamin supplements don't include minerals.

This improved food selection is more "ideal" as it is closer to the recommended dietary goals for human nutrition (see Figure 9–3). In addition, the vitamin and mineral deficiencies were largely corrected except for vitamin D intake (60 percent RDA) and zinc intake (63 percent RDA) (see Tables 9–4 and 9–5).

Even though the amount of zinc in this diet is insufficient, we do not recommend additional vitamin and mineral preparations but would add food sources high in zinc (meat, beef, eggs). In fact, most standard multivitamin preparations do not include any minerals. Therefore, their use may give health professionals and parents a false sense of security when it comes to assuring adequate intakes of zinc, calcium, phosphorus, magnesium, and other essential trace minerals. A standard chewable multivitamin preparation for children supplementing the above menu would result in excess intakes of all vitamins from 160 to over 400 percent above the RDAs (see Fig. 9–4).

Although these levels of nutrient intakes may not be associated with toxic side effects (see Table 9–9), they are certainly far above what is generally recommended for a healthy toddler. Moreover, it should be kept in mind that vitamin A toxicity may result from long-term intake of as little as 14,000 IU per day (Olsen 1987). This potentially toxic level of intake is only twice the level of a child receiving a regular diet as described above plus a standard multivitamin for children.

A typical menu for an older child of 11 years weighing 83 pounds (38 kg) might include the following choices:

MENU 3

Breakfast
¾ cup sweetened cereal with ½ cup whole milk
1.5 ounces raisins
1 cup fruit drink

Lunch
cheeseburger
1 serving french fries
diet soda

Snack
1 cup whole milk
3 chocolate sandwich cookies with vanilla creme

Dinner
3 ounces breaded chicken
½ cup broccoli with margarine
½ cup noodles with margarine
diet soda

Snack
chocolate popsicle
1 cup fruit juice

Although this diet includes fast food items, cookies, and ice cream, it is a well-balanced meal pattern in many respects. The caloric contribution (1851 calories) of this diet is appropriate for this average-weight 11-year-old girl (Fig.

9–5). It will not promote obesity but will allow her to maintain normal weight. Moreover, note that this diet is relatively low in fat, providing 30 percent of the calories from fat, even though whole milk and a cheeseburger are consumed. The cholesterol intake is only 50 milligrams per 1000 calories (94 mg/d), and it does not exceed 300 milligrams per day, which is the maximum recommended intake. Also, the sodium intake of 1.34 grams is not excessive.

The goals of reducing consumption of refined sugars and increasing unrefined complex carbohydrates in the diet are not achieved by this typical dietary intake of schoolaged children. This did not occur even though this child was ingesting "diet" carbonated drinks to avoid sugar. Sweets such as presweetened cereals, carbonated drinks, and frozen desserts are favorite foods and their disappearance from our children's diets may be difficult to attain (see Chapter 15).

Insufficient dietary intakes of zinc, calcium, iron, and folacin are quite common among schoolaged children. These deficiencies are present in the typical diet that this child likes to eat (Fig. 9–6). The food preferences of sweetened fruit drinks and refined carbohydrates rather than milk and whole grains partially account for such dietary deficiencies.

If the child would consume a whole grain cereal instead of a presweetened one; salad instead of french fries; an apple for dessert; and a lean pork chop with enriched noodles instead of breaded chicken, the vitamin and mineral deficiencies in the diet would be corrected while preserving the flavor of the diet and maintaining the appropriate fat and cholesterol intake.

MENU 4

Breakfast
¾ cup raisin bran with ½ cup milk
½ cup orange juice

Lunch
cheeseburger
lettuce/tomato salad with dressing
1 apple

Snack
1 cup milk
3 chocolate chip cookies

Dinner
3 ounces lean pork chop
½ cup enriched noodles with 1 tsp. margarine
½ cup broccoli with 1 tsp. margarine
1 cup cranberry juice

Snack
fudgesicle

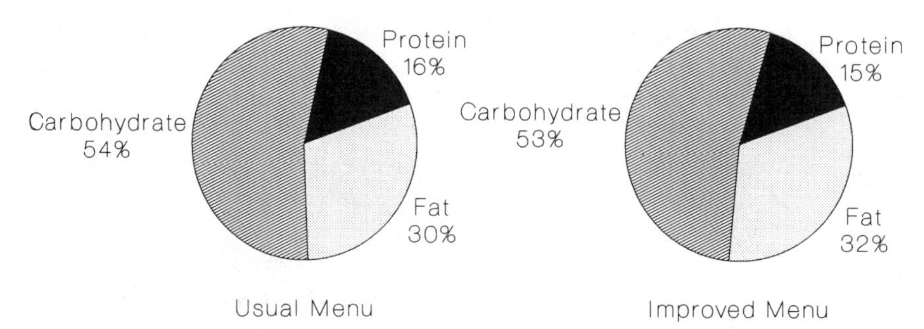

Figure 9–5. Caloric distribution of menus for an 11-year-old girl. Usual menu = menu 3; improved menu = menu 4.

Moreover, simply increasing the use of whole grain cereals and breads, fresh fruits, and vegetables in combination with the food preferences of the child would improve the overall nutritional quality of the diet. Caloric intake of this improved menu is adequate to maintain normal growth with an appropriate caloric distribution (see Figure 9–5). All nutrient requirements have been met with the exception of copper (28 to 57 percent of estimated adequate intake) (see Fig. 9–6). This menu incorporates most of the principles of good nutrition and meets the nutrition goals that are considered by most experts as ideal for a child.

CLINICAL INTERVENTION

Parents are very concerned about providing their children the best nutrition and optimal diets. The pursuit of better health is one of the prime reasons for individual food choices (Key 1987, Worsley & Leditch 1981). Often the main determinant of our food choices is a desire for a healthy diet that will foster longevity and prevent the devastating consquences of chronic degenerative diseases (Norton & Gillespie 1988). However, unlike nutritional deficiencies, which undoubtedly afflict anyone who consumes an inadequate diet, the underlying causes of these chronic disorders are complex and poorly understood. Thus, no one can predict at present what the effects of the current recommendations will be, particularly when implemented in childhood. But by implying that such nutritional strategies against chronic diseases of the elderly are necessary and should be applicable to the population at large and even to growing children, health officials have shaken confidence in our Western diets and have created a widespread fear of food.

Parents worry about what to feed their children. The same food consump-

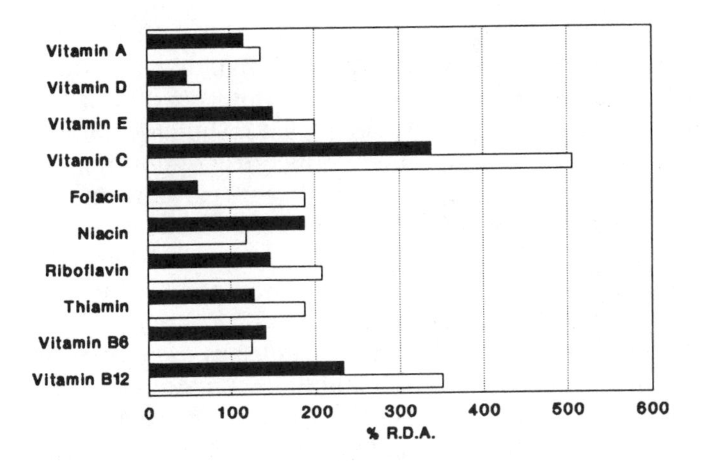

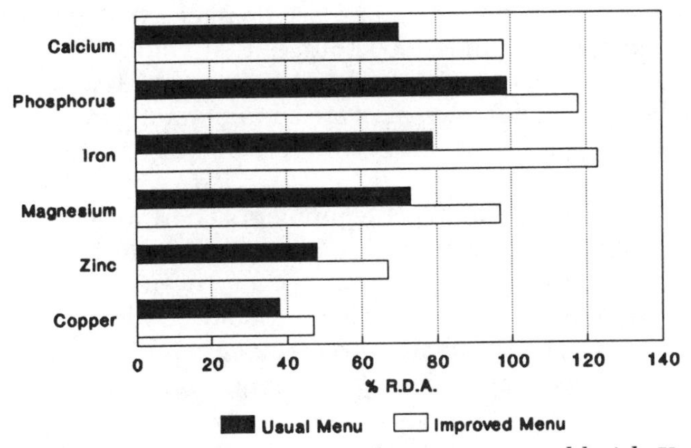

Figure 9–6. Nutrient analysis of menus for an 11-year-old girl. Usual menu-menu 3; improved menu-menu 4.

tion that allowed them and their parents to reach longevity in larger numbers than ever before is now being questioned and blamed for the chronic degenerative diseases of old age. Many parents have come to believe that diet is mainly responsible for various maladies and that an alteration of the diets of their children will protect them against these chronic illnesses. This thinking may be faulty and even hazardous, especially for growing children. In fact, some affluent parents have been undernourishing their small children by feeding them snacks of raw vegetables and skim milk rather than cookies and whole milk in an attempt to protect them from heart disease, obesity, and "junk food" dependence (Pugliese et al 1987). Similarly, older children and adolescents have come to our attention because of nutritional dwarfing related to poor intake due to health beliefs that are currently in vogue and often recommended by some health care professionals (Lifshitz et al 1987, Lifshitz & Moses 1988 & 1989).

Children and adolescents need a large number of calories and essential nutrients to grow and develop normally. Eating a variety of foods containing certain amounts of sugar and animal products is the easiest way to ensure that they will get sufficient nutritional intake. Children should be fed in accordance with the general nutrition rules that parents and health professionals have followed for many years. The basic feeding guide for children and adolescents is shown in Table 9–10. The major food groups are represented to supply all the nutrients needed for normal growth and development. Eating a variety of foods within each group is the best way to ensure that all nutritional needs are met. However, babies need to be gradually introduced to a variety of foods at an appropriate time (see Chapter 13). A well-balanced diet is one derived from multiple food sources that children like. These foods should be given throughout the day; usually three meals and two snacks are needed for growing children. Snacks are an important part of children's diet; they cannot eat enough carrots and broccoli in a day to get all the nourishment they need!

This chapter does not address the problem of how to get babies, children, and adolescents to eat a healthy diet to meet all their nutritional needs. Some topics on feeding behaviors and strategies are covered more specifically in other chapters of this book. However, it should be remembered that fussy eaters aren't born, they're made. And they're usually made by parents who can't learn to accept their children's changing food habits throughout their life cycle.

A mother who uses pressure to get her child to eat can cause general feeding problems. Parents should not tease or use tricks to get food into the child's mouth. It's not only cruel, but it can result in real resistance and eating difficulties later in life (see Chapter 17). In other words, it just makes a fussy eater. Another good way to create a fussy eater is to feed sweets such as candy or soda between meals. That curbs the appetite for more nourishing foods, ensuring that the child will surely pick and fuss at mealtime.

The important thing to remember is that it is normal for children to sometimes show a real slow-down in their desire for food. For example, when growth slows down after one year of age less food is required and the appetite decreases. The reverse is also true: adolescents need enormous quantities of food during their growth spurt and they need a large supply of high-energy

Table 9–10. Basic Feeding Guide for Children and Adolescents.

FOOD GROUP	SERVINGS PER DAY	FOOD ITEMS	SERVING SIZE			
			Toddlers (1–3 yr)	Preschooler (4–6 yr)	Preadolescents (7–10 yr)	Adolescents (11–18 yr)
Milk and milk products	4	Milk	½–¾ cups	¾ cup	¾–1 cup	1 cup
		or				
		Cheese	¾–1 ounce	1 ounce	1–1.5 ounces	1.5 ounces
		or				
		Yogurt	½–¾ cup	¾ cup	¾–1 cup	1 cup
Fish, poultry, meat, and beans	2 or more	Meat products	1–2 ounces	1–2 ounces	2–3 ounces	3–4 ounces
		or				
		Cooked dried beans, peas, or lentils	¼–½ cup	½–¾ cup	¾–1 cup	1–1½ cup
		or				
		Peanut butter	1 tablespoon	2 tablespoons	4 tablespoons	4 tablespoons
		or				
		Egg	1	1–2	1	1
Vegetables and fruits (2 choices from high vitamin C foods every day; 1 choice from high vitamin A foods every other day)	4 or more	Cooked vegetables or fruit	2–4 tablespoons	¼–½ cup	½ cup	½ cup
		or				
		Raw vegetables or fruit	¼–½ cup	½–1 cup	1 cup	1 cup
		or				
		Juice	¼–½ cup	½ cup	½ cup	½ cup

Table 9–10. Basic Feeding Guide for Children and Adolescents. *(cont.)*

FOOD GROUP	SERVINGS PER DAY	FOOD ITEMS	SERVING SIZE			
			Toddlers (1–3 yr)	Preschooler (4–6 yr)	Preadolescents (7–10 yr)	Adolescents (11–18 yr)
Breads and cereals	4 or more	Bread	½ slice	1 slice	1 slice	1 slice
		or				
		Ready-to-eat cereal	½ cup	¾ cup	¾ cup	¾ cup
		or				
		Cooked cereal	¼–⅓ cup	½ cup	½ cup	½ cup
		or				
		Pasta	¼–⅓ cup	½ cup	½ cup	½ cup
Fats and sweets	The amount of these foods that can be included in a child's diet depends on their individual caloric needs. A child who is overweight or gaining weight too quickly may need to restrict these items, whereas an underweight child should not limit their intake of these food items.					

products to keep up with their growth demands and activity. It is a good idea to give the child relatively small portions at each meal. If the child finishes everything on the plate, more can always be added. This is much more effective than loading up a child's plate with an overwhelming amount of food that cannot, and should not, be eaten.

Eating is one of life's greatest pleasures, yet too many people today are unsuccessful with eating and unsuccessful with feeding their children. Eating is more than meeting the nutritional needs of the child; it is a complicated, dynamic process. Feeding difficulties often result from complex psychosocial, behavioral interactions. The reader is referred elsewhere to deal with feeding problems and how to get children to eat (Satter 1987). Meanwhile, parents and health care professionals can be reassured that children's diets are better than ever before. When given as mixed, well balanced, varied meals, they will most likely provide all the necessary nutrients to promote good health and meet all the human nutrition needs. The only rational approach to children's nutrition is to feed them a variety of foods and to allow them to savor the foods fully.

REFERENCES

American Academy of Pediatrics, Committee on Nutrition. Pediatric nutrition handbook 2nd ed. Elk Grove Village, IL: American Academy of Pediatrics, 1985:53–65.

American Academy of Pediatrics, Committee on Nutrition. Prudent life-style for children: Dietary fat and cholesterol. Pediatrics 1986; 78:521–525.

American Cancer Society. Nutrition and cancer: Cause and prevention. New York: American Cancer Society, 1984.

American Heart Association, Nutrition Committee. Dietary guidelines for healthy American adults. Circulation 1986; 74:1465A.

American Medical Association Statement. Dietary goals for the US—supplemental views. Select Committee on Nutrition and Human Needs 1977:670–677.

Byrne G. Surgeon General takes aim at saturated fats. Science 1988; 241:651.

Committee on Dietary Allowances, Food and Nutrition Board, National Research Council. Recommended dietary allowances. 10th ed. Washington, D.C.: National Academy of Sciences, 1989.

Dairy Council. A national nutrition policy: Current and emerging issues. Dairy Council Digest 1977; 48:31–36.

Dallman PR, Yip R, Johnson C. Prevalence and causes of anemia in the United States 1976 to 1980. Am J Clin Nutr 1984; 39:437–445.

Eastwood M. Dietary fiber. In Olson RE, Broquist HP, Chickester CO, Darby WJ, Kolbye AC, Staney RM, eds. Nutrition reviews: Present knowledge in nutrition. 5th ed. Washington, D.C.: Nutrition Foundation, 1984.

Eaton SB, Shostak M, Konner M. The Paleolithic prescription. New York: Harper & Row, 1988.

Farrow JA, Rees JM, Worthington-Roberts BS. Health, developmental, and nutritional status of adolescent alcohol and marijuana abusers. Pediatrics 1987; 79:218–223.

Gortmaker SL, Dietz WH, Sobol AM, Wehler CA. Increasing pediatric obesity in the United States. Am J Dis Child 1987; 141:535–540.

Hallberg L. Iron. In Olson RE, Broquist HP, Chichester CO, Darby WJ, Kolbye AC, Stawey RM, eds. Nutrition reviews: Present knowledge in nutrition. 5th ed. Washington, D.C.: Nutrition Foundation, 1984:459–478.

Hennon DK, Stookey GK, Beiswanger BB. Fluoride-vitamin supplements: Effects on dental caries and fluorosis when used in areas with suboptimum fluoride in the water supply. J Am Dental Assoc 1977; 95:965–971.

Kelsay JA. A review of research on effects of fiber intake in man. Am J Clin Nutr 1978; 31:142–159.

Key CJ. Health factors in food choices: Risk avoidance or health seeking? Clin Nutr 1987; 6:163–167.

Kovar MG. Use of medications and vitamin-mineral supplements by children and youths. Public Health Report 1985; 100:470–473.

Lifshitz F, Moses N. Growth failure—a complication of hypercholesterolemia treatment. Am J Dis Child 1989; 143:537–542.

Lifshitz F, Moses N. Nutritional dwarfing: Growth, dieting, and fear of obesity. J Am Coll Nutr 1988; 7:367–376.

Lifshitz F, Moses N, Cervantes C, et al. Nutritional dwarfing in adolescents. Sem Adolesc Med 1987; 3:255–266.

Mehansho H, Kanerva RL, Hudepohl GR, Smith KT. Calcium bioavailability and iron-calcium interaction in orange juice. J Am Coll Nutr 1989; 8:61–68.

National Research Council Board on Agriculture. Designing foods: Animal products in the marketplace. Washington, D.C.: National Academy Press, 1988:18–44.

Norton BS, Gillespie A. A review of dietary recommendations. Professional Perspectives No. 3. Ithaca, NY: Cornell University, Division of Nutritional Sciences, 1988.

Olsen JA. Recommended dietary intakes (RDA) of vitamin A in humans. Am J Clin Nutr 1987; 45:704–716.

Pugliese MT, Weyman-Daum M, Moses N, Lifshitz F. Parental health beliefs as a cause of nonorganic failure to thrive. Pediatrics 1987; 80:175–182.

Satter E. How to get your kid to eat . . . but not too much. Palo Alto, CA: Bull Publishing Co., 1987.

Semlitz K, Gold MS. Adolescent drug abuse—Diagnosis, treatment and prevention. Psychiatr Clin North Am 1987; 9:455–473.

U.S. Department of Agriculture, U.S. Department of Health and Human Services. Nutrition and your health: Dietary guidelines for Americans. Home and Garden Bulletin No. 232. Washington, D.C.: Government Printing Office, 1985.

Wolinsky H. Talking heart. Science 1980; 21:6–10.

Worsley A, Leditch D. Students' perceptions of favorite and disliked foods. J Hum Nutr 1981; 35:173–187.

10

How to Measure Children's Nutrition

George was driving his car and was pulled over by the police to check his papers, again. This was the fourth time in the one month since he had received his license. He was a good driver but he looked so young that the police would not believe he was over 16 years old. He looked like a 12-year-old boy. George decided to do something about his appearance, and his parents took him to see a pediatric endocrinologist to help him grow and develop. What a surprise it was to him and his family to find out that inadequate nutrition was the cause of his short stature and lack of adolescent development. No one ever told him that he was malnourished. He even thought he was chubby, and his own doctor had not suspected malnutrition. Grudgingly, he followed the endocrinologist's advice to eat more, despite great fears about becoming a "fat dwarf." It made such a difference after he started eating. He grew like a weed and within 6 months he began having pimples and was never bothered by the police again.

Measuring children's nutrition is not a simple task. There are a number of measurements which vary in their level of sophistication, that must be done to determine whether a child is or is not well nourished. Certainly, most observers would be able to identify subjectively a severely malnourished child (Baker et al 1982). However, especially in the United States, the expression of nutritional deficiency is more subtle and requires special attention to nutritional assessment to be identified. Nutritional deficits and excesses are forms of malnutrition that need to be recognized for prompt treatment. For example, obesity among schoolaged children increased more than 50 percent from the mid-1960s to the late 1970s (Gortmaker et al 1987). This problem of excess nutrition sometimes goes unrecognized and untreated until the child is quite obese (see Chapter 18). In addition, the indiscriminant use of vitamin and mineral supplementation may go unnoticed and result in toxicity associated with specific excessive nutrient intakes. The reverse is also true. A child who is malnourished might escape detection, as in George's case, when even the doctor failed to identify the inadequate nutrition that led to poor growth and delayed puberty. Similarly, iron deficiency, which is the most frequent nutritional deficiency in the United States, might not be detected unless it is specifically looked for (Dallman, Yip & Johnson 1984).

NUTRITIONAL MEASUREMENTS

Height and Weight

Assessment of nutritional status can be most easily and accurately accomplished by evaluating the child's growth pattern. During the first 16 years of life, a child's weight increases twentyfold; final adult height after the adolescent growth spurt can be three to four times the birth length. In order to accomplish this increase in weight and height, the child must be healthy and be adequately nourished. Therefore, growth is a very useful yardstick of nutritional status in children. If a child is growing properly in both weight and height, chances are that his or her nutrition is adequate. It is important to note that size alone at any particular time does not necessarily reflect the child's nutritional status; rather, the rate of growth is the key parameter to monitor. All height and weight measurements should be accurately obtained (Morgan, Hill & Burkinshaw 1980) (Fig. 10–1) and plotted on a graph that shows the range of normal values for children of the same sex and age (Fig. 10–2). A child's growth may be compared with these reference growth standards as established by the National Center for Health Statistics.

Inadequate nutrition during infancy and short-term or acute undernutrition leads to alterations in body weight with little or no change in linear growth (Bray, Greenway, Molitch et al 1978). These children become underweight for height, and might be described as "wasted." However, in children who are undernourished for long periods of time, the nutritional deficits may affect the linear growth to a greater extent than weight (Suskind and Varma 1984). These children have been described as "stunted" or as having nutritional dwarfing (Lifshitz et al 1987), and may not necessarily be underweight for height (Trowbridge et al 1987) (Fig. 10–3). On the other hand, overnutrition during infancy usually results in accelerated growth in both weight and height; as the child grows older, however, persistent overnutrition expresses itself as weight excess for length or height (see Chapter 18).

In general, a weight-for-height deficit or excess of 10 percent or less is considered to be within a normal range, whereas a deviation from expected weight for height of greater than 10 percent is considered abnormal. A child with a weight-for-height deficit of 10 to 20 percent is classified as having

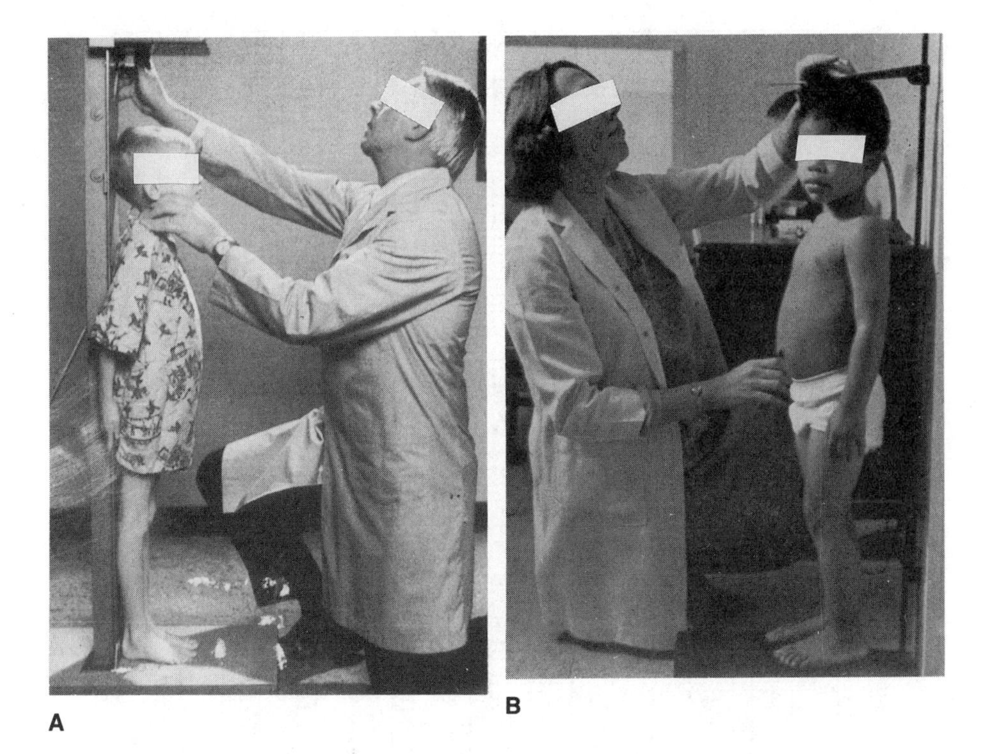

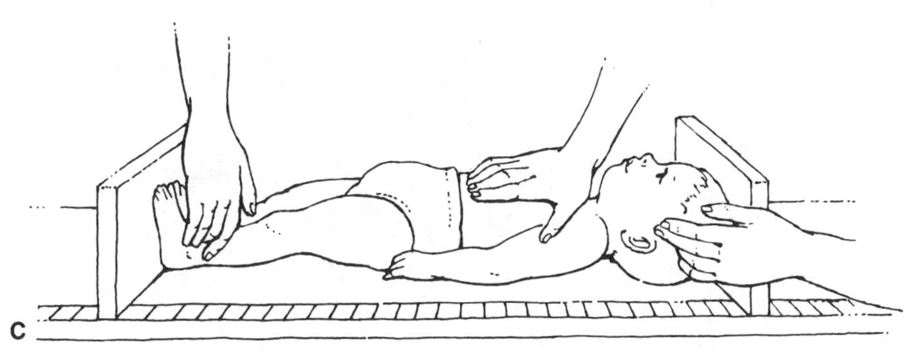

Figure 10–1. **A.** Appropriate height measurement. **B.** Wrong height measurement. **C.** Appropriate length measurement. Measurement of infant length involves supine placement on a flat measuring board with a stationary headboard and sliding footboard. The child should be flat with heat abutting headboard and eyes gazing vertically. The shoulders should be held firmly, legs extended, and feet held against footboard. The reading should be to the nearest 0.1 cm.

Reprinted with permission from LeLeiko, Benkov. Nutritional support for hospitalized children. Hosp Prac 1986; April 15:179–190.

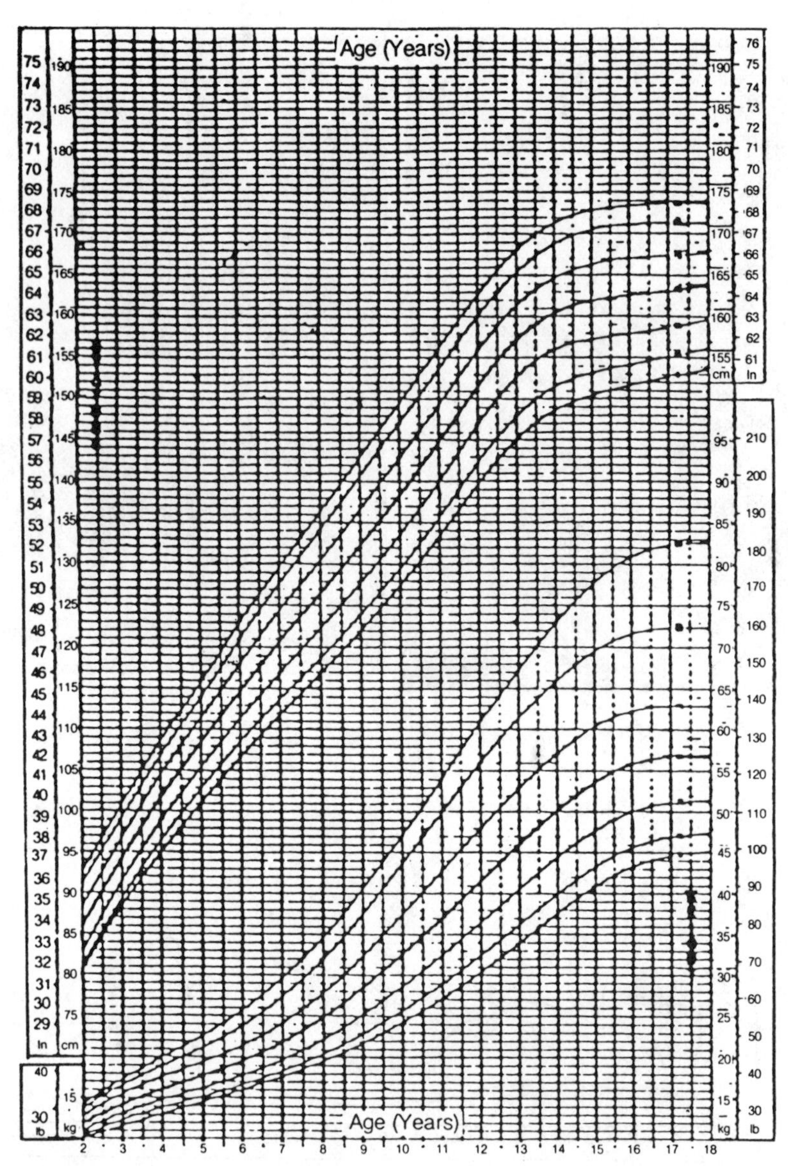

Figure 10–2. Percentiles of typical growth for females (A) and males (B) from ages 2 through 18.

From Hamill PVV, Drizd PA, Johnson CL, Reed RV, Roche AS, Moore WM. Physical growth; National Center for Health Statistics Percentiles. Am J Clin Nutr 1987; 36:607–629. © Am J Clin Nutr. American Society for Clinical Nutrition.

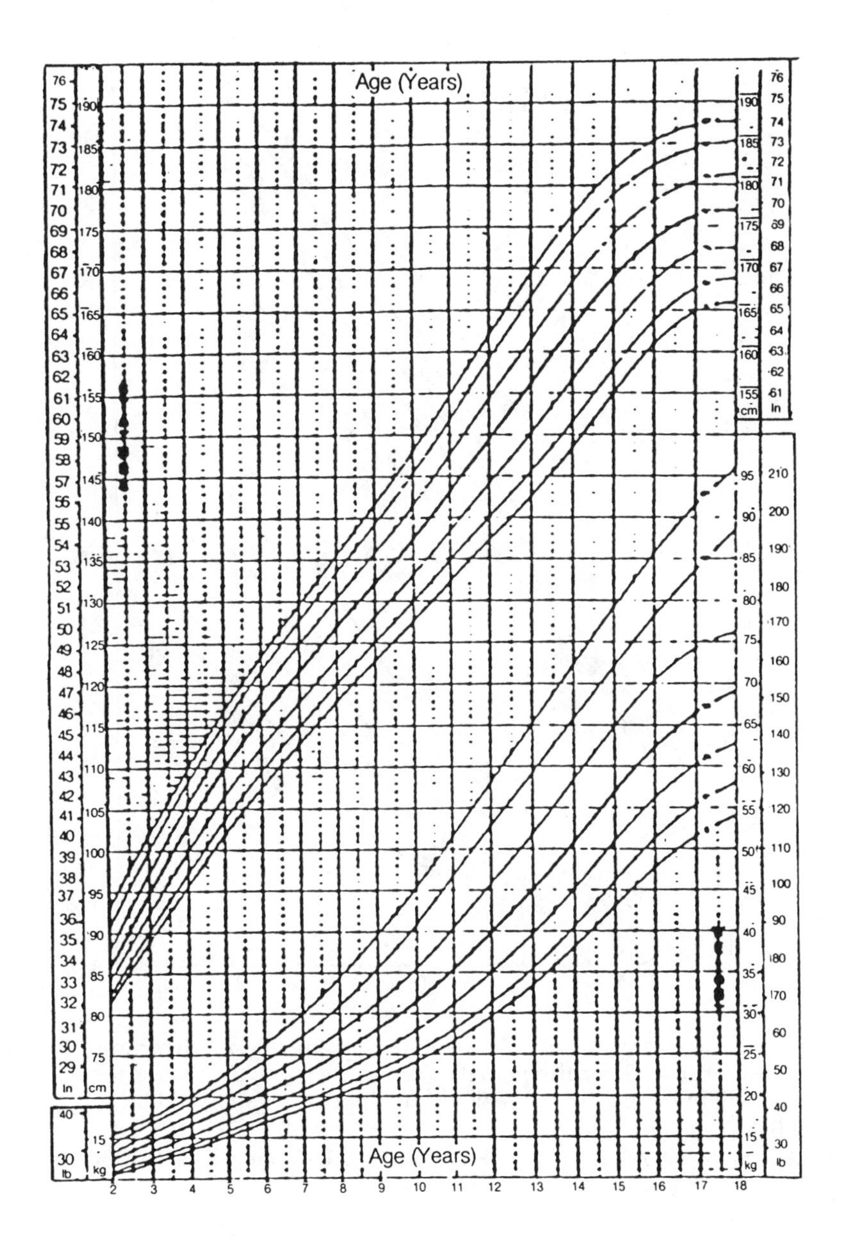

B

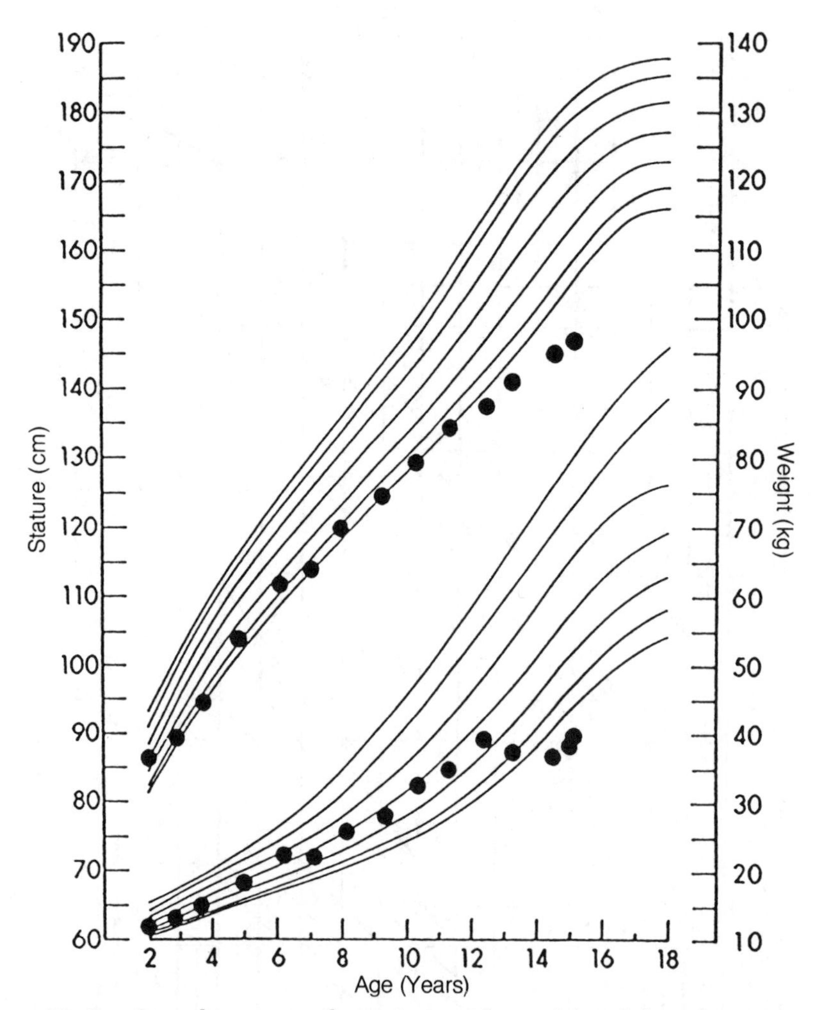

Figure 10–3. Growth pattern of a patient with nutritional dwarfing. Note that growth slowed down after the patient began a diet at age 12 years to avoid obesity. Body weight increments ceased, although he never showed body weight deficits for height.

From Lifshitz F, Moses N, Cervantes C, et al. Nutritional dwarfing in adolescents. Sem Adolesc Med 1987; 3:255–266.

"mild," or first-degree malnutrition. A digression from the expected of between 20 and 40 percent is "moderate," or second-degree malnutrition, and differences greater than 40 percent represent "severe," or third-degree malnutrition. However, not every child who has a body weight deficit for height is malnourished (Fig. 10–4). Thus, it is more important to evaluate the progression of weight and height over time to assess the nutritional status of an individual. Also, in children who retain fluids (edema) because of protein

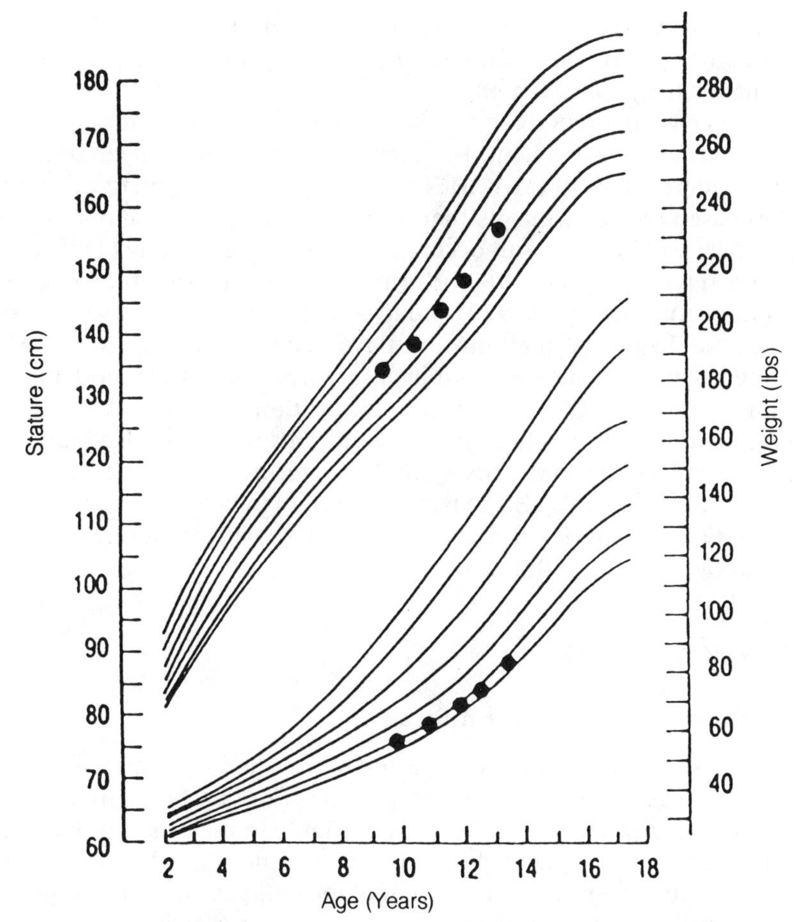

Figure 10–4. Growth pattern of a patient with constitutional underweight for height. Note the constant progression of both height and weight on the same percentile for at least 6 years.

From Lifshitz F. Nutrition and growth. Clin Nutr 1985; 4:40–47.

malnutrition, weight measurements alone are misleading. The presence of edema in a child by itself indicates that he or she is unquestionably suffering from severe undernutrition.

Head Circumference

During the first 3 years of life, a child's head circumference is a good indicator of growth and nutritional status. Malnutrition during critical stages of brain development can result in reduced brain cell numbers (Winick & Rosso 1969), which may correlate with diminished growth of the head (Dobbing

1974). Reference standards are available to monitor head circumference, and changes in the measurement should progress along similar growth percentiles as the infant's height and length.

The head circumference can also be compared with other measures of the body for nutritional assessment. For example, upper mid-arm circumference: head circumference ratio (MAC:HC) is a good index of protein-calorie malnutrition based on the principle that during times of marginal malnutrition, relative sparing of head growth occurs compared with wasting of muscle and fat reserves (Freedman et al 1980). Normative data are available for older infants (Kanawati & McLaren 1970) and for children (Frisancho 1981). Classification for the degrees of malnutrition have been developed using MAC:HC ratios: mild malnutrition is defined by a ratio less than 0.31; moderate malnutrition less than 0.27; and severe malnutrition less than 0.25. In well-nourished children, the ratio is at least 0.33. This ratio was also found to be useful in identifying newborns with intrauterine nutritional alterations (Georgieff et al 1986). MAC:HC may also be useful to determine loss or gain of muscle and fat. This index is more sensitive than weight alone because it is unaffected by changes in fluid.

BODY COMPOSITION

Why Is Body Composition Important?

Body composition is the ultimate measure of nutritional adequacy. There are methods to measure every single component of the body in the laboratory with great accuracy. However, the tools available to measure body composition cannot always be used in children. Only simple clinical tools are usually available to judge the body composition of the child as an index of his or her nutritional state; most of these methods are indirect at best.

Since body composition may vary without altering body weight, there are concerns regarding appropriateness and validity of the weight-for-height "cut-off" criteria described above to assess nutritional status. For example, a group of Peruvian children with short stature and high weight-for-height index was recently studied (Trowbridge et al 1987). Although the increased weight-for-height in these children suggested obesity, body composition evaluation revealed reduced body fat and undernutrition. Other studies have demonstrated this type of growth pattern in the United States (Lifshitz et al 1987) as well as in other undeveloped nations (Trowbridge 1983).

CLINICAL ANTHROPOMETRY

At the present time, the most widely used practical anthropometric measurements for assessing body fat and lean body mass are triceps skinfold thickness and arm circumference. The triceps skinfold thickness (TSF) measurement is an index of available fat or energy stores, while arm circumference measurements are used to determine both fat and lean body mass. The technique for measuring skinfold thickness uses a constant-tension caliper such as Lange Skinfold Caliper (Cambridge Scientific Industries) or Harpenden Skinfold Caliper (Pfister Import-Export, Inc.). To obtain an accurate, reliable TSF measurement, it is important to locate and mark the back of the arm at the midpoint between the tip of elbow (olecranon process) and the tip of the shoulder blade (acromion process of the scapula) (Fig. 10–5). This midpoint is located while the arm is bent at a 90-degree angle. The skinfold should be grasped (pinched) with the fingers approximately 1 to 2 centimeters (½–1 in.) above the midpoint, and the jaws of the caliper placed at the midpoint. The reading should be taken three times and the average of these measurements recorded. Mid-arm circumference is simply measured at the midpoint level mark used for the TSF measurement. The tape measure should encircle the arm without any gaps and without compressing the underlying tissue. Tables for skinfold thickness of different ages are available (Frisancho 1981) and percentiles for these measurements have been established for infants during the first year of life (Sann et al 1988).

However, there are several limitations to this methodology. The first set of references, developed over 20 years ago, was based on an international population in which age was not taken into consideration (Jeliffe 1966). More recent reference data have become available for use in children, but the survey population includes only Caucasians (Frisancho 1981). Another problem with these measurements is that the TSF thickness is difficult to reproduce. If the TSF measurement is taken properly, the measurement should be twice the thickness of the layer of subcutaneous fat (Fig. 10–6). However, the varying compressibility of fat makes the precision of the measurement questionable, particularly when measuring obese children (Bray et al 1978).

The use of arm fat and arm muscle areas calculated from the TSF thickness and arm circumference measurements are thought to be better indicators of energy and protein nutritional status than the individual measurements (Himes, Roche & Webb 1980). Mathematical calculations of arm muscle area (AMA) and arm fat area (AFA) based on mid-arm circumference and TSF measurements are made as follows:

$$\text{AMA} = \frac{[\text{mid-arm circumference (mm)} - [3.14 \times \text{TSF (mm)}]]^2}{12.6}$$

$$\text{AFA} = \frac{[\text{mid-arm circumference (mm)}]^2}{3.14} \times 0.79 - \text{AMA}$$

Table 10–1 gives the standard percentiles for estimates of upper AFA and upper AMA for children 1 to 19 years of age (Frisancho 1981).

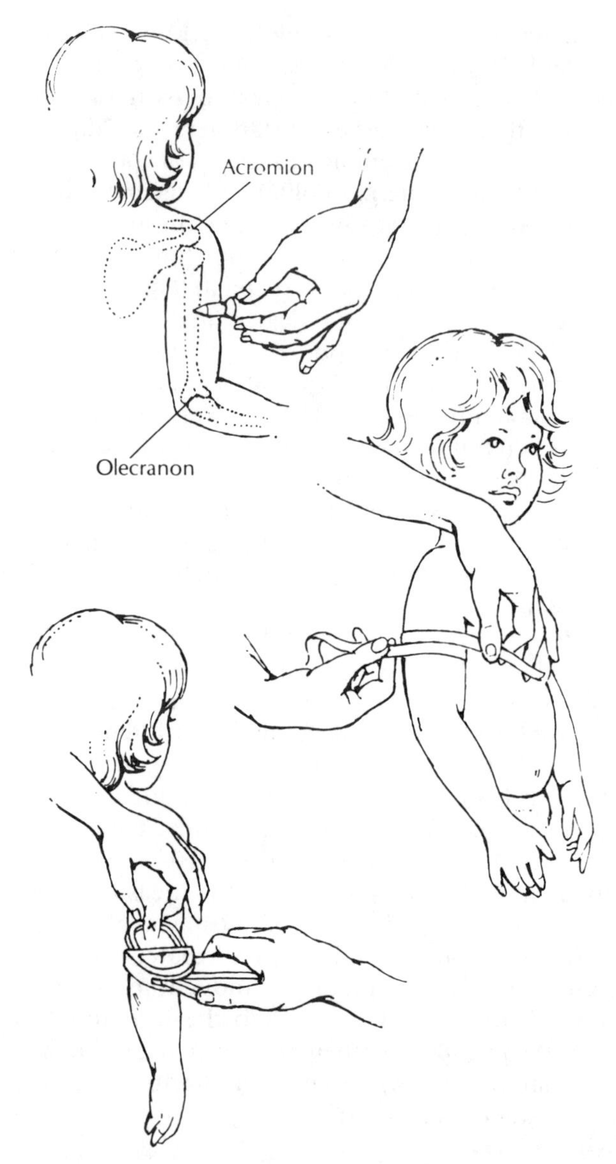

Figure 10–5. Measurement of mid-upper arm circumference (see text).
Reprinted with permission from LeLeiko NS, Benkov KJ. Nutritional support for hospitalized children. Hosp Prac 1986; April 15:179–190.

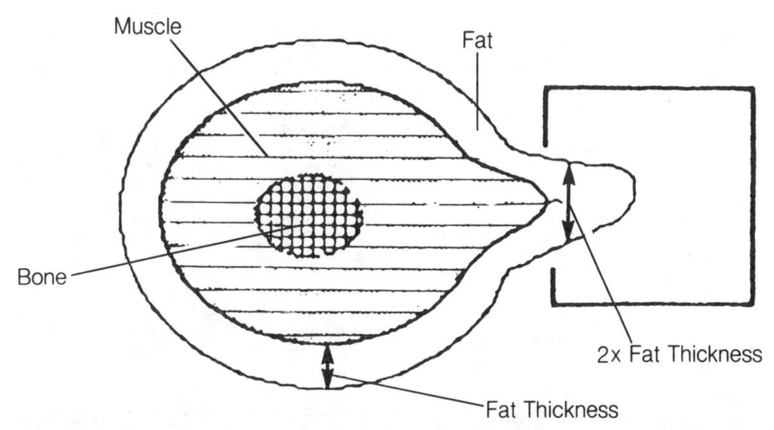

Figure 10–6. The triceps skin fold thickness should be two times the thickness of the layer of subcutaneous fat. However, this measurement is often difficult to reproduce, even by the same observer. The varying compressibility of fat, and the inherent distortion of the arm involved in taking this measurement, make the precision of this measurement very questionable.

RADIOLOGIC METHODS

An alternative method of determining subcutaneous fat thickness is the use of soft-tissue radiography, sonography, or ultrasound. Radiography of the soft tissue is more accurate than skinfold measurement of subcutaneous fat, but it is not generally used in children because of the undesirable radiation exposure. With sonography or ultrasound, either sound waves or high-frequency ultrasonic energy, respectively, is directed at the midpoint of the nondominant arm, the same site as TSF thickness measurement. The sound or ultrasonic waves are deflected off the fat/muscle interface owing to the differences in impedance between the two tissue types. The sonographic method is very accurate and in skilled hands may be more reliable than the caliper method, especially in obese children (Fried, Coughlin & Griffen 1986). However, comparisons between ultrasound and skinfold methods at the same site to predict body fatness give conflicting results (Borkan et al 1982, Fanelli & Kuczmarski 1984). Due to the high cost of ultrasound and sonography, as well as the lack of reference standards of subcutaneous fat thickness for children, these methods may not be useful to assess body composition in a typical clinical setting. It is important to note that regardless of the technique, single-site measurements of fat thickness are not very sensitive indicators of changes in total body fat.

Table 10–1. Percentiles for Estimates of Upper Arm Fat Area and Upper Arm Muscle Area.*

	ARM MUSCLE AREA PERCENTILES (mm²)							ARM FAT AREA PERCENTILES (mm²)						
AGE GROUP	5	10	25	50	75	90	95	5	10	25	50	75	90	95
							Males							
1–1.9	956	1014	1133	1278	1447	1644	1720	452	486	590	741	895	1036	1176
2–2.9	973	1040	1190	1345	1557	1690	1787	434	504	578	737	871	1044	1148
3–3.9	1095	1201	1357	1484	1618	1750	1853	464	519	590	736	868	1071	1151
4–4.9	1207	1264	1408	1579	1747	1926	2008	428	494	598	722	859	989	1085
5–5.9	1298	1411	1550	1720	1884	2089	2285	446	488	582	713	914	1176	1299
6–6.9	1360	1447	1605	1815	2056	2297	2493	371	446	539	678	896	1115	1519
7–7.9	1497	1548	1808	2027	2246	2494	2886	423	473	574	758	1011	1393	1511
8–8.9	1550	1664	1895	2089	2296	2628	2788	410	460	588	725	1003	1248	1558
9–9.9	1811	1884	2067	2288	2657	3053	3257	485	527	635	859	1252	1864	2081
10–10.9	1930	2027	2182	2575	2903	3486	3882	523	543	738	982	1376	1906	2609
11–11.9	2016	2156	2382	2670	3022	3359	4226	536	595	754	1148	1710	2348	2574
12–12.9	2216	2339	2649	3022	3496	3968	4640	554	650	874	1172	1558	2536	3580
13–13.9	2363	2546	3044	3553	4081	4502	4794	475	570	812	1096	1702	2744	3322
14–14.9	2830	3147	3586	3963	4575	5368	5530	453	563	786	1082	1608	2746	3508
15–15.9	3138	3317	3788	4481	5134	5631	5900	521	595	690	931	1423	2434	3100
16–16.9	3625	4044	4352	4951	5753	6576	6980	542	593	844	1078	1746	2280	3041
17–17.9	3998	4252	4777	5286	5950	6886	7726	598	698	827	1096	1636	2407	2888
18–18.9	4070	4481	5066	5552	6374	7067	8355	560	665	860	1264	1947	3302	3928
19–24.9	4508	4777	5274	5913	6660	7606	8200	594	743	963	1406	2231	3098	3652
25–34.9	4694	4963	5541	6214	7067	7847	8436	675	831	1174	1752	2459	3246	3786
35–44.9	4844	5181	5740	6490	7265	8034	8488	703	851	1310	1792	2463	3098	3624
45–54.9	4546	4946	5589	6297	7142	7918	8458	749	922	1254	1741	2349	3245	3928
55–64.9	4422	4783	5381	6144	6919	7670	8149	658	839	1166	1645	2236	2976	3466
65–74.9	3973	4411	5031	5716	6432	7074	7453	573	753	1122	1621	2199	2876	3327

Females

1–1.9	885	973	1084	1221	1378	1535	1621	401	466	578	706	847	1022	1140
2–2.9	973	1029	1119	1269	1405	1595	1727	469	526	642	747	894	1061	1173
3–3.9	1014	1133	1227	1396	1563	1690	1846	473	529	656	822	967	1106	1158
4–4.9	1058	1171	1313	1475	1644	1832	1958	490	541	654	766	907	1109	1236
5–5.9	1238	1301	1423	1598	1825	2012	2159	470	529	647	812	991	1330	1536
6–6.9	1354	1414	1513	1683	1877	2182	2323	464	508	638	827	1009	1263	1436
7–7.9	1330	1441	1602	1815	2045	2332	2469	491	560	706	920	1135	1407	1644
8–8.9	1513	1566	1808	2034	2327	2657	2996	527	634	769	1042	1383	1872	2482
9–9.9	1723	1788	1976	2227	2571	2987	3112	642	690	933	1219	1584	2171	2524
10–10.9	1740	1784	2019	2296	2583	2873	3093	616	702	842	1141	1608	2500	3005
11–11.9	1784	1987	2316	2612	3071	3739	3953	707	802	1015	1301	1942	2730	3690
12–12.9	2092	2182	2579	2904	3225	3655	3847	782	854	1090	1511	2056	2666	3369
13–13.9	2269	2426	2657	3130	3529	4081	4568	726	838	1219	1625	2374	3272	4150
14–14.9	2418	2562	2874	3220	3704	4294	4850	981	1043	1423	1818	2403	3250	3765
15–15.9	2426	2518	2847	3248	3689	4123	4756	839	1126	1396	1886	2544	3093	4195
16–16.9	2308	2567	2865	3248	3718	4353	4946	1126	1351	1663	2006	2598	3374	4236
17–17.9	2442	2674	2996	3336	3883	4552	5251	1042	1267	1463	2104	2977	3864	5159
18–18.9	2398	2538	2917	3243	3694	4461	4767	1003	1230	1616	2104	2617	3508	3733
19–24.9	2538	2728	3026	3406	3877	4439	4940	1046	1198	1596	2166	2959	4050	4896
25–34.9	2661	2826	3148	3573	4138	4806	5541	1173	1399	1841	2548	3512	4690	5560
35–44.9	2750	2948	3359	3783	4428	5240	5877	1336	1619	2158	2898	3932	5093	5847
45–54.9	2784	2956	3378	3858	4520	5375	5974	1459	1803	2447	3244	4229	5416	6140
55–64.9	2784	3063	3477	4045	4750	5632	6247	1345	1879	2520	3369	4360	5276	6152
65–74.9	2737	3018	3444	4019	4739	5566	6214	1363	1681	2266	3063	3943	4914	5530

*Data collected from whites in the United States Health and Nutrition Examination Survey I (1971–1974)

From Frisancho AR. New norms of upper limb fat and muscle areas for assessment of nutritional status. Am J Clin Nutr 1981; 34:2540–2545. Am J Clin Nutr. American Society for Clinical Nutrition.

HIGH-TECH METHODS

More sophisticated methods for estimating body composition do not use site-specific measurements but rather involve an estimation of total body water, which is a good index of the fat-free mass of the body. Total body water can be accurately measured by isotope-dilution techniques using radioactive tracers such as tritium, but their use is contraindicated for clinical use in children. Total body electrical conductivity (TOBEC) has also been used to estimate body composition. This method is based on the determination of resistance and reactance to the electrical current, which differ in accordance to the composition of the tissue. The electrical current moves with greater ease through fat-free tissues, which contain virtually all the water. However, due to the lack of standards in children and the high cost of the instrument (over $70,000), the TOBEC's usefulness is limited in many clinical settings.

Bioelectrical impedance analysis of body composition is a rapid, noninvasive, and simple means of assessing lean body mass with a system that is a small version of the TOBEC. This system delivers a small electrical current through aluminum foil spot electrodes attached to the top (dorsal) surfaces of the hands and feet. The amount of fat measured with this method correlates strongly with the measurements of total body water as determined by isotope dilution and densitometry (Segal et al 1988, Lukaski et al 1986). It has also been shown that bioelectrical impedance is a more reliable indicator of fat mass than skinfold measurements in adult populations (Lukaski et al 1985). A major drawback of this methodology is the lack of standards for children as well as limited investigation of this instrumentation in terms of reliability and accuracy in young children and in children with various disease processes.

Another research method available to determine body composition is underwater weighing. The underwater weighing system is based on the Archimede's principle: the volume of an object submerged in water equals the volume of the water the object displaces. This method determines an individual's body density, which is inversely proportional to the percent of body fat. In younger children or those afraid of being submerged in the water, this is not a very acceptable method to determine body composition. Also, the ability of the child to cooperate and exhale most of the air out of their lungs to obtain only residual lung volume may interfere with the ability to use this method effectively.

Computerized tomography (CT) is a modern, radiographic technique that is able to differentiate between bone, adipose, and fat-free tissue. Although CT scanners may be a sensitive method to assess body composition, their usefulness may be limited by the undesirability of exposure to ionizing radiation as well as the cost and general reduced availability of this instrumentation.

The latest in the forefront of medical technology is magnetic resonance imaging (MRI). This new instrument has been applied to body composition assessment. MRI is able to develop an accurate image based on the different physical properties of the tissue, fat and muscle, and their response to exposure to a magnetic field. Unlike soft-tissue radiography or CT, MRI does not require ionizing radiation. However, despite the advantages of this safe, non-invasive method, the cost of the procedure and the limited availability of the apparatus may thwart its acceptance as a standard component of nutritional assessment.

Neutron activation analysis is a technique that goes beyond merely differentiating between fat and muscle; it can determine the human body's content of specific elements such as calcium, sodium, chloride, phosphorus, and nitrogen. A beam of fast neutrons is directed at a subject, and unstable isotopes of the forementioned elements emit characteristic gamma rays. Each specific emission can be quantified to determine the body's absolute composition of these elements. Through mathematical calculations, estimation of muscle and fat mass can also be made. However, the machinery required for neutron activation analysis costs more than $400,000 and requires skilled technicians to run. Additionally, the use of ionizing radiation limits its practical use in young children.

The determination of total body potassium can give a very accurate estimate of lean body mass or fat-free mass. Potassium is an electrolyte that is found throughout the body except in fat. It is naturally present and emits a characteristic gamma ray that can be detected and counted. However, a total body potassium counter is needed, and this technology is not readily available for clinical purposes. Another method available to determine body composition uses sophisticated mass spectrophotometers. Scientists can now measure the stable isotopes within a child's body without giving any radioactive material. This will surely be the way to measure children's nutrition in the future, once the cost and techniques are more accessible.

BIOCHEMICAL MEASUREMENTS

Biochemical investigation is a very practical tool for nutritional assessment as it will facilitate early detection of nutritional inadequacies before clinical signs and symptoms of malnutrition become apparent. However, the type of laboratory tests that should be undertaken varies with the child's clinical presentation as well as with the type of nutritional problem that needs to be tested.

An important criteria for the diagnosis of malnutrition has traditionally been the determination of the visceral protein status by measuring circulating serum protein levels. Ideally, a sensitive serum protein for the assessment of nutritional status should have a short biologic half-life and decreased storage to reflect quickly changes in protein intake (Haider & Haider 1984).

Serum albumin is synthesized by the liver, and is the most abundant of all the serum proteins. Low serum albumin levels (hypoalbuminemia) have been documented in conditions of severe malnutrition such as kwashiorkor and chronic protein deficiency. However, a similar reduction does not occur in marasmus, a severe form of malnutrition due to insufficient calorie intake despite adequate protein intake. Also, serum albumin is not very responsive to acute changes in protein intake; it has a relatively long half-life of approximately 14 to 20 days.

Low plasma albumin levels in kwashiorkor have been correlated with a reduction in muscle mass based on anthropometric assessment (Bistrian et al 1976), but reduced serum albumin levels may also develop as a result of low protein intake even before anthropometric parameters suggest protein depletion (Whitehead, Frood & Poskitt 1971). In general, serum albumin measurements have been used to classify degrees of protein depletion from mild to severe (Table 10–2) (Weisberg 1983). However, due to the many nonnutritional factors that may influence serum albumin concentrations, clinicians have often questioned the usefulness of this laboratory measurement in diagnosing malnutrition (Golden 1982, Craig 1986). Many conditions other than low protein intake affect serum albumin levels, including chronic liver disease, nephrotic syndrome, infection, immunologic diseases, protein-losing gastrointestinal diseases such as inflammatory bowel disease, and changes in hydration status. Serum albumin levels also fall during times of stress such as surgery, trauma, and burns because albumin moves from the intravascular to the extravascular spaces. Blood albumin levels may be increased by dehydration, steroid or insulin therapy, and transfusions of blood products.

Serum transferrin is a somewhat better indicator of visceral protein status and is more sensitive to nutritional depletion than serum albumin because of its shorter half-life (8–10 days) and its smaller body storage level. However, transferrin levels also fluctuate with nonnutrition-related conditions as serum albumin levels do, thereby limiting transferrin's usefulness as a marker for nutritional status. Also, iron deficiency has been shown to induce transferrin

Table 10–2. Biochemical Assessment of Protein Malnutrition.

		DEGREE OF MALNUTRITION		
SERUM PROTEIN	**NORMAL LEVEL**	**Mild**	**Moderate**	**Severe**
Serum albumin (g/dL)	3.8–5.0	2.8–3.5	2.1–2.7	<2.1
Serum transferrin (mg/dL)	200–400	150–200	100–150	<100
Retinol binding protein (mg/dL)	3–7	—*	—	—
Prealbumin (mg/dL)	20–36	10–15	5–10	<5
Total lymphocytes (mm^3)	5000–7000	1200–2000	800–1200	<800

*Not determined.

synthesis, while iron overload is associated with low transferrin levels. Normal ranges for transferrin values representative of mild, moderate, and severe protein depletion are shown in Table 10–2.

Prealbumin (PA) and retinol-binding protein (RBP) appear to be even more sensitive to protein malnutrition than albumin and transferrin (Goffery 1978). These two carrier proteins have a very short half life of 2 to 3 days and 12 hours, respectively. Therefore, they seem to more accurately reflect rapid changes in the protein status of a patient. Since PA is four to five times more concentrated in the serum than RBP, PA is recommended for routine clinical use. Also, the levels of these proteins are rapidly increased with nutritional rehabilitation (Weisberg 1983, Large et al 1980). However, both PA and RBP are influenced by other conditions, as are serum albumin levels. Therefore, interpretation of any of these serum protein levels should be done with an understanding that clinical factors other than nutrition may affect their circulating concentrations. PA and RBP may circulate in the plasma bound together, and unbound RBP undergoes glomerular filtration and is reabsorbed by the kidney. Thus, in conditions of renal insufficiency, RBP levels in the serum can be elevated while PA, which is not catabolized in the kidney, remains relatively unchanged. However, both RBP and PA are synthesized in the liver, and reduced levels are observed in conditions of liver disease.

Urinary creatinine can be a useful indirect measure of lean body mass. Creatine, a precursor of creatinine, is found in active muscle tissue and is metabolized and excreted in the urine as creatinine. Therefore, urinary creatinine is a reflection of muscle mass. Normal levels of expected creatinine excretion based on age, height, and sex are available for comparison (Table 10–3). Creatinine height index (CHI) is calculated by dividing actual urinary creatinine excretion over a 24-hour period by expected urinary creatinine excretion as listed in the table. A value close to 1.0 indicates a well-nourished child, whereas a CHI below 0.8 suggests depleted lean body mass. Results may be invalid if the patient suffers from renal dysfunction or fever or is taking medications such as steroids. Also, accuracy of the CHI clearly is dependent on the ability to collect a complete 24-hour sample. This may be difficult in infants and younger children.

Chronic protein–calorie malnutrition and isolated vitamin and mineral deficiencies result in compromised immune status. This partially explains why malnourished children are at greater risk of becoming sick with infections or other illnesses, and why the severity of the illness is usually worse in malnourished children (Sherman 1986). For example, measles may become a life-threatening illness for a child who is malnourished, while it is usually a mild problem for the well-nourished child. Therefore, the total lymphocyte count in the blood, which represents one type of defense system of the body to protect itself against infections, may be used as a measurement of malnutrition. Absent, reduced, or delayed cutaneous hypersensitivity response (skin

Table 10–3. Normal 24-Hour Creatinine Excretion (mg/24 hr).

HEIGHT (cm)	CHILDREN 0–9 yr	HEIGHT (cm)	CHILDREN 0–9 yr	HEIGHT (cm)	MALE	FEMALE
50.0	35.5	92.8	219.9	130.0	448.1	525.2
53.5	44.9	94.1	231.5	135.0	480.1	589.2
56.9	55.2	95.5	244.5	140.0	556.3	653.1
60.4	66.4	96.8	256.5	145.0	684.3	717.2
62.4	72.4	98.0	263.6	150.0	812.2	780.9
64.4	78.6	99.2	272.8	155.0	940.3	844.8
66.4	85.0	100.4	281.1	160.0	1068.3	908.8
68.0	90.4	101.6	287.5	165.1	1386.0	1006.0
69.6	96.1	102.8	293.0	170.2	1467.0	1076.0
71.2	101.8	104.0	299.5	175.3	1555.0	1141.0
72.5	107.3	105.1	305.8	180.3	1642.0	1206.0
73.8	112.9	106.2	311.2	182.9	1691.0	1240.0
75.2	118.8	107.1	318.1	185.4	1739.0	
76.3	123.6	108.0	329.4	188.0	1785.0	
77.4	128.5	111.0	359.6	190.5	1831.0	
78.5	132.7	112.2	379.2	193.0	1891.0	
79.6	137.7	113.2	384.9			
80.7	142.8	114.1	390.2			
81.8	147.2	115.9	399.9			
82.8	156.4	117.2	407.9			
83.7	159.0	118.6	431.7			
84.7	165.2	120.0	456.0			
85.6	171.2	121.5	477.5			
86.6	177.5	123.0	499.4			
87.5	183.8	124.5	527.9			
88.5	189.4	126.0	556.9			
89.8	198.5	127.5	586.5			
91.5	209.5	129.0	616.6			

Adapted from Viteri FE, Awarad J. The creatinine height index: Its use in the estimation of the degree of protein depletion and repletion in protein calorie malnourished children. Pediatrics 1970; 96:696-706; Graystone JE; Creatinine excretion during growth. In Cheek DB, ed. Human growth, body composition, cell growth, energy and intelligence. Philadelphia: Lea and Febiger, 1968:182–197; and Blackburn G et al. Nutritional and metabolic assessment of the hospitalized patient. JPEN 1977; 1:11-21.

tests) to common microbial antigens such as *Candida* extract and tuberculin preparations are also indices of chronic malnutrition.

While a deficiency in essential fatty acids also causes reduced immunocompetence, excessive intake of fat, particularly polyunsaturated fatty acids, suppresses immunity as well. Therefore, overweight and underweight children are at risk for an impaired immune system owing to nutrient imbalances. In fact, obesity and associated hyperlipidemias may also adversely affect immune function (Watson 1984). Large intakes of iron, zinc, and vitamin E may also be immunosuppressive.

WHAT IS IN CHILDREN'S DIETS

A very important part of measuring children's nutrition is to gather information about what foods they eat, how much they eat, and when and where they eat. It is also important to understand why they eat or refuse certain foods as changes and diet plans are made to meet their likes or dislikes. To find out how a child has been fed throughout life, a dietary history should be taken. A trained interviewer should ask about feeding practices during infancy and childhood with specific questions aimed at identifying long-standing nutrition problems.

Another method of determining what kinds of food a child eats is to ask how often different foods are eaten in a day, week, or month. This is called a food frequency inventory and will only yield descriptive data about the child's recent past food intake (Sampson 1985). Deficit or excessive intakes of certain individual foods or food groups or a lack of overall variety in the diet will be detected by this type of dietary information.

In some settings it is important to have more precise information regarding what and how much a child eats during the day. Food records that list the foods eaten as well as the amount consumed can be kept by the parent and/or child over a given period of time. The quantity of food consumed can be determined by weighing all food by using common household measures or by estimating amounts. Food weighing will provide the most precise information but it is also the most costly and requires a lot of effort on the part of the family. When household measures are used to estimate the amount of food eaten by the child, the accuracy of the information will depend on the parent's or child's ability to do this task well. Food records can be kept for varying lengths of time, usually for 1, 3, or 7 days.

The most common method for measuring what a child eats is the so-called 24-hour dietary recall. With the assistance of a trained interviewer, the parent and/or child is asked to remember what they ate during the previous day. It is necessary to do this type of interview in a systematic, nonjudgmental way, with food models and measuring bowls, cups, and spoons. These are used as memory aids to help get the most accurate information about quantities of food eaten. Although this method of assessing dietary intake is quick and inexpensive, the information obtained may not represent the child's usual diet. However, under ordinary circumstances, a 24-hour dietary recall is an appropriate, valid tool to measure what children eat (Klesges et al 1987).

Once the diet information is collected, the next task is to analyze the nutrient quality of the child's intake. Before the age of computers, this information was tediously analyzed by hand, looking up the nutrient composition of each food in extensive tables. Now, computers facilitate the process. There are many computer nutrient analysis systems available to analyze diets. However, these are only as good as the information in their data bases. It must also be kept in mind that the quality of food may vary based on the soil it was grown in, the feed given to the cattle, the method and duration of storage, and the type of preparation. Thus, the food that was analyzed by the laboratory for input into the data base of the computer program may not be the same as the food on the child's plate. More work needs to be done to determine the complete nutrient composition of the food we eat and standardize it for a computer program in accordance with specific factors for local use. However, personal computer programs are quite useful for deriving quick information about a patient's dietary intake as long as trained health personnel are available to interpret the data appropriately. There are many sophisticated data bases available (Byrd-Bredbenner & Pelican 1984).

CLINICAL INTERVENTION

Measuring children's nourishment could be simple or very cumbersome, but most children who grow and develop appropriately receive all the necessary calories and protein and are well nourished. This applies even to children who are thin and may be thought of as undernourished. Children who grow in height and who gain weight at a constant rate are not usually undernourished even if they have body-weight deficits for height (see Fig. 10–4). The growth chart of the child shown in this figure demonstrates very convincingly that the child might be constitutionally thin but growing normally. Thus, this patient is getting all the fuel necessary for growth. However, there is a body-weight deficit for height at any one point in time. Since weight and growth charts do not include "body frame," this type of child may have what is commonly known as a small body frame.

To assess for specific nutrient deficiencies or excesses, more sensitive tests might be needed. However, an accurate dietary history gives good clues for potential nutritional problems. By knowing a child's usual menu and food preferences, we may be able to determine that the child is not getting some nutrients. Indeed, this dietary information may be more enlightening than blood testing. For example, a child who does not get sufficient iron in the diet might become iron deficient, but when the blood is tested, he or she might not show anemia. Iron stores (ferritin levels) must be depleted before the child has anemia, yet the child might be suffering from iron deficiency with symptoms such as irritability and poor appetite (Dallman 1982).

Other mineral deficiencies also might be difficult to diagnose with a simple blood test. Most of these elements change very little in the blood despite great changes in intake and body stores. For example, zinc and magnesium are located mainly inside the cells, and blood tests do not show low serum zinc and magnesium levels unless there are marked body deficits. Many at-

Table 10–4. Pertinent Clinical and Biochemical Aspects of the ABCDs of Nutritional Assessment.

NUTRITIONAL DEFICIT	CLINICAL FINDINGS	BIOCHEMICAL MARKERS
Protein malnutrition (kwashiorkor)	Edema Muscle wasting with preserved fat Hair dyspigmentation, thin and sparse Skin depigmentation and flaky paint Moonface Enlarged liver Irritability	Levels of protein as in Table 10–2
Protein-energy malnutrition (marasmus)	Muscle and fat wasting ("skin and bones") Sunken cheeks Skin and hair: sparse, thin, and dry Apathetic	Normal to low visceral protein levels
Vitamin A	Bitot's spots Night blindness Eye changes: roughened appearance (conjunctivae verosis) and corneal softening (keratomalacia)	Serum carotene, retinol, and retinol binding proteins Liver retinol stores
Thiamin	Edema Cardiac enlargement/failure Rapid heart beat (tachycardia) Loss of reflexes, weakness Calf-muscle tenderness Sensory loss Convulsions	RBC transketolase activity Urinary thiamin
Riboflavin	Cracks at sides of mouth and eyelids Swollen lips Scaling around nostrils Magenta-color tongue Scrotal dermatosis	Plasma riboflavin RBC glutathione reductase and riboflavin
Niacin	Red, inflamed tongue with cracks Cracks at sides of mouth Scaling nostrils Dry skin and pigmentation "Four Ds": dermatosis, dementia, diarrhea, and death	Urinary N^1-methylnicotinamide and 2-pyridone (ratio) RBC nicotinamide mononucleotide
Vitamin B_6	Swollen lips and tongue with cracks Scaling nostrils Anemia	Tryptophan load test (xanthurenic and kynurenic acids in urine) Plasma and RBC pyridoxal phosphate
Vitamin B_{12}	Inflamed, smooth tongue Peripheral neuropathy Megaloblastic anemia	Serum B_{12} and thimidylate synthetase RBC B_{12}

Table 10–4. Pertinent Clinical Aspects of the ABCDs of Nutritional Assessment. *(cont.)*

NUTRITIONAL DEFICIT	CLINICAL FINDINGS	BIOCHEMICAL MARKERS
		Urinary methylmalonic acid* Macrocytic anemia
Folate	Red, fissured, swollen tongue Hyperpigmentation Megaloblastic anemia	Serum and RBC folate Schilling test Urinary FIGLU Macrocytic anemia
Vitamin C	Petechiae (purplish spots) Ecchymoses (black/blue marks) Painful joint swelling Bleeding gums Diarrhea	Serum and WBC ascorbic acid Vitamin C saturation
Vitamin D, calcium, and phosphorus	Rickets Muscle weakness Pneumonia Joint enlargement Frontal bossing Chest beading Anorexia Malaise	Serum $25OHD_3$ and $1,25\ (OH)_2D_3$ Alkaline phosphatase Urinary calcium and phosphorus excretion
Vitamin E	Neuromuscular alterations Anemia	Hydrogen peroxide RBC hemolysis test Serum or plasma vitamin E RBC vitamin E
Iron	Anorexia Irritability Lethargy Pale, smooth tongue Spoon-shaped, brittle nails Cold sensitivity	Serum iron, TIBC, and ferritin % saturation of transferrin Protoporphyrin heme Mycrocytic hypochromic anemia
Zinc	Poor growth Delayed sexual development Poor wound healing Hyperpigmentation Pica	Serum zinc Urine zinc WBC zinc Zinc tolerance test
Magnesium	Neuromuscular hyperirritability Convulsions GI disturbances	Serum magnesium Urine magnesium Magnesium tolerance test

The ABCD of nutrition assessment stands for: Anthropometry, Biochemical, Clinical, and Dietary. In most nutritional diseases there is growth retardation and specific biochemical alterations denoting the nutrient deficit.

*Necessary to distinguish vitamin B_{12} and folate deficiency.

tempts have been made to evaluate these mineral deficiencies by using readily available tissue such as hair and nail clippings, but unfortunately the results of such analyses have been unreliable (Klevay et al 1987). Only by using a variety of urine, blood, and tolerance tests can clinicians obtain more solid evidence of specific mineral alterations.

Since most children in America do not have major vitamin or mineral deficiencies, we do not recommend vitamin/mineral supplementation. More is not necessarily better. In other chapters of this book we discuss some of the specific problems that could develop from vitamin/mineral supplements added to an already rich diet. For example, zinc in excess might suppress the immune functions (Chandra 1984). Too much iron can cause iron intoxication (hemosiderosis). Excess vitamin C does not prevent colds but may cause kidney stones. A wholesome, healthy diet with selection from all food groups is a better investment of a parent's time and money.

The nutrient analysis of the diet might not be fully representative of the child's actual nutrient supply, as no information is given about bioavailability of nutrients, quality of the products, and interactions between nutrients. This information may be more important than the amount taken in the diet. For example, the typical American breakfast of cereal and milk might be a good source of zinc. However, the phosphates in milk and the phytates in cereal may set the stage for interference with zinc absorption. So, even when the diet contains all the necessary zinc, if the foods eaten in a meal which interfere with its bioavailability, zinc deficiency could occur. Therefore, all aspects of the nutritional assessment of a child must be interpreted in accordance with the clinical condition of the child (Table 10–4).

REFERENCES

Baker JP, Detsky AS, Wesson AS, et al. Nutrition assessment: A comparison of clinical judgment and objective measurements. N Engl J Med 1982; 306:969–972.

Bistrian BR, Blackburn GL, Vitale J, Cochran D, Nayler J. Prevalence of malnutrition in general medical patients. JAMA 1976; 235:1567–1570.

Borkan GA, Hults DE, Cardarelli J, Burrows BA. Comparison of ultrasound and skinfold measurements in assessment of subcutaneous and total fatness. Am J Phys Anthropol 1982; 58:307–313.

Bray GA, Greenway FL, Molitch ME, et al. Use of anthropometric measures to assess weight loss. Am J Clin Nutr 1978; 31:769–773.

Byrd-Bredbenner C, Pelican S, eds. Software programs reviews. J Nutr Educ 1984; 16:80–98.

Chandra RK. Excessive intake of zinc impairs immune responses. JAMA 1984; 252:1443–1446.

Craig RM. Criteria for the diagnosis of malnutrition. JAMA 1986; 256:866–867.

Dallman PR. Manifestations of iron deficiency. Semin Hematol 1982; 19:19–30.
Dallman PR, Yip R, Johnson C. Prevalence and causes of anemia in the United States 1976 to 1980. Am J Clin Nutr 1984; 39:437–445.
Dobbing J. Later growth of the brain: Its vulnerability. Pediatrics 1974; 53:2–6.
Fanelli MT, Kuczmarski RJ. Ultrasound as an approach to assessing body composition. Am J Clin Nutr 1984; 39:703–709.
Freedman LS, Samuels S, Fish I, et al. Sparing of the brain in neonatal undernutrition: Amino acid transport and incorporation into hair and muscle. Science 1980; 207:902–904.
Fried AM, Coughlin K, Griffen WO. The somographic fat/muscle ratio. Invest Radiol 1986; 21:71–75.
Frisancho AR. New norms of upper limb fat and muscle areas for assessment of nutritional status. Am J Clin Nutr 1981; 34:2540–2545.
Georgieff MK, Sasanow SR, Mammel MC, Pereira GR. Mid-arm circumference/head circumference ratios for identification of symptomatic LGA, AGA, and SGA newborn infants. J Pediatr 1986; 109:316–321.
Goffery H. Prealbumin and retinol-binding protein—highly sensitive parameters for the nutritional state in respect of protein. Med Lab 1978; 5:38–44.
Golden MHN. Transport proteins as indices of protein status. Am J Clin Nutr 1982; 35:1159–1165.
Gortmaker SL, Dietz WH, Sobol AM, Wehler CA. Increasing pediatric obesity in the United States. Am J Dis Child 1987; 141:535–540.
Haider M, Haider SQ. Assessment of protein-calorie malnutrition. Clin Chem 1984; 30:1286–1299.
Himes JH, Roche AF, Webb P. Fat areas as estimates of total body fat. Am J Clin Nutr 1980; 33:2093–2100.
Jeliffe DM. The assessment of the nutritional status of the community. Geneva: World Health Organization Monograph No. 53, 1966.
Kanawati AA, McLaren DS. Assessment of marginal malnutrition. Nature 1970; 228:573–575.
Klesges RC, Klesges LM, Brown G, Frank GC. Validation of the 24-hour dietary recall in preschool children. J Am Diet Assoc 1987; 87:1383–1385.
Klevay LM, Bistrian BR, Fleming CR, Neumann CG. Hair analysis in clinical and experimental medicine. Am J Clin Nutr 1987; 46:233–236.
Large S, Neal G, Glover J, Thanangkul O, Olson RE. The early changes in retinol-binding protein and prealbumin concentrations in plasma of protein-energy malnourished children after treatment with retinol and an improved diet. Br J Nutr 1980; 43:393–402.
Lifshitz F, Moses N, Cervantes C, et al. Nutritional dwarfing in adolescents. Sem Adolesc Med 1987; 3:255–266.
Lukaski HC, Johnson PE, Bolonchuk WW, Lykken GI. Assessment of fat-free mass using bioelectrical impedance measurements of the human body. Am J Clin Nutr 1985; 41:810–817.
Lukaski HC, Bolonchuk WW, Hall CB, Siders WA. Validations of tetrapolar bioelectrical impedance method to assess human body composition. J Appl Physiol 1986; 60:1327–1332.
Morgan DB, Hill GL, Burkinshaw L. The assessment of weight loss from a single

measurement of body weight: The problems and limitations. Am J Clin Nutr 1980; 33:2101–2105.

Sampson L. Food frequency questionnaires as a research instrument. Clin Nutr 1985; 4:171–178.

Sann L, Durand M, Picard J, Lasne Y, Bethenod M. Arm fat and muscle areas in infancy. Arch Dis Child 1988; 63:256–260.

Segal KR, Loan MV, Fitzgerald PI, Hodgden JA, Van Itallie TB. Lean body mass estimation by bioelectrical impedance analysis: A four-site cross-validation study. Am J Clin Nutr 1988; 47:7–14.

Sherman AR. Alterations in immunity related to nutritional status. Nutrition Today 1986; July/Aug:7–13.

Suskind RM, Varma RN. Assessment of nutritional status of children. Pediatr Rev 1984; 5:195–202.

Trowbridge FL. Prevalence of growth stunting and obesity: Pediatric nutrition surveillance system, 1982. CBC Surveillance Summaries, 1983; 32:23–26.

Trowbridge FL, Marks JS, de Romana GL, Madrid S, Boulton TW, Klein PD. Body composition of Peruvian children with short stature and high weight for height. II. Implications for the interpretations for weight-for-height as an indicator of nutritional status. Am J Clin Nutr 1987; 46:411–418.

Watson RR, ed. Nutrition, disease resistance, and immune function. New York: Marcel Dekker, 1984.

Weisberg HF. Evaluation of nutritional status. Ann Clin Lab Sci 1983; 13:95–106.

Whitehead RG, Frood JDL, Poskitt EME. Value of serum-albumin measurements in nutritional surveys. Lancet 1971; 2:287–289.

Winick M, Rosso P. Head circumference and cellular growth of the brain in normal and marasmic children. J Pediatr 1969; 74:774–778.

11

Feeding the Low-Birth-Weight Baby

She was so small that it was scary to touch her. Mary was born prematurely and she only weighed 2 pounds (a bit less than 1 kg). A few years ago she would have died soon after birth, but in the intensive-care nursery, doctors and nurses were working hard to keep her alive. They even gave her a fair chance of survival and of normal development. Mary could not be bottle-fed because she couldn't even suck. She needed gavage feedings, which required a tube to be inserted through her nose into her stomach. Moreover, her mother's breast milk had to be enriched and supplemented. This was needed so she could get all the nutrition to complete the development that was interrupted by her premature birth. It was a trying time for all, but when Mary finally doubled her birth weight she was feeding normally, and her parents had a big party for all personnel in the intensive-care unit who helped her reach discharge day in good health and properly nourished.

The low-birth-weight (LBW) infant must receive an optimal nutrient intake to survive and to complete growth and development. Infants with a birth weight of 5.5 pounds (2500 g) or less are classified as low-birth-weight (LBW) and may be of premature, term, or postterm gestation (see Chapter 1). However, birth weight by itself does not denote maturity of the infant; it simply reflects growth in utero. Both the length of gestation and the adequacy of intrauterine growth are factors that alter the infant's nutrient needs, nutrient tolerance, and the selection of the most effective feeding modality (Galeano & Roy 1985, Anderson 1987).

Premature infants—that is, those infants born at less than 37 weeks' gestation (full-term infants are born at 37 to 42 weeks' gestation)— are at greater risk for malnutrition. Nutrients that are stored and deposited during the last trimester of pregnancy are diminished owing to the shortened gestation period. Additionally, the rate of growth after birth is relatively greater in these infants and their nutrient requirements are increased above those of full-term infants. This growth may result in rapid depletion of poor nutrient stores, particularly when they cannot eat sufficient food to sustain these needs. The gastrointestinal (GI) tract and renal system are immature in LBW babies. Thus, the amounts and types of feedings these babies are able to tolerate are often insufficient to support growth. Moreover, these infants often suffer from a variety of illnesses common to the newborn period, which may delay the introduction of enteral feedings and further alter their nutrient needs. In short, these babies are in a quandary; they require the most and can tolerate the least.

NUTRITION AND FEEDING CONSIDERATIONS

Optimal nutrition is critical in the management of the ever-increasing number of surviving LBW infants. Although the most appropriate goal of nutrition of such babies is not definitively known, having the baby grow after birth as it would have grown in the mother's womb (an approximation of the in utero growth of a normal fetus at the same postconception age) appears to be the most logical approach at present (AAP 1977). In uncomplicated cases, growth usually begins by the second week after birth (Fig. 11–1).

Body composition changes radically throughout gestation, and while many substances accumulate at a fairly constant rate (e.g., sodium, potassium, magnesium, and water), many other substances accumulate at exponential rates between the 25th and 35th week of gestation (Table 11–1). Rapid skeletal mineralization requires increasing amounts of calcium and phosphorus as the fetus approaches term. Similarly, the rate of fat accretion also rises very fast near term. However, the quality of fetal growth differs from that of LBWs. For example, weight gain of a premature infant given milk formula produces more fat gain than that in a fetus of the same maturity (Reichman et al 1981). Therefore, an ideal objective should be to duplicate both fetal growth rates and fetal body composition when planning the feedings of a LBW infant. It needs to be kept in mind that bigger may not necessarily be better.

The ability of LBW babies to digest, absorb, and utilize the given nutrients differs from that of full-term infants. Gastrointestinal immaturity alters both GI motility and enzyme availability and may decrease the effectiveness of feedings in promoting growth in the LBW baby. GI motility disturbances of the LBW infant most often involve the upper gastrointestinal tract. They have a limited gastric capacity, which is often complicated by delayed or incomplete gastric emptying. This results in many of the common deterrents to feed-

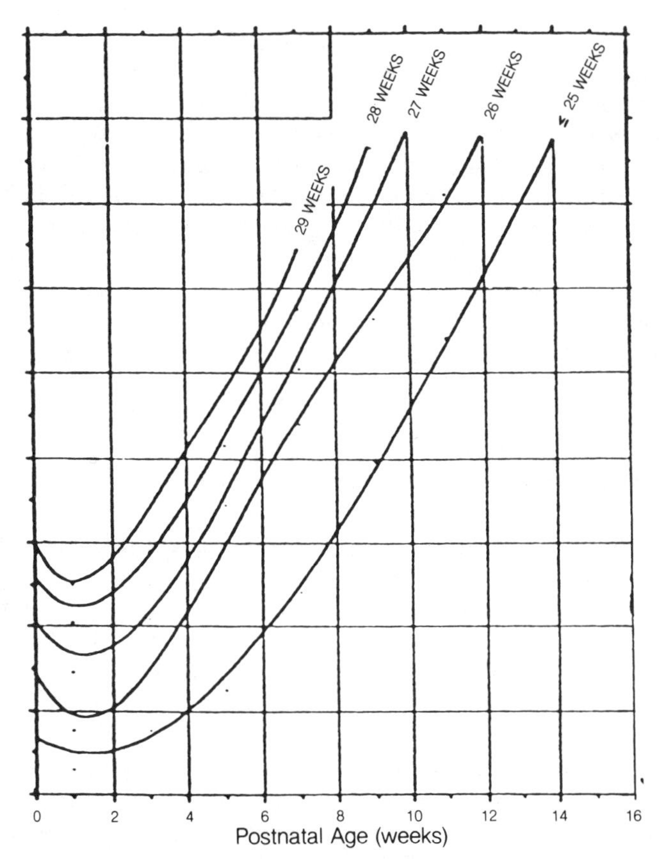

Figure 11–1. Percentiles of body weight of premature infants of varying gestational ages for the first 16 weeks of life (A) and growth record for weight, length, and head circumference for LBW infants from 25 to 40 weeks of gestation and up to 12 months of age (B). Both charts are applicable to both sexes.

(A) Adapted from Gill A, Yu VYH, Aspbury J. Postnatal growth in infants from before 30 weeks gestation. Arch Dis Child 1986; 61:549; (B) Adapted from Babson SG, Benda GI. Growth graphs for the clinical assessment of infants of varying gestational age. J Pediatr 1976; 89:814–820.

ing LBW babies: satiety with a small feeding, abdominal distention, gastric residuals that remain in the stomach and interfere with the next feeding, and regurgitation. In the presence of these symptoms, it is quite common for a doctor to respond by restricting feedings.

The small stomach capacity and impaired gut motility that cause delayed gastric emptying are more of a problem in the LBW baby weighing less than 1000 grams than in those weighing more than 1400 grams (Calabio et al

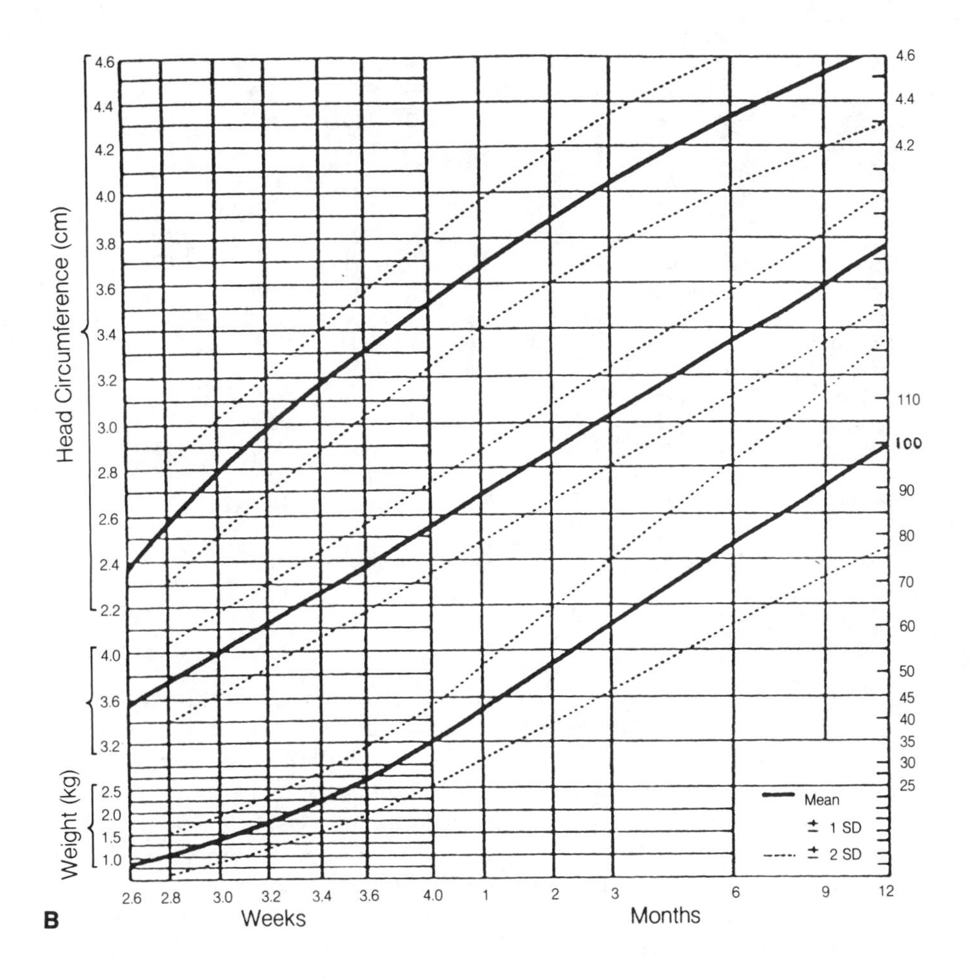

1988). Poor and unsustained suck is also a frequent problem since coordination of sucking, swallowing, and respiration does not occur until about 32 to 34 weeks' gestation. Prior to this developmental stage, the risk of food being aspirated into the lungs is high. Additionally, the rapid respiration that occurs in the LBW baby can lead to feeding aspiration.

More subtle, but of equal importance to motility disorders, are problems that may result in intestinal malabsorption. LBW babies have both quantitative and qualitative deficiencies of many enzymes and bile salts that are necessary for the digestion and absorption of foods. Most notably, deficiencies of intestinal lactase, pancreatic lipase, and bile acids may make it difficult to

Table 11–1. Calculated Daily Rates of Accumulation of Various Substances by the Fetus at Different Periods of Gestation.

	WEEKS OF GESTATION						
SUBSTANCE	**24**	**26**	**28**	**30**	**32**	**34**	**36**
Nitrogen (mg/d)	159	207	269	349	452	587	761
Protein (g/d)	1	1.3	1.7	2.2	2.8	3.7	4.8
Sodium (mg/d)	15	18	23	28	33	43	53
[mEq/d]	[0.65]	[0.78]	[1.0]	[1.22]	[1.43]	[1.87]	[2.30]
Potassium (mg/d)	15	19	24	31	39	50	64
[mEq/d]	[0.38]	[0.49]	[0.62]	[0.79]	[1.0]	[1.28]	[1.64]
Calcium (mg/d)	59	79	105	140	186	248	330
Phosphorus (mg/d)	36	47	62	82	108	142	188
Magnesium (mg/d)	1.9	2.4	3.1	3.9	5.0	6.4	8.1
Iron (mg/d)	0.8	1.1	1.4	1.9	2.5	3.3	4.3
Copper (μg/d)	39	52	67	88	116	151	199
Zinc (μg/d)	169	208	256	316	389	480	591
Fat (g/d)	0.25	0.43	0.75	1.32	2.31	4.0	7.1
Water (g/d)	7.6	9.7	12.3	15.7	20.0	25.6	32.6

Adapted from Shaw JCL. Parenteral nutrition in the management of sick low birth weight infants. Pediatr Clin North Am 1973; 20:333.

achieve normal absorption of fat and lactose. However, premature infants are a heterogeneous group. The enzymatic and functional deficiencies of immaturity exist as a spectrum, which changes as the infant grows and ages. For example, intestinal lactase activity in the premature infant remains at less than 30 percent of the normal term infant through 34 weeks' postconception. Afterwards, it increases rapidly to reach normal levels at 38 to 40 weeks (Lifshitz 1985). While the problems associated with GI tract immaturity suggest restrained progression of enteral feeding, critically needed energy and essential substrates must be provided. Ideally, the LBW infant should be nourished by enteral means, but for practical reasons, parenteral nutrition may be necessitated either as a result of food intolerance or malabsorption (see Chapter 28).

NUTRIENT NEEDS

To achieve appropriate growth, the LBW infant's requirements for energy, protein, minerals, and selected vitamins are usually higher than that of a term infant. The nutritional guidelines for LBW babies of different ages and birth weight as per the American Academy of Pediatrics (1985a) are shown in Table 11–2.

The enterally fed LBW infant usually requires 125 to 130 calories per kilogram of body weight per day to obtain satisfactory weight gain (Reichman,

Table 11–2. Estimated Requirements and Advisable Intakes for Protein and Major Minerals by Infant's Weight as Derived by Factorial Approach.*

	TISSUE INCREMENT (/d)	DERMAL LOSS (/d)	URINE LOSS (/d)	INTESTINAL ABSORPTION (% intake)	ESTIMATED REQUIREMENT (/d)	ADVISABLE INTAKE Per day	ADVISABLE INTAKE Per kg†	ADVISABLE INTAKE Per 100 kcal‡
800–1200 grams (26–28 weeks' gestation)								
Protein (g)	2.32	0.17	0.68	87‡	3.64	4.0	4.0	3.1
Sodium (mEq)	1.63	0.06	1.21	90	3.22	3.5	3.5	2.7
Chloride (mEq)	1.23	0.10	1.18	90	2.79	3.1	3.1	2.4
Potassium (mEq)	0.87	0.12	1.11	83	2.52	2.5	2.5	1.9
Calcium (mg)	116	2	4	65	188	210	210	160
Phosphorus (mg)	75	1	25	80	126	140	140	108
Magnesium (mg)	3.2	—	2.0	60	8.7	10.0	10.0	7.5
1200–1800 grams (29–31 weeks' gestation)								
Protein (g)	3.01	0.25	0.90	87	4.78	5.2	3.5	2.7
Sodium (mEq)	1.77	0.09	1.81	90	4.08	4.5	3.0	2.3
Chloride (mEq)	1.30	0.15	1.77	90	3.47	3.8	2.5	2.0
Potassium (mEq)	1.03	0.18	1.66	83	3.45	3.4	2.3	1.8
Calcium (mg)	154	3	6	85	251	280	185	140
Phosphorus (mg)	98	2	37	80	171	185	123	95
Magnesium (mg)	4.0	—	3.0	60	11.7	13.0	8.5	6.5

*The estimated dietary guidelines for additional minerals (Anderson 1987) are zinc 0.5; iron 2.0–3.0 mg/100 kcal/d; manganese 5.0; copper 90; and iodine 5.0 μg/100 kcal/d. The estimated guidelines for vitamins are folacin 50, vitamin K 12+, biotin 35 μg/kg/d; pantothenic acid 2 mg/kg/d; vitamin E 1.7/100 kcal/d (though 5 and 25 IU supplements have been suggested). A 35 mg/d additional vitamin C supplement has been suggested to be given in addition to the 35 mg contained in the infant formula. Vitamin A and D guidelines are 1400 and 500 IU/d, respectively. For thiamin 0.3, riboflavin 9.4, niacin 6.0, and vitamin B_6 0.3 mg/d and for vitamin B_{12} 0.5 μg/d are recommended (AAP 1985b).

†Assuming body weight of 1000 and 1500 g, respectively, for the 800- to 1200-g infants and 1200- to 1800-g infants.

‡Assuming calorie intake of 130 kcal/kg/d.

From Ziegler EE, Biga RL, Fomon SJ. Nutritional requirements for the premature infant. In Suskind RM, ed. Textbook of pediatric nutrition. New York: Raven Press, 1981.

Chessex, Putet et al 1981). Higher energy intakes for the healthy premature infant do not necessarily result in greater weight gain. Excessive formula feedings may overtax the absorptive capacity of the premature infant and result in increased fecal nutrient losses (Pereira & Barbosa 1986). However, many premature or LBW infants who suffer from respiratory illnesses or other problems have increased energy needs due to increased basal metabolic rates and activity levels. Higher energy needs make it necessary to increase calories beyond 120 to 130 calories per kilogram of body weight per day.

The amount of protein intake needs to be sufficient for tissue accretion without the development of protein overload (AAP 1985ab). Protein intakes of 4.5 grams per kilogram have resulted in azotemia, acidosis, and increased plasma amino acid levels (Raiha et al 1976). Decreased I.Q. scores were shown in infants who received 6 to 7 grams of protein per kilogram during the neonatal period (Goldman et al 1974). Preterm infants demonstrate low liver enzyme concentrations and poor oxidation of selected amino acids, which could cause the above-mentioned problems. For example, the amount of liver enzyme needed for the oxidation of phenylalanine and tyrosine (para-hydroxyphenylpyruvic acid oxidase) is decreased in LBW babies. Therefore, high levels of these amino acids may develop in blood, which could be toxic to the LBW baby as is the case in children with phenylketonuria (PKU) (see Chapter 25).

The type of protein the LBW infant receives is also important. The most suitable protein is contained in whey-predominant formulas with whey:casein protein ratios (60:40) similar to breast milk. These protein feedings were associated with metabolic indices and plasma amino acid levels closest to infants fed pooled mature human milk (AAP 1977).

The fat of human milk is well absorbed by the LBW infant, but the predominantly saturated triglycerides of cow's milk are poorly digested and absorbed. The recognition of the magnitude of fat malabsorption led in the 1940s and 1950s to the use of low-fat formulas for feeding premature infants. However, medium-chain triglycerides are well absorbed, presumably because their digestion and absorption are not dependent on duodenal intraluminal bile salt levels, which are low in the premature infant. Thus, the recently developed special formulas for premature infants contain a mixture of medium-chain triglycerides and predominantly unsaturated long-chain triglycerides (Table 11–3). The essential fatty acid requirement (at least 3 percent of total calories in the form of linoleic acid) is amply met by this fat mixture. However, the gain in energy through improved absorption of medium-chain triglycerides may be offset by an increased frequency of intestinal disturbances (abdominal distention, loose stools, vomiting) attributable to the medium-chain triglycerides (Okamoto et al 1982).

The LBW infant may also have difficulty in digesting the lactose in cow's milk formulas during the first days of life, because of low intestinal mucosal lactase activity (AAP 1977, MacLean & Funk 1980). Lactose in breast milk is better tolerated regardless of the infant's diminished intestinal enzyme activity (Okuni, Okinaga & Baba 1972). In the absence of adequate lactase activity, undigested lactose may cause intestinal distention, diarrhea and/or metabolic acidosis (Lifshitz et al 1971, Lifshitz 1985). However, enzymes necessary for digestion of glucose polymers are active in small premature infants (Cicco et al 1981). Thus, the carbohydrate portions of the various special formulas for premature infants now contain approximately 40 to 50 percent lactose and 50 to 60 percent glucose polymers.

Premature infants begin life with low vitamin E stores. Moreover, if a diet high in polyunsaturated fatty acids (PUFA) and/or high in iron is consumed, the needs for vitamin E are increased. Without additional vitamin E, the red blood cells are more susceptible to oxidation and hemolytic anemia. Therefore, current LBW infant formulas have been altered to contain less PUFA and iron and more vitamin E (see Table 11–3). Pharmacologic dosing of vitamin E at 100 milligrams per kilogram (IU) has been advocated to prevent retinopathy of prematurity (ROP) and bronchopulmonary dysplasia (Pereira & Barbosa 1986, Hilter et al 1981). Although benefits from such treatment are questionable (Pereira & Barbosa 1986), cases of vitamin E toxicity have been reported, with the development of liver failure, GI damage, necrotizing enterocolitis (NEC), infection (sepsis), or bleeding in the brain (intracranial hemorrhage) (Phelps 1984). The American Academy of Pediatrics placed a hold on pharmacologic vitamin E treatment, particularly with the intravenous preparation of the acetate ester (AAP 1985b).

Clinical symptoms of folate deficiency in LBW infants may not be present, but folacin supplements of 50 micrograms per day are often given to prevent the drop in serum folacin levels that occurs during the neonatal period. Results of folacin supplementation studies have varied in regard to the infant's weight gain and hemoglobin levels (Pereira & Barbosa 1986). It is important to note that the liquid multivitamin preparations usually do not contain folic acid, owing to the instability of this substance in solutions.

Vitamin C supplementation to LBW babies has been suggested as a means to improve the oxidation of phenylalanine, an amino acid that can cause brain damage at high concentrations in the blood. This is of particular concern in LBW babies because of their decrease in liver enzyme for phenylalanine oxidation. Dosages as high as 100 milligrams of vitamin C per day have been shown to be effective in lowering amino acid levels in the blood (Light, Berry & Sutherland 1966) of premature babies, but others have not substantiated these observations (Bakker et al 1975). Because of the absence of compelling evidence for a high vitamin C requirement in LBW infants, the American Academy of Pediatrics Committee on Nutrition does not recommend a supplement in addition to the 35 milligrams of vitamin C contained in the daily oral multivitamin mixture (AAP 1985b).

It is difficult to supply the small LBW infant with adequate amounts of calcium and phosphorus for normal bone growth and mineralization (Table 11–2). LBW babies often do not ingest enough milk to meet their calcium and phosphorus requirements for adequate bone mineralization. Even parenteral nutrition may have limited effectiveness since calcium and phosphorus in sufficient amounts to meet the babies' needs may precipitate out in IV solutions. As a result, osteopenia (rickets and bone fractures) are frequent features in small premature infants.

Human milk and infant formulas designed for term infants are both deficient in calcium and phosphorus relative to fetal accretion rates (AAP 1977). The bone mineral content of the LBW infants receiving such feedings is therefore far below normal fetal values (Minton, Steichen & Tsang 1979). But when calcium and phosphorus intakes are increased the bone mineral content of LBW infants increases at the fetal rate (Steichen, Gratton & Tsang 1980). Although more calcium and phosphorus is good for bone accretion, this is not accomplished without added risk. Tolerance to feedings may decrease, calcium phosphate may precipitate in the stomach or in the kidneys (Venkataraman & Blick 1988), and/or aluminum toxicity may occur (see Chapter 28). At present, the prevention of severe bone disease in LBW infants is based on high oral intake of calcium and phosphorus and at least 400 IU of vitamin D per day.

The LBW baby should also be considered at risk for developing other mineral deficiencies (Tsang 1985). The needs of zinc and copper are of particular importance. Zinc metabolism is complex in the LBW infant. Theoretically, the fetal retention rate of 250 micrograms per kilogram per day for zinc could be met by the LBW infant's consumption of mother's milk (Mendelson, Anderson & Bryan 1982). However, when consuming heat-treated human milk, LBW infants are in negative zinc balance until about 70 days of age (Parker, Helinek, Meneely et al 1982), apparently because of limitations in intestinal absorption of zinc. The AAP Committee on Nutrition has proposed (AAP 1976, 1977) that infant formulas for full-term infants supply 0.5 milligrams of zinc per 100 calories. There is no reason, at present, to modify these recommended levels for LBW infants.

Copper balances are also negative in premature infants until the fifth week after birth (Manser et al 1980), and copper deficiency may occur in these babies (Shaw 1980). Copper available from the breast milk of mothers of premature infants is appropriate, ranging from 58 to 72 micrograms per deciliter during the first month after birth (Mendelson, Anderson & Bryan 1982). However, increases in copper concentration in formula from 50 micrograms per deciliter to 160 micrograms per deciliter did not lead to increased serum copper levels in LBW infants (Hillman, Martin & Fiore 1981). Only with a higher, nonphysiologic dose of 1500 micrograms per deciliter could this be achieved. Therefore, the copper intake recommended by the AAP Committee on Nutrition (1985) (90 micrograms per 100 calories) continues to be appropriate.

The amount of iron needed by LBW infants is controversial despite extensive information on this subject (AAP 1979). It is well known that the iron stores of prematurely born infants is lower at birth than that of full-term infants. Additionally, these babies lose this mineral in large quantities owing to the frequent blood samplings required for their medical care. To top it all off, the dietary supply may be inadequate, while their growth needs are high. However, the early physiologic anemia of prematurity is not benefited by iron therapy (AAP 1977). Also, there are common clinical conditions for which LBW infants receive transfusions of red blood cells (e.g., apnea of prematurity), which supply plenty of iron. In addition, high levels of oral iron supplementation can interfere with vitamin E metabolism in the small premature infant and may interfere with zinc absorption (Parker et al 1982). Thus, while there is no clear indication for iron supplementation before 1 to 2 months of age, it has been suggested that oral iron supplements be started at about 2 weeks of age, or when enteral feedings are tolerated, at a dose of 2 to 3 milligrams per kilogram per day (Ziegler, Biga & Fomon 1981, Lundstrom, Siimes & Dallman 1977). If iron is administered this early, vitamin E supplements should be given.

Once the LBW infant reaches about 2000 grams and/or goes home, iron supplementation is definitely needed. Infants fed human milk should receive 2 to 3 milligrams per kilogram per day of elemental iron, as ferrous sulfate drops. Formulas with iron usually contain sufficient supplemental iron (AAP 1979). Premature formulas (Table 11–3), however, are low in iron and supplementation is indicated. Iron supplementation for all LBW infants should be continued to age 12 to 15 months.

In LBW babies, the excretion of sodium in the urine is high for the first 10 to 14 days after birth. Thus, feedings of mature human milk, which is low in sodium, or of some commercial formulas designed for the feeding of term infants may lead to low levels of sodium in the blood (hyponatremia). Special formulas for LBW infants should provide 2.5 to 3.5 milliequivalents per kilogram per day (57.5–80.5 mg/kg/d) of sodium at full feeding levels (Fomon, Ziegler & Vazquez 1977). Very LBW infants (<1500 g), however, may require even higher levels of 4 to 8 milliequivalents per kilogram per day (92–184 mg/kg/d) of sodium to prevent hyponatremia (Kumar & Sacks 1978).

Water is another important nutrient of concern to LBW babies. In practice, fluid is often given at 100 milliliters per kilogram per day. However, breast milk provides 180 milliliters per kilogram per day in order to deliver 120 calories per kilogram per day. This is different from the amount of water available in LBW formulas, which provide 81 calories per 100 milliliters of formula (Table 11–4). Thus, 148 milliliters per kilogram per day of milk formula would be necessary to provide 120 calories per kilogram per day. These

Table 11–3. Formulas for LBW Infants per 100 mL.

	BREAST MILK FORTIFIERS		COMPLETE INFANT FORMULAS				
	Similac Natural Care	Enfamil Human Milk Fortifier (4 packets/100 mL breast milk)	Similac PM 60:40	Similac Special Care 20	Similac Special Care 24	Enfamil Premature Formula 20	Enfamil Premature Formula 24
Protein (g)	2.20	0.7	1.58	1.83	2.20	2	2.4
Whey:casein	60:40	60:40	60:40	60:40	60:40	60:40	60:40
Fat (g)	4.41	0.04	3.76	3.67	4.41	3.4	4.1
MCT (%)	50	—	—	50	50	40	40
LCT (%)	50	—	—	50	50	60	60
Carbohydrate (g)	8.61	2.7	6.90	7.17	8.61	7.4	8.9
Lactose (%)	50	25	100	50	50	40	40
Glucose polymers (%)	50	75	—	50	50	60	60
Vitamins							
A (IU)	552	—	203	460	552	800	952
D (IU)	122	—	40.6	101.4	122	220	262
E (IU)	3.2	—	2.0	2.7	3.2	3.1	3.6
C (mg)	30	—	6.1	25	30	23	27.8
B_1 (μg)	203	—	67.6	169	203	167	198
B_2 (μg)	503	—	101.4	419	503	233	277
Niacin (mg)	4.06	—	7.10	3.38	4.06	2.67	3.17
B_6 (μg)	203	—	40.6	169	203	167	198
B_{12} (μg)	0.45	—	0.17	0.37	0.45	0.2	0.24
Folic acid (μg)	30	—	10	25	30	23	27.8
K_1 (μg)	9.7	—	5.4	8.1	10	8.7	10.3

Minerals							
Calcium (mg)	170	60	56	122	146	78	92.9
Phosphorus (mg)	85	33	18.9	60.8	73	39	46.8
Magnesium (mg)	9.7	4	4.1	8.1	10	3.3	3.9
Sodium (mg)	40.6	7	16.2	33.8	41	26	31
Potassium (mg)	113.7	15.6	58.1	94.6	114	74	88
Chloride (mg)	73.1	17.7	39.9	60.8	73	56.7	67.5
Zinc (mg)	1.2	0.8	0.5	1.01	1.22	0.67	0.8
Iron (mg)	0.3	—	0.1	0.25	0.3	0.17	0.2
Copper (μg)	203	—	60.8	169	203	106.7	127
Osmolality							
mOsm/kg water	300	—	280	250	300	244	300
Calories/oz	24	—	20	20	24	20	24
Comments	To be mixed with human breast milk or be fed alternately with human milk	To be added to mother's milk for premature infants	For LBW infant <1500 g, additional calcium, phosphorus, and sodium may be necessary during periods of rapid growth; low iron	For LBW infant <2000 g; low iron	For LBW infant <2000 g requiring high-calorie formula; low iron	For LBW infant; low iron	For LBW infant requiring high-calorie formula; low iron

Table 11–4. Approximate Water Content of Standard and Concentrated Infant Formulas.

	WATER CONTENT	
Formula	**mL/L**	**oz/qt**
20 calories/oz	900	29.5
24 calories/oz	880	29.3
27 calories/oz	865	28.8

infants also have a limited kidney capacity to excrete high solute loads and to concentrate urine. Therefore, water balance is critical and when water is not given in sufficient quantities it may lead to dehydration and/or to inadequate use of the calories supplied, with resultant poor growth. In contrast, when more water is given, there may be lower sodium levels in blood, and a higher incidence of complications such as NEC or persistence of patent ductus arteriosus (Bell & Oh 1983).

There are concerns about carnitine needs in LBW babies who may become deficient in this nutrient because of poor intake of carnitine and increased losses due to immature kidney function. However, the effects of carnitine deficiency in these babies are not clear (Borum 1988).

HUMAN MILK

Human milk is the most ideal food for infants (see Chapter 12), but it is not as perfect for the LBW infant. Nonetheless, premature babies should be given their own mothers' milk when it is available. However, human milk often contains insufficient nutrients for the premature infant and may be inadequate to support growth as the infant matures. It may be low in energy, protein, calcium, phosphorus, and sodium. The clinical consequences of these inadequacies may be poor growth (Fomon & Ziegler 1977, Heird 1977, Fleischman & Finberg 1979, Atkinson, Bryan & Anderson 1981), hyponatremia (Kumar & Sacks 1978, Engelke et al 1978), hypoproteinemia (Ronnholm, Sipila & Siimes 1982) and rickets (Greer, Steichen & Tsang 1982). Several investigators have reported that milk from mothers who deliver prematurely contains greater amounts of these nutrients than milk from mothers who deliver at term, but the increased concentration of nutrients is not always consistent (AAP 1985b, Tsang 1985). Therefore, even when milk from the premature infant's own mother is given, breastfeeding supplements are needed. Mixing human milk with premature infant formula is one means of supplementing the diet. Other suggestions include the use of fortifiers designed for human milk or the addition of specific nutrient supplements (see Table 11–3).

Human milk contains taurine, a sulfur-containing amino acid present in low concentrations in cow's milk (AAP 1977). The role of this amino acid in the human infant is not clear, and its essential nature to the LBW infant has not been established. Recent studies of premature babies receiving taurine-supplemented, whey-protein–predominant commercial formula have shown that the added taurine did not enhance growth, production of taurine-conjugated bile acids, or fat absorption (Jarvenpaa et al 1983a, b & c). However, others claim that fat absorption is improved (Galeano & Roy 1985).

The antiinfectious properties of human milk are important attributes, which cannot be duplicated in infant formulas. The secretory immunoglobulin A (IgA) in the milk inhibits adherence and proliferation of bacteria and has an important role in controlling the microbial environment of the GI tract. The secretory IgA is present in a higher concentration in milk from mothers of preterm infants than in milk from mothers of term infants (Gross et al 1981), but its role in preventing disease in LBW babies is less clear. In some studies, however, human milk was considered beneficial in preventing NEC. However, a note of caution has been raised regarding feedings of mothers' milk to premature infants. Forbes (1982) is concerned by the marked variability in the composition of human milk and thus the difficulty of assuring an adequate nutrient intake for the infant. It is important to reemphasize that most advantages are obtained when fresh milk from the premature infant's own mother is used. The advantages are most obvious during the first month of life. Pooled human milk does not necessarily provide all the benefits and may indeed add risks, such as the transmission of viral infections to the infant (see Chapter 12).

INFANT FORMULAS FOR LBW BABIES

The past few years have seen the introduction of proprietary infant formulas designed expressly for the premature infant (see Table 11–3). The compositions of these formulas reflect both the special nutritional requirements of these babies and the functional immaturity of their small intestines. A premature formula is characterized by these main aspects. It contains an increased calorie density (24 kcal/oz) to allow higher calorie intake in a smaller volume. Whey protein has been added to duplicate the whey:casein ratio (60:40) found in human milk and to provide more digestible protein. In LBW formulas, medium-chain triglyceride (MCT) oil replaces a portion of the fat content to improve absorption and retention of fat, and glucose polymers replace a portion of lactose. The exact vitamin and mineral concentrations of premature formulas vary among the preparations, but in general are increased to compensate for decreased volume intake.

Ideally, the osmolarity of infant formulas, as well as any other products given to these babies, should be kept isotonic, <300 milliosmoles per kilogram water (Ernest et al 1983) because hypertonic solutions (> 300 mOsm/kg water) fed to LBW babies may lead to the development of feeding intolerances and NEC. These problems may not be due to formula feedings but may result from the high osmotic activity of medications given for the treatment of illnesses common in LBW infants.

The use of soy formula is not recommended for premature infants. The soy protein composition may not be of sufficient biologic quality to meet the needs of the premature baby (Hall et al 1984).

Often, LBW infants are given dietary supplements such as MCT or glucose polymers to increase their caloric intake and nutrient absorption. For example, in babies with jaundice, a higher MCT content may facilitate fat absorption. In infants who are not able to ingest sufficient formula, supplements may be used to increase the calorie supply. However, feedings of high caloric density formulas may lead to a decreased daily intake (Brooke & Kinsey 1985), and the addition to the formula of modular supplements may lead to GI problems and to imbalances in the total amounts of nutrients given. MCT oil and glucose polymers may cause abdominal distention, loose stools, and even vomiting (Okamoto et al 1982), and the addition of these products to the formula may result in dilution of essential nutrients such as protein, vitamins, and minerals (Fig. 11–2 and 11–3). The addition of 20 calories by a modular supplement increases the calorie density of a formula but decreases the amount of calories derived from protein to an unsafe level (see Fig. 11–2). In a study

Composition of 3 Formulas Containing Fat or Carbohydrate Supplements

Premature Formula *	100 ml PF +2.6 cc MCT Oil	100 ml PF +10 cc CHO
193 ml (6.4 oz)	159 ml (5.3 oz)	153 ml (5.1 oz)
24 kcal/oz	29.4 kcal/oz	30.3 kcal/oz
81 kcal/dl	98 kcal/dl	101 kcal/dl
Carbohydrate 42%	Carbohydrate 33%	Carbohydrate 53%
Protein 11%	Protein 8%	Protein 9%
Fat 48%	Fat 59%	Fat 38%

* Similac Special Care, Ross Laboratories

Figure 11–2. Composition of three types of feedings for LBW babies. Premature formula alone is compared with feedings of such formulas containing fat or carbohydrate supplements as described in legend of Figure 11–3.

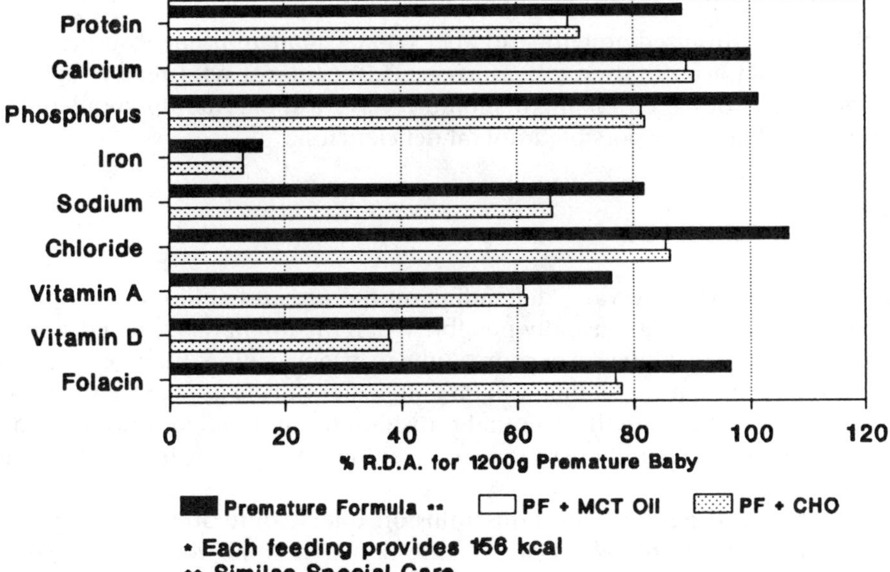

Figure 11–3. Nutrient composition of three feedings for LBW infants. The nutrients shown are those that do not meet 100 percent of RDAs; the nutrients that exceeded the daily requirements when supplementation was added are not shown. Feedings given were premature formula (PF) 193 mL (6.4 oz); PF and MCT oil 159 mL (5.3 oz)–2.6 mL MCT oil with 100 mL of formula; and PF and CHO 153 mL (5.1 oz)–10 mL CHO (Polycose) with 100 mL of formula. In all instances the type of feedings provided 100 percent of the caloric requirement (see Fig. 11–2).

by Kashyap et al (1986), LBW babies who were given a formula that provided only 7.8 percent of the calories from protein grew more slowly than those receiving 9.4 percent or 12.5 percent of calories from protein. Similarly, the proportion of the vitamins and minerals provided by the diet would be diluted by the extra calories provided, and the intake of these elements would therefore be below the recommended nutrient requirements for premature babies (see Fig. 11–3). Therefore, when a formula is supplemented with either fat or carbohydrate to increase calories, the intake of all other nutrients becomes unbalanced and the LBW infant's requirements may not be met. Also, the amount of water may become insufficient when the caloric density is increased by modular supplements of fat or carbohydrate (see Table 11–4). To ensure adequate water intake when a baby is receiving a concentrated formula, their hydration status should be checked regularly, although small babies may not concentrate urine well.

The use of other special infant formulas is indicated when infants develop complications such as NEC or short gut syndrome or when they cannot tolerate milk formula (see Chapters 19 and 20). Formulas that contain glucose polymers, hydrolyzed protein, and MCT will facilitate nutrient absorption by the infant with an injured gut. However, LBW infants who receive special formulas not designed for them should receive a multivitamin supplement and be evaluated for possible mineral deficiencies.

FEEDING METHODS

Feeding methods may vary, depending on the age and abilities of the LBW infant. Nipple feeding is usually possible when the infant has reached a postconception age of 34 weeks or more. Tube (gavage) feedings may be required by younger premature infants. Offering a pacifier during gavage feedings has been found to facilitate the eventual transition to full nipple feedings. A soft rubber nipple is generally used for early feedings to allow the infant to obtain milk with less effort.

Gavage feeding by continuous infusion offers some advantages in the smallest of premature babies (see Chapter 27). The small volume infused at any given time presents a minimal volume load to the stomach, reducing the likelihood of large gastric residuals, vomiting, and aspiration of formula. The infusion rate may be increased as the infant's stomach capacity and tolerance of formula dictate. Infants should be fed via a perfusion pump, which can be adjusted to deliver accurately volumes as small as 1 milliliter per hour when continuous infusion is employed.

Gastric bolus feedings of milk can lead to breathing disturbances in infants with respiratory problems (Patel et al 1977). Thus, continuous jejunal (transpyloric) feedings by nasal or oral tubes may be better tolerated (AAP 1977). Clinical results of this feeding mode have been excellent in many centers, but there has been some criticism that bypassing the stomach and duodenum with a jejunal tube may cause inefficient utilization of the nutrients in the formula (Whitfield 1982). Bolus feedings into the stomach via gavage tube or nipple, every 2 to 3 hours, is the goal once the LBW infant clears the respiratory distress associated with prematurity and gastric emptying is improved.

Parenteral feeding is often the main source of nutrition for LBW babies. As a general rule, any neonate who is incapable of tolerating oral feeding for more than 3 days is a candidate for intravenous nutrition. The preterm newborn is much more sensitive to fasting than the full-term newborn, and one should not delay in providing nutrition to these babies (Sutphen 1981). In fact, for the full-term newborn partial parenteral nutrition, consisting of only a 10 percent glucose solution with electrolytes, will be sufficient for a short period (Anderson 1987), whereas the amount of calories that the premature newborn can receive with 5 percent, 7.5 percent, or 10 percent dextrose solutions is not at all adequate (Sutphen 1981). Peripheral parenteral nutrition guidelines for LBW infants are shown in Tables 11–5 and 11–6. The reader is referred to the discussion in Chapter 28 regarding the intravenous nutrition by peripheral-vein infusion for a complete discussion of this subject.

Administration of nutrients via a peripheral vein is probably preferable when intravenous nutrition is expected to be necessary for less than 2 weeks. In addition, the calories supplied via peripheral vein can be provided in a proportion similar to that of the oral route. Central intravenous nutrition is preferable for long-term treatment, but this procedure requires highly trained, experienced personnel (see Chapter 28). Central vein-fed infants can receive more calories and gain more weight on a daily basis. However, it should be kept in mind that LBW infants frequently develop high blood glucose levels (hyperglycemia) because of their limited ability to metabolize glucose given in the intravenous nutrition solution.

CLINICAL INTERVENTION

Enteral feeding can be introduced once the LBW infant is clinically stable with normal respiration, body temperature, cardiovascular function, and the presence of bowel sounds (Galeano & Roy 1985, Anderson 1987). Bottle feedings may be given if the infant is medically stable, has a respiration rate less than 60 breaths per minute, and is of at least 32 weeks' gestation.

Those infants who lack developmental skill or who are too ill to nurse should receive feedings via tube (gavage). Either nasogastric or orogastric tube feedings can be used in the LBW baby, and bolus feedings or continuous infusion can be given.

Standard infant formulas are often well tolerated by the LBW baby who is over 4 pounds (1700 g). Premature infants less than 4 pounds should be fed special LBW formulas almost exclusively or in combination with breast milk. Considering the content and net retention of nutrients for infants under 2 pounds (1000 g), it becomes abundantly clear that despite its advantages, breast milk alone is inadequate. However, when breast milk is available, it should be given alternately or mixed with 24-calories-per-ounce premature formula. When human milk is not available infants in this weight group may be fed initially with half-strength (12 kcal/oz) premature formula, to be advanced to full strength after 24 hours.

Whatever the mode of feeding, the formula volume should be advanced slowly—over at least 10 to 14 days in infants weighing less than 2 pounds (1000 g) and over 6 to 8 days in infants weighing more than 3 pounds (1500 g). This allows adaptation of the intestinal tract to enteral feeds, without the development of vomiting, distention, and diarrhea.

Feeding problems are common in the intensive-care nursery. Formula intolerance frequently results from difficulties in achieving normal gut motility

Table 11–5. Peripheral Parenteral Nutrition for Low-Birth-Weight Infants.

	DAYS OF LIFE								
PREMATURE NEWBORNS WITH GESTATIONAL AGE >33 WEEKS AND FULL-TERM NEWBORNS	**1**	**2**	**3**	**4**	**5**	**6**	**7**	**8**	**9**
10% Intralipid									
mL	0	10	15	20	25	30	35	40	
kcal	0	11	16.5	22	27.5	33	38.5	44	
Freamine III									
mL	0	15	20	25	30	30	30	30	
kcal	0	5	7	8	10	10	10	10	
10% Dextrose									
mL	70	80	90	100	105	110	115	120	
kcal	28	32	36	40	42	44	46	48	
Fluid									
mL/d	70	105	125	145	160	170	180	190	
kcal/d	28	48	59.5	70	79.5	87	94.5	102	
PREMATURE NEWBORNS WITH GESTATIONAL AGE ≤33 WEEKS AND SGA NEWBORNS									
10% Intralipid									
mL	0	5	10	15	20	25	30	30	30
kcal	0	5.5	11	16.5	22	27.5	33	33	33
Freamine III									
mL	0	15	20	25	30	30	30	30	30
kcal	0	5	7	8	10	10	10	10	10
10% Dextrose									
mL	80	80	90	100	110	120	130	140	150
kcal	32	32	36	40	44	48	52	56	60
Fluid									
mL/d	80	100	120	140	160	175	190	200	210
kcal/d	32	42.5	54	64.5	76	85.5	95	99	103

From Rubaltelli FF, Carnielli V, Orzali A. Parenteral nutrition of the newborn. In Stern L, ed. Feeding the sick infant. New York: Raven Press, 1987: 241–256.

Table 11–6. Daily Intravenous Nutrition Guidelines for the LBW Infant.

NUTRIENT	AMOUNT*
Calcium (mg/kg/d)	30–40
Phosphorus (mg/kg/d)	30–60
Magnesium (mg/d)	15–25
Zinc (μg/kg/d)	300–438
Copper (μg/kg/d)	20–63
Chromium (μg/kg/d)	0.14–0.20
Manganese (μg/kg/d)	2–10
Sodium (mEq/kg/d)	2–4
Potassium (mEq/kg/d)	2–3
Chloride (mEq/kg/d)	2–3
Vitamin A (IU/kg/d)	1230–2490
Vitamin D (IU/kg/d)	250–500
Vitamin E (IU/kg/d)	0.7–1.2
Vitamin K (mg/kg/d)	0.02
Vitamin C (mg/kg/d)	20.0–40.0
Folacin (μg/kg/d)	80.0
Niacin (mg/kg/d)	2.4–4.8
Riboflavin (mg/kg/d)	0.24–0.48
Thiamin (mg/kg/d)	0.24–0.48
Vitamin B_6 (mg/kg/d)	0.12–0.24
Vitamin B_{12} (μg/kg/d)	300–700
Pantothentic acid (mg/kg/d)	0.24–0.48
Biotin (μg/kg/d)	2.0–4.0
L-carnitine (mg/kg/d)	10.0

*The lower ranges are for preterm and the higher ranges are for full-term neonates.

Adapted from Rubaltelli FF, Carnielli V, Orzali A. Parenteral nutrition of the newborn. In Stern L, ed. Feeding the sick infant. New York: Raven Press, 1987:241–255.

and intestinal absorption. However, signs of poor gastric emptying and abdominal distention are symptomatic of both abnormal gut motility, and, more seriously, early sepsis. Slowing infusion rates or discontinuing the feedings for a short time may be sufficient to alleviate formula intolerance, but medical intervention is necessary if there is infection. When formula intolerance is persistent, or coupled with blood in the stools (guaiac-positive stools), bilious residuals, apnea, or lethargy, further investigation is imperative. When these signs and symptoms occur, NEC may be present. This life-threatening complication was first shown to be related to feedings in infants with diarrhea who had lactose intolerance and malnutrition (Coello-Ramirez, Gutierrez-Topete & Lifshitz 1970). LBW infants, particularly those weighing less than 1500 grams, were also shown to be at high risk for this ominous complication (Lifshitz 1981). However, fear of NEC should not lead to insufficient nutrient intake.

Another complication related to feedings in newborns may be the development of lactobezoars. Abdominal distention, vomiting, and diarrhea are frequent symptoms in premature babies who develop milk curd balls within the stomach (lactobezoars), which can be identified by an abdominal roentgenogram. These lactobezoars have been found to occur in babies fed concentrated formulas, particularly those high in casein, perhaps due to the higher curd tension. If recognized promptly, and if they are of small size, withholding feedings for a day or two may lead to improvement. Large lactobezoars must be surgically removed.

The achievement of adequate growth in the premature infant is evaluated by serial measures of body weight, length, and head circumference. Plotting these measurements on an infant growth chart will identify whether growth is occurring consistently along a normal curve (see Fig. 11–1). Growth may not, however, occur at the expected percentile when compared with term infants. Therefore, the use of fetal growth curves is preferred until the infant reaches a postconceptional age of 40 weeks. After this point, chronologic age should be corrected for prematurity when assessing growth and weight gain. When growth and/or ability to take nourishment enterally falls below established minimum standards, alternative feeding modalities may be required (see Chapters 27 and 28).

Mothers should be encouraged to provide milk for their infants to aid in maternal-infant attachment. Assistance should be offered to the mother who wishes to breast feed. She should be provided a place that is fairly quiet and private. Talking to the infant, removing outer clothing, or stroking can help awaken the infant for nursing. The mother may need to hand-express some milk to erect the nipple. This allows the premature infant with a small mouth and weak suck to begin milk flow. The infant should be placed in the chest-to-chest position to establish direct attachment. The number of opportunities for nursing will depend on the infant's clinical status, but parents must always participate.

Rooming-in arrangements often help the mother gain confidence and experience in caring for her premature infant. A health care team member should talk with the mother after each feeding to monitor the success of nursing for both the mother and infant. The mother should be reminded that nursing is a learned skill for the infant. There is no agreement on the recommended time the LBW infant should be allowed to nurse, but allowing the baby the opportunity to try to nurse will soon lead to success after the infant has developed the skills to do so. It should always be kept in mind that developmental delays occur in infants kept off oral feedings and nursing for long periods of time.

Meeting the nutritional requirements of small premature babies is a big challenge. Limiting feedings of the LBW infant at a time of critical brain growth might be very risky, yet enteral feeding might not be well tolerated. Thus, the nutritional rehabilitation of LBW infants is a challenge for all who care for these small babies.

REFERENCES

American Academy of Pediatrics, Committee on Nutrition. Commentary on breast feeding and infant formulas, including proposed standards for formulas. Pediatrics 1976; 57:278–289.

American Academy of Pediatrics, Committee on Nutrition. Iron deficiency. In Pediatric nutrition handbook. Evanston, IL: American Academy of Pediatrics, 1979.

American Academy of Pediatrics, Committee on Nutrition. Nutritional needs of low-birth-weight infants. Pediatrics 1977; 60:519–530.

American Academy of Pediatrics, Committee on Nutrition. Nutritional needs of the low-birth-weight infant. Pediatrics 1985a; 75:976–986.

American Academy of Pediatrics, Committee on the Fetus and Newborn. Vitamin E and the prevention of retinopathy of prematurity. Pediatrics 1985b; 76:315–316.

Anderson DM. Nutrition care for the premature infant. Top Clin Nutr 1987; 2:1–9.

Atkinson SA, Bryan MH, Anderson GH. Human milk feeding in premature infants: Protein, fat, and carbohydrate balances in the first two weeks of life. J Pediatr 1981; 99:617–624.

Bakker HD, Wadman SK, Van Sprang FJ, et al. Tyrosinemia and tyrosinuria in healthy prematures: Time courses not vitamin C dependent. Clin Chim Acta 1975; 61:73–90.

Bell EF, Oh W. Water requirements of premature newborn infants. Acta Paediatr Scand (Suppl) 1983; 305:21–26.

Borum PR. Primary and secondary carnitine deficiencies. Am Coll Nutr 1988; 7:426 (abstract).

Brooke OG, Kinsey JM. High energy feeding in small for gestational age infants. Arch Dis Child 1985; 60:42–26.

Calabio R, Myers M, Sunaryo F, Zarafu I, Sisson T, Cohen M. The developmental maturation of gastric emptying in premature infants. J Am Coll Nutr 1988; 7:408.

Cicco R, Holzman IR, Brown DR, et al. Glucose polymer tolerance in premature infants. Pediatrics 1981; 67:498–501.

Coello-Ramirez P, Gutierrez-Topete C, Lifshitz F. Pneumatosis intestinalis. Am J Dis Child 1970; 120:3–8.

Engelke SC, Shah BL, Vasan U, et al. Sodium balance in very low birth weight infants. J Pediatr 1978; 93:837–841.

Ernest JA, Williams JM, Glick MR, et al. Osmolality of substances used in the intensive care nursery. Pediatrics 1983; 72:347–352.

Fleischman AR, Finberg L. Breast milk for term and premature infants—Optimal nutrition? Semin Perinatol 1979; 3:397–405.

Forbes GB. Human milk and the small baby. Am J Dis Child 1982; 136:577–578.

Fomon SJ, Ziegler EE. Protein intake of premature infants: Interpretation of data. J Pediatr 1977; 90:504–506.

Fomon SJ, Ziegler EE, Vazquez HD. Human milk and the small premature infant. Am J Dis Child 1977; 131:463–467.

Galeano NF, Roy CC. Feeding the premature infant. In Lifshitz F, ed. Nutrition for special needs in infancy: Protein hydrolysates. New York: Marcel Dekker, 1985:213–228.

Goldman HI, Goldman JS, Kaufman I, et al. Late effects of early dietary protein intake on low-birth-weight infants. J Pediatr 1974; 85:764–769.

Greer FR, Steichen JJ, Tsang RC. Calcium and phosphate supplements in breast milk related rickets. Am J Dis Child 1982; 136:581–583.

Gross SJ, Buckeley RH, Wakil SS, et al. Elevated IgA concentration in milk produced by mothers delivered of preterm infants. J Pediatr 1981; 99:389–393.

Hall RT, Callenbach JC, Sheehan MB, et al. Comparison of calcium- and phosphorus-supplemented soy isolate formula with whey-predominant premature formula in very low birth weight infants. J Pediatr Gastrointest Nutr 1984; 3:571–576.

Heird WC. Feeding the premature infant: Human milk an artificial formula? Am J Dis Child 1977; 131:468–469.

Hillman LS, Martin L, Fiore B. Effect of oral copper supplementation on serum copper and ceruloplasmin concentrations in premature infants. J Pediatr 1981; 98:311–313.

Hilter HM, Godio LB, Rudolph J, et al. Retrolental fibroplasia: Efficacy of vitamin E in a double-blind clinical study of preterm infants. N Engl J Med 1981; 305:1365–1371.

Jarvenpaa A-L. Feeding the low birth weight infant. IV. Fat absorption as a function of diet and duodenal bile acids. Pediatrics 1983a; 72:684–689.

Jarvenpaa A-L, Raiha NCR, Rassin DK, et al. Feeding the low birth weight infant. I. Taurine and cholesterol supplementation of formula does not affect growth metabolism. Pediatrics 1983b; 71:171–178.

Jarvenpaa A-L, Rassin DK, Kuitunen P, et al. Feeding the low birth weight infant. III. Diet influences bile acid metabolism. Pediatrics 1983c; 72:677–683.

Kashyap S, Forsyth M, Zucker C, et al. Effects of varying protein and energy intakes on growth and metabolic response in low-birth weight infants. J Pediatr 1986; 108:955–963.

Kumar SP, Sacks LM. Hyponatremia in very low birth weight infants and human milk feedings. J Pediatr 1978; 93:1026–1027.

Lifshitz F. Carbohydrate intolerance: A result of inborn errors of carbohydrate absorption. In Wapnir RA, ed. Congenital metabolic diseases: Diagnosis and treatment. New York: Marcel Dekker, 1985:347–374.

Lifshitz F. Necrotizing enterocolitis and feedings. In Lifshitz F, ed. Pediatric nutrition. New York: Marcel Dekker, 1981:513–530.

Lifshitz F, Diaz-Bensussen S, Martinez-Garza V, Abdo-Bassols F, Diaz del Castillo F. The influence of disaccharides in the development of systemic acidosis in the premature infant. Pediatr Res 1971; 5:213–225.

Light IJ, Berry HK, Sutherland JM. Ammoacidemia of prematurity: Its response to ascorbic acid. Am J Dis Child 1966; 112:229–236.

Lundstrom U, Siimes MA, Dallman PR. At what age does iron supplementation become necessary in low birth weight infant? J Pediatr 1977; 91:878–883.

MacLean WC, Funk BB. Lactose malabsorption by premature infants: Magnitude and clinical significance. J Pediatr 1980; 97:383–388.

Manser JI, Crawford CS, Tyrala EE, et al. Serum copper concentrations in sick and well preterm infants. J Pediatr 1980; 97:795–799.

Mendelson RA, Anderson GH, Bryan MH. Zinc, copper and iron content of milk from mothers of preterm and full term infants. Early Hum Dev 1982; 6:145–151.

Minton SD, Steichen JJ, Tsang RC. Bone mineral content in term and preterm appropriate-for-gestational age infants. J Pediatr 1979; 95:1037–1042.

Okamoto E, Muttart CR, Zucker CL, et al. Use of medium-chain triglycerides in feeding the low birth weight infant. Am J Dis Child 1982; 136:428–431.

Okuni M, Okinaga K, Baba K. Studies in reducing sugars in stools of acute infantile diarrhea, with special reference to differences between breast fed and artificially fed babies. Tohoku J Exp Med 1972, 107:395–402.

Parker PH, Helinek GL, Meneely RL, et al. Zinc deficiency in a premature infant fed exclusively human milk. Am J Dis Child 1982; 136:77–78.

Patel BD, Dinwiddie R, Kuman SP, et al. The effects of feeding on arterial blood gases and lung mechanics in newborn infants recovering from respiratory disease. J Pediatr 1977; 90:435–438.

Pereira GR, Barbosa NMM. Controversies in neonatal nutrition. Pediatr Clin North Am 1986; 33:65–89.

Phelps DL. E-Fesol: What happened and what now? Pediatrics 1984; 74:1114–1116.

Raiha NCR, Heinonen K, Rassin DK, et al. Milk protein quantity and quality in low-birthweight infants. I. Metabolic responses and effects in growth. Pediatrics 1976; 57:659–674.

Reichman B, Chessex P, Putet G, et al. Diet, fat accretion, and growth in premature infants. N Engl J Med 1981; 305:1495–1500.

Ronnholm KAR, Sipila I, Siimes MA. Human milk protein supplementation for the prevention of hypoproteinemia without metabolic imbalance in breast milk fed, very low birth weight infants. J Pediatr 1982; 101:243–247.

Shaw JCL. Trace elements in the fetus and young infant. II. Copper, manganese, selenium, and chromium. Am J Dis Child 1980; 134:74–81.

Steichen JJ, Gratton TL, Tsang RC. Osteopenia of prematurity: The cause and possible treatment. J Pediatr 1980; 96:528–534.

Sutphen JL. Nutritional support of the pediatric patient. Clin Consult Nutr Support 1981; 1:1–21.

Tsang RC, ed. Vitamin and mineral requirements in preterm infants. New York: Marcel Dekker, 1985.

Venkataraman PS, Blick KE. Renal status in preterm infants ingesting high mineral content formulas: Studies with renal sonograms, serum chemistries and urine minerals. J Am Coll Nutr 1988; 7:418.

Whitfeld MF. Poor weight gain of the low birth weight infant fed nasojejunally. Arch Dis Child 1982; 57:597–601.

Ziegler EE, Biga RL, Fomon SJ. Nutritional requirements for the premature infant. In Suskind RM, ed. Textbook of pediatric nutrition. New York: Raven Press, 1981:29.

12

Breastfeeding and Lactation

Like magic it happened. With a surge, 3 days after the birth of my first child, my breasts became distended with milk. I had naively assumed throughout my pregnancy that when the infant arrived I would automatically be ready to feed him, and that it was as simple as that. But my joy turned to anguish as the baby screamed angrily when there was not enough milk. Little did I know that I had begun the terrifying cycle so familiar to many mothers who had tried for the first time to breastfeed.

When the baby was but a week old, I became really anxious. The baby cried louder. I strained to feed. The baby got nothing and I got more frightened. Finally, screaming with frustration, the baby turned away. Panic-stricken, I did the one thing I had promised myself I would never do. I prepared a bottle.

The "magic" of breastfeeding? As far as I was concerned, it was more like sorcery, for without warning, a short time later my milk disappeared altogether (Raphael 1973).

The past decade has seen a renewed interest in breastfeeding in this country (Fomon 1987). Tragically, it is often a token of good wishes. Women often wean their babies of breastfeedings during the first week of life, and most during the first 3 weeks of life (Ryan & Gussler 1981) (Fig. 12–1). The most common reason for stopping is the mother's belief that she has "insufficient milk" (Eastham et al 1976). In addition to not having "enough milk," even highly selected "educated" women are often unable to overcome the difficulties of breastfeeding. They stop prematurely because they "always felt tired" and/or the "doctor said to stop" (Cole 1977).

In societies where breastfeeding is the cultural norm, the great majority of

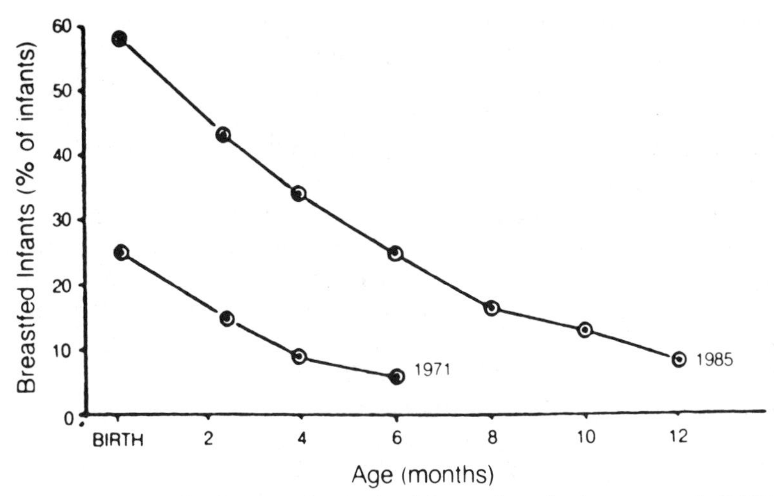

Figure 12–1. Breastfeeding in the United States in relation to age in 1971 and 1985.

From Fomon SJ. Reflections on infant feeding in the 1970s and 1980s. Am J Clin Nutr 1987; 46:171–182. © Am J Clin Nutr. American Society for Clinical Nutrition.

mothers are able to nurse their babies successfully and continue to do so beyond 6 months of age. Mothers in the United States are no different from mothers in other cultures or throughout history, but it seems that many of them have lost the art of successful breastfeeding.

THE IMPORTANCE OF HUMAN MILK

Human milk is best! Nature provided us with a product that has been perfected over a million years of evolution, prepackaged in an ideal container ready to be fed with maximum ease. Breast milk has the unique capacity to change to match the baby's needs at each particular stage of growth and development. There is no other food or milk formula that is comparable to human milk, and for the infant-formula industry, mother's milk is the gold standard. Infant formulas will never be able to provide a product that meets all the qualities of mother's milk; at best they can be a substitute when human milk is not available (see Chapter 13).

Many comprehensive reviews have been written about the many advantages of human milk (Jelliffe & Jelliffe 1978, Hanson 1988). Therefore, we will only review some of the most important clinically relevant aspects of this milk. Anthropologists have observed that infant skeletons throughout human history are relatively large when compared with their adult counterparts. Infant skeletons in most parts of the world and at different stages of history are of comparable size to our present-day norms (Washburn & Lancaster 1967). This occurred despite the most diverse climatic and adverse conditions through the millenia. The similarities of growth of infants throughout human history is most likely due to the fact that babies at all times have been given an ideal nutritional intake, human milk.

Human milk has provided all needs for maximum growth in the first few months of life throughout human evolution, regardless of many biologic factors or environmental circumstances. Mothers from all over the world and from different generations, races, and cultures were able to feed their babies the best food available, and therefore infants grew to their maximum genetic potential (Montagu & Brace 1977). Later on in life, when human milk is not sufficient to sustain growth at its maximum, there may be a stature reduction when adverse circumstances prevail; adult heights then fall below our current standards (Nilkens 1976). We now know that even mothers who are malnourished and live under impoverished conditions produce milk that is sufficient to provide all the nutrients infants need for the first few months of life, and such breast-fed babies maintain growth at our current standards for up to 6 months of life (Brown, Robertson & Akhtar 1986). Thus, no other food that can offer so much, and no writings can ever do justice in describing all the benefits of human milk.

Nutritional Advantages

Human milk is ideally adapted to the human infant. The approximate composition of mature human milk as compared to cow's milk is shown in Figures 12–2 and 12–3 and in Table 12–1. Human milk contains over 100 constituents, which are present in different proportions and in different chemical forms than those found in complex milks from other species (Jelliffe & Jelliffe 1978). In the past few years several hundred scientific papers have been published to describe the biochemical properties of human milk and yet there is still an incompleteness of knowledge. Human milk is usually a thin bluish-appearing liquid that differs markedly from the appearance of formulas based on cow's milk. The composition and volume of mature human milk varies among mothers and among ethnic groups. It also changes throughout the day and at different times during lactation.

Human milk is the best digested and absorbed of all available infant feeds. This is evident to the mother in the stools of breast-fed babies, which are sweet-smelling because they lack the undigested protein and fat present with other infant feeds. The feces are loose and seedy as compared with the firmer, larger stools of the formula-fed baby. Constipation is rarely a problem, whereas it is a frequent occurrence in the formula-fed infant. Diarrhea and other illnesses are also less frequent in the breast-fed baby (see below).

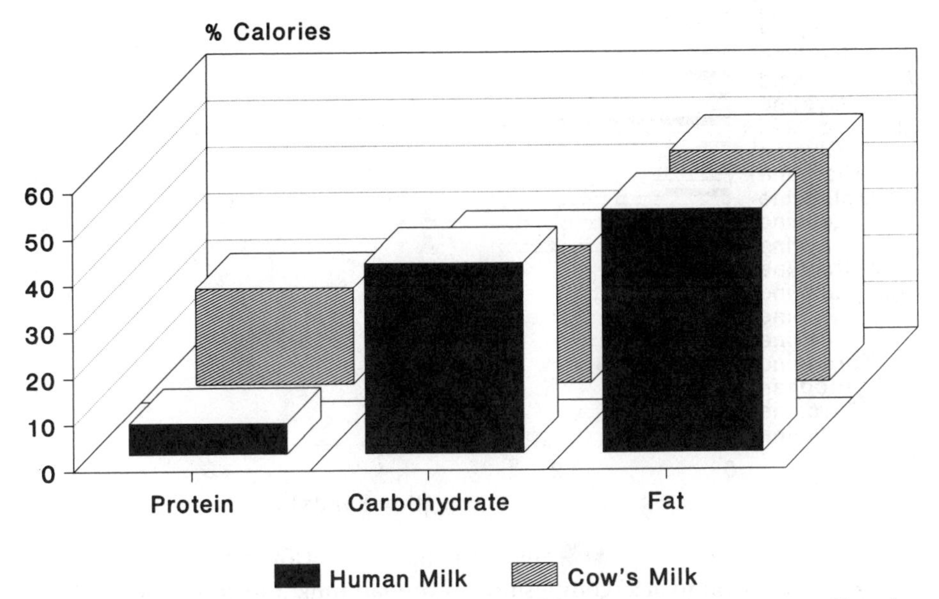

Figure 12–2. Macronutrient composition of human versus cow's milk. The protein content of human milk is casein (3.4 g/L) and whey (4.8 g/L), whereas cow's milk contains 27 g/L of casein and no whey. The carbohydrate content is lactose in both, but the fat content varies as follows:

	HUMAN MILK*	COW'S MILK†
Fat (g)	38.4	36.3
Saturated fatty acids (g)	18.2	21.2
Monounsaturated fatty acids (g)	13.9	9.9
Polyunsaturated fatty acids (g)	3.9	1.2
Linoleic acid (g)	3.6	0.9
Linolenic acid (g)	0.2	0.2
Arachidonic acid (g)	0.04	—
Cholesterol (mg)	238	119

*Mature milk from the tenth day postpartum.
†3.5% fat content.

Adapted from Souci SW, Fachmann W, Kraut H. Food composition and nutrition tables 1986/87. 3rd ed. Stuttgart: Wissenschaftliche Verlagsgesellschaft, 1986.

Breast milk is a more efficient nutrient source than cow's-milk formula. With breast milk, the amount of energy babies need to consume to maintain health is less than previously thought and less than when cow's-milk formula is fed (White, Paul & Cole 1981, Whitehead & Paul 1984). Breast-fed babies consume about 95 to 105 calories per kilogram per day as compared with the 120 calories per kilogram per day needed by babies fed cow's-milk formula during the first 3 months of life. Similarly, the amount of protein required by breast-fed babies is less than that needed by infants fed cow's-milk formulas.

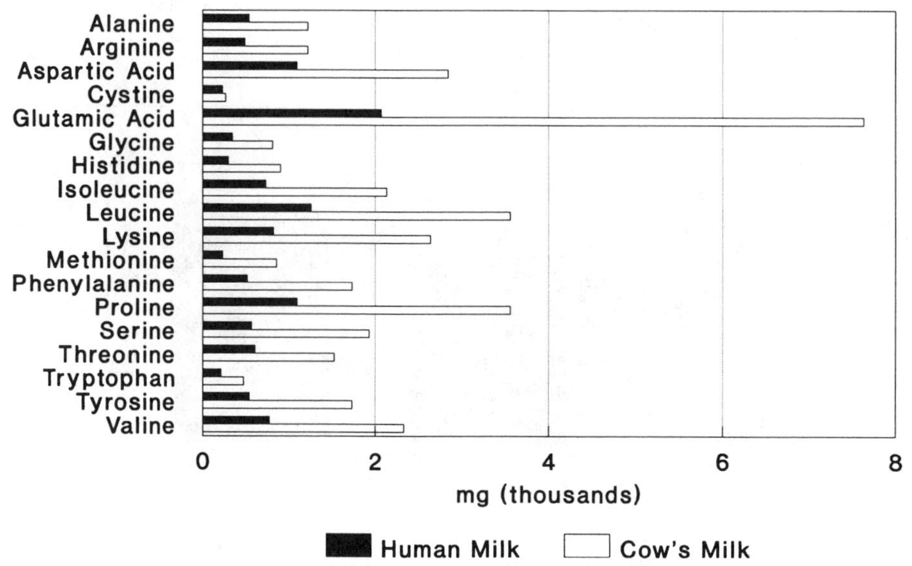

Figure 12–3. Amino acid composition of human milk and cow's milk (1 L).

Human milk contains proteins such as IgA, lysozymes, and lactoferrin in higher concentrations than cow's milk (Hanson 1988). In contrast, cow's milk has high IgG and beta-lactoglobulin; the latter is not found in human milk. Also, there are differences in the type of protein; whey represents more than 70 percent of the total protein in human milk, whereas casein is the main component of the protein in cow's milk. In the past few years the protein composition (whey:casein) of several cow's-milk formulas has been changed to resemble that of human milk (see Chapter 13). However, these improvements in cow's-milk formulas have not resulted in equal performance to human milk as the protein in cow's-milk formulas is not as well digested and absorbed and the serum amino acid levels still differ from those of babies fed breast milk.

Human milk provides all the protein needed by babies for the first 6 months of life (see Fig. 12–2). Breast-fed babies usually consume 1.6 to 1.9 grams of protein per kilogram per day during the first month of life, 1.0 gram per kilogram per day at 3 months of life, and 0.9 gram per kilogram per day at 4 and 6 months (Beaton & Chery 1988). In contrast, infants fed cow's-milk formula consume much more protein, between 2.6 and 4.1 gram per kilogram per day (Axelson et al 1987). The metabolic effects of this high protein intake and the possible long-term consequences are discussed elsewhere (see Chapter 13).

The amino acid composition of breast milk is also different from cow's milk (see Fig. 12–3). The glutamine content of human milk is four to five

Table 12–1. Vitamin and Mineral Composition of Human and Cow's Milk Per Liter (33.3 oz).

	HUMAN MILK*	WHOLE COW'S MILK†
Vitamin		
Vitamin A (μg)	514	285
Carotene (μg)	228	173
Vitamin D (ng)	476	610
Vitamin E activity (mg)	4.95	0.85
α-Tocopherol (mg)	4.95	0.85
Vitamin K (μg)	29	41
Vitamin B_1 (μg)	143	376
Vitamin B_2 (μg)	362	1830
Nicotinamide (mg)	1.62	0.91
Pantothenic acid (mg)	2.00	3.60
Vitamin B_6 (μg)	5.52	35.6
Folic acid (μg)	48	60
Vitamin B_{12} (ng)	476	427
Vitamin C (mg)	42	17
Minerals/Trace Elements		
Calcium (mg)	295	1220
Phosphorus (mg)	143	935
Iron (μg)	276	468
Magnesium (mg)	36	122
Zinc (mg)	2.1	3.9
Copper (μg)	333	173
Sodium (mg)	152	488
Potassium (mg)	505	1596
Chloride (mg)	381	1037
Manganese (μg)	13.3	25.4
Cobalt (μg)	13.3	0.8
Nickel (μg)	9.5	10.2
Chromium (μg)	638	17.3
Molybdenum (μg)	9.5	—
Vanadium (μg)	4.8	—
Iodine (μg)	60.0	112
Fluoride (μg)	162	173
Selenium (μg)	31.4	—
Bromine (mg)	0.95	1.0
Nitrate (mg)	—	0.8

*Mature milk from the tenth day postpartum.
†3.5% fat content.

Adapted from Souci SW, Fachmann W, Kraut H. Food composition and nutrition tables 1986/87. 3rd ed. Stuttgart: Wissenschaftliche Verlagsgesellschaft, 1986.

times less than that of cow's milk, and the levels of tyrosine and phenylalanine in breast milk are three times less than in cow's milk. These differences are critical in feeding babies, particularly newborns who may show a transient elevation of serum amino acid levels such as hypertyrosinemia, and hyperphenylalaninemia, with potential consequences on mental development (see Chapter 25) (Mamunes et al 1976). Human milk is rich in taurine, whereas cow's milk contains virtually none. Taurine may be an essential nutrient for the newborn, as the human infant cannot synthesize this amino acid. Deficiency of taurine has been shown to result in retinal dysfunction (Wright & Gaull 1988).

Fat is the main source of calories in human milk and it supplies essential fatty acids and fat-soluble vitamins. The fat content varies with the time of suckling; there is a threefold increase in fat content with the last milk of the feed. During the day the amount of fat rises two to five times from early morning to a plateau about midday. The overall fat content of human and cow's milks appears to be similar but there are marked differences in composition. Of particular importance are the greater levels of essential polyunsaturated fatty acids, notably linoleic acid, which is three times higher in breast milk. These substances may play a significant role in the biochemical development of the brain, since they are found in high concentrations in the human central nervous system.

The fat of human milk is also more efficiently digested and absorbed than that of cow's-milk fat (Milner et al 1975). The cholesterol levels in human milk are also higher than in cow's milk and even more so than in adapted infant formulas (see Chapter 13). The larger amounts of cholesterol in human milk may be necessary to facilitate myelinization of the central nervous system and brain, which has a high lipid and cholesterol content. A high cholesterol intake through breastfeeding during infancy may also ensure the development of enzyme systems to maintain appropriate levels of blood cholesterol in adulthood (Kark et al 1984).

Almost all the carbohydrate in human milk is lactose, which is present in concentrations of around 7 percent. In contrast, in cow's milk, this sugar is found in much lower quantities, 4 to 5 percent. The high lactose content in breast milk ensures the baby a readily available source of galactose (a component of lactose), which is a necessary fuel for the rapidly growing human brain. Lactose also enhances calcium absorption and thus plays a role in enhancing bone calcification and prevention of rickets. Together with the bifidus factor of human milk, the relatively high lactose content of breast milk promotes the growth of protective bacteria in the intestine, which decreases the chances of infection with pathogenic organisms (see below). Of interest is that even when the infant is sick and has difficulties tolerating lactose, the baby can better tolerate the high quantity of lactose in breast milk than the lower amount of lactose in cow's milk (see Chapter 19).

Human milk also has higher quantities of vitamins A, C, and E than those found in cow's milk (see Table 12–1). In addition, the ratio of vitamin E to polyunsaturated fatty acids is different in human milk. The ratio of these elements is essential for the metabolism and utilization of these nutrients. The heat treatment used in preparing processed cow's milk–based formulas could potentially reduce or destroy heat-labile vitamins such as vitamin C and folate. The vitamin B_{12} present in cow's milk may also be different from that of human milk. In contrast, vitamin K and vitamin D are lower in human milk than in cow's milk.

The concentration of minerals is over three times higher in cow's milk than in human milk (see Table 12–1). Cow's milk contains three to four times more sodium, and the renal solute load is much greater than that of breast milk. Sodium retention and/or sodium poisoning (hypernatremia) occurs more easily in cow's milk–fed babies. Thus, babies fed cow's milk may need additional water to quench thirst. By contrast, human milk is a low-solute fluid that appears to be designed as a perfect supply of fluid and electrolytes; therefore, human milk–fed babies do not need additional water feedings even on hot summer days.

Cow's milk has four times more calcium and six times more phosphorus than human milk. Paradoxically, this is associated with a much greater incidence of low serum calcium levels (neonatal hypocalcemia) and convulsions in babies fed cow's milk. Calcium absorption is diminished by the poor digestion of bovine fat, which results in calcium precipitation and unabsorbable calcium soaps in the lumen of the intestine. In addition, the higher phosphorus load of cow's milk may lead to a diminished calcium uptake and hypocalcemia (Hanson 1988).

Both human and cow's milk are low in iron, but the iron from human milk is better absorbed than that from cow's milk (McMillan, Landaw & Oski 1976). Thus, iron-deficiency anemia is not common in breast-fed babies. While the daily intake of iron in the breast-fed baby can be estimated to be as low as 1 milligram per day, it is enough to prevent anemia in the normal newborn baby who is born with appropriate iron stores. In contrast, the iron in cow's-milk formulas is of a lower bioavailability and often there is additional iron loss in cow's milk–fed babies due to gastrointestinal microhemorrhages (occult blood loss). Thus, the recommended dietary allowance of iron of 6 milligrams per day for the first 6 months of life seems necessary only for infants not fed human milk. Some authors suggest that extra iron given to breast-fed babies may be detrimental because it can inactivate the transport protein lactoferrin in human milk and thereby interfere with its antiinfective properties and perhaps inadvertently provide the necessary iron for the growth of some intestinal pathogens (Masawe, Muindi & Swai 1974). However, some others have found a high incidence of iron deficiency anemia in breast-fed babies of poor socioeconomic groups (Herterampf et al 1986); thus suggesting that such high-risk babies require supplements even when breast-fed.

Human milk contains fluoride in varying levels (Grossman 1975) depending to a certain extent on the amount in the drinking water. Cow's milk has been found to contain much more fluoride than human milk (up to 50 times more) in certain areas of the country. However, to date no ill effects have been shown due to the differences in concentration of this element. Fluoride supplementation in early infancy in areas where there is insufficient fluoride in drinking water (less than 1 ppm) appears necessary for both human- and cow's milk–fed babies. Such supplements reduce the incidence of dental cavities in children by 50 percent.

Other trace elements differ in concentrations between human milk and cow's-milk formulas, with potential nutritional advantages for breast milk. For example, zinc deficiency does not occur in breast-fed babies even when there is a congenital malabsorption of this element (acrodermatitis enteropathica). In contrast, it has been suggested that cow's-milk formulas be supplemented with 4 milligrams of zinc per liter to improve the growth performance of babies (Walravens & Hambidge 1976). In addition, copper levels are higher in human milk than in cow's milk. This may be of importance; it has been noted that mortality rates from coronary heart disease are correlated with diets having a high zinc:copper ratio. These ratios are very low in human milk.

Protective Effects

Human milk offers a wide variety of protective effects during the critical time the baby becomes adapted to the risks of extrauterine life. Recent evidence suggests that the protective effects of human milk are not only antiinfective, but may also help protect against the development of many other problems later on in life. Included are diseases such as celiac disease (gluten sensitivity) (Auricchio et al 1983), diabetes mellitus (Mayer et al 1988), coronary artery disease and atherosclerosis (Kark et al 1984), and the development of several forms of allergies (Saarinen et al 1979).

The protective effects of human milk against infections have been known for centuries (Cussen 1980). It has long been known that non–breast-fed babies had a higher risk of dying from infectious diseases than breast-fed babies. More recent observations revealed that breast-fed infants have a remarkable resistance to infection, especially diarrhea, otitis, and respiratory disease (Mata 1982). This has been attributed to the cleanliness and lack of opportunity for contamination of human milk, whereas bottle-fed babies often drink milk that has been contaminated with bacteria, especially in hot climates where refrigeration is not available. Thus, artificially-fed babies often have diarrhea, malnutrition, and a high infant mortality rate in conditions of poor hygiene and in developing countries. However, human milk and colostrum are never strictly sterile, and there may be a significant number of microorganisms reaching the breast-fed baby. Yet disease rates, even in babies in developed countries, are much lower compared with those of babies not fed human milk (Fallot, Boyd & Oski 1980). Thus, it is not only cleanliness but more importantly the antiinfective properties of human milk that play a role in preventing disease.

There are humoral and cellular factors in human milk that confer protection to the baby (Table 12–2) (Hanson 1988). Human milk imparts protection mainly at the intestinal level because it contains substances such as immunoglobulins, lysozymes, bifidus factor, lactoferrin, and so on, all of which

Table 12–2. Protective Factors in Human Milk.

FACTOR	ROLE
Secretory IgA	High concentration in colostrum; specific activity against microorganisms and infectious agents (rotaviruses and bacterial enterotoxins)
IgM and IgG Antibodies	Specific activity against allergens; neutralize toxins and viruses
Complement factors (C_3, C_4)	Low levels in milk; permit bacteria or other cells to be destroyed (opsonization)
Lactoferrin	Inhibition of bacterial growth (bacteriostasis)
Lysozyme	Destroys bacteria (bacterolysis); limits inflammatogenic activity of the immune system
Milk lipids	Neutralize viruses
Antioxidants α-Tocopherol, cystein, ascorbic acid	Counteract inflammatory activity of the immune system
Antistaphylococcal factor	Inhibits staphylococcal infection in the blood
Bifidus factor	Promotes growth of bifidobacteria in the intestinal flora, limits the growth of disease-producing microorganisms (enteric pathogens)
Antiviral RNAase	Inhibits viral activity
Interferon	Inhibits viral infection
Lymphocytes	Synthesis of immunoglobulins (IgA, IgM, IgG)
Macrophage and polymorph	Bacterial killing and phagocytosis
Catalase, glutathione peroxidase	Destroy peroxides
Protease inhibitors α_1-Antitrypsin, α_1-Antichymotrypsin	Inhibit proteases, decrease inflammation
Histaminase	Catabolizes histamine, decreasing inflammation
Prostaglandins E_2, F_2a	Inhibit neutrophil degranulation, noninflammatogenic
α_2-Glycoprotein	Inhibits lymphocytes, noninflammatogenic

Adapted from Goldman AS, Thorpe LW, Goldblum RM, Hanson LA. Antiinflammatory properties of human milk. Acta Paediatr Scand 1986; 75:689–695; and Mata L. Breast feeding, diarrheal disease, and malnutrition in less developed countries. In Lifshitz F, ed. Pediatric nutrition. Infant feedings, deficiencies, diseases. New York: Marcel Dekker, 1982:355–372.

are natural defense mechanisms. The most important immunoglobulin present in breast milk is secretory IgA, although immunoglobulins such as IgG, IgM, and IgD are also present. IgA is especially high in colostrum (2–4 mg/mL), supplying an initial bolus of this protective coat to the baby's intestine. After 2 to 4 days this excretion rate falls to lower levels, but substantial amounts are given to the infant as long as breastfeeding is continued. In contrast, IgA is present in very small amounts in cow's milk, allowing for potential infections during the early weeks of life before the intestinal epithelial surfaces mature and begin making their own IgA. Secretory IgA has proven antibacterial, antiparasitic, and antiviral effects (see Table 12–2) (Hanson 1988).

Human milk and colostrum also contain a variety of cells that give immunologic advantages to breast-fed babies at a time when they are most vulnerable (Hanson 1988). In human milk, the highest concentration of cells (up to 10 million cells per milliliter) are observed during the first 3 to 4 days after the onset of lactation. By 4 to 6 weeks postpartum this number declines to less than 100,000 cells per milliliter. These cells include macrophages and phagocytes, which are the transport vehicles for the large quantities of immunoglobulin present in human milk. The lymphocytes in breast milk account for about 10 to 15 percent of the cells. They are primarily of the T cell variety and appear to transfer systemic immunity from the mother to the baby via breast milk. Also, breast milk contains B lymphocytes, which appear to transfer the mother's local gut mucosal immunity to the baby. Additionally, breast milk and colostrum contain other cells with a variety of functions. Some of these cells modulate and process microbial antigens and their immune response (Hanson 1988). Also found are large amounts of epithelial cells, especially after 2 to 3 weeks of lactation, but their role remains to be determined.

Human milk contains many enzymes, hormones, and growth factors in concentrations higher than milk from other species (Hanson 1988). These may have important physiologic and protective effects, and may have a role in stimulating gut growth and gut immunity. That is, human milk is not only a passive vehicle for transmission of immune factors but it also stimulates the baby's own immune production (Jensen et al 1988). Human milk stimulates the functional maturation of the gastrointestinal tract as well as other tissues in the newborn. These enzymes, hormones, and other factors in human milk carry messages of great physiologic importance to the nursing infant that help him or her adapt to the outside world and to mature more appropriately than with any other substitute feeding. In the Koran, breast milk is referred to as "white blood." What a good comparison, since human milk is as live a fluid as blood.

Psychologic Benefits

The psychologic advantages of breastfeeding are often more difficult to define and document than the nutritional or immunologic benefits, although they are no less significant. The successful breastfeeding mother gives comfort, love, and cuddling to the baby. The interactions between mother and child during breastfeeding are a fail-safe system to ensure proximity of mother and child. Breastfeeding provides a synchronous giving and taking, an emotional attachment and physical pleasure to both mother and child (Klaus & Kennel 1976). All these needs may be met in other ways, but breastfeeding is uniquely suited to meeting most of the infant's emotional needs in one act.

Many studies have assessed the relationship between childhood intelligence and psychologic performance as it pertains to human milk feedings. Higher scores for intelligence, reading and mathematical attainment, and verbal ability were obtained by the breast-fed children (Rodgers 1978). These differences persisted in all measures even when comparisons were made between groups that were matched for all recognized socioeconomic variables. Other studies have also confirmed much higher intelligence scores among exclusively breast-fed children (Fergusson, Beautrais & Silva 1982). Babies fed human milk read and speak better than bottle-fed infants (Whittlestone 1983). Differences in amino acid composition between human milk and cow's-milk formula could be factors that influence the ultimate intellectual performance of the child; for example, high phenylalanine levels that may be damaging to the developing brain (see Chapter 25). In addition, the percentage of patients with learning disorders who were fed human milk was significantly less than in an appropriate control group (Menkes 1977). However, this study does not elucidate whether the children with learning disabilities had feeding problems as infants and were therefore not breast-fed.

Maternal Effects

Breastfeeding is not only good for babies, it is also beneficial to the mother. Breastfeeding can be considered to have a slimming effect, which is usually very desirable to mothers in our society. Mothers who breast-feed their babies may lose 2 pounds (1kg) excess weight as compared with those who bottle-feed their infants. Successful lactation with adequate emptying of the breasts also decreases the probability of cracked nipples, infective mastitis, or breast abscess. Breastfeeding may also lower the incidence of breast cancer (Ing, Petrakis & Ho 1977), but its role in this disease is not yet completely clear.

A very important effect of lactation is contraception, since breastfeeding appears to delay the onset of fertility. The pregnancy-spacing effect of lactation appears to be hormonal, primarily due to the effects of pituitary prolactin in the inhibition of ovulation. This hormone is much higher during breastfeeding and, when lactation is partial or reduced by supplemental feedings, the prolactin levels decrease and the contraceptive effect diminishes (Van Balen & Ntabomvura 1976). In poorly fed communities, maternal malnutrition may also add to the prolactin effect in extending the length of postpartum amenorrhea (Delgado et al 1975). Lactation seems to be nature's prescription designed to ensure an optimal period for the child to mature between births.

There are psychologic benefits to the mother from breastfeeding. Lactation has been related to coitus and orgasm, and there is a sensuous nature to nursing. Most women describe the time spent nursing an infant as pleasurable; sometimes, those are the only moments of peace and tranquility in an otherwise hectic day. It has been said that "for a baby who cannot be breast-fed there is a substitute food, however imperfect. For the mother who cannot breast feed, there is no real substitute" (Lloyd 1976).

Economics and Convenience

In addition to the biologic consequences of breastfeeding there are economic and other social considerations that must be addressed. The breast-fed baby is portable; he or she travels easily, and requires only the mother. Nourishment and nurturing are ever-ready. Human milk has an economic significance of major proportion at a national level. It has been calculated that human milk comprises about one quarter of total milk production in developing countries (Helsing 1976). When breastfeeding declines, an expensive industry is necessary to produce, process, and distribute infant formula as a replacement. In developing countries this is often impossible to accomplish and prohibitive in cost. Importing formulas aggravates the fiscal problems and the limited foreign exchange balance of such nations. Furthermore, there is an increased cost for the health services needed to provide care for the increased number of infants with infections and malnutrition that occur with premature weaning.

The family cost of feeding an infant is also important, and economic considerations go beyond the simple cost of buying the formula versus the relative lack of cost for human milk. Some have calculated that the cost of feeding the mother is greater than that of purchasing the formula. This is certainly not correct, as the conversion of nutrients by lactating women is very efficient. A simple increase of 500 calories per day and a base of 20 grams per day of protein will suffice to provide for the maternal needs of lactation (see below). A simple peanut butter sandwich and a glass of milk would provide the above for mothers in the United States, and a serving of the local popular food, for example, rice and tempeh (fungus-digested soya) would allow for the increased needs during lactation in other countries.

The financial savings to families who breastfeed could be substantial even without considering the other costs, such as the medical care for increased infections. In the American economic context it has been calculated that breastfeeding a 3-month-old infant costs about one third as much as the cost of bottle-feeding (Jelliffe & Jelliffe 1975). In well-to-do circumstances, these are only theoretic calculations. However, even in resource-rich countries like ours the cost of milk formulas is a concern, necessitating corrective measures among the disadvantaged sections of the population. The Women, Infants, and Children Food Supplemental Program (WIC) now requires special pricing to purchase infant formula for distribution to disadvantaged populations (see Chapter 13). In technically less-developed countries without resources, the situation is infinitely more serious. Often, over 50 percent of the minimum wage is spent for infant formula by poor families, and at times up to 93 percent of the basic wages are needed to feed an infant (Cameron & Hofvander 1975). The results are often disastrous as baby formulas are overdiluted or "stretched" to extend their use and save some of the cost. The cost of the resultant malnutrition of poorly fed infants goes beyond the considerations of this chapter.

On the other hand, the cost of breastfeeding must also be evaluated from the point of view of the working mother, who may not return to her job until she stops nursing. The net loss of earnings of the mother needs to be related to the cost of breastfeeding. In urban circumstances some studies have shown that up to 36 percent of the mother's income was needed to purchase adequate amounts of infant formula for the baby for the first year of life (Popkin & Solon 1976). Thus, the increased net income may not offset other factors that may be more important, such as the decreased time to child care and home production because the mother is away at work.

Convenience is in the eye of the beholder. In our culture, ready-to-eat convenience foods are highly desirable. Thus, human milk should be the ideal feeding for those who seek convenience. There is no need to buy it, make it, or worry over whether there is enough in the house or for travel. There is no need to worry over details about bottles and nipples. There is no need to warm it or cool it. Human milk is always right and is always there. However, in our culture, breastfeeding is often neither easy, convenient, or desirable, and for working mothers lactation is often an impossibility. Also, there may be more interference with parents' sleep than with bottle-feedings, and some mothers have complaints about "tennis elbow" while breastfeeding or using hand-operated breast pumps (Williams, Auerbach & Jacobi 1989). More often than not, the end result is the loss of this valuable natural resource for infant feedings.

THE CONSEQUENCES OF NOT BREASTFEEDING

If the advantages of breastfeeding mentioned above are not sufficient to point out that human milk is best for the baby, the following brief description of some of the consequences that have been associated with artificial feedings should convince even the skeptic. In well-developed countries such as the United States, cow's-milk formula feedings are the usual way of feeding babies, though there is a recent increased trend toward breastfeeding (Fomon 1987). Under the economic, hygienic, and social conditions found in these countries, bottle feedings are considered safe and effective, but even here potential consequences cannot be ignored. The two most frequent nutritional alterations in our country—obesity and iron deficiency—may have roots in the lack of breastfeeding. Weight gain in formula-fed babies is more rapid than that achieved by breast-fed babies (Neumann & Alpaugh 1976), and obesity has been reported to be more common by some investigators, but not by others, among artificially-fed babies (see Chapter 11). Iron-deficiency anemia has been found in up to one third of young children 3 to 36 months of age, particularly in infants who are not breast-fed. This is largely due to the low iron content of most formulas, the poor bioavailability of iron from cow's milk, and the increased losses of this mineral from intestinal microhemorrhages in artificially-fed infants. However, this problem has been somewhat improved by the iron fortification of infant formulas (see Chapter 13).

Nutritional problems such as hypocalcemia, hyponatremia, and other deficiency syndromes are now only rarely seen owing to improvements in the formula composition and manufacturing process, but they may still occur. Alimentary consequences of bottle feedings may include malocclusion, an inappropriate bite that may require expensive orthodontic repair (Simpson & Cheung 1976), and/or the "nursing-bottle syndrome," which results in severe tooth decay in children who sleep with bottles.

The most common allergy in infants and young children is to cow's milk (see Chapter 20). There are over 20 proteins in cow's milk to which the child may become allergic, the most common being β lactoglobulin, which is not present in breast milk. The current estimates of cow's milk protein intolerance vary, but up to a 7.5 percent prevalence rate has been reported (Bahna 1988). In contrast, breastfeeding decreases the chance of developing allergies to cow's milk. It is rare for a very sensitive infant to develop problems with cow's milk protein while being breast-fed by a mother who ingests milk (Host, Husby & Osterballe 1988).

Babies who are not breast-fed may be affected by more frequent infections, even if they live in relatively rich resource communities. Respiratory illnesses in bottle-fed infants occur more often than in breast-fed infants. Also, otitis, vomiting, and diarrhea appear to be three times more common in bottle-fed babies (Cunningham 1979). The prevalence of hospitalization with gastrointestinal and respiratory infections is higher among infants who are not breast-fed during the first 3 months of life (Leventhal et al 1986).

The goodness of breast milk is even more apparent in conditions of poverty and poor hygiene, as is prevalent in the developing world. In these countries weaning the child results in a progressive acquisition of intestinal enteropathogens and onset of recurrent diarrheal disease (Mata 1982). Diarrhea is the main contributor to stunting and malnutrition in less-developed countries; and there is no doubt that diarrheal disease is the most important contributor to the high infant mortality rate throughout the world. Thus, human-milk feedings are essential under those conditions. Breast milk cannot be contaminated, as may occur with bottle feedings. Also, human milk cannot be diluted, as is done with milk formula. In 1973 a journalistic war began in London to minimize the promotion and use of cow's-milk formula as a substitute for human milk and thereby reduce the problems of malnutrition and diarrhea worldwide (Muller 1974). It has been calculated that several million children would be saved from malnutrition and diarrhea by human milk feedings (Jelliffe & Jelliffe 1978). Hopefully, the current trend toward increasing breastfeeding among some groups (Fomon 1987) will prevail and be expanded in countries where they are most needed, though there is little evidence to suggest that this is occurring. Even in the United States, breastfeeding rates among poor and minority women have plateaued.

LACTATION

Maternal health and nutrition are critical determinants to ensure successful lactation. The nutritional requirements for lactating women at different stages are shown in Table 12–3. The effects of maternal nutritional status on lactation performance have been reviewed extensively (Rasmussen 1988). There are great variations in the major nutritional components and the micronutrients of human milk of women from different countries, social groups, and socioeconomic status. Generally, there are lower concentrations of all nutrients in the milk of underprivileged women as compared with that of well-nourished populations.

Dietary alterations can be responsible for changes in human milk composition. Dietary fat can be responsible for influencing the fatty acid composition. A diet elevated in polyunsaturated fats such as corn or soybean oil will result in milk with an increased content of polyunsaturated fats. Under conditions of dietary restriction, the fatty acid profile of human milk will reflect the fat that has been mobilized by the mother to compensate for the energy deficit. The converse is also noted—that an increase in energy intake will result in an increase of short- and medium-chain fatty acids. Its implication for the human infant, if any, remains to be elucidated.

In poorly nourished mothers the amount of milk and the fat content may be less than in well-fed mothers. However, even breast-fed infants from undernourished women usually receive sufficient nutrient intake to grow at appropriate rates for the first 6 months of life (Brown, Robertson & Akhtar 1986). Also, human milk may lack certain vitamins, particularly in mothers who have vitamin deficiencies or did not receive appropriate dietary intake during pregnancy. The micronutrients of particular concern are vitamin A, thiamin, riboflavin, vitamin B_{12}, folate, vitamin B_6, and vitamin C.

The calcium levels of human milk of poorly nourished mothers have also

Table 12–3. Nutritional Requirements of Breastfeeding Women.

RECOMMENDED DAILY REQUIREMENTS		
	1st 6 months	2nd 6 months
Energy (kcal)*	+500	+500
Protein (g)	65	62
Vitamin A (μg RE)†	1300	1200
Vitamin D (μg)‡	10	10
Vitamin E (mg)§	12	11
Vitamin K (μg)	65	65
Vitamin C (mg)	95	90
Folic Acid (μg)	280	260
Niacin (mg)	20	20
Riboflavin (mg)	1.8	1.7
Thiamin (mg)	1.6	1.6
Vitamin B_6 (mg)	2.1	2.1
Vitamin B_{12} (μg)	2.6	2.6
Calcium (mg)	1200	1200
Phosphorus (mg)	1200	1200
Iron (mg)ǁ	15	15
Magnesium (mg)	355	340
Zinc (mg)	19	16
Iodine (μg)	200	200
Selenium (μg)	75	75

*Energy needs are increased above normal needs by 500 calories per day during lactation.
†Retinol equivalents.
‡1 μg of vitamin D = 40 IU.
§1 mg of vitamin E = 1.49 IU.
ǁAlthough iron needs during lactation are not increased above normal (15 mg iron/d), continued iron supplementation for 2 to 3 months after the baby is born is recommended to replenish stores depleted during pregnancy.

Adapted from the Committee on Dietary Allowances, Food and Nutrition Board, National Research Council. Recommended dietary allowances. 10th ed. Washington, D.C.: National Academy of Sciences, 1989.

been found to be low, but in well-nourished mothers lactation does not seem to produce undue losses of bone mineral (Byrne, Thomas & Chan 1987). The calcium content of human milk appears to be maintained at normal levels despite low maternal dietary calcium intake, although there is increased maternal bone resorption (Moser et al 1988a). In terms of trace elements, copper, iron, and zinc concentrations are fairly constant over a wide range of maternal dietary intakes. However, maternal dietary selenium intake seems to directly influence selenium concentration in human milk (Moser et al 1988b).

A few studies have examined whether the concentrations of protective and antiinfective elements in human milk are affected by maternal malnutrition. Reduced immunoglobulin, cells, and complement values are seen in colostrum of malnourished women, but the differences become insignificant in mature milk, and their ability to produce antibodies in milk in response to oral immunization is not impaired (Rasmussen 1988). These data provide evidence for the benefits of breast milk in protecting infants from diarrheal illness even among malnourished populations.

Improvement of lactation performance and the nutritional composition of human milk can be accomplished with maternal dietary supplementation. The message is clear. As with so much else concerning the health and nutrition of children, the emphasis should be in large measure on the mother. The individual needs of the baby may best be met if he or she is allowed to take as much as wanted, preferably from the mother only. Feed the mother: thereby the baby!

PITFALLS OF HUMAN MILK

Human milk is best for babies, and its importance and beneficial effects have been described above. However, it is not perfect in every regard. Human milk is not appropriate for premature and low-birth-weight babies (see Chapter 11). Even for the normal newborn infant, human milk can be complemented by the supplementation of vitamin K to avoid hemorrhagic disease of the newborn (Kries et al 1987). This was first recognized about 40 years ago, but was more recently confirmed by identification of cases of intracranial hemorrhage that occurred more frequently in exclusively breast-fed infants (Lane & Hathaway 1985). Vitamin D supplementation is necessary to avoid rickets and to achieve adequate bone mineralization, especially in Northern climates where babies are not exposed to sunlight for long periods of time. Thus, it is advisable to provide 400 IU per day of vitamin D to breast-fed babies, particularly during winter months. The amounts of calcium and phosphorus contained in human milk are insufficient, particularly for small, low-birth-weight infants (see Chapter 11). There is no evidence that additional vitamins are needed for the solely breast-fed baby in the first 6 months of life, but when maternal malnutrition exists the levels of vitamins in human milk could be affected, especially water-soluble vitamins such as C and A. Vitamin supplements may be indicated for the offspring of such women.

Breastfeeding has also been associated with neonatal jaundice (hyperbilirubinemia) in the great majority of infants (Maisels & Gifford 1986). High bilirubin levels in newborn babies are of concern since they have been associated with potentially serious problems (kernicterus). There are several reasons why human milk can contribute to neonatal jaundice. The most likely mechanisms include slight caloric deprivation and more weight loss in human milk-fed babies compared with bottle-fed babies (Fig. 12–4). Also, breast-fed babies excrete less bilirubin in their stools, have a delayed passage

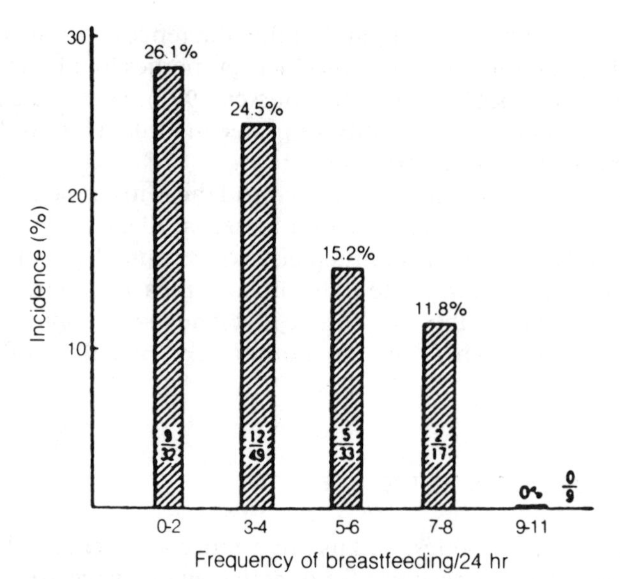

Figure 12–4. Correlation between breastfeeding frequency during the first 24 hours after birth and incidence of hyperbilirubinemia. There was a strong correlation between frequency of nursing and decreased incidence of hyperbilirubinemia. Increasing the frequency of breastfeeding decreases nipple pain and breast tenderness; significantly increases milk output and neonatal weight gain; decreases peak serum bilirubin levels; increases the success of lactation; and decreases ovulation, markedly improving the contraceptive effects of breastfeeding. From Yamauchi Y, Yamunouchi I. Breastfeeding frequency during the first 24 hours after birth in full-term neonates. Pediatrics 1990; 86:171–175. Copyright 1990. Reproduced by permission of Pediatrics.

of meconium, and pass less feces (by weight) than bottle-fed infants in the first few days of life. However, the elevation of serum bilirubin, which produces the jaundice in the breast-fed babies, is usually small and well within the limits of tolerance. Few infants reach bilirubin levels above 14 milligrams per deciliter, a level that could be of concern, and those who do can easily be treated by offering extra water. Other treatments may be necessary for babies with higher bilirubin levels, but they require further medical assessment to ensure that no other problems exist and that human milk was responsible for the jaundice. It should be noted that phototherapy, the common treatment of hyperbilirubinemia in infants, will not be effective if the baby's calorie intake is insufficient. Early introduction and more frequent feedings with human milk have been associated with lower serum bilirubin levels.

Human milk may also contain potentially toxic substances or infective organisms that could be transmitted to the infant, with potential harmful effects. Most drugs taken therapeutically are transferred into the breast milk in different concentrations. Often scientific information is either inadequate or is lacking regarding certain drugs and their excretion in human milk. The duration and dosage of the medication may also influence the levels found in maternal milk and the possible toxicity to the newborn baby. For example, the simple occasional use of aspirin for a headache is different from its long-term use for the treatment of conditions such as rheumatoid arthritis. An occasional aspirin may have no consequences to the baby, but high continuous dosages may induce metabolic acidosis, rash, and alterations in platelet function (Erickson & Oppenheim 1979, Clark & Wilson 1981). The reader is advised to check regularly for possible drug effects and contraindication for use of a drug during lactation, as new knowledge and information usually alters current recommendations (AAP 1989). However, only the use of a few types of drugs are thought to be real contraindications to breastfeeding.

Mothers are exposed to social and environmental toxins that may have deleterious effects on the breast-fed baby. For example, caffeine is quite popular in our society. The effects of this drug are often related to body size or weight. For an adult weighing 70 kilograms (150 lb), a cup of instant coffee or a can of a cola beverage provides about 1 milligram of caffeine per kilogram of body weight. A nursing mother should be aware that caffeine passes into her breast milk and that this could have a stimulating effect on her infant. Some pediatricians have expressed concern over caffeine use in children. Restlessness, irritability, sleeplessness, and nervousness are some of the symptoms resulting from caffeine, and the same could occur in a human milk-fed baby if the mother ingests caffeine in large quantities. However, a recent study showed that maternal ingestion of a single cup of caffeinated beverage does not appear to present a significant dose of caffeine to the nursing infant (Berlin et al 1984).

Nicotine and alcohol are drugs of concern for the lactating woman. Indeed, smoking 20 cigarettes daily can lead to relatively high levels of fat-soluble nicotine in the breast milk, which could be harmful to the baby as well as reduce the amount of milk secretion in the mother. The passive-smoker effect also should be kept in mind, as babies may suffer the harmful effects of smoke when the mother or father smokes. Ethanol (alcohol), even in small amounts, could also affect the baby if the mother drinks, but it takes moderate amounts of alcohol to inhibit the mother's let-down reflex. Heroin abuse by the mother is a contraindication for breastfeeding since this drug is passed to the infant, who may suffer from the drug effects as well as from withdrawal symptoms with uncoordinated and ineffective suckling.

Environmental toxins may also be present in human milk. Toxic substances such as polychlorinated biphenyl (PCB) or DDT, which are used as pesticides, have contaminated both human and cow's milk. Testing of breast milk for these contaminants is recommended for nursing mothers who have potentially high exposure to those substances. For example, mothers in areas where antimalaria campaigns are used should be concerned. Women who consume meat from cattle raised in areas using pesticides might also need to have their breast milk tested. Limiting breastfeedings would be advisable if high toxins are found (Wickizer & Brilliant 1981). Infective organisms may also be present in breast milk. When hepatitis, cytomegalovirus, or streptococcal organisms are present in human milk, the milk should not be used. In recent years the problem of contamination of human milk has taken on a new dimension. The use of human milk from breast-milk banks or from previously expressed milk has become more common, and this could easily become contaminated. It should be kept in mind that most of the goodness of human milk may be lost if it is not used fresh. The protective factors are rapidly lost in the process of banking of the product as well as with storage, refrigeration, or heating. Additionally, the cost of breast milk from breast milk banks may be prohibitive.

Finally, breastfeeding could be a problem when appropriate lactation is not established. Regardless of the cause, a breast-fed infant who is not thriving and gaining weight should be evaluated and lactation checked. In the majority of instances there may be insufficient milk secreted by the mother due to inadequate breastfeeding. The main factors responsible for decreased production of milk are disturbed reflex behavior of the ejection of milk or the let-down reflexes. Rarely, there may be inadequate milk production due to a variety of other causes, such as smoking or environmental stress. Inadequate maternal nutrition usually yields sufficient milk production for the infant to grow and develop (Brown, Robertson & Akhtar 1986), but at times there may be specific nutrient deficits that render human milk ineffective. In recent years chloride-deficient human milk was recognized as a cause of failure to thrive in breast-fed infants. In all instances, if growth is not resumed after an appropriate trial to improve breastfeedings, supplemental infant formula should be initiated. We usually recommend it at once if the infant has lost weight. However, under adverse environmental circumstances of most resource-poor, less-developed countries, a more moderate approach is recommended and further efforts be made to initiate adequate lactation (Mata 1982). Interestingly, some mothers who consider themselves "naturalists" persist and refuse to try infant formula even when their efforts to give breast milk are not successful and their babies fail to thrive (Pugliese et al 1987).

CLINICAL INTERVENTION

Although there is complete agreement that human milk is the best food for babies, it is often not given because mothers find it difficult to initiate and maintain successful nursing. This often occurs with the first-born child. Throughout history, the art of breastfeeding was passed from one generation to the next. Mothers now need education and emotional support both during the pregnancy and throughout lactation in order to breast feed their babies. Instinct alone is simply not enough.

In preparation for breastfeeding, the pregnant woman should take steps to learn about the process of lactation, to prepare her breasts for feeding, and to establish a support system for help with problems and questions as they arise. The prenatal classes where expectant parents learn about labor and delivery is an ideal time to begin to explore the topic of breastfeeding. The relaxation techniques used to make labor more bearable can also be applied during breastfeeding. The woman's breasts and nipples should be examined to identify any problems with their structure that may interfere with successful breastfeeding. Special nipple preparation can be undertaken for women with inverted nipples who want to breastfeed.

Although nipple preparations such as massaging with a rough cloth or exposing them to the sun to "toughen" the nipples is often recommended, the effectiveness of such methods in preventing soreness during breastfeeding has not been demonstrated (Brown & Hurlock 1975). However, nipple preparation may help the woman become more accustomed to handling her own breasts and may reduce some anxiety about breastfeeding.

Once the baby is born, efforts should be made by the health care professionals in the hospital to teach the mother how to breastfeed. Mothers need instruction on relaxation techniques such as a warm shower, breast massage, comfortable positioning for feeding, and listening to relaxing music. These are just a few of the ways to initiate the let-down reflex necessary for breastfeeding. For many women, nursing in public places makes relaxation difficult, and they should avoid feeding their babies then. Information on how to care for the breasts to avoid and alleviate soreness and prevent and relieve engorgement may be discussed with the mother. There are many handbooks on breastfeeding, and organizations such as the La Leche League provide support and practical guides for the woman who wishes to breastfeed (Goldfarb & Tibbetts 1980, Kamen & Kamen 1986). There are also a variety of lactation consultants as a resource in hospital settings or in the community. The benefit of such resources, as well as friends and family members who have breast-fed their own babies, should not be underestimated.

Many women who return to work may still wish to continue to give their babies human milk. Breast pumps should be made available at the hospital for purchase or rental. Insurance companies often will cover the cost of breast-pump supplies. Many women find the electric pump to be the easiest method of expression. Mothers who cannot afford an electric pump can use the hospital equipment to supplement hand-pump expression.

Mothers using breast pumps need instructions on proper methods of milk expression and equipment sterilization. Mothers should be encouraged to express milk every 3 to 4 hours during the day to establish a milk supply. The same relaxation techniques to initiate the let-down reflex with breastfeeding can be practiced prior to milk expression. Sometimes, placing a picture of the infant on the milk pump can be reassuring to the mother. Sleeping through the night is encouraged unless the mother awakens because of breast engorgement.

As we have discussed, it is not enough to know that breast milk is the ideal food and to want to breast feed; the art of successful nursing must be mastered. For those women who are unable to breastfeed, or choose not to breastfeed, there are many alternative feedings available to promote a healthy baby (see Chapter 13). Ultimately, whether or not to breastfeed is a personal decision to be made by the mother; it should be respected, and "commerciogenic" temptations should not interfere. The American Academy of Pediatrics has issued several policy statements against directly promoting commercial infant formulas to the consumer via mass media (AAP 1982, 1986, 1988). This stand was taken so that mass media advertisement of infant formula would not have a negative effect on mothers and their decision to breastfeed. Despite these efforts, more companies are now engaging in public advertising campaigns to promote infant formula. These new marketing strategies undermine the efforts to encourage breastfeedings; they therefore should be condemned.

REFERENCES

American Academy Pediatrics, Committee on Drugs. The transfer of drugs and other chemicals into human breast milk. Pediatrics 1989; 84:924–936.

American Academy of Pediatrics, Policy Statement. The promotion of breastfeeding. Pediatrics 1982; 69:654–661.

American Academy of Pediatrics, Policy Statement. The pediatrician's responsibility for infant nutrition. AAP News, October 1986:7.

American Academy of Pediatrics, Policy Statement. Follow-up formula. AAP News, October 1988:6.

Auricchio S, Follo D, de Ritis, et al. Does breast feeding protect against the development of clinical symptoms of celiac disease in children? J Pediatr Gastroenterol Nutr 1983; 2:428–433.

Axelson I, Borulf S, Righard R, et al. Protein and energy intake during weaning. I. Effects on growth. Acta Paediatr Scan 1987; 76:321–327.

Bahna SL. Milk allergy. In Chiaramonte LT, Schneider AT, Lifshitz F, eds. Food allergy: A practical approach to diagnosis and management. New York: Marcel Dekker, 1988:107–116.

Beaton GH, Chery A. Protein requirements of infants: A reexamination of concepts and approaches. Am J Clin Nutr 1988; 48:1403–1412.

Berlin CM, Denson HM, Daniel CH, Ward RM. Disposition of dietary caffeine in milk, saliva and plasma of lactating women. Pediatrics 1984; 72:59–63.

Brown KH, Robertson AD, Akhtar NA. Lactational capacity of marginally nourished mothers: Infants' milk nutrient consumption and patterns of growth. Pediatrics 1986; 78:920–927.

Brown MS, Hurlock JT. Preparation of the breast for breastfeeding. Nurs Res 1975; 24:448–451.

Byrne J, Thomas MR, Chan GM. Calcium intake and bone density of lactating women in their late childbearing years. J Am Diet Assoc 1987; 87:883–887.

Cameron M, Hofvander Y. Manual on feeding infants and young children. 2nd ed. New York: Protein Advisory Group of the U.N., 1975.

Clark JH, Wilson WG. A 16-day-old breast-fed infant with metabolic acidosis caused by salicylate. Clin Pediatr 1981; 20:53–54.

Cole JP. Breastfeeding in the Boston suburbs in relation to personal-social factors: Are pediatricians thoughtlessly influencing the outcome in their postpartum care? Clin Pediatr 1977; 16:352–356.

Cunningham AS. II. Morbidity in breast-fed and artificially-fed infants. J Pediatr 1979; 95:685–689.

Cussen GH. Breast feeding and infant mortality. In Wharton B, ed. Topics in perinatal medicine. Kent, England: Pitman Medical, 1980:79–87.

Delgado H, Lechtig A, Yarbrough C, Marshall R, Klein RE. The effect of marginal malnutrition in the duration of post partum amenorrhea in moderately malnourished communities. Proceedings of the 4th International Congress of Nutrition, Kyoto, Japan, 1975.

Eastham E, Smith D, Poople D, et al. Further decline of breast-feeding. Br Med J 1976; 1:305–307.

Erickson SH, Oppenheim GL. Aspirin in breast milk. J Fam Pract 1979; 8:189–190.

Fallot ME, Boyd II JL, Oski FA. Breast feeding reduces incidence of hospital admissions for infection in infants. Pediatrics 1980; 65:1121–1124.

Fergusson DM, Beautrais AL, Silva PA. Breast-feeding and cognitive development in the first seven years of life. Soc Sci Med 1982; 16:1705–1708.

Fomon SJ. Reflections on infant feeding in the 1970s and 1980s. Am J Clin Nutr 1987; 46:171–182.

Goldfarb J, Tibbetts E. Breast feeding handbook. Hillside, NJ: Enslow Publishers, 1980.

Grossman ER. Letter: More on the prophylactic dose of fluoride. J Pediatr 1975; 87:840–842.

Hanson LA. Biology of human milk. New York: Raven Press, 1988.

Helsing E. Lactation education: The learning of the "obvious." In Breastfeeding and the mother. Elsevier, Amsterdam: Ciba Foundation Symposium No. 45, 1976.

Herterampf E, Cayazzo M, Pizarro F, Stekel A. Bioavailability of iron in soy-based formula and its effect on iron nutriture in infancy. Pediatrics 1986; 78:640–645.

Host A, Husby S, Osterballe O. A prospective study of cow's milk allergy in exclusively breast-fed infants. Acta Paediatr Scand 1988; 77:663–670.

Ing R, Petrakis NL, Ho JH. Unilateral breast-feeding and breast cancer. Lancet 1977; 2:124–127.

Jelliffe DB, Jelliffe EFP. Human milk, nutrition and the world resource crisis. Science (NY) 1975; 188:557–561.

Jelliffe DB, Jelliffe EFP. Human milk in the modern world. Oxford: Oxford University Press, 1978.

Jensen RG, Ferris AM, Lammikeefe CJ, Henderson RA. Human milk as a carrier of messages to the nursing infant. Nutr Today 1988; 23:20–25.

Kamen B, Kamen S. Total nutrition for breast-feeding mothers. Boston: Little, Brown & Company, 1986.

Kark JD, Troya G, Friedlander Y, Slater PE, Stein Y. Validity of maternal reporting of breast feeding history and the association with blood lipids in seventeen-year-olds in Jerusalem. J Epidemiol Comm Health 1984; 38:218–225.

Klaus M, Kennel J. Maternal-infant bonding. St. Louis: C.V. Mosby Co., 1976.

Kries RV, Shearer M, McCarthy PT, Haug M, Harzer G, Gobel U. Vitamin K content of maternal milk: Influence of the stage of lactation, lipid composition, and vitamin K supplements given to the mother. Pediatr Res 1987; 22:513–517.

Lane PA, Hathaway WE. Vitamin K in infancy. J Pediatr 1985; 106:351–359.

Leventhal JM, Shapiro ED, Aten CB, Berg AT, Egerter SA. Does breast-feeding protect against infections in infants less than 3 months of age? Pediatrics 1986; 78:896–903.

Lloyd JK. Chairman's introduction. CIBA Found Symp 1976; 45:1.

Maisels MJ, Gifford K. Normal serum bilirubin levels in the newborn and the effect of breast-feeding. Pediatrics 1986; 78:837–843.

Mamunes P, Prince PE, Thortton NH, et al. Intellectual deficits after transient tyrosinemia in the term neonate. Pediatrics 1976; 57:675–680.

Masawe AE, Muindi JM, Swai GB. Infections in iron deficiency and other types of anaemia in the tropics. Lancet 1974; 2:314–317.

Mata L. Breast feeding, diarrheal disease, and malnutrition in less developed countries. In Lifshitz F, ed. Pediatric nutrition: Infant feedings, deficiencies, diseases. New York: Marcel Dekker, 1982:355–372.

Mayer EJ, Hamman RF, Gay EC, Lezotte CD, Savitz AD, Lingenshith GJ. Reduced risk of IDDM among breast-fed children. Diabetes 1988; 37:1625–1632.

McMillan JA, Landaw SA, Oski FA. Iron sufficiency in breast-fed infants and the availability of iron from human milk. Pediatrics 1976; 58:686–691.

Menkes JH. Early feeding history of children with learning disorders. Dev Med Child Neurol 1977; 19:169–171.

Milner RD, Deodhar AD, Chard CR, et al. Fat absorption by small babies fed two filled milk formulae. Arch Dis Child 1975; 50:654–656.

Montagu A, Brace CL. Human evolution. 2nd ed. New York: Macmillan Co., 1977:470.

Moser PB, Reynolds RD, Achanya S, Howard P, Andon MB. Calcium and magnesium dietary intakes and plasma and milk concentrations of Nepalese lactating women. Am J Clin Nutr 1988a; 47:735–739.

Moser PB, Reynolds RD, Achanya S, Howard P, Andon MB, Lewis SA. Copper, iron, zinc and selenium dietary intake and status of Nepalese lactating women and their breast-fed infants. Am J Clin Nutr 1988b; 47:729–734.

Muller M. The baby killer. London: War on Want, 1974.

Neumann CG, Alpaugh M. Birthweight doubling time: A fresh look. Pediatrics 1976; 57:469–473.

Nilkens PR. Stature reduction as an adaptive response to food production in mesoamerica. J Arch Soc 1976; 3:21–41.

Popkin BM, Solon F. Income, working mothers and infant nutrition. J Trop Pediatr Env Child Health 1976; 22:156.

Pugliese MT, Daum-Weyman M, Moses N, Lifshitz F. Parental health beliefs as a cause of non-organic failure to thrive. Pediatrics 1987; 80:171–182.

Raphael D. The tender gift: Breastfeeding. Englewood Cliffs, NJ: Prentice Hall, 1973.

Rasmussen KM. Maternal nutritional status and lactational performance. Clin Nutr 1988; 7:147–155.

Rodgers B. Feeding in infancy and later ability and attainment: A longitudinal study. Dev Med Child Neurol 1978; 20:421–426.

Ryan AS, Gussler JD. The international breast-feeding compendium. 3rd ed rev. Columbus, OH: Ross Laboratories, 1981.

Saarinen UM, Backman A, Kojosaari M, Siimes MA. Prolonged breast feeding as prophylaxis for atopic disease. Lancet 1979; 2:163–166.

Simpson WJ, Cheung DK. Developing infant occlusion: Related feeding methods and oral habits. I. Methodology and results at 4 and 8 months. J Can Dent Assoc 1976; 42:124–132.

Van Balen H, Ntabomvura V. Methods of birth spacing, maternal lactation and post partum abstinence in relation to traditional African culture. J Trop Pediatr 1976; 22:50–52.

Walravens PA, Hambidge KM. Growth of infants fed a zinc-supplemented formula. Am J Clin Nutr 1976; 29:1114–1121.

Washburn SL, Lancaster CS. Estimated early man's height range. In Korn N, Thompson F, eds. Human evolution. New York: Holt, Reinhardt & Winston, 1967:67–83.

White RG, Paul AA, Cole TJ. A critical analysis of measured food energy intakes during infancy and early childhood in comparison with current international recommendations. J Hum Nutr 1981; 35:339–348.

Whitehead RG, Paul AA. Growth charts and the assessment of infant feeding practices in the Western world and in developing countries. Early Hum Dev 1984; 9:187–207.

Whittlestone WG. Breast feeding: A foundation of preventive medicine. Nutr Health 1983; 1:133.

Wickizer TM, Brilliant LB. Testing for polychlorinated biphenyls in human milk. Pediatrics 1981; 68:411.

Williams JM, Auerbach KG, Jacobi A. Lacteral epicondylitis (tennis elbow) in breastfeeding mothers. Clinical Pediatrics 1989; 28:42–43.

Wright LE, Gaull GE. Taurine in human milk. LA Hanson, ed. New York: Raven Press, 1988:95–109.

13

Formula Choices and the Introduction of Solid Foods

Joyce was only 5 weeks old and had already spent 10 days in the hospital because of her difficulty with feeding. Joyce started spitting up at 1 week of age while receiving a cow's milk–based infant formula. The pediatrician then prescribed a number of soy-based formulas which, were "not tolerated" either. Joyce began to have a little diarrhea and thus she was admitted to the community hospital for evaluation. There, she was treated with a special predigested infant formula but continued to spit up and have abnormal stools. Because of her persistent condition Joyce was transferred to the university hospital where she was initially treated with a glucose-electrolyte solution and was kept fasting. However, when the professor reviewed Joyce's case, he promptly noticed that her problem was not due to formula intolerance but rather a result of overfeeding. Joyce had gained more than sufficient weight since she was born, and that was the main clue to making the correct diagnosis. At birth, Joyce weighed 3 kilograms (6.6 lb) and she gained 1.5 kilograms (3.3 lb) during the first 5 weeks of life despite spending a lot of time in the hospital. She was taking as much as 1½ quarts of infant formula a day; almost 8 ounces at each feeding! It was no wonder that Joyce could not "tolerate" any formula in such large amounts. When the formula intake was reduced, she dramatically improved and was able to go home on a standard infant formula.

INFANT FORMULA FEEDINGS

Until 200 to 300 years ago, the only source of feeding available for infants was human milk. In the past, when the mother was unable to breastfeed, the use of wet nurses was essential during the first month of life for the survival of the baby. After the first month of life, substitute feedings for breast milk such as beer, gruel, and paps made from bread and water were used, but even at an older age, as many as 50 percent of these babies died (Radbill 1981). It was not until the late eighteenth century that cow's milk was widely used as a substitute for breast milk feedings and the value of cereals and sugars in infant feedings was first recognized. The onset of the industrial revolution, with a move toward women in the workplace, was the impetus for the development of alternate feeding methods for babies. Although these developments gave women greater freedom, the switch from breastfeeding to cow's milk had disastrous consequences, particularly in developing countries (Mata 1982). Initial attempts at artificial feedings resulted in almost 100 percent mortality (Radbill 1981).

Over the past decade, there has been a trend to return to breastfeeding. This movement has been supported by continued documentation that human milk is best for babies (see Chapter 12). In 1971, only 25 percent of infants were breast-fed, and by 4 months of age fewer than 10 percent of those babies continued to receive breast-milk feedings (Martinez & Nalezienski 1979). In contrast, in 1985, 60 percent of babies were breast-fed at birth and as many as 35 percent were still given breast milk at 4 months of age (Ryan & Gussler 1986). Even though breastfeeding has increased, the consumption of infant formulas has also risen (Fomon 1987b). This trend is a result of the decreased use of cow's milk for infant feeding and a more prolonged period of feeding with infant formula (AAP 1983a, Anderson et al 1985) (Fig. 13–1 and 13–2).

Infant formulas must be used when breast milk is either unavailable or insufficient to meet a baby's needs. Also, if the mother is sick or receiving medications, breastfeeding may be undesirable (see Chapter 12). Commercially prepared infant formulas have been manufactured to mimic the nutrient composition of human milk, and standards have been developed to ensure the provision of all the necessary nutrients including vitamins and minerals within a given range for all infant formulas (AAP 1976) (Table 13–1).

COW'S-MILK FORMULAS

The first choice for feeding babies who are not fortunate enough to be breast-fed is a cow's-milk formula (Table 13–2). Milk-based formulas are made from nonfat milk with added demineralized whey, soy protein isolate, or buttermilk, depending on the particular product. Taurine supplementation is often provided to simulate the amino acid composition of human milk. The most commonly used fats for infant cow's-milk formulas are soybean, corn, and coconut oils. The carbohydrate source is lactose (milk sugar).

The protein content of a standard cow's-milk formula typically has a

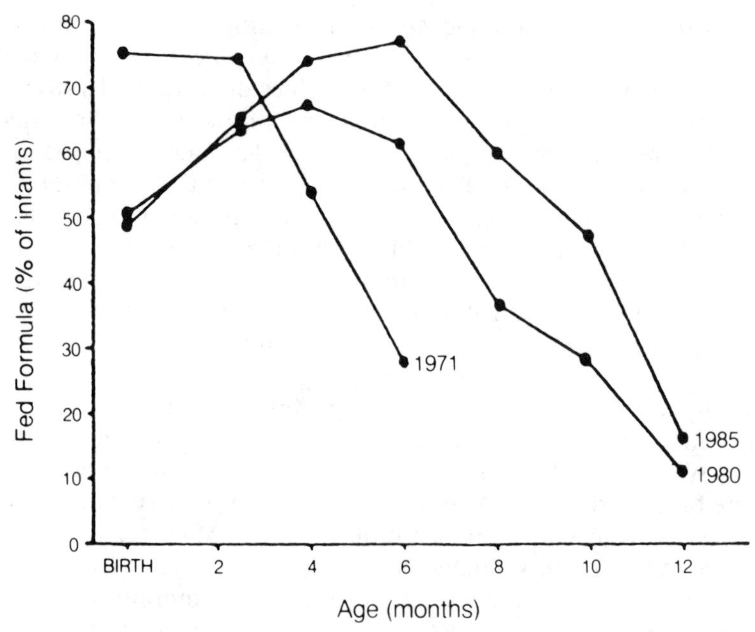

Figure 13–1. Percentage of U.S. infants fed commercially available formulas at various ages. Data from Martinez and Nalezienski for 1971, Martinez et al for 1980, and Martinez (personal communication) for 1985.

From Fomon SJ. Reflections on infant feeding in the 1970s and 1980s. Am J Clin Nutr 1987b; 46:171–182. © Am J Clin Nutr. American Society for Clinical Nutrition.

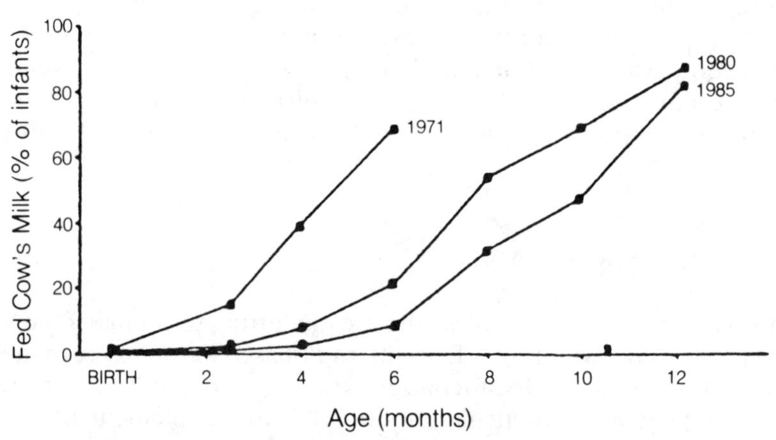

Figure 13–2. Percentage of U.S. infants fed cow's milk at various ages in 1971, 1980, and 1985. Data from Martinez and Nalezienski for 1971, Martinez et al for 1980, and Martinez (personal communication) for 1985.

From Fomon SJ. Reflections on infant feeding in the 1970s and 1980s. Am J Clin Nutr 1987b; 46:171–182. © Am J Clin Nutr. American Society for Clinical Nutrition.

Table 13–1. Nutrient Specifications for Infant Formulas (per 100 Calories).

	MINIMUM	MAXIMUM
Protein (g)	1.8	4.5
Fat (g)	3.3	6.0
Linoleic acid (g)	0.3	—
Vitamin A (IU)	250	750
Vitamin D (IU)	40	100
Vitamin E (IU)	0.7	—
Vitamin K (μg)	4	—
Thiamin (μg)	40	—
Riboflavin (μg)	60	—
Vitamin B_6 (μg)	35	—
Vitamin B_{12} (μg)	0.15	—
Niacin (μg)*	250	—
Folic acid (μg)	4	—
Pantothenic acid (μg)	300	—
Biotin (μg)†	1.5	—
Vitamin C (mg)	8	—
Choline (mg)†	7	—
Inositol (mg)†	4	—
Calcium (mg)	60	—
Phosphorus (mg)	30	—
Magnesium (mg)	6	—
Iron (mg)	0.15	3.0
Zinc (mg)	0.5	—
Manganese (μg)	5	—
Copper (μg)	60	—
Iodine (μg)	5	75
Sodium (mg)	20	60
Potassium (mg)	80	200
Chloride (mg)	55	150

*Includes nicotinic acid and niacinamide.
†Required only for non-milk-based infant formulas.

Adapted from the Food and Drug Administration. Rules and regulations. Nutrient requirements for infant formulas. Fed Reg 1985; 50:45106-8 (21 CFR Part107).

whey:casein ratio of 20:80. In some infant formulas demineralized whey has been added to the cow's milk to provide a whey:casein ratio of 60:40; the latter protein composition is more akin to the amino acid composition of human milk and forms a smaller curd, which may be more easily digestible (George & Lebenthal 1981). Studies in premature infants have shown a nutritional benefit of whey-predominant formulas with less metabolic abnormalities such as high urea and ammonia levels (azotemia and hyperammonemia), or acidosis (Raiha et al 1976). However, for full-term infants who are better able to handle an increased protein load there is no nutritional or metabolic basis for selecting whey- versus casein-predominant formulas (Jarvenpaa et al 1982). Similarly there is no currently available formula that is ideal for the changing needs of the infant as he or she grows older, though manufacturers are producing milk formulas designed for older babies (see Table 13–2).

Soy Formulas

Soy-based infant formulas (see Table 13–2) are alternatives to cow's-milk formula for babies with conditions such as lactose intolerance and/or milk protein intolerance (see Chapters 19 and 20). These milk-free formulas have been available for more than 40 years and their use as infant feedings has increased dramatically in the United States. The American Academy of Pediatrics estimates that 10 to 15 percent of all formula-fed babies receive soy-based infant formulas (AAP 1983b). Pediatricians and parents often switch from milk-based to soy-based formulas when the baby demonstrates any gastrointestinal abnormality such as frequent regurgitation, colic, or other poorly defined problems. However, there is no scientific basis for this practice.

Unlike cow's milk–based formula, soy formulas are lactose-free and contain sucrose (table sugar), corn syrup solids, or tapioca dextrins as their carbohydrate source; the fat source is a blend of vegetable oils similar to the milk-based formulas. The protein source in these formulas is soy-protein isolate, to which the essential sulfur-containing amino acid methionine has been added to compensate for the relatively lower concentration of the amino acid in vegetable protein. Since soy-based formulas have a higher total protein concentration than milk-based formulas (1.5 g vs 2.0 g per oz), the need for additional methionine fortification has been questioned (Fomon et al 1986). Regardless of the protein quantity and quality, soy-based infant formulas have been shown to promote adequate weight gain and growth in healthy full term infants (AAP 1983b), although there are questions about its effectiveness and safety in premature infants (see Chapter 11).

Some concerns have been raised regarding the bioavailability of minerals in soy formulas owing to the protein-phytic acid mineral complex formed during the processing of the soy-protein isolate (AAP 1983b). Full-term healthy babies fed soy-based formulas were shown to have a lower bone mineral content than babies fed cow's milk–based formula, although rickets was not reported (Steichen & Tsang 1987). These findings suggest that there is lower calcium and phosphorus absorption/retention with soy-based infant formula than with cow's-milk formula or human milk. This occurs even though soy formulas contain at least 25 percent more calcium and 50 percent more phosphorus than cow's-milk infant formulas.

Iron and zinc are other minerals that may have compromised bioavailability in the presence of the high phytate content of soy formulas (Cook, Morck & Lynch 1981). Recent attempts have been made to reduce the phytate content of soy formula to improve mineral bioavailability (Lonnerdal et al 1988). However, from a clinical standpoint, iron-fortified soy-based infant formulas have been shown to be as effective as the iron-fortified cow's-milk formulas in preventing iron deficiency in infants (Hertrampf et al 1986).

In the early 1950s soy protein was considered less allergenic than cow's-milk protein and perhaps to have some preventive role against protein intolerance (Glaser & Johnstone 1953). However, soy protein is now known to be as antigenic as cow's-milk protein. As many as one fifth to one third of infants who are intolerant of cow's-milk protein are also allergic to soy protein (see Chapter 20). Therefore, the practice of managing the cow's-milk protein–intolerant infant by changing to a soy-based formula is incorrect. Such action does not eliminate antigens from the diet but simply exposes the infant to another potential allergen—soy protein. The American Academy of Pediatrics (1983b) recommends the use of protein hydrolysate formulas instead of soy formulas if there is sensitivity or intolerance to intact cow's-milk protein, which produces persistent diarrhea or severe infantile colic (Lifshitz 1985).

Protein Hydrolysate Formulas

Protein hydrolysate formulas (see Table 13–2) are very useful for feeding babies with special needs. These formulas are predigested and have incorporated into their formulation a variety of changes that give them special characteristics for the treatment of conditions such as chronic diarrhea, malabsorption, cow's-milk and/or soy-protein intolerance, and food allergies. The state of the art in the preparation and clinical use of these formulas is reviewed elsewhere (Lifshitz 1985).

Protein hydrolysate infant formulas contain hydrolyzed casein or whey that has been specially treated to reduce allergenicity (Lifshitz 1985). In these formulas the protein is subjected to a series of hydrolyses, which simulate the process of intestinal protein digestion to yield small peptides and amino acids. To further reduce the allergenicity of the hydrolysate, it is treated with activated charcoal. The final protein hydrolysate is of excellent nitrogen quality to meet the nutritional needs of growing infants. A new "hypoallergenic infant formula," manufactured by the Carnation Company, is a whey-protein hydrolysate formula. To date there is insufficient experience to know whether there are any advantages or disadvantages to using whey protein instead of casein hydrolysates, but it appears that this formula is not necessarily a "hypoallergenic" one. Babies with milk allergy may be sensitive to this preparation also.

The casein hydrolysate formulas do not contain lactose, but it is present in whey-predominant formulas. This is important as infants with diarrhea who receive these special formulas are usually intolerant of disaccharides, particularly lactose (Lifshitz 1982). Thus, the amount and type of carbohydrate may be important in deciding which formula to use. The glucose polymers are carbohydrates, which are better tolerated by sick infants and are found in varying proportions in all the protein hydrolysate infant formulas.

The fat source varies among these special products and may include vegetable oils or a blend of medium-chain triglycerides (MCT) and corn oil. MCT oil is an important source of fat for babies with fat malabsorption (steatorrhea). MCT is absorbed and utilized more easily than long-chain fats, and these formulas are useful in the treatment of patients with malabsorption. However, because of their special, predigested formulations, they tend to be more costly and their smell and taste may be unpleasant, particularly for the adult who is feeding the child.

Special Infant Formulas

There are formulas (see Table 13–2) that have been designed for the treatment of specific problems, such as monosaccharide malabsorption. Special infant formulas are also available for the treatment of infants with specific metabolic problems in whom complete formulas will not be tolerated. These types of formulas are considered modular formula feedings; these formula powders omit either protein or carbohydrate while they provide all other nutrient requirements for a growing baby. In this form, these infant formula powders can be individually designed to meet a baby's special metabolic needs. Other formulas available for the treatment of infants and children with metabolic disorders are described in Chapter 25.

Table 13–2. Infant Formulas.

FORMULA	MANUFACTURER
Milk-based	
Enfamil	Mead Johnson
Gerber	Gerber
Milumil	Milupa
Similac	Ross Laboratories
Similac with Whey	Ross Laboratories
Similac PM 60/40	Ross Laboratories
Pedia Sure	Ross Laboratories
Advance	Ross Laboratories
SMA	Wyeth
Soy-based	
Prosobee	Mead Johnson
Isomil	Ross Laboratories
Isomil SF	Ross Laboratories
Nursoy	Wyeth
Protein Hydrolysate	
Nutramingen	Mead Johnson
Pregestimil	Mead Johnson
Good Start HA	Carnation
Alimentum	Ross Laboratories
Special Infant Formulas	
Portagen	Mead Johnson
Mono- and Disaccharide Free Diet Powder (Product 3232A)	Mead Johnson
Protein Free Diet Powder (Product 80056)	Mead Johnson
RCF (Ross Carbohydrate Free)	Ross Laboratories
Calcilo X D (Vitamin D free, low calcium)	Ross Laboratories

The reader is referred to lists provided by the manufacturers for complete and ever-changing compositions of each of the formulas. A comprehensive list is available elsewhere (Lifshitz 1985).

HOW MUCH FORMULA?

Good nutrition for a growing baby requires the intake of enough nutrients and calories to ensure normal growth and development and meet all the baby's needs. For infants below 6 kilograms (13.2 lb), all nutritional needs can be met with either breast milk or infant formula (Table 13–3). However, when the baby is 6 kilograms (13.2 lb), the calories provided by 1 liter of formula begins to fall slightly below the estimated requirements for normal growth and development. Increasing the formula intake beyond 1 liter a day in attempts to meet the baby's nutrient needs is generally not recommended, as the volume of milk may overcome the capacity of the infant's stomach and the baby's fluid tolerance. When the infant is more than 7 kilograms (15.4 lb), milk alone does not provide adequate energy, protein, and essential minerals.

WHY NOT COW'S MILK?

The use of pasteurized cow's milk during infancy was a frequent practice in the early 1970s, with as many as 70 percent of infants fed cow's milk by 6 months of age (Martinez & Nalezienski 1979). However, there are many medical and nutritional concerns regarding the use of cow's milk as a component of infant feedings during the first 6 months of life. Early exposure to cow's

Table 13–3. Formula Intake (1 Liter) to Meet Nutrient Needs of Growing Babies.*

	5-kg BABY† (2–3 mo)	6-kg BABY (3–4 mo)	7-kg BABY (4–5 mo)	9-kg BABY (9–12 mo)
Volume (mL) [oz]	1000 [33.3]	1000 [33.3]	1000 [33.3]	1000 [33.3]
Calories (kcal)	667	667	667	667
kcal/kg	133	111	95	74
% Requirements‡	124	103	88	76
Protein (g)	15	15	15	15
g/kg	3.0	2.5	2.1	1.7
% Requirements	136	114	97	104
% Vitamin requirements	all ≥ 100	all ≥ 100	all ≥ 100	all > 100
% Mineral requirements	all > 100	all > 100	all > 100	all > 100 except: 86% magnesium 77% calcium 63% phosphorus

*Enfamil with Iron (20 kcal/oz). Mead Johnson & Company, Evansville, IN 47721.

†Average male baby boy gaining weight along the 50th percentile for age and sex, birth weight 3.3 kg (7 lb, 4 oz).

‡Requirements based on the Committee on Dietary Allowances, Food and Nutrition Board, National Research Council. Recommended dietary allowances. 10th ed. Washington, D.C.: National Academy of Sciences, 1989.

milk (before the age of 4 months) has been associated with increased risk of food sensitivity to milk protein (Foucard 1985). Iron-deficiency anemia in young infants has also been reported, owing to the low concentration and poor bioavailability of iron in cow's milk; anemia may be further exacerbated by gastrointestinal blood loss that occurs in infants fed cow's milk (Martinez, Ryan & Malec 1985, Oski 1985). However, occult blood loss from the gastrointestinal tract was typically reported in very young babies or in infants receiving large amounts of cow's milk feedings (Andersen et al 1985). In older infants (140 days) fed whole cow's milk with iron and vitamin C supplementation, no adverse effects on iron status or gastrointestinal blood loss were noted (Fomon et al 1981).

The higher renal solute load of whole cow's milk compared with human milk or commercially prepared formula also is a concern. This may be more important in younger infants who have a greater risk of dehydration; there is no evidence to suggest that the kidneys of healthy full-term infants over 6 months of age are unable to handle the renal solute load of whole cow's milk as long as other foods and adequate amounts of water are offered. However, if the infant is sick with diarrhea or fever, or if the baby lives in a hot climate or in heated rooms, additional water intake may be necessary.

Another important problem with cow's-milk feedings is the potential for developing essential fatty acid deficiency. Linoleic acid, an essential fatty acid, must provide about 3 percent of the energy intake to prevent essential fatty acid deficiency (AAP 1985). Breast milk provides approximately 8 to 10 percent of calories from this essential fatty acid. Commercially available infant formulas generally provide 10 percent of the calories as linoleic acid. However, whole cow's milk does not provide sufficient amounts of this essential fatty acid, and certainly low-fat dairy products contain even lower amounts of this important nutrient (Table 13–4). Feeding low-fat milk to babies will certainly increase the risk of such deficiency and may lead to malnutrition and poor myelinization of the central nervous system.

WHEN TO SWITCH TO COW'S MILK?

The age at which to switch from infant formula to pasteurized cow's milk remains controversial (AAP 1985a, Martinez, Ryan & Malec 1985). As discussed previously, cow's milk must not be fed to younger infants. However, it has been shown that babies can safely tolerate whole-fat cow's milk when they are older, have gained more than 6 kilograms in body weight, and are ingesting supplemental feedings to account for one third of their daily calories (AAP 1983a). However, because it is unknown whether iron deficiency may develop in older infants consuming excessive amounts of cow's milk with no

Table 13–4. Macronutrient and Essential Fatty Acid Composition of Cow's Milk.

	INFANT FORMULA*	3.5% WHOLE COW'S MILK	1.5–1.8%-FAT COW'S MILK	SKIM COW'S MILK
Caloric Distribution				
Protein (%)	9	21	28	38
Carbohydrate (%)	41	30	42	57
Fat (%)	50	49	30	5
Linoleic acid				
mg/100 g	785.5	92	60	0.20
mg/245 g (1 cup)	1924.96	225.4	147	0.49
% Total Amount of Fat	21.5	2.6	0.2	0.05
% Total Energy	10.6	1.26	1.18	0

*Enfamil Infant Formula (20 kcal/oz). Mead Johnson & Company, Evansville, IN 47721.

iron supplements, the American Academy of Pediatrics Committee on Nutrition recommends that no more than 1 liter of cow's milk per day should be fed to any infant and that a well-balanced mixture of iron-fortified cereals, fruits, vegetables, and meats be fed to ensure adequate intakes of iron and vitamin C (AAP 1983a). Moreover, if infant formula is readily available and the increased cost of this feeding is not a burden for the family, providing infant formula throughout the first year of life would be a prudent recommendation. Thereafter, introduction of whole-fat cow's milk is appropriate. However, the cost factor must be seriously considered. Infant formula has increased in price at a rate greater than inflation. From 1980 to 1987 the price increase amounted to well over 100 percent, a figure that is particularly impressive since the consumer price index for milk, the major ingredient in formulas, rose only 9 percent during the same period. Women, Infants, and Children Supplemental Food programs for families in need are now obtaining special discounts from formula manufacturers to provide these products at a lower cost.

UNCONVENTIONAL INFANT FEEDINGS

Low-Fat Milk

Reduced-fat milks such as 2 percent, 1 percent, or skim milk are not recommended for infants during the first 2 years of life (AAP 1986). In addition to the inadequate essential fatty acid content of these milks (see Table 13–4) (AAP 1983a, 1985, Fomon et al 1977, 1979), babies fed low-fat milk have to consume larger volumes to meet their energy needs. Failure to thrive and depleted body fat stores have occurred when these types of feedings are given (Fomon et al 1977, Pugliese et al 1987). In addition, the protein intake of babies fed low-fat milk may become excessive: skim milk provides about 9 grams of protein per 100 calories, 1 percent–fat milk has 7.8 grams per 100 calories, and 2 percent–fat milk contains 6.6 grams per 100 calories, while the maximum concentration of protein permitted in infant formulas is 4.5 grams per 100 calories (see Table 13–1). The higher renal solute load of low-fat cow's-milk products increases an infant's risk of dehydration, especially under conditions of excessive fluid loss such as high temperature, diarrhea, or vomiting.

These types of milk are often prescribed for infants who are considered obese, to reduce the amount of fat in the diet. However, feeding skim milk usually does not decrease the total calorie intake as the baby ends up ingesting a larger amount of low-fat milk yielding an equal number of calories. Thus, overweight babies should not be treated with skim-milk feedings. If excess weight gain is occurring, a comprehensive approach to the problem of obesity must be followed (see Chapter 18).

Although low-fat types of milk have been used to prevent the potential problems of high cholesterol, the results may be less than desirable; these babies may fail to thrive (Pugliese et al 1987). It should be remembered that breast milk, which is the ideal food for infants, is neither low in fat nor low in cholesterol (see Chapter 12), and that the American Academy of Pediatrics as well as the American Heart Association do not recommend low-fat feedings before 2 years of age (see Chapters 16 and 24).

Other Milks

Other types of milk, such as goat's milk and raw milk, have been promoted as "health" food and may be used as alternative feedings for infants. However, neither one is considered to be nutritionally superior to cow's milk and both can be dangerous to the well-being of the baby. Goat's milk is deficient in vitamins C and D and iron and is inadequate in folic acid and vitamin B_{12} (Sawaya, Khalil & Al-Shalhat 1984, AAP 1985). In addition, goat's milk has a higher renal solute load than cow's milk. Any milk that is "raw" or unpasteurized may contain harmful pathogenic microorganisms, which can cause serious infections. All milks should be pasteurized to ensure their safety and quality.

CONTAMINANTS OF INFANT FORMULAS

Nonnutritive substances may be present in commercially available formulas because of contamination or processing techniques. For example, lead was a frequent contaminant of infant formulas in the early 1970s due to the use of lead-seamed cans. The change to nonsoldered cans resulted in a dramatic decrease in lead content, with present concentrations in standard infant formulas meeting acceptable limits (Miles 1982). To date, a baby taking 150 milliliters per kilogram of a 20 calorie per ounce infant formula will receive 1.5 micrograms of lead per kilogram of body weight, which is within the acceptable level of less than 3 micrograms per kilogram (Ryu et al 1983).

Aluminum is another contaminant of highly processed infant formulas (Koo & Kaplan 1988a). Although aluminum absorption from the GI tract is limited in adults, some concerns have been raised regarding increased absorption from a more immature intestine during infancy (Jakobsson & Lindberg 1985). Nutritionally based aluminum toxicity has been associated with the development of infant bone disorders, particularly in infants receiving parenteral nutrition contaminated with aluminum (see Chapter 28). However, infants receiving high levels of aluminum from formulas may also be at risk and there is a need to monitor the aluminum content of infant formulas (Koo & Kaplan 1988b).

VITAMIN AND MINERAL SUPPLEMENTS

The vitamin and mineral composition of infant formulas is regulated by the Food and Drug Administration and therefore is designed to meet the nutritional requirements of infants. A liter (33.3 oz) of infant formula will contain at least 100 percent of the Recommended Daily Dietary Allowances for most nutrients for babies until the baby's weight reaches 7.0 kilograms (15.4 lb) between 6 to 9 months of age (see Table 13–3). However, younger infants do not usually ingest such large quantities of formula. Thus, a vitamin supplement may be necessary for babies who do not consume 1 liter of milk formula per day (Table 13–5). These nutrient deficits become less marked as the baby begins to take more formula; thus, continued supplementation may not be necessary after the baby receives all the daily requirements from the formula alone.

The usual vitamin/mineral supplements provided to babies include vitamins A, D, and C, with or without fluoride and/or iron. The need to include vitamin C in the vitamin supplements is not clear. Vitamin C is already provided in the formula in amounts far in excess of normal requirements. Any baby who takes as little as 600 milliliters (20 oz) of milk formula will ingest all the vitamin C he or she needs. The vitamin supplements frequently given to infants contain 35 milligrams of vitamin C per dose (1 milliliter), and this would increase the percentage of RDA to 255 percent if the baby takes 1 liter of formula.

Healthy, full-term babies are born with iron stores adequate to last until

Table 13–5. Nutritional Adequacy of Milk Formula Feedings.

	24-oz COW'S-MILK FORMULA*	REQUIREMENTS FOR A 1-MONTH-OLD BABY†	% REQUIREMENTS
Calories (kcal)	480	464	103
Protein (g)	10.8	9.5	114
Vitamin A (IU)	1500	1875	80‡
Vitamin D (IU)	300	300	100
Vitamin E (IU)	15	4.5	333
Vitamin K (μg)	<41	<5	<820
Vitamin C (mg)	39	30	130
Folic acid (mg)	75	25	300
Thiamin (mg)	0.5	0.3	167
Riboflavin (mg)	0.75	0.4	188
Niacin (mg)	6.0	5.0	120
Vitamin B_6 (mg)	0.4	0.3	133
Vitamin B_{12} (μg)	1.5	0.3	500
Calcium (mg)	330	400	83‡
Phosphorus (mg)	225	300	75‡
Iron (mg)	0.75	6	13§
Magnesium (mg)	37.5	40	94
Iodine (μg)	49	40	109
Sodium (mg)	131	120	109

*Enfamil without iron, 20 kcal/oz. Mead Johnson & Company, Evansville, IN 47721.
†Recommended dietary requirements for a 1-month-old baby boy weighing 9 lb 7 oz (4.3 kg) and length of 21¼″ (54 cm).
‡Intake <90% of the recommended dietary allowance.
§Intake <67% of the recommended dietary allowance.

the fourth to sixth month of life. Thus, the need for iron supplementation during the first few months of life has been questioned. Moreover, many pediatricians and parents believe that babies fed iron-fortified formulas may experience fussiness, colic, and GI problems such as spitting up, diarrhea, and/or constipation (Fomon 1987a). However, when this concern has been evaluated in a scientific, standardized fashion, iron-fortified formulas have been shown to be as well-tolerated as non–iron-fortified formulas and to have a positive impact on iron status (Nelson et al 1988). The American Academy of Pediatrics Committee on Nutrition (1976) has recommended that all non–breast-fed infants receive the iron-fortified (12–13 mg iron/L) infant formulas.

Fluoride supplementation during infancy is recommended for breast-fed babies and infants receiving ready-to-use formulas that do not contain this element. The recommended dose of fluoride for infants up to 2 years of age to prevent dental caries is 0.25 milligrams per day (AAP 1979). However, if the formula is prepared from either concentrated liquid or powder, the fluoride supplementation is dependent on the fluoride content of the water used to make the final infant feeding. When the fluoride concentration of drinking water is less than 0.3 ppm, 0.25 milligrams fluoride per day can be given as a supplement, but if the fluoride concentration of the water is higher, additional fluoride supplementation should be avoided to prevent dental fluorosis (see Chapter 9).

PROGRESSION OF FOODS

When to Start Solid Foods?

In the early 1970s, babies were given supplemental foods such as cereal as early as 6 weeks of age. It is now recommended that the introduction of baby foods be delayed until later in infancy, after the infant has doubled his or her birth weight. Food sensitivities or intolerances may result if introduction of solid food occurs early in life, before the baby is more physically and developmentally mature. Before babies attain about 6 kilograms (13.3 lb) in body weight they have an immature digestive system, with insufficient pancreatic enzymes and other GI deficits. Thus, foods may not be well digested, which can lead to malabsorption and sensitization to allergenic proteins.

Today, most baby foods are commercially manufactured and are readily available for use by parents without any need for preparation. Baby foods are prepared to meet current standards. For example, addition of salt and sugar to baby foods to meet adult taste preferences has been minimized over the past 15 years (Filer 1971a). Other additives, such as modified food starches, have also been restricted in commercially available baby foods (Filer 1971b). For easy transportation, convenience, and economy, dehydrated baby foods are currently available as the latest advancement in baby foods.

From the example in Table 13–5, it is clear that the introduction of solid foods to an infant's diet is not arbitrary, nor is it totally age-dependent. Progression to solid foods to supplement formula intake should be undertaken when the baby's nutrient needs can no longer be met by the usually tolerated amount of formula (1 L). This occurs about when the baby weighs 6 kilograms (13.3 lb). When this takes place, it is time to introduce solid foods to the baby's diet.

Moreover, if the introduction of solid foods is delayed until the baby's weight is around 6 kilograms, the order of introduction of the various types of baby foods seems to be of little importance (Fomon et al 1979). At this stage it is more important to introduce high-calorie foods rather than high-protein foods, since the need for calories is very marked. In these rapidly growing infants the protein requirements can easily be met by formula alone. The caloric intake is the first nutrient to become inadequate when an infant is fed formula alone, whereas the intake of protein and other nutrients remains sufficient (see Table 13–3).

An additional iron source might be needed before the baby reaches 6 kilograms if a non-iron-fortified infant formula is given (see Table 13–5). Although many professionals have advocated the role of iron-fortified infant cereals in meeting the nutritional needs of babies (AAP 1985, Fomon et al 1979, Rees, Monsen & Merrill 1985), more recent studies have suggested that iron in infant cereals is not very bioavailable (Fomon 1987a). Moreover, cereal fibers and phytates may interfere with iron absorption and further exacerbate the underlying concern with iron deficiency (Hurrell 1984). In contrast, iron-fortified infant formulas will meet the baby's requirements for this mineral with ease.

Cereals

Infant cereals are generally the first solid food introduced (Table 13–6). The texture of baby cereal makes it easier for a baby to learn to swallow food taken from a spoon as a step forward from taking liquid from a nipple. Cereals, rice cereal in particular, are readily digested by the young infant and are considered to be the least likely to cause an allergic reaction. There are a variety of ready-to-serve dry cereals available for infants. They include single-grain cereals such as rice, oatmeal, and barley, as well as mixed grain cereals and cereals with added fruit. Single-grain foods should always be introduced as the baby's first foods to allow for identification of any problem or intolerance. High-protein cereals, which contain five times the protein content of regular infant cereals, are also available. However, babies receiving a liter of infant formula will be consuming adequate protein intake until they are 7 kilograms (15.4 lb) (see Table 13–3). Therefore, these high-protein cereals are not necessary for normal babies.

Fruits and Vegetables

After a baby has accepted single-grain infant cereals, fruits and vegetables can be offered. These foods should be given one at a time and given at least 3 or 4 days apart to identify any possible individual food sensitivity or intolerance (see Chapter 20). There are a variety of strained fruit products available for feeding the young infant. These include single-ingredient fruits such as applesauce, peaches, and pears, which are usually referred to as first foods and are designed for the baby first starting to take pureed foods. They contain only the specified fruit and enough water necessary to make a smooth textured product. Fruit combinations like apple-blueberry and fruits with tapioca are more appropriate for the older infant. Citrus fruits and juices are considered to be the leading offenders in food allergies, and their use should be delayed until after 1 year of age.

Wet-packed cereal-fruit combinations are also available. These products are iron-fortified and, because they are enclosed in jars without exposure to air, ferrous sulfate may be used. This form of iron supplement is a more bioavailable form of iron as compared with that found in dry infant cereals. Therefore, it is a much better source of iron for infants, but care must be taken when offering infants just starting foods combination foods such as cereal mixed with fruit. Most medical professionals agree that each new food should be introduced slowly and separately, so that the baby can become accustomed to it and any undesirable reaction recognized.

Vegetable baby food products include single-ingredient vegetable purees such as carrots, green beans, peas, squash, and sweet potatoes, which are made only from the pure vegetable and added water. Any of these single-item strained vegetable products (except peas) can be given as the baby's first vegetable. Peas are a member of the legume family and may be more allergenic than the other vegetable choices (Chiaramonte & Rao 1988). Moreover, pureed peas have the highest protein content of any single vegetable product, and, as mentioned before, extra protein intake may not be necessary for the young infant. Other strained vegetable products, such as creamed vegetables and mixed vegetables, contain ingredients other than vegetables. They may include nonfat milk, rice, oat or wheat flour, and tomato puree. These products should not be given as the baby's first foods since care must be taken when introducing these items before all the individual ingredients have first been given to the infant. In addition, spinach, beets, turnips, and collard greens are not good choices for early infancy because of their high nitrate composition, which may lead to methemoglobinemia (AAP 1980).

Meats

Single-ingredient strained meat foods, including egg yolk, are available from various baby-food companies. In general, the introduction of baby meats is not necessary even when the baby's intake of formula is reduced to 24 ounces a day and the baby is given adequate amounts of cereal, fruits, and vegetables (see Table 13–6). Eggs are a very common food allergen and their introduction into a baby's diet should be delayed, especially in children with a history of food allergies. Egg white contains most of the major allergens, whereas the allergenic components in egg yolk are considered minor (Chiaramonte & Rao 1988). Other meat products for infants include lean meat dinners with vegetables or with vegetables and starch. These combination foods should not be given to babies just beginning to eat solid foods. Mixed foods should be introduced separately. Combination foods do not allow the baby to develop a sense of the individual taste of foods, and the unit price is often greater than for single food items.

By the time the baby weighs 10 kilograms (22 lb), the intake of cow's milk should be a minimum of 24 ounces a day, and a variety of iron-fortified cereals, fruits, vegetables, and meats may be offered. In the amounts listed in Table 13–6, the daily meal pattern will provide all the nutrition needed for

Table 13–6. Progression of Foods.

Weight kg [lb]	6 [13.2]	7 [15.4]	9 [19.8]	10 [22]
Age (mo)	3–4	4–5	9–10	12–13
Infant formula (mL) [oz]*	1000 [33.3]	960 [32]	900 [30]	720 [24]
Iron-fortified infant cereal (T)†	1	8	12	16
Fruits (T)	1	8	12	16
Vegetable (T)	0	4	6	8
Meats (T)	0	0	4	8
Teething biscuit	0	0	1	0
Nutrient Composition				
Total calories	688	828	972	998
kcal/kg	115	118	108	100
% Requirements‡	106	110	110	98
Protein (g)	15.37	17.4	26.9	36.5
g/kg	2.5	2.5	3.0	3.7
% Requirements	116	113	187	304
% Vitamin requirements	100	≤95	100	100; >two thirds RDA for B_6 and D
% Mineral requirements	100	100	100 ? magnesium§	100; >two thirds RDA for calcium, phosphorus, ? magnesium, and zinc§

*Enfamil with iron, 20 kcal/kg. Mead Johnson & Company, Evansville, IN 47721.
†Nutrient composition of baby foods based on Gerber products. Nutrient values, 1988, Gerber Product Company, Tremont, MI 49412.
‡From the Committee on Dietary Allowances, Food and Nutrition Board, National Research Council. Recommended dietary allowances. 10th ed. Washington, D.C.: National Academy of Sciences, 1989.
§Nutrient analysis of baby foods are not complete for magnesium, zinc, vitamin B_{12}, vitamin D, vitamin E, and folacin.

normal growth and development. The stage will be set for healthy eating practices with a diet providing 15 percent of calories from protein, 55 percent from carbohydrate, and 30 percent from fat (see Chapter 9).

The Toddler Years

As the infant progresses into the toddler years, ages 1 to 5, feeding skills mature and a gradual transition to the family's regular diet takes place. However, the family's diet may not always be appropriate for the growing child. For example, low-fat milk and other reduced-fat dairy products are not recommended for children under the age of 2 years (AAP 1986) (see Chapters 9 and 24). Other attempts at reducing fat and cholesterol in the diets of young children as well as restricting high-energy foods and in-between meal time snacks can lead to inadequate nutrition and failure to thrive (Pugliese et al 1987). Children must receive three meals and frequent snacks of nutrient-dense foods daily to ensure an adequate diet. It is important for families to remember that what is good for adults may not always be good for babies and children because of their special nutritional needs.

A decrease in appetite is to be expected as the growth rate slows after 1 to 2 years of age. The average preschooler from 2 to 5 years of age may gain 7.0 kilograms (15.4 lb), whereas the same child will have gained this same amount of weight during the first year of life alone! Guidelines for promoting good nutrition during the preschool years include providing a variety of nutritious foods that will foster appropriate eating behaviors (see Chapter 9). Battles about food should be avoided and the use of food as a reward or punishment discouraged. Physical activity is to be maintained for normal development and to help establish a balance between caloric intake and energy expenditure.

CLINICAL INTERVENTION

The amount of breast milk or formula necessary to meet a healthy baby's nutrient requirements will vary from infant to infant. Breast-fed babies usually nurse until satisfied, and are much less likely to be pressured by mom into taking more nutrition than is needed (see Chapter 12). However, babies fed from a bottle may be encouraged to drink every last drop, whether they want to or not . . . an early version of those dreaded parental instructions to "clean your plate." Forcing those extra calories on the baby is simply overfeeding, which leads to fat babies, excessive regurgitation, spitting up, and even diarrhea. A healthy baby should always be allowed to set the limits on how much food to take and when to stop feeding. As described in Chapter 10, there is no need to worry about a baby being underfed as long as the infant takes the food that is necessary to sustain normal growth and development.

During the nursing period, up to 4 to 6 months of age, oral and neuromuscular development allow the infant to suck and swallow only liquids. The intestinal tract and kidney functions are immature during the first months of life, and foods other than breast milk or specially designed infant formulas may not be well tolerated. Moreover, babies do not need and should not be fed solid foods during this nursing period. Most solid foods are not nutritionally complete, and when they replace breast milk or formula to any extent the nursing baby's nutritional needs may not be satisfied.

Since this is the age of the microwave oven, it is necessary to point out that although they are convenient, microwave ovens should not be used to heat baby bottles. Heating formula in the microwave may cause changes in its composition and decrease its nutritional value. More importantly, using the microwave oven to warm a baby's bottle may be dangerous. The formula may become very hot while the bottle remains cool to the touch. This may lead to inadvertently feeding hot liquid to infants, thereby burning the baby's mouth, throat, or esophagus! Also, heating liquid in a closed container like a baby's bottle can cause pressure to build up and an explosion might occur (Puczynski, Rademaker & Gatson 1983). If warmed formula is desired, the bottle can be held under warm tap water and then gently shaken to redistribute the warm liquid. The temperature of the formula should always be tested before offering the bottle to a baby.

Babies give off definite signals when they are ready to start solid foods, usually at about the time they double their birth weight (age 4 to 6 months). The baby's weight, appetite, and activity will be the clinical guidelines to initiate the gradual introduction of solid food. At that time formula intake will exceed a quart a day, or the breast-fed baby will demand nursing more frequently than every 2 hours and the baby will still seem hungry. Also, the baby's oral and neuromuscular development allows him or her skills for chewing and swallowing nonliquid foods (Table 13–7). The extrusion reflex is one of the first things to disappear to allow for introduction of solid foods. This reflex helps infants nurse properly by causing the tongue to push against anything that is placed in the mouth. So, until this reflex disappears, the baby will automatically push out any solid foods entering the mouth. Introducing solid foods before this reflex decreases can lead to a lot of frustration and a very messy meal time. Another basic sign to start solid foods is an increased interest in family food. The older infant may even lean forward with mouth open and perhaps drool in anticipation of food. Until these behaviors are demonstrated, feeding of solid foods may represent a type of force-feeding (Fomon et al 1979). Baby foods should only be offered from a spoon; never from a bottle. A baby may choke on food or thickened liquids sucked through a nipple. Also, taking baby foods from a bottle will lead to the development of inappropriate eating habits and will not permit the infant to develop spoon-feeding skills.

From birth an infant has a preference for sweets. As a baby is introduced to solid foods, the sugar intake changes from the lactose of mother's milk and most formulas to sucrose (table sugar), the standard sweetener and source of empty calories in the American diet. As the baby is introduced to new foods, he or she naturally shows a preference for the sweetened varieties. However, since these sweeter foods can supply significant amounts of calories, and little in the way of nutrients, they should be given in moderation (see Chapter 1).

Juice is an item that babies usually like because of its sweetness. Excessive consumption of juice instead of milk has often been seen as a cause of failure to thrive in infants (see Chapters 16 and 17). Although juice is a very nutritious food, it cannot be a substitute for milk in babies or young children. Each bottle of juice contains only 80 to 100 calories, has no protein, and is defi-

Table 13–7. Dietary Recommendations and Feeding Guidelines During the First 6 Months of Life.

	0–2 WEEKS	2–8 WEEKS	2 MONTHS	3 MONTHS	4–5 MONTHS	5–6 MONTHS
Formula						
Ounces per feeding	2–3	3–5	4–6	5–7	5–7	5–7
Average total ounces	22	28	30	32	32	30
No. of feedings	6–8	5–6	4–5	4–5	4–5	4–5
Food texture	Liquid	Liquid	Liquid	Liquid	Liquid	Liquid
Food addition per day						
Juice from cup (oz)					1	2–4
Baby cereal					1 tsp, B & S†	2 T, B & S
Strained fruit					1 tsp, B & S	2 T, B & S
Strained vegetables					—	1–2 T, L
Strained meats					—	—
Teething biscuit					—	—
Total calories	440	475	600	640	670	800
Requirements (115 kcal/kg)*	390	414–540	540	610	690–760	760–830
Oral/neuromuscular development	Rooting, sucking, swallowing Extrusion reflex Turns mouth toward nipple Posterior tongue swallowing			Anterior tongue swallowing	No extrusion reflex Voluntary sucking	Chewing

*Estimated requirements based on a baby girl growing along the 50th percentile in weight. Smaller babies would require less while bigger babies have greater caloric and nutrient needs.

†B, L, and S stand for breakfast, lunch, and supper meals.

cient in many nutrients including calcium, vitamin D, and the B-complex vitamins. Whole milk, on the other hand, is an excellent source of calories and protein, providing 160 calories and 8 grams of protein in each cup. It is also rich in many of the vitamins and minerals that are insufficient in fruit juices. Using the newly marketed calcium-fortified juice will only replace one of the many nutritional qualities that milk has to offer growing children. Therefore, juice should be given to children only after sufficient milk has been consumed. Also, nursing-bottle syndrome with dental erosion is associated with the use of juice bottles as pacifiers, especially at bedtime (Fomon et al 1979, Loesche 1985). To avoid this dental health problem, some professionals recommend that juice be introduced only after the infant can drink from a cup.

During the latter half of the first year of life, a baby will begin to pick up bits of food with the thumb and first two fingers of the hand, and from that point on, mealtimes can be messy. With limited dexterity, the baby can't be too accurate in transferring food from the plate to the hand, and from the hand to the mouth. Often, much of the food ends up mashed back into the high-chair or onto the floor. But parents should still encourage their infant to pursue the messy process of self-feeding. It is an important time for exploration and experimentation for the baby, and this learning process is every bit as important as the actual consumption of the food. Self-feeding, starting with finger foods and advancing to utensils, is to be emphasized and supported (Satter 1987).

As babies learn to self-feed, they also learn more about the family environment, and these experiences with the taste and feel of foods tend to develop constructive eating habits. However, they may be reluctant to try new foods. Offering more highly textured foods is usually advisable as the older infant becomes more skilled with chewing and begins to have eruption of teeth. A move toward table foods can be accomplished by giving soft fruits and vegetables that are well-cooked and are mashed or blended. Canned fruits and vegetables are not recommended for the infant because of potential lead contamination. With canned vegetables, the high sodium content is undesirable and with fruit, light or heavy syrup should be avoided.

It has been suggested that early feeding practices during infancy and childhood may lead to the development of chronic diseases of adulthood such as hypertension, obesity, food allergy, and atherosclerosis (Udall & Kilbourne 1988). The tendency toward elevated blood pressure can begin in early childhood by parents exposing their babies to excessive quantities of salt in their diets (Dahl 1968, Hofman, Hazebroek & Valkenburg 1983). Thus, commercially prepared baby foods no longer contain added salt. In the early 1970s, a subcommittee of the Food Protection Committee of the Food and Nutrition Board (NRC, NAS) reported that the average dietary intake of salt by infants exceeded the minimum requirement by four to six times (Filer 1971a), and recommendations were made to reduce the salt content of infant foods. Young children do not have a natural preference for salt, so parents must realize that babies will easily accept foods with no added salt. However, infants fed greater amounts of salted food have been shown to continue to consume larger quantities of sodium later in life (Yeung, Leung & Pennell 1984). Therefore, the practice of adding extra salt to baby food to meet the parents' taste preferences should be discouraged.

There is no relationship between body fatness and type of milk feeding during infancy, whether it be breast or bottle feedings or the time of introduction of solid foods. Additionally, parents should not worry if their baby is chubby; obese babies do not necessarily become obese adults (see Chapter 18).

How an infant is fed during the first year of life also has been implicated in the development of food allergies (see Chapter 20). Babies at risk of developing food allergies are those with a strong family history. These babies may benefit if breast-milk feedings are given while the mother eats an allergen-avoidance diet (Wittig et al 1978, Saarinen et al 1979). However, other studies have reported no prolonged benefit of breast-milk feeding in preventing the development of food allergies (Halpern et al 1973, Hide & Guyer 1985). Moreover, recent studies have shown that breast milk is not completely hypoallergenic (Jakobsson & Lindberg 1983, Lake, Whitington & Hamilton 1982). Allergenic substances that can cause allergic reactions in the baby have been shown to be present in human breast milk.

The most recent nutritional controversy is whether dietary manipulation during infancy and childhood will have any impact on the development of atherosclerosis in adulthood (see Chapter 24). It is clear that atherosclerosis begins in childhood. However, no conclusive evidence shows that modifying the cholesterol intake of babies has any effect on the serum cholesterol levels of older children (Friedman & Goldberg 1975, Hodgson et al 1976). Breast milk, which is the ideal food for infants, contains 40 to 50 percent of its calories as fat, and about 150 milligrams per liter of cholesterol (Barness 1986), and usually produces a higher serum cholesterol level than that in babies fed milk formula (Friedman & Goldberg 1975). This may underline the importance of cholesterol and fat in the diet of growing infants; they are necessary for adequate energy intake as well as for the development of the central nervous system. The energy requirement for newborn babies is about three times higher than for adults based on body weight. Moreover, infancy is the time for critical brain development, especially during the first 6 to 12 months of life. Of the materials required for brain growth, approximately 60 percent is structural fat. It may also be that a high cholesterol intake during infancy may facilitate the induction of enzymes necessary for cholesterol metabolism later in life (Sanjurjo, Rodriguez-Alarcon & Rodriguez-Soriano 1988). Thus, current recommendations advise that dietary reduction in fat and cholesterol should not be undertaken in children less than 2 years of age. In general, the best diets for growing children are the ones that avoid extremes.

REFERENCES

American Academy of Pediatrics Committee on Nutrition. Commentary in breast-feeding and infant-formulas, including proposed standards for formulas. Pediatrics 1976; 57:278–285.

American Academy of Pediatrics Committee on Nutrition. Fluoride supplementation: Revised dosage schedule. Pediatrics 1979; 63:150–152.

American Academy of Pediatrics Committee on Nutrition. On the feeding of supplemental foods to infants. Pediatrics 1980; 65:1178–1181.

American Academy of Pediatrics Committee on Nutrition. The use of whole cow's milk in infancy. Pediatrics 1983a; 72:253–255.

American Academy of Pediatrics Committee on Nutrition. Soy-protein formulas: Recommendations for use in infant feeding. Pediatrics 1983b; 72:359–363.

American Academy of Pediatrics Committee on Nutrition. Forbes GB, Woodruff CW, eds. Pediatric nutrition handbook. 2nd ed. Elk Grove Village, IL: American Academy of Pediatrics, 1985.

American Academy of Pediatrics Committee on Nutrition. Prudent life-style for children: Dietary fat and cholesterol. Pediatrics 1986; 78:521–525.

Andersen GH, Morson-Pasut LA, Bryan H, et al. Age of introduction of cow's milk to infants. J Pediatr Gastroenterol Nutr 1985; 4:692–698.

Barness LA. Cholesterol and children. JAMA 1986; 256:2871.

Chiaramonte LT, Rao YAK. Common food allergens. In Chiaramonte LT, Schneider AT, Lifshitz F, eds. Food allergy: A practical approach to diagnosis and management. New York: Marcel Dekker, 1988:89–106.

Cook JD, Morck TA, Lynch SR. The inhibitory effect of the soy products on nonheme iron absorption in man. Am J Clin Nutr 1981; 34:2622–2629.

Dahl LK. Salt in processed baby foods. Am J Clin Nutr 1968; 21:787–792.

Filer LJ Jr. Salt in infant foods. Nutr Rev 1971a; 29:27–30.

Filer LJ Jr. Modified food starches for use in infant foods. Nutr Rev 1971b; 29:55–59.

Fomon SJ. Bioavailability of supplemental iron in commercially prepared dry infant cereals. J Pediatr 1987a; 110:660–661.

Fomon SJ. Reflections on infant feeding in the 1970s and 1980s. Am J Clin Nutr 1987b; 46:171–182.

Fomon SJ, Filer LJ Jr, Andersen TA, et al. Recommendations for feeding normal infants. Pediatrics 1979; 63:52–59.

Fomon SJ, Filer LJ Jr, Ziegler EE, Bergmann KE, Bergmann RL. Skim milk in infant feeding. Acta Paediatr Scan 1977; 66:17–30.

Fomon SJ, Ziegler EE, Nelson SE, Edwards BB. Cow milk feeding in infancy: Gastrointestinal blood loss and iron nutritional status. J Pediatr 1981; 98:540–545.

Fomon SJ, Ziegler EE, Nelson SE, Edwards BB. Requirements for sulfur-

containing amino acids in infancy. J Nutr 1986; 116:1405–1422.
Foucard T. Development of food allergies with special reference to cow's milk allergy. Pediatrics 1985; 75(Suppl):177–181.
Friedman G, Goldberg SJ. Concurrent and subsequent serum cholesterols of breast- and formula-fed infants. Am J Clin Nutr 1975; 28:42–45.
George DE, Lebenthal E. Human breast milk in comparison to cow's milk. In Lebenthal E, ed. Textbook of gastroenterology and nutrition. New York: Raven Press, 1981:295–320.
Glaser J, Johnstone DE. Prophylaxis of allergenic disease in the newborn. JAMA 1953; 153:620–622.
Halpern SR, Sellars WA, Johnson RB, et al. Development of childhood allergy in infants fed breast, soy or cow milk. J Allergy Clin Immunol 1973; 51:139–151.
Hertrampf E, Cayazzo M, Pizarro F, Stekel A. Bioavailability of iron in soy-based formula and its effect on iron nutriture in infancy. Pediatrics 1986; 78:640–645.
Hide DW, Guyer BM. Clinical manifestations of allergy related to breast and cow's milk feeding. Pediatrics 1985; 76:973–975.
Hodgson PA, Ellefson RD, Elvebach LR, et al. Comparison of serum cholesterol in children fed high, moderate or low cholesterol milk diets during the neonatal period. Metabolism 1976; 25:739–746.
Hofman A, Hazebroek A, Valkenburg HA. A randomized trial of sodium intake and blood pressure in newborn infants. JAMA 1983; 250:370–373.
Hurrell RF. Bioavailability of different iron compounds used to fortify formulas and cereals: Technological problems. In Stekel A, ed. Iron nutrition in infancy and childhood. New York: Raven Press, 1984:147–178.
Jakobsson I, Lindberg T. Cow's milk protein cause infantile colic in breast-fed infants: A double-blind crossover study. Pediatrics 1983; 71:268–271.
Jakobsson I, Lindberg T, Benediktsson B, Hansson BG. Dietary bovine B lactoglobulin is transferred to human milk. Acta Pediatr Scand 1985; 74:342–345.
Jarvenpaa AL, Raiha NCR, Rassin DK, Gaull GE. Milk protein quantity and quality in the term infant. I. Metabolic responses and effects on growth. Pediatrics 1982; 70:214–220.
Koo WWK, Kaplan LA. Aluminum contamination of infant formulas. JPEN 1988a; 12:170–173.
Koo WWK, Kaplan LA. Aluminum and bone disorders: With specific reference to aluminum contamination of infant nutrients. J Am Coll Nutr 1988b; 7:199–214.
Lake AM, Whitington PF, Hamilton SR. Dietary protein-induced colitis in breast-fed infants. J Pediatr 1982; 101:906–910.
Lifshitz F. Perspectives of carbohydrate intolerance in infants with diarrhea. In Lifshitz F, ed. Carbohydrate intolerance in infancy. New York: Marcel Dekker, 1982:3–20.
Lifshitz F. Nutrition for special needs in infancy: Protein hydrolysates. New York: Marcel Dekker, 1985.
Loesche WJ. Nutrition and dental decay in infants. Am J Clin Nutr 1985; 41:423–435.
Lonnerdal B, Bell JG, Hendrickx AG, Burns RA, Keen CL. Effect of phytate re-

moval in zinc absorption from soy formula. Am J Clin Nutr 1988; 48:1301–1306.

Martinez GA, Nalezienski JP. The recent trend in breast-feeding. Pediatrics 1979; 64:686–692.

Martinez GA, Ryan AS, Malec DJ. Nutrient intakes of American infants and children fed cow's milk or infant formula. Am J Dis Child 1985; 139:1010–1018.

Mata L. Breast feeding, diarrheal disease, and malnutrition in less developed countries. In Lifshitz F, ed. Pediatric nutrition: Infant feedings, deficiencies, diseases. New York: Marcel Dekker, 1982:355–372.

Miles JP. Analytical methods used by industry for lead in infant formula. J Assoc Off Anal Chem 1982; 65:1016–1024.

Nelson SE, Ziegler EE, Copeland AM, Edwards BB, Fomon SJ. Iron-fortified formula: Lack of adverse reactions. Pediatrics 1988; 81:360–364.

Oski FA. Is bovine milk a health hazard? Pediatrics 1985; 75(Suppl):182–186.

Puczynski M, Rademaker D, Gatson RL. Burn injury related to the improper use of a microwave oven. Pediatrics 1983; 72:714.

Pugliese MT, Weyman-Daum M, Moses N, Lifshitz F. Parental health beliefs as a cause of nonorganic failure to thrive. Pediatrics 1987; 80:175–182.

Radbill SX. Infant-feeding through the ages. Clin Pediatr 1981; 20:613–621.

Raiha NCR, Heinonen K, Rassin DK, Gaull GE. Milk protein quantity and quality in low-birthweight infants. I. Metabolic responses and effects on growth. Pediatrics 1976; 57:659–674.

Rees JM, Monsen ER, Merrill JE. Iron fortification of infant foods: A decade of change. Clin Pediatr 1985; 24:707–710.

Ryan AS, Gussler JD. The international breast-feeding compendium. 3rd ed rev. Columbus, OH: Ross Laboratories, 1986.

Ryu JE, Ziegler EE, Nelson SE, Fomon SJ. Dietary intake of lead and blood lead concentration in early infancy. Am J Dis Child 1983; 137:886–891.

Saarinen UM, Kajosaari M, Backman A, et al. Prolonged breast-feeding as prophylaxis for atopic disease. Lancet 1979; 2:163–166.

Sanjurjo P, Rodriguez-Alarcon J, Rodriguez-Soriano J. Plasma fatty acid composition during the first week of life following feeding with human milk or formula. Acta Paediatr Scand 1988; 77:202–206.

Satter E. How to get your kid to eat . . . but not too much. Palo Alto, CA: Bull Publishing Co., 1987.

Sawaya WN, Khalil JK, Al-Shalhat AF. Mineral and vitamin content of goat's milk. J Am Diet Assoc 1984; 84:433–435.

Steichen JJ, Tsang RC. Bone mineralization and growth in term infants fed soy-based or cow milk-based formula. J Pediatr 1987; 110:687–692.

Udall JN Jr, Kilbourne KA. Selected aspects of infant feeding. Nutrition 1988; 4:409–417.

Wittig HJ, McLaughlin ET, Leifer KL, Belloit JD. Risk factors for the development of allergic disease: Analysis of 2,190 patient records. Ann Allergy 1978; 41:84–88.

Yeung DL, Leung M, Pennell MD. Relationship between sodium intake in infancy and at 4 years of age. Nutr Res 1984; 4:553.

14

Fuel for Exercise*

Peggy loved to dance! She can still remember how excited she was to get her first pair of ballet slippers. Peggy would forever be jumping, stretching and turning—it seemed as if she never sat still. Peggy always wanted to become a professional dancer, and on her 11th birthday her dream was to be realized. She was offered a summer scholarship at a prestigious ballet company in New York City where she would be participating in three 1½-hour ballet classes a day for 8 weeks. On her first day, she could not believe how thin the dancers were. They always wore plastic sweat suits to help them "lose weight" and they would hardly eat anything all day. They drank special beverages with added electrolytes and took salt tablets. When they did eat, they would choose high-protein foods; they told Peggy it would help build muscles instead of fat. Peggy was embarrassed to show the other dancers the lunches and snacks her mother had lovingly packed for her, which included two sandwiches, pretzels, two pieces of fruit, and two thermoses filled with juice. Her teacher told her that if she was going to be a ballet dancer, her diet would certainly have to change.

Obtaining fuel for exercise is not really very different from providing nourishment for other purposes. There are no magical foods or supplements to be given to the athlete. Given the increased expenditure associated with physical activity, it is important that all nutrient requirements be met. To date, we know of no specific nutrient, whether it be protein, vitamins, or minerals, that will enhance physical performance. Contrary to the scientific facts, adults and children in training often embark on different diets or take food supplements purported to enhance their skills or to meet their altered nutri-

*Ms. Pat Larsen made significant contributions to the final version of this chapter.

tional standards. The competitive atmosphere in athletics, even among school sporting events, makes the child and teenager very susceptible to the lure of diets and other medications that are advocated to give the "winning edge." An enormous number of athletes use nutrient supplements without any knowledge of why, how, and when to use them. The nutritional practices of 2977 athletes in the United States, including high-school adolescents, revealed that a large number of them used vitamin, mineral, and protein supplements (Parr, Porter & Hodgson 1984). Although it may not be very glamorous or exciting, the best nutrition for peak athletic performance is a well-balanced diet that provides all the nutrient needs for the individual child or teenager (see Chapter 9).

NUTRITION GUIDELINES FOR EXERCISE

Energy

A well-balanced diet that provides 55 to 60 percent of total calories from carbohydrate is generally recommended for all healthy children to provide all their energy needs (see Chapter 9). Energy requirements for the physically active child are increased substantially, and dietary intakes should be modified to meet the energy cost of the sport. Based on the type, intensity, and duration of exercise, energy requirements could increase by 35 to 85 percent as a result of exercise training (Tables 14–1 and 14–2). Thus, a child involved in a high-intensity or long-duration exercise training program would have higher energy requirements than a more sedentary child of the same age. In a study of ballet dancers it was found that their diet did not fulfill the requirements for protein, carbohydrate, and some of the micronutrients (Cohen et al 1985). However, normal vitamin status was found, probably because of high intake of vitamin supplements. Most determinations of energy expenditure are based on studies in adults, not growing children. Therefore, the best clinical tool to ensure that the athletic child is receiving an adequate caloric intake over time is to monitor growth. Maintaining normal weight gain and linear growth will indicate that the athletic child has been able to increase dietary intake to meet the greater energy needs (see Chapter 10).

Certain sports make demands on the weight of the participants. Limited-weight sports such as wrestling, gymnastics, dancing, and skating stress a low body weight for competition and maximum performance. These athletes may participate in inappropriate eating behaviors to control their weight (Steen 1988, Brownell, Steen & Wilmore 1987). Severe caloric restrictions and intermittent fasting, laxative and diuretic abuse, and vomiting may be employed to reduce weight to meet set goals at a given time or throughout the duration of the child's involvement in the activity. The result of such practices

Table 14–1. Energy Demands of Various Activities.

ACTIVITY	INTENSITY	KCAL/LB/MIN
Badminton	Average	0.044
Dancing	Fast	0.075
Table tennis	Average	0.080
Tennis	Average	0.049
Swimming (crawl)	20 yd/min	0.032
	45 yd/min	0.058
	50 yd/min	0.070
Bicycling	13 mph	0.045
	15 mph	0.049
	19 mph	0.076
	21 mph	0.090
	23 mph	0.109
	25 mph	0.139
Running	11:30 min/mi— 5.2 mph	0.061
	9:00 min/mi— 6.7 mph	0.088
	8:00 min/mi— 7.5 mph	0.094
	7:00 min/mi— 9.0 mph	0.103
	6:00 min/mi—10.0 mph	0.114
	5:30 min/mi—11.0 mph	0.131

Modified from the American College of Sports Medicine, Encyclopedia of sports sciences and medicine. New York: Macmillan 1971:1128–1129.

is inadequate nutrition to support normal growth and sexual development. Moreover, these practices may also result in impaired performance and endangerment of physical health. Numerous negative metabolic and performance effects of this cyclical behavior have been reported, including loss of lean body mass, dehydration, decreased muscle glycogen content, lowered blood volume, greater electrolyte losses, impaired temperature regulation, tachycardia, decreased muscular strength and/or endurance, more frequent fractures, and disturbed reproductive function.

Other sporting events, such as football and sumo wrestling, believe that "bigger is better." These athletes may practice binging behavior and consume excessive calories to promote rapid weight gain, which is often mostly un-

Table 14–2. Average Daily Energy Demands of Various Sports for Males.

ACTIVITY	KCAL/LB/DAY
Nonathlete	107
Cross-country skier	198
Marathon runner	191
Weight lifter	167
Shotput, discus thrower	149

Modified from the American College of Sports Medicine, Encyclopedia of sports sciences and medicine. New York: Macmillan 1971:1128–1129.

wanted fat. Excess weight may be associated with serious health consequences including diabetes, heart disease, and hypertension (see Chapter 18). Regardless of the goal weight for a particular athletic endeavor, children should compete in their "weight category" in accordance with their genetic endowment . . . it's foolish to try to trick nature!

For the athlete who is involved in endurance activities that may last for more than 1 hour, maximizing carbohydrate storage in the body as muscle glycogen has been recommended to improve performance (Costill 1985). To maximize muscle glycogen, different types of "carbohydrate loading" techniques have been popular among athletes and their trainers. Among the most dramatic regimens is a day of exhaustive exercise to "deplete glycogen stores" followed by a high-fat, high-protein, low-carbohydrate diet. After 2 to 3 days of this diet, a second exhaustive training program is undertaken. Then, the individual rests and consumes a high-carbohydrate diet (80–95 percent of calories) for 3 to 7 days until the competition. This regimen can be harmful and is not recommended for anybody, especially growing children. Some negative side effects associated with "carbohydrate loading" include excessive weight gain and fat accumulation, water retention, and gastrointestinal discomfort. In addition, individuals consuming such diets may show abnormal blood tests, including increased serum triglycerides, glucose, and urea nitrogen, and may have cardiac disturbances (Wright 1988). During the low-carbohydrate-diet phase, there may be fatigue as well as irritability and reduced cognitive functioning (Gollnick & Matoba 1984). Moreover, the low-carbohydrate phase of "carbohydrate loading" regimens is not necessary to achieve supercompensation of muscle glycogen stores following glycogen-depleting exercise (Sherman et al 1981).

A modified approach to enhance glycogen stores may be more appropriate for the young athlete (Sherman et al 1981, Hargreaves et al 1984). Because of the importance of carbohydrate as an exercise fuel (Costill 1988, Sherman & Lamb 1988), and because glycogen stores in the body are limited, most of the increased energy intake associated with exercise training presumably should be in the form of carbohydrate. It is generally recommended that athletes (especially endurance athletes) increase their carbohydrate intake from 55 to 60 percent to 60 to 70 percent (Costill 1988, Costill & Miller 1980). Under special circumstances a higher carbohydrate diet (up to 70 percent of calories from carbohydrate) may be offered for 3 days before a very intense competition. The type of carbohydrate, simple or complex, does not seem to affect the body's capacity to make glycogen (Costill & Miller 1980). Simultaneously, exercise training is modified to be maximal at the beginning of the high-carbohydrate dietary regimen and gradually be reduced until the match. This method yields an increase in body glycogen stores without the disadvantages of the dramatic variations described above. However, care must be taken to provide all the necessary nutrients during carbohydrate loading. A reduced intake of any essential dietary component may hamper aerobic oxidative pathways and decrease the athlete's endurance and performance (Jette et al 1978).

Carbohydrate loading is not necessary for most young athletes, but a moderate increase in carbohydrate intake may be advisable for those involved in athletic competition that requires endurance and high energy demands for more than 1 hour at a time. A large quantity of carbohydrate can add excessive bulk to the diet. This may be difficult for young athletes to consume (more so if most of the carbohydrate is in the form of starch). Eating 4 to 6 meals a day will reduce the impact of the bulk; however, it may be necessary to add simple carbohydrate snacks or liquid carbohydrate supplements to maintain energy balance. Long-term ingestion of a high-carbohydrate diet (one that provides 80 percent of the calories as carbohydrate) should be discouraged. This type of dietary intake leads to changes in insulin secretion and elevated triglyceride levels with reduced high-density lipoprotein (HDL) levels (Coulston, Liv & Reaven 1983) and consequently increases the risk of atherosclerotic disease (see Chapter 24). Although in sedentary individuals intake of carbohydrate above the recommended for age and sex is associated with elevated blood triglyceride concentrations, this may not be the case with more active individuals who take excess sugar in accordance with their energy expenditures. This is probably because the carbohydrate is used to restore liver and muscle glycogen rather than to synthesize fat (Costill et al 1979).

Protein

On the surface, it makes sense that if exercise builds muscle and muscle is made from protein, then physical activity must increase protein requirements (Young & Torun 1981, Lemon 1987). This type of thinking has led body builders competing in physique contests to consume 255 to 400 grams of protein a day and induce negative health consequences (Darden & Schendel 1971). Although most studies suggest that exercise increases protein requirements, the actual protein need is difficult to determine and will depend on the type of activity, degree of training, and exercise intensity (Fig. 14–1). Based on nitrogen balance measures, Tarnopolsky and colleagues (1988) reported that the protein intake for zero nitrogen balance was greater in both young adult body-builders (around 24 years of age) and endurance athletes than for sedentary subjects of the same age. From these data, they estimated the recommended or safe protein intake to be 112 percent and 162 percent of the current protein RDA for body builders and endurance runners, respectively.

Protein requirements also depend on overall energy and nutrient intake. If energy intake is increased to maintain normal weight during exercise, the

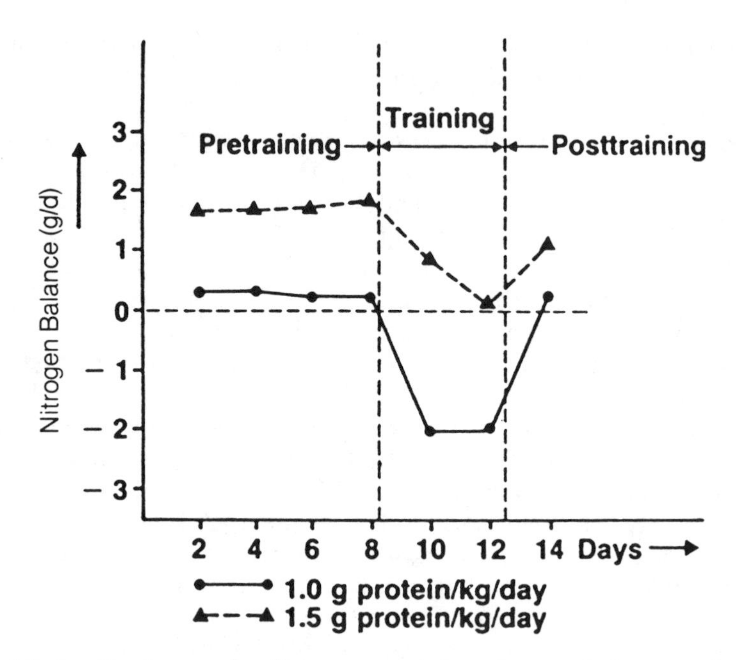

Figure 14–1. Gontzea and colleagues used the nitrogen balance technique to determine dietary protein needs. His group observed that nitrogen balance became negative when untrained subjects (21–29 years) began an endurance exercise program while consuming 125 percent of the RDA for protein. A continued negative nitrogen balance would lead to decreased muscle mass and presumably impaired athletic performance. When the experiment was repeated at 188 percent of the RDA for protein, nitrogen balance remained positive, indicating the the protein intake was sufficient to maintain muscle mass.

From Gontzea I, Sutzescu P, Duitrache S. The influence of muscular activity on the nitrogen balance and on the need of man for protein. Nutrition Reports International. J Nutr Biochem 1974; 10:33–43. Copyright 1974, Butterworth-Heinemann. Reproduced by permission of the publisher.

established recommended dietary allowance for protein intake will be adequate to promote positive nitrogen balance (Butterfield & Calloway 1984, Dohm 1984). In contrast, if energy intake is insufficient, negative nitrogen balance will occur unless additional protein is provided. An energy deficit, whether it is caused by decreased intake or increased energy expenditure, will lead to negative nitrogen balance (Goranzon & Forsum 1985) and subsequent losses of lean body mass. To preserve muscle mass, it is therefore necessary to at least match any increase in energy expenditure with an increase in dietary intake. Maintaining muscle mass in athletes is extremely important because reduced muscle mass will negatively affect performance due to a loss in strength. If energy intake decreases, the chances of incurring a nutritional deficiency are greatly increased. This may also have a negative effect on growth (see Chapters 9 and 10). This is especially important for adolescent athletes because of their accelerated growth requirements. During adolescence it is extremely important to balance energy intake and energy expenditure carefully to minimize losses of lean body mass. Since American children usually consume more than the recommended amount of dietary protein (see Chapter 9), additional protein supplements are not usually necessary for the athletic child.

However, athletes, specifically weight-lifters and body-builders, continue to use protein supplements to improve exercise performance and build bigger muscles. The underlying mechanism responsible for the potentially beneficial effects of additional dietary protein on muscle strength and size is unclear. As mentioned before, Tarnopolsky and associates (1988) found that the protein requirement of body-builders was elevated relative to sedentary controls. However, the increase in protein needs was very modest relative to what typical-strength athletes routinely consume or to the intake that produced substantial gains in strength and size in the study by Dragan and colleagues (1985). Many studies have shown that there is no improvement in muscle size (hypertrophy), muscle strength, or physical performance with high-protein diets (Rasch, Hamby & Burns 1969, Marable et al 1979). Only training will increase muscle size within the limitations of the individual's genetic potential. Protein intake in excess of requirements will be used for energy or converted to fat. In either case, metabolism of excess protein will require more water and may exacerbate dehydration, which is a more important problem during exercise. Also, high-protein diets have been associated with other complications; for example, there may be increased urinary calcium excretion (Allen, Oddoye & Margen 1979). This may be of particular concern in growing children who may already have insufficient dietary calcium intakes (see Chapter 9). High-protein diets may also compromise renal function over time (see Chapters 22 and 23). There is no scientific evidence to justify use of protein supplements.

Fat

Adipose tissue in the body acts as a storage for fatty acid fuel, which is used during aerobic exercise. Since body fat stores are greater than carbohydrate (glycogen) stores, fatty acids provide most of the muscle's fuel as the duration of exercise is extended. Depending on a person's nutritional status and level and duration of physical activity, 30 to 80 percent of the energy for aerobic work is usually derived from fat molecules. One pound of fat provides enough energy to support 30 to 40 miles of long-distance running. However, as glycogen stores are reduced and fatty acids begin to contribute energy, reduced muscle performance and fatigue will occur (Gollnick & Matoba 1984). Without any carbohydrate present, there is a deficiency of metabolic intermediates necessary to make the energy cycle turn (TCA cycle), and severe ketoacidosis may occur. This is referred to by runners as "hitting the wall."

Exercise training will improve fatty acid utilization for energy (Gollnick 1985). Fat is the preferred fuel for aerobic endurance activities, but it is the fat from adipose tissue that is utilized, not dietary fat. Although the use of ketogenic (high-fat, low-carbohydrate) diets under strict medical supervision has been shown to increase utilization of fatty acids and decrease glycogen depletion during exercise (Phinney et al 1980), the efficacy of high-fat diets in improving exercise performance has not been clearly demonstrated, and such diets are not recommended for the young athlete. Ensuing electrolyte imbalances can lead to cardiac and renal dysfunction. In addition, diets that provide fat in excess of 35 percent of the total calorie intake may be associated with increased risk of coronary heart disease (see Chapter 24).

Water and Electrolytes

Exercise increases the child's need for water. Water is needed for the metabolism of the nutrients used for fuel and to replace the extra losses of water through sweat (Costill et al 1984). Dehydration is a major enemy of the athlete. Children's thermoregulatory efficiency is lower than adults (Bar-Or 1980). Therefore, the young athlete has a potentially higher risk of contracting heat-related illnesses. Children expend more chemical energy per unit mass than do adults while performing similar tasks. As a result, they produce greater metabolic heat per kilogram of body weight which, during intense exercise, subjects their thermoregulatory system to a greater strain. Some authors have reported that as little as 3 percent dehydration of total body weight can interfere with athletic endurance and performance by decreasing cardiovascular and thermoregulatory capacity (Bijlani & Sharma 1980). However, there is research (Guastella et al, unpublished data) that shows that dehydration of less than 4 percent does not affect anaerobic power. Dehydration of more than that amount causes severe reduction in muscle strength and endurance (Senay & Pivarnik 1985), and dehydration greater than 6 percent of total body weight can be life-threatening. It is therefore extremely important to achieve positive water balance during exercise by consuming adequate fluid intake before, during, and after exercising.

Extensive literature emphasizes the importance of maintaining water, electrolyte, and energy (carbohydrate) balance in order to maintain optimal performance capacity and to reduce the risk of complete exhaustion (Blom et al 1987, Costill & Miller 1980). Plain water is the best fluid to drink to avoid exercise-induced dehydration, since the body loses much more water than electrolytes during exercise.

The osmolarity of ingested fluid may determine gastric motility and emptying (Table 14–3). A solution containing 20 milliequivalents of salt per liter,

Table 14–3. Replacement Fluids.

PRODUCT	FLUID OUNCES	CALORIES (KCAL)	CARBOHYDRATE (G)	SODIUM (MG)	POTASSIUM (MG)	FAT (G)	PROTEIN (G)
Cola (regular)	12	164	41	18	7	0	0
	8	96	20.5	9	3.5	0	0
Gatorade Thirst							
Quencher	8	50	14	110	25	0	0
Orange	8	50	14	45 mg/100 g	10 mg/100 g	0	0
Lemon/Lime	8	50	14	45 mg/100 g	10 mg/100 g	0	0
Citrus	8	50	14	45 mg/100 g	10 mg/100 g	0	0
Fruit Punch	8	50	14	45 mg/100 g	10 mg/100 g	0	0
Lemonade from concentrate	8	94	23	26	100	Tr*	Tr*
Orange juice (raw)	8	94	26	20	496	0	2
Recharge Tropical Thirst							
Quencher	8	70	18	35	85	0	0
Orange	8	50	13	15	25	0	0
				5.9 mg/100 g			
Lemon	8	72	17.6	30	86.9 mg	0	0
				15 mg/100 g			
Rubykist lemonade	6	100	25	10	—	0	0
Sprint fresh lime	8	72	17.6	110	150	0	0

*Tr = trace. Data as given on product labels.

for example, will be emptied faster than water. Fluids with high-salt content, however, will retard gastric emptying, as will sugar solutions that exceed 25 grams of glucose per liter. Addition of salt in liberal quantities to the regular diet is practiced by many athletes, often in the form of salt tablets. Such a habit is not beneficial for children and may even be detrimental. The American College of Sports Medicine Position Statement on Prevention of Heat Injuries During Long Distance Running recommends that adult runners periodically drink fluid that includes not more than 10 milliequivalents of sodium per liter, 5 milliequivalents of potassium per liter, and 2.5 grams of glucose per liter. Children, because of the low salt content of their sweat, should have drinks that do not exceed 5 milliequivalents of sodium per liter (0.3 g/L NaCl), 4 milliequivalents of potassium per liter (0.28 g/L KCl), and 2.5 grams of glucose per liter.

How Much Fluid Is Enough? For athletic children, a simple and reliable gauge is thirst and body weight. One should strive to attain a postactivity body weight identical to that of the preactivity level. However, special drinks with sugar and electrolytes are often selected by athletes to replace fluid losses because of their advertised "beneficial effect" (see Table 14–3). Sugar and electrolyte solutions may slow the rate of absorption of water owing to delayed emptying from the stomach (Costill & Saltin 1974), although drinks containing moderate levels of carbohydrate (6 percent) and low-carbohydrate electrolyte-containing beverages (2.5 percent glucose) are similar to water in fluid replenishment capacity (Davis et al 1988). There is no advantage in performance or endurance associated with ingestion of moderate-carbohydrate-containing drinks as compared with water (Coyle et al 1986). Therefore, concentrated sugar waters are generally considered to be poor and unnecessary choices to replace water lost during exercise (see Table 14–3). The idea that cold water causes cramps is a fallacy. In fact, cold drinks (<20° C; 60° F) empty more quickly from the stomach than warm drinks and therefore reduce the gastric distress associated with abdominal distention (Costill & Saltin 1974). In addition, cold drinks cool off the body!

Salt tablets and potassium supplements are generally not necessary for the young athlete. Excessive salt intake may further compound dehydration by accelerating water loss. There is limited evidence to support the concept that potassium depletion will develop while exercising (Costill et al 1984). Low serum sodium concentration (hyponatremia) is a concern during athletic activities of long duration (>5 hours) in warm weather and during the first 1 to 2 weeks of training. Under these conditions the athlete may lose large quantities of sodium in sweat and/or drink excessive amounts of water (Frizzeu et al 1986, Williams 1985). When strenuous exercise leads to excessive water losses of more than 5 to 10 pounds a day (more than 3 percent loss of body weight), one salt tablet (7 g) or teaspoon of salt (5 g) per quart of water is recommended (Wright 1988, O'Neil, Hynak-Hankinson & Gorman 1986). However, others have suggested that because salt tablets can be gastric irritants and cause nausea and vomiting, their use should be avoided entirely (ACSM 1975).

Vitamins and Minerals

Vitamins have been thought to have the ability to give an "energy boost," to "maximize performance," and to "alleviate the extra stress of competition." Vitamin manufacturers have even gone so far as to invent "new vitamins," such as "vitamin B_{15}," to enhance exercise capacity. This type of propaganda is very enticing to a young athlete who is seeking the competitive edge. Clearly, nutrient deficiency states, such as iron-deficiency anemia (Edgerton et al 1979), and restriction of water-soluble vitamins (van der Beek et al 1988) have been shown to have a negative affect on physical endurance. Van der Beek (1985) has reviewed the need for vitamins in relation to athletic performance. He concluded that the intake must meet the recommendations, but that higher intake does not increase athletic performance. At present, there is no evidence to support the notion that vitamin and mineral supplementation in already well-nourished individuals improves athletic performance (Weight, Myburg & Noakes 1988).

Some studies suggest that there may be an increased need for vitamins and minerals during exercise (Belko 1987) (Table 14–4). There has been a suggestion of increased requirements for vitamin C (Buzina et al 1984) and riboflavin (Belko et al 1983, 1984), and reduced plasma concentrations of B vitamins, copper, magnesium, and zinc have been reported in long-distance runners (Van Dam 1978, Haralambie 1981, Dressendorfer et al 1982). Also, a greater incidence of iron deficiency, especially among women athletes, has been noted (Clement & Sawchuck 1984, Haymes 1987). However, a more recent evaluation of male long-distance runners revealed normal biochemical status of the forementioned nutrients and no need for additional supplementation if the athletes consumed a well-balanced diet (Weight et al 1988). Further investigation of nutrient requirements during exercise in young people is required to address the question of altered vitamin and mineral needs.

CLINICAL INTERVENTION

Children and teenagers are often disappointed when they are told that there are no magic foods to enhance their athletic aims and that they should eat a well-balanced diet for exercise training. Special protein drinks to build muscles, high-potency vitamin and mineral supplements for the additional "stress" of exercise, exotic colored liquids to replace electrolyte losses in sweat, and fad diets to maximize athletic performance may add glamour and

Table 14–4. Theoretic and Actual Roles of Vitamins During Exercise.

VITAMIN	THEORETIC BENEFIT	ACTUAL BENEFIT
A	Glycogen biosynthesis	None
Biotin	Gluconeogenesis	None
Thiamin (B_1)	Carbohydrate metabolism Hemoglobin synthesis	Increased requirement with increased energy expenditure and increased carbohydrate intake
Riboflavin (B_2)	Fatty acid oxidation	None
B_6	Protein metabolism Hemoglobin synthesis Breakdown of glycogen to glucose	None
B_{12}	Red blood cell synthesis	None
C	Oxygen consumption	None
D	None	None
E	Protect red blood cell integrity	None except in high altitudes
Folic acid	DNA synthesis Red blood cell synthesis	None
Niacin	Anaerobic energy cycle	Deficiency may occur in high-carbohydrate diets with resultant reduced endurance
Pantothenic acid	Fatty acid oxidation	None

Adapted from Belko AZ. Vitamins and exercise—an update. Med Sci Sports Exer 1987; 19:5191–5196.

excitement for the young athlete, but these practices are ineffective and may even be harmful to the health of the child. Examples of the negative impact of nutrition practices on athletic performance are often found among wrestlers who compete in a weight category in which they do not belong and who starve to lose weight. After "weighing in" for the match they overeat to get back their strength. However, high-protein, high-fat meals do not provide a ready source of energy and are difficult to digest, often leaving the athlete feeling full and bloated. Protein and extra salt could also serve to exacerbate dehydration due to increased fluid loss. Ingestion right before the match of "quick" energy, such as chocolates and "Gatorade," may also be detrimental since carbohydrate ingestion within 30 minutes of a physical activity causes insulin secretion, which interferes with fatty acid utilization, the major fuel for exercise.

A more appropriate pregame strategy for an athlete should include competing in an appropriate weight category and ingesting an adequate diet that promotes good nutritional health throughout life (see Chapter 9). Wrestlers might not benefit from high carbohydrate intake for 3 days before the competition, as is recommended for longer endurance athletes such as marathon runners. For them, a light, high-carbohydrate meal 2 to 3 hours before competing, or a more substantial meal 3 to 4 hours before the match, would be recommended. Excessive fat, protein, and fiber intake should be avoided as these substances will lead to delayed gastric emptying, intestinal residue, and abdominal distention.

Adequate fluid intake of 8 to 16 ounces of water or juice is recommended to promote hydration. Often, liquid meal replacements can be used 1 to 2 hours before an event (see Chapter 19). These supplements are low in fiber and increase fluid intake. Liquid meals are beneficial for young athletes who are participating in all-day competition, when there is little time for or interest in eating. A high carbohydrate intake should be avoided less than 30 minutes before the event, but providing carbohydrates during the activity may have a positive influence.

For competitive and recreational athletes and for all those who search for fuel for exercise it must be remembered that nutritional health does not depend on consumption of specific foods or food products but on meeting all the nutrient needs from a variety of foods in a mixed, well-balanced diet (Hecker 1984, Wilmore & Freund 1984, Williams 1985). Athletes are at increased risk for the development of eating disorders (see Chapter 17), cessation of normal menstrual periods (Green, Weiss & Daling 1988), and the consequences of inadequate nutrition.

REFERENCES

Allen LH, Oddoye EA, Margen S. Protein-induced hypercalcuria: A longer term study. Am J Clin Nutr 1979; 32:741–749.

American College of Sports Medicine. Encyclopedia of sports sciences and medicine. New York: Macmillan 1971:1128–1192.

American College of Sports Medicine. Position statement on prevention of heat injuries during distance running. Med Sci Sports 1975; 7(1):vii–viii.

Bar-Or O. Climate and the exercising child—a review. Int J Sports Med 1980; 1:53–65.

Belko AZ. Vitamins and exercise—an update. Med Sci Sports Exerc 1987; 19:5191–5196.

Belko AZ, Obarzanek E, Kalkarf HJ, et al. Effects of exercise on riboflavin requirements of young women. Am J Clin Nutr 1983; 37:509–517.

Belko AZ, Obarzanek E, Roach R, et al. Effects of aerobic exercise and weight loss on riboflavin requirements of moderately obese, marginally deficient young women. Am J Clin Nutr 1984; 40:553–561.

Bijlani RL, Sharma KN. Effect of dehydration and a few regimens of rehydration on human performance. Indian J. Physiol Pharmacol 1980; 24:255–266.

Blom PCS, Hostmark AT, Vaage O, Kardel KR, Maehlum S. Effect of different post-exercise sugar diets on the rate of muscle glycogen synthesis. Med Sci Sports Exerc 1987; 19:491–496.

Brownell KD, Steen SN, Wilmore JH. Weight regulation practices in athletes: Analysis of metabolic and health effects. Med Sci Sports Exerc 1987; 19:546–556.

Butterfield GE, Calloway DH. Physical activity improves protein utilization in young men. Br J Nutr 1984; 51:171–184.

Buzina K, Buzina R, Brubacker G, Sapunar J, Christeuer S. Vitamin C status and physical working capacity in adolescents. Int J Vit Nutr Res 1984; 54:55–60.

Clement DB, Sawchuck LL. Iron status and sports performance. Sports Med 1984; 1:65–74.

Cohen JL, Potosnak L, Frank O, Baker H. A nutritional and hematologic assessment of elite ballet dancers. Phys Sportsmed 1985; 13(5):43–54.

Costill DL. Carbohydrate nutrition before, during and after exercise. Fed Proc 1985; 44:364–368.

Costill DL. Carbohydrates for exercise: Dietary demands for optimal performance. Int J Sports Med 1988; 9:1–18.

Costill DL, Fink WJ, Ivy JL, Getchell LH, Witzmann M. Lipid metabolism in skeletal muscle of endurance-trained males and females. Diabetes 1979; 28:818–822.

Costill DL, Miller JM. Nutrition for endurance sport: Carbohydrate and fluid balance. Int J Sports Med 1980; 1:2–14.

Costill DL, Saltin B. Factors limiting gastric emptying during rest and exercise. J Appl Physiol 1974; 37:679–683.

Costill F, et al. Acid-base balance during repeated bouts of exercise: Influence of HCO_3. Int J Sports Med 1984; 5:228–231.

Coulston AM, Liu GC, Reaven GM. Plasma glucose, insulin, and lipid responses to high-carbohydrate low-fat diets in normal humans. Metabolism 1983; 32:52–66.

Coyle EF, Coggan AR, Hemmert MD, Ivy JL. Muscle glycogen utilization during prolonged strenuous exercise when fed carbohydrate. J Appl Physiol 1986; 611:165–172.

Darden E, Schendel HE. Dietary protein and muscle building. Scholastic Coach 1971; 40:70–76.

Davis JN, Lamb DR, Pate RR, Slentz CA, Burgess WA, Bartoli WP. Carbohydrate-electrolyte drinks: Effects on endurance cycling in the heat. Am J Clin Nutr 1988; 48:1023–1030.

Dohm GL. Protein nutrition for the athlete. Clin Sports Med 1984; 3:595–604.

Dragan GI, Vasiliu A, Georgescu E. Effect of increased supply of protein on elite weight-lifters. In Galesloot TE, Tinbergen BJ, eds. Milk proteins. Wageninger, Netherlands: Pudoc, 1985:99–103.

Dressendorfer RH, Wade CE, Keen CL, Scaff JH. Plasma mineral levels in marathon runners during a 20-day race. Phys Sportsmed 1982; 10:113–118.

Edgerton VR, Gardner GW, Ohira V, Gunawardena KA, Senewiratne B. Iron-deficiency anaemia and its effect on worker productivity and activity patterns. Br Med J 1979; 2:1546–1549.

Frizzeu RT, et al. Hyponatremia and ultramarathon running. JAMA 1986; 255:772–774.

Gollnick PD. Metabolism of substrates: Energy substrate metabolism during and as modified by training. Fed Proc 1985; 44:353–357.

Gollnick PD, Matoba H. Role of carbohydrate in exercise. Clin Sports Med 1984; 3:583–594.

Goranzon, H, Forsum E. Effect of reduced energy intake versus increased physical

activity on the outcome of nitrogen balance experiments in man. Am J Clin Nutr 1985; 41:919–928.
Green BB, Weiss NS, Daling JR. Risks of ovulatory infertility in relation to body weight. Fertil Steril 1988; 50;721–726.
Guastella PC. The effects of rapid weight loss on anaerobic power in high school wrestlers. (unpublished data)
Haralambie G. Serum zinc in athletes in training. Int J Sports Med 1981; 2:135–138.
Hargreaves M, Costill DL, Coggan AR, Fink WJ, Nischibata I. Effect of carbohydrate feedings on muscle glycogen utilization and exercise performance. Med Sci Sports Exer 1984; 16:219–222.
Haymes EM. Nutritional concerns: Need for iron. Med Sci Sports Exerc 1987; 19:5197–5200.
Hecker AL. Nutritional conditioning for athletic competition. Clin Sports Med 1984; 3:567–582.
Jette M, Pelletier O, Parker L, Thoden J. The nutritional and metabolic effects of a carbohydrate-rich diet in a glycogen supercompensation training regimen. Am J Clin Nutr 1978; 31:2140–2148.
Lemon PWR. Protein and exercise: Update 1987. Med Sci Sports Exerc 1987; 19:5179–5190.
Marable NL, Hickson JF, Korslund MK, et al. Urinary nitrogen excretion as influenced by a muscle-building exercise program and protein intake variation. Nutr Rep Int 1979; 19:795–805.
O'Neil FT, Hynak-Hankinson MT, Gorman J. Research and application of current topics in sports nutrition. J Am Diet Assoc 1986; 86:1007–1015.
Parr RB, Porter MA, Hodgson SC. Nutrition knowledge and practice of coaches, trainers and athletes. Phys Sportsmed 1984; 12(3):127–138.
Phinney SD, et al. Capacity for moderate exercise in obese subjects after adaptation to a hypocaloric, ketogenic diet. J Clin Invest 1980; 66:1152–1161.
Rasch PJ, Hamby JW, Burns HJ Jr. Protein dietary supplementation and physical performance. Med Sci Sports 1969; 1:195–199.
Senay LC Jr, Pivarnik JM. Fluid shifts during exercise. Exerc Sport Sci Rev 1985; 13:335–387.
Sherman WM, et al. Effects of exercise-diet manipulation on muscle glycogen and its subsequent utilization during performance. Int J Sports Med 1981; 21:114–118.
Sherman WM, Lamb DR. Nutrition and prolonged exercise. In Lamb DR, Murray R, eds. Perspectives in exercise science and sports medicine. Vol. 1. Prolonged exercise. Indianapolis: Benchmark Press, 1988:213–280.
Steen SN. Metabolic effects of repeated weight loss and regain in adolescent wrestlers. JAMA 1988; 260:560–561.
Tarnopolsky MA, MacDougall JD, Atkinson SA. Influence of protein intake and training status on nitrogen balance and lean mass. J Appl Physiol 1988; 64:187–193.
Van Dam B. Vitamins and sport. Br J Sports Med 1978; 12:74–79.
van der Beek EJ. Vitamins and endurance training: Food for running and faddism claims. Sports Med 1985; 2:175–197.
van der Beek EJ, van Dokkum W, Schrijver J, et al. Thiamin, riboflavin, and

vitamins B_6 and C: Impact of combined restricted intake on functional performance in man. Am J Clin Nutr 1988; 48:1451–1462.

Weight LM, Noakes TD, Labadarios D, Graves J, Jacobs P, Berman PA. Vitamin and mineral status of trained athletes including the effects of supplementation. Am J Clin Nutr 1988; 47:186–191.

Weight LM, Myburgh KH, Noakes TD. Vitamin and mineral supplementation: Effect on the running performance of trained athletes. Am J Clin Nutr 1988; 47:192-195.

Williams MH. Nutritional aspects of human physical and athletic performance. Springfield, IL: Charles C. Thomas, 1985.

Wilmore JH, Freund BJ. Nutritional enhancement of athletic performance. Nutr Abstr Rev 1984; 54:1–16.

Wright ED. Nutrition and exercise. In Paige DM, ed. Clinical nutrition. Toronto: C.V. Mosby Co., 1988:677–717.

Young VR, Torun B. Physical activity: Impact on protein and amino acid metabolism and implications for nutritional requirements. In Harper AE, Dairs GK, eds. Nutrition in health and disease and international development. New York: Alan R. Liss, 1981:57–85.

15

Alternative Eating Styles

What a struggle! Sheila bought the best food and prepared it herself so her family would benefit from the healthiest, most wholesome foods. But her son Benjamin would sneak out with his friends to eat "junk" at a fast food place 2 miles from home. He would even take his allowance and walk there to have a hamburger and other "junk foods" that were going to "harden his arteries" and shorten his life span. Sheila brought him to the best nutritionist in New York so she would tell him how bad "junk food" was and how he was endangering his life.

FAST FOODS UPDATE

Fast foods have become a large part of the Western dietary lifestyle, with older adolescents consuming "junk" and "fast" food more often than any other age group (AAP 1985). The tremendous growth of the fast-food industry is, in part, due to the convenience and taste of fast foods, their reasonable cost, and the improved economy that allows more free time for recreation (Young et al 1986). With the increased number of women working outside the home, approximately 7 percent of U.S. children aged 5 to 13 years (approximately 2 million children) must care for themselves after school and may avail themselves of the convenience of fast foods (Hofferth & Phillips 1987).

These highly prevalent dietary choices are unfortunately labeled by terms that place guilt on the consumers. The term "junk food" is usually a misnomer; indeed, there is no such thing as junk food (Lifshitz 1989). A child could eat a "junky diet" by eating any single type of food in excess, which violates the general principle of good nutrition of including a varied food selection from the basic food groups. For example, Ding Dongs (sweet rolls) may complement a well-balanced meal, whereas a child who drinks excessive quantities of a nutritious, natural food such as fruit juice may not drink sufficient water and milk or consume other foods in sufficient amounts to achieve a well-balanced diet (see Chapters 9 and 12). This diet would qualify as a "junky diet" despite not including any of the so called "junk" foods.

Nutrient Quality of Fast Foods

Fast foods tend to be high in calories because they are usually fried or made from fatty meats. However, the excess fat content of these foods is largely responsible for their good taste. The fat content of fast food may provide up to 45 grams of fat per serving (e.g., a hamburger), and may yield as much as 62 percent of its calories from fat (e.g., a fried chicken thigh). Moreover, most fat in fast foods is of animal origin and is, therefore, predominantly of the saturated type. In addition, the high temperature used in frying foods increases the degree of saturation of frying oils and fats. This is a matter of particular concern to health care professionals (see Chapters 9 and 24), and some establishments have made attempts to modify the menu choices to include low-calorie items and to use vegetable shortening. For example, McDonald's recently altered its method of processing some menu items, namely Chicken McNuggets and Filet-O-Fish, to use 100 percent vegetable shortening.

Although fast foods are excellent sources of protein, they tend to be low in important nutrients such as iron, calcium, and vitamins A and C; high in sodium (Young et al 1986); and low in dietary fiber. Good sources of vitamins and fiber, including fruits, vegetables, and whole grain cereals, have not traditionally been available in "fast" food establishments. The trend toward salad bars, however, is encouraging. Salads are good sources of these nutrients and are relatively low in calories, provided that high-calorie dressings are not used. Salad bars attract many customers, but they tend to be costly and are low-profit items.

The reader is referred to specific tables describing the nutrients of individual "fast" food items (Young et al 1986). It should be kept in mind that the fast-food industry may vary the preparation and ingredients of their foods; therefore, the analysis of the nutrient composition of fast foods needs to be updated frequently.

Fast Food Choices

Fast food is an integral part of our lives. Children like these foods and will eat them regardless of what health care professionals or parents think. Therefore, it is important to put the matter of the nutrient quality of fast food into proper perspective, which varies in the context of the menu that children like to eat.

In Figure 15–1 the nutrient intake of a 13-year-old teenage girl who ate all

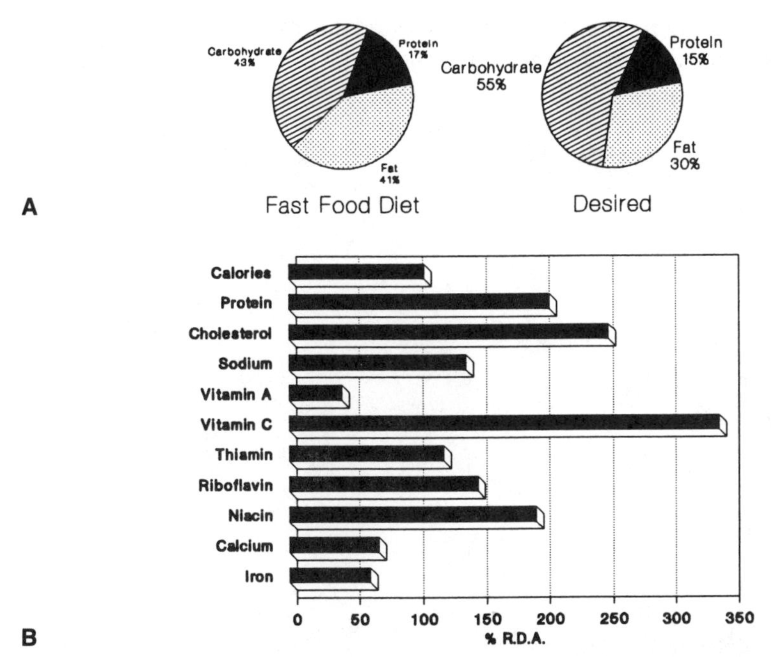

Figure 15–1. **A.** Caloric distribution of a fast-food diet. **B.** Percent of requirements for a 13-year-old girl met by a fast-food diet. The diet consisted of breakfast at McDonald's (Egg McMuffin, hashbrown potatoes, orange juice [6 oz]); lunch at Burger King (cheeseburger, regular french fries, medium vanilla shake); and dinner at Roy Rogers (fried chicken breast and wing, biscuit, cole slaw, cola [12 oz]).

her meals at fast-food restaurants is presented. Breakfast at McDonald's, lunch at Burger King, and dinner at Roy Rogers—what a nutritional nightmare! The food choices that this adolescent selected for these three meals provided her with sufficient calories to maintain her growth and development. However, the amount of fat in the diet was quite high, with most of the fat coming from animal sources. Consequently, the cholesterol intake was over twice the recommended level and it can be assumed that the amount of saturated fat in this diet was more than two times the amount of polyunsaturated fat.

This menu also was very high in salt. Several fast-food entree sandwiches contain 1500 to 1750 milligrams of sodium, more than three times the minimum daily recommended sodium intake. Some children add even more salt to the meal. With the selection of salted french fries, onion rings, or a milkshake, the sodium intake would increase even more. This menu was also insufficient in essential nutrients, particularly vitamin A, iron, and calcium. The needs of these nutrients are not easily met by fast foods.

More often, children will have a menu that includes fast-food selections but is not exclusively composed of these items. Joe, a 14-year-old teenager, was eating the following menu, which included a lunch in a fast food restaurant with breakfast and dinner offered at home.

MENU 1

Breakfast
1 cup sweetened cereal
1 cup 2% milk
1 cup orange juice

Lunch
2 cheeseburgers
large order of french fries
vanilla shake

Snack
1 cup 2% milk
4 chocolate cookies

Dinner
1½ cup pasta with meat sauce
1 cup salad with vegetable oil and vinegar-type dressing
garlic bread made with margarine
1 cup soda

Snack
1 cup ice cream with 1 sliced banana

In addition to his fast-food lunch, this menu also contained other foods that are quite high in sugar. Yet his caloric intake was appropriate for his age (2990 calories, 109 percent RDAs), and the distribution of calories from protein, carbohydrate, and fat was not too far from the ideal nutrition goals (Figure 15–2) (see Chapter 9). Cholesterol intake was appropriate at 100 milligrams per 1000 calories consumed, but saturated fat and sodium were high. The nutrient quality of this diet was good except that zinc and copper intakes were low (less than 65 percent RDAs).

By changing the type of cereal for breakfast (Special K), adding a salad at lunch, using tomato sauce instead of meat sauce at dinner, and changing the evening dessert to ice milk instead of ice cream, this menu was improved in accordance with the basic nutrition principles (see Chapter 9). The caloric content was not affected but the amount of fat in the diet was reduced to one third of the total calories and polyunsaturated fat was increased from 8.1 to 12.6 grams. The zinc content of the diet was improved and was no longer deficient for a 14-year-old boy.

These two examples shed the right perspective on the role of fast-food

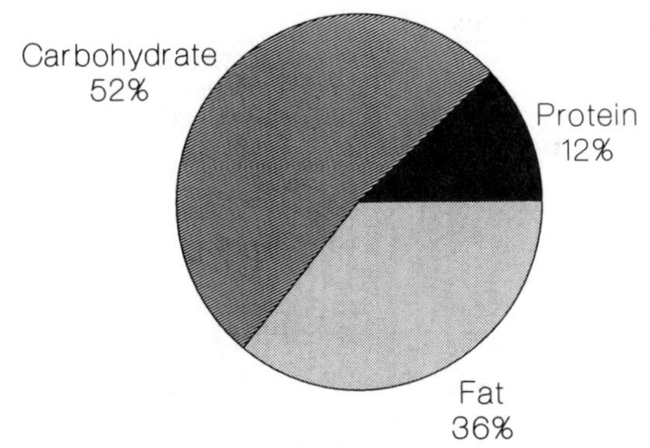

Figure 15–2. Caloric distribution of a fast-food menu. This fast-food menu of a 14-year-old boy included lunch with two cheeseburgers and a milk shake (see Menu 1), yet his daily intake was not far from ideal.

menus. There should be no doubt that the nutrient quality of these foods is often suboptimal, especially if they are consumed to the exclusion of other foods. On the other hand, the avoidance of these foods is not easy, nor will it guarantee that the diet will be nutritious and/or healthier.

VEGETARIANISM

Approximately 7 million Americans adhere to some form of vegetarian diet (Zeman & Ney 1988). A person may become vegetarian for a variety of reasons, including cultural, religious, and economic considerations. In developing countries, people are partly vegetarian out of poverty and the unaffordability of animal foods. In the United States the cost of a vegetarian diet is usually not a motivating factor, as the exclusion of meat does not necessarily reduce the cost. People may become vegetarians because of opposition to killing animals. There are also those who cite concerns about the purity of the food supply and the desire to maintain and improve health. Indeed, studies in various vegetarian groups have shown that they have decreased rates of obesity, high blood pressure, high blood cholesterol levels, coronary heart disease, osteoporosis, and some forms of cancer (Dwyer 1988). However, the extent to which these benefits are related to the avoidance of animal products is not clear. The intake of specific forms of fats or carbohydrates as well as the differences in lifestyle that these people follow may influence the rates of these illnesses. For example, vegetarians may have other habits such as decreased alcohol, caffeine, and nicotine consumption, which would improve health independent of dietary habits.

Most of us in our society refuse to eat some animal foods (Table 15–1). For

Table 15–1. Types of Vegetarian Food Patterns.

	RED MEAT	FISH AND FOWL	DAIRY	EGGS	VEGETABLES, FRUIT, GRAINS, NUTS
Traditional American	x	x	x	x	x
Partial vegetarian		x	x	x	x
Lacto-ovo vegetarian			x	x	x
Ovo vegetarian				x	x
Lacto vegetarian			x		x
Vegan					x

example, Americans avoid insects, dogs, cats, and horses, which are considered delicacies in some other cultures. However, partial vegetarians are people who avoid an entire category of animal food that is generally well-accepted in our culture. There are vegetarians who eat poultry or fish but not other types of meat. Lacto-ovo vegetarians will accept milk, milk products, and eggs, but more restrictive vegetarians (vegans) will avoid all animal products and eat only plant foods. There are also those who only eat fruit, so-called fruitarians, whose diets are largely composed of fruits, nuts, honey, and olive oil (ADA 1980, Vyhmeister 1984).

Nutrient Quality of Vegetarian Diets

Given the variations in the degree of dietary restriction in vegetarian diets, coupled with the variation in nutrient requirements, problems may or may not occur. Certain groups, such as pregnant and lactating women, infants, and children, are particularly at risk when ingesting a vegetarian diet. For any person the risk of malnutrition or specific nutrient deficiencies from poorly planned vegetarian diets increases with greater restrictions on varieties of foods eaten. Thus, the risk of malnutrition is greater for a vegan than for a lacto-ovo vegetarian.

For example, Kathy is a 5-year-old, 41-pound (18 kg) girl who followed a lacto-ovo-vegetarian diet. Her typical menu consisted of the following.

MENU 2

Breakfast
1 scrambled egg
1 slice whole wheat toast with 1 teaspoon margarine
½ cup orange juice

Lunch
1 slice pizza
¾ cup whole milk
½ sliced apple

Snack
½ cup rice pudding with raisins

Dinner
½ cup macaroni and cheese
½ cup string beans with 1 tsp. margarine
½ cup apple juice

Snack
½ cup milk
1 tablespoon peanut butter
4 crackers

This menu provided all the energy needs of this child to grow and develop (1560 kcal, 102 percent RDAs) with an appropriate distribution of calories (Fig. 15–3A). However, despite relatively little restriction of this diet there are certain deficiencies like zinc, copper, vitamin B_6, and vitamin D, as well as nutrient excesses (Fig. 15–3B).

These dietary deficiencies may result when meat is not ingested. Although the addition of fruits and vegetables may compensate for these deficiencies, very large quantities would have to be ingested. Eggs and milk in larger quantities would supply the minerals that are deficient, but with an increased risk of ingesting a totally inadequate unbalanced diet. Thus, a vitamin and mineral supplement in this case could facilitate nutritional adequacy of the diet.

Unlike Kathy's diet, which contains milk and eggs, her friend Mary was given a vegan diet that consisted of only grains, fruits and vegetables:

MENU 3

Breakfast
2 slices white toast with 2 tsp. margarine and 1 tsp. jelly
½ cup orange juice

Lunch
½ peanut butter and jelly sandwich
1 cup apple juice
carrot sticks

Snack
1 cup canned pears
1 cup apple juice

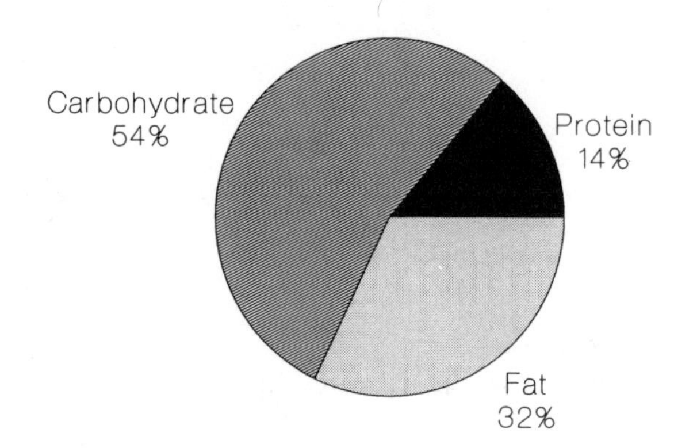

A

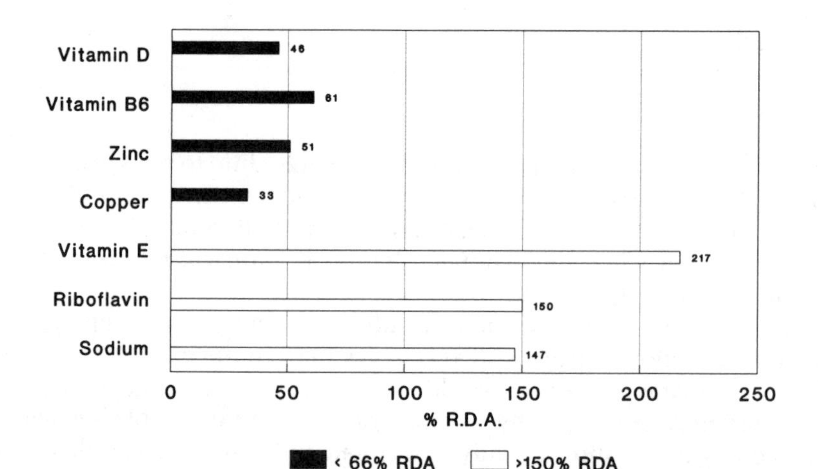

B

Figure 15–3. **A.** Caloric distribution of a lacto-ovo-vegetarian menu. This diet (Menu 2) of a 5-year-old girl provided adequate energy for growth. **B.** Inappropriate nutrient intakes of a lacto-ovo-vegetarian menu. The vitamin and mineral deficits are the result of avoidance of nutrients such as meat. Vitamin D deficiency can easily be compensated for by sunlight and/or by vitamin D-fortified milk.

Dinner
1 cup macaroni with tomato sauce
½ cup green beans with 1 tsp. margarine
1 cup apple juice

Snack
3 sandwich cookies
1 cup apple juice

This menu was of poor nutrient quality even though it provided all the calories (1539 calories, 95 percent RDAs) Mary needed (Fig. 15–4). However,

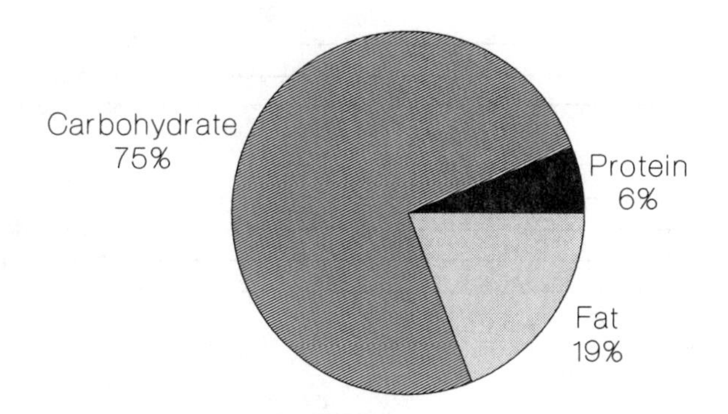

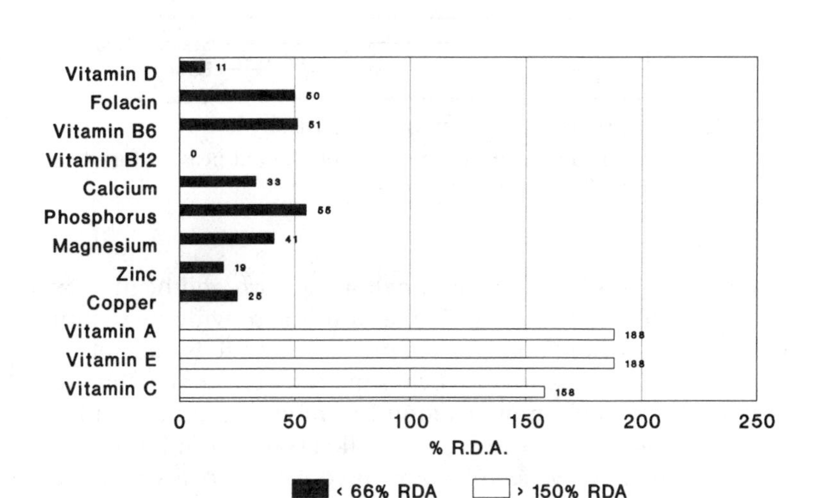

Figure 15–4. **A.** Caloric distribution of a vegan menu. This diet (Menu 3) of a 5-year-old girl provided all the energy needed but was inadequate in many respects. **B.** Inappropriate nutrient intakes of a vegan menu. Multiple vitamin and mineral deficiencies are apparent. Of particular concern is vitamin B_{12}, which is not found in plant foods. Iron deficiency may also occur even though the intake of iron from the diet is adequate, due to the poor absorption of iron from vegetables sources.

there were concerns about the fact that plant proteins were not appropriately balanced to provide all the amino acids needed. Vegetable proteins are incomplete because they do not provide all the essential amino acids necessary for growth. The most limiting amino acids in plant proteins are lysine, methionine, and tryptophan. In general, grains are low in lysine and high in methionine, while legumes are low in methionine and tryptophan and high in lysine. Most nuts and seeds are lysine-deficient. Thus, combining different legumes, nuts, and grains could provide an appropriate quality of protein intake, accounting for all the essential amino acids (Figure 15–5). For example, Mexi-

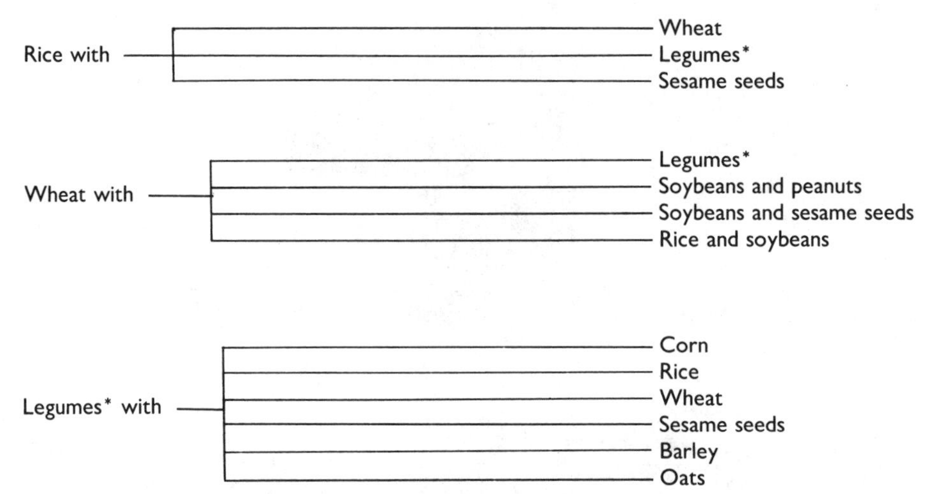

Figure 15–5. Complementary vegetable proteins.

*Appropriate legumes include soybeans, peanuts, black-eyed peas, kidney beans, chick-peas, navy beans, pinto beans, and lima beans.

can Indians have subsisted on combinations of corn and beans. Corn is low in lysine, tryptophan, and threonine; and beans provide these amino acids but do not have sufficient quantities of methionine and isoleucine, which are abundant in corn. Thus, corn and beans make a perfect match! Care must be taken with the vegetable proteins found in raw soybeans, lima beans, and mung beans, which contain an enzyme called trypsin inhibitor. This enzyme is present when these vegetables are uncooked and it can decrease the bioavailability of protein in food. Therefore, these vegetable proteins should not be fed to infants with immature gastrointestinal tracts unless they are well cooked.

The diet in Menu 3 also contained inadequate quantities of several minerals and vitamins; less than two thirds of the RDA for calcium, phosphorus, magnesium, zinc, copper, and vitamins D, B_2, and B_{12} (see Fig. 15–4B). Vitamin B_{12} is not found in plant foods. Therefore, vegans must obtain vitamin B_{12} by using a vitamin supplement or by eating B_{12}-fortified foods, such as yeast, soy milk, cereals, and other meat analogues. Although adults may take 7 to 8 years to develop vitamin B_{12} deficiency, infants of vegan mothers have smaller stores, and may develop a deficiency rapidly. In fact, vitamin B_{12} deficiency has even been described in infants born to strictly vegetarian mothers who were breastfeeding their babies (Higgenbottom, Sweetman & Nyhan 1978).

Vitamin D is also not present in plant foods and supplementation should be provided for vegetarian children and pregnant or lactating women. Vitamin D may be obtained from fortified cow's milk or fortified soy milk. This is particularly important in winter climates where sunlight for endogenous synthesis of vitamin D is limited.

In addition to the decreased nutrient quality of vegan diets, nutrient absorption may also be a problem because of the high fiber content of the diet and/or the poor bioavailability of certain nutrients. Vegan preschoolers have been shown to ingest an average of 18 grams of fiber daily (Sanders & Purves 1981). In contrast, the general preschooler population (aged 1 to 5 years) were reported to consume approximately 10 grams of dietary fiber daily. High fiber intakes bind iron, calcium, zinc, and other trace minerals in the intestine, preventing their maximum absorption (Reinhold et al 1976, Mercurio & Betim 1981).

Iron deficiency may be present in children on vegan diets even though they appear to ingest iron in appropriate quantities (Dwyer et al 1982). Although iron exists in foods of vegetable origin it is present in the non-heme-iron form, which is not as well absorbed as the heme form found in animal foods. In general, foods high in non-heme iron are dark green leafy vegetables, beans, and whole grain or enriched cereals and eggs. Since iron absorption can be increased by the concurrent ingestion of ascorbic acid, fruits and vegetables that contain vitamin C should be encouraged in these children.

Nutrient deficiencies may be encountered in vegan children (Sanders & Purves 1981, Shull et al 1977, Zmora, Gorodischer & Bar-Ziv 1979, Fulton, Hutton & Stitt 1980, Dwyer et al 1982), and their growth may be compromised (Sanders 1988). However, their diets can be improved and they may grow well in sophisticated vegan communities (O'Connell et al 1989). Strict vegans must carefully select plant foods that are high in minerals and vitamins. Calcium is present in dark green leafy vegetables, broccoli, brussel sprouts, legumes, dried fruits, and almonds. Calcium may also be obtained from calcium-fortified soy milk and calcium-precipitated tofu. Zinc is contained in whole grain, cereals, peas, oatmeal, dried yeast, and wheat germ. Riboflavin is derived from milk and milk products; therefore, vegetarians who eliminate milk should include in their diets two servings of alternative riboflavin sources such as enriched grains, dark green leafy vegetables, legumes, nuts, broccoli, or avocado.

Nonnutritional Hazards of Vegetarian Products

Avoidance of animal products and use of vegetables and fruits is no guarantee of ingesting a healthy diet. Vegetarians who depend on nuts and seeds for a large portion of their protein intake must remember that these products can become contaminated with aflatoxins. These toxins are produced by malt that grow on nuts and seeds when stored at humidities above 70 percent. Aflatoxins are a cause of liver cancer and may play a causal role in the development of protein malnutrition (kwashiorkor) (Hendrickse 1988). Vegetarians who eat large quantities of nuts and seeds should avoid long-term storage at high humidity and roast them before eating to reduce these toxins in these foods.

Even in our society of advanced medical technology, there is a widespread appeal of herbal preparations. Total herb sales from health-food stores in the United States grossed $167 million in 1980 and $360 million in 1987 (Price & Brown 1984). The use of herbal preparations has been advocated because these "natural" products are considered to be safer and healthier than synthetic chemicals (Kaufman & Siek 1980, Larkin 1983). However, their use can be dangerous (Table 15–2). These herbal preparations lack quality control and their purity, safety, and pharmacologic effectiveness must be questioned (Gazella & Pinto 1987). The time of harvest may influence the amount of active compound in the herb (Mitchell 1984), whereas some herbs are edible when immature but are poisonous if allowed to mature before harvesting (Cooper 1982). In addition, accidental contaminants such as insect parts, pollen, mold, and allergens may be found in these preparations. For example, yellow-root herbal tea contaminated with arsenic was reported in the southern United States due to soil and stream contamination in the fields where the plant was grown (Parsons 1981). Thus, parents and children who substitute herbal teas for caffeine-containing beverages should be cautioned of the potentially hazardous effects of herbs. They should also be aware that honey and corn syrups, which might be considered "healthy" and "natural" additions to a vegetarian meal plan, may be the source of botulism, thereby making these products unacceptable and dangerous for the infant (Midura et al 1979, Kaulter et al 1982).

FOOD FADS AND HEALTH FOODS

Good nutrition requires no single food intake; man requires specific nutrients, not specific food items. As simple as this concept may be, individuals are still susceptible to the lure of faddism. Our society's current awareness of health promotion, combined with the desire to reduce the risk of disease, make a fertile environment for the "health hustler" (Herbert 1976). These are individuals or industries that focus on the needs and fears of people and exploit the hypotheses of science. For example, a scientific suggestion that a particular nutrient such as vitamin C or vitamin A may slow tumor growth will lead the health hustlers to promote their own megadose vitamin supplement to prevent or cure cancer.

In general, there are three basic types of food fads: (1) those in which special virtues of a particular food are exaggerated and purported to cure a specific disease; (2) those in which certain foods are eliminated from the diet

Table 15–2. Toxicity Associated with Herbal Preparations.

PREPARATIONS	FOLKLORE USE	TOXIC EFFECTS
Alfalfa leaves	Treatment of arthritis, pain relief	Gas and diarrhea; toxic analogue of the amino acid arginine produces severe lupus erythematosus-like syndrome
Aloe vera	Treatment of burns; laxative; physicians in India use it to control hyperlipidemia and hyperglycemia	Skin irritation; nausea, vomiting, diarrhea; red urine; large doses lead to kidney failure (nephritis)
Apple, apricot, bitter almond, cherry, peach, pear, plum (seeds or pits, bark and leaves)	—	Cyanide ion is produced; fatal poisoning
Catnip	Induction of euphoria, stimulation; used to treat colic; presently used as a marijuana substitute	Hallucinations
Cayenne pepper	Improvement in circulation; to normalize blood pressure (high or low)	Nausea, vomiting, diarrhea
Chamomile	Treatment of "female complaints"; cramps; diarrhea; teething; for sedation; in infants used to replace milk to treat diarrhea	Allergic reaction in persons sensitive to ragweed, asters, and chrysanthemums; skin irritation; in infants can cause water intoxication associated with hyponatremia and seizure disorders
Cohosh, black and blue	Treatment of dyspepsia; induces menses	Causes tonic contractions of the uterus and abortion
Devil's claw root tea	Treatment of rheumatism, arthritis, gout, lumbago	Causes abortion
Eucalyptus oil	Treatment of upper respiratory infections, asthma, cough	Gastroenteritis, seizure, coma, kidney irritation, cardiovascular collapse, cyanosis
Ginseng	Treatment of impotence, anemia, depression, diabetes, edema, hypertension	Breast development due to high content of estrogens; excitation, arousal, nervousness, tension, hypertension
Juniper berries	Diuretic, hallucinogen, euphoriant, stimulant	Gastrointestinal irritability
Laetrile	Treatment of cancer	Cyanide poisoning
Licorice root	Treatment of dyspepsia and ulcers	Sodium and water retention, hypertension, heart failure
Nutmeg tea	Aphrodisiac; treatment of GI disorders and rheumatism; promotes menstruation	Hallucinogen; induces abortion; headache; cramps; nausea, vomiting; large amount can cause liver damage and death
Peppermint tea	Treatment of diarrhea in infants	Causes water intoxication associated with hyponatremia and seizures
Sassafras root	Treatment of mumps, pneumonia, bronchitis, head cold	Contains a hepatoxin and hepatocarcinogen in rats; banned by the FDA
Starch blockers	Weight loss	Nausea, vomiting, diarrhea, abdominal pain

Adapted from Gazella JG, Pinto JT. Herbs: Use and abuse. Current concepts and perspectives in nutrition. New York: New York Hospital–Cornell Medical Center, Memorial Sloan–Kettering Cancer Center 1987; 6(2):1–20.

because of a belief that harmful constituents are present; and (3) those in which emphasis is placed on "natural" food. Food faddism often includes the false promises of superior health and freedom from disease, which may delay individuals from obtaining appropriate medical care. Economic extravagance is another consequence of food faddism. Foods that are associated with the word "health" imply health-giving or curative properties and are more expensive than their counterparts.

The use of organically grown foods (food grown without the use of chemicals or additives) is an important aspect of the health food movement. Claims have been made that organically grown foods are nutritionally superior to and/or better tasting than foods grown under standard agricultural conditions using chemical fertilizers. There is no scientific basis for these claims. Plants use only inorganic food, and there are no organic forms of plant food. Therefore, it is relatively immaterial whether traditional agricultural methods using chemical fertilizers or organic farming practices are followed. Moreover, the latter farming techniques have the added disadvantage of possible contamination with infectious organisms (Arnon 1980).

Claims are also made that our food supply is being poisoned with pesticides and food additives; lists have been published that contain over 250 toxic compounds normally present in common foods. However, the use of additives and pesticides is regulated by law. The Food and Drug Administration regularly conducts "market basket" studies in several regions of the United States, and these substances are usually present in amounts that do not cause any known adverse effects. In contrast, little is known about naturally occurring toxicants in organically grown foods.

Natural foods are considered to be those foods that are in their original state or have minimal refinement and processing. Some examples of such foods are fresh fruits and vegetables, milk, unrefined sugar, honey, and whole grain flour and cereals. Part of the movement toward natural foods is expressed by the increased demand for unpasteurized milk. Raw certified milk is basically pure and nutritious in its natural state. Unfortunately, this type of milk is costly and may easily become contaminated with pathogenic organisms. The requirements and quality control systems that regulate "health food" standards may not be optimal, whereas pasteurization of milk as performed by the dairy industry offers good control of infective organisms.

The Zen macrobiotic philosophy, which was quite popular in the 1960s, accepted the concept that the path to health and happiness consisted of no medicine, no surgery, and a diet of natural food (Ohsawa 1965). This diet consists of stages that place emphasis on whole grain cereals and avoidance of sugar. In the most extreme situation, cereals constitute 100 percent of the daily Zen diet. Of course, these very restricted diets resulted in cases of scurvy, hypocalcemia, malnutrition, anemia, and so on. Therefore, adherents of this philosophy have recently been encouraged to eat a greater variety of foods including dairy products, eggs, and fish.

Nutritional fad treatments are often followed for many diseases or complaints (see Chapter 18). For example, for premenstrual syndrome (PMS), vitamin B_6, essential fatty acids, magnesium, vitamin E, and/or elimination of caffeine have been prescribed (Casey & Dwyer 1987). However, there is no evidence that PMS results from dietary inadequacies or that it can be treated effectively by dietary management or vitamin or mineral supplementation. Regardless, health food stores continue to market specific products containing vitamins and minerals and oils for the treatment of many ailments. Often, these ''cures'' are of no benefit to the patient; they may, in fact, be harmful. The FDA recently suspended the sales of L-tryptophan, a naturally occurring amino acid, because it was linked to an unusual disease known as eosinophilia myalgia syndrome (EMS 1989).

CURRENT EATING PRACTICES

Concern with the type and quality of food often transcends parent's preoccupation with the eating habits of their children and adolescents. However, skipping meals, particularly breakfast, has become a hallmark of our industrial culture. Missed meals often occur among schoolaged children owing to a lack of time or the priority of other activities over eating. In general, older adolescents are more likely to display this pattern of skipping meals than children under 11 years of age (Evans & Cronin 1986). In addition, most meals children eat are unsupervised by an adult. Meal skipping and the lack of structure at meal time may contribute to dietary inadequacies and inappropriate food selection.

Children are also beset with a fear of obesity and a desire to control weight (Moses, Banilivy & Lifshitz 1989, Maloney et al 1989), and these eating attitudes may interfere with the child's ability to eat an appropriate diet and to grow and develop (Lifshitz et al 1987). A large proportion of high-school students engage in dieting to avoid obesity, and they frequently skip meals and/or engage in other inappropriate eating behaviors to achieve their goals (Lifshitz & Moses 1988) (see Chapter 17).

Snacking between meals is generally perceived as undesirable; however, contrary to this opinion held by many parents and health care professionals, snacking is an important part of children's eating patterns. Data from the USDA's Nationwide Food Consumption Survey reveal that snacking accounts for up to one third of the total calories ingested by children, and snacks are responsible for increased intakes of calcium, magnesium, vitamin B_6, and iron (Morgan & Goungetas 1986). For physically active adolescents, or those in a growth spurt, between-meal snacking may help to meet their high daily energy needs (Evans & Cronin 1986).

Therefore, the eating patterns of a child might be as important as the food selected to attain optimal nutritional intake. The judicious selection of nutritious snacks and avoidance of meal skipping is important to help children meet their nutritional requirements. In fact, low-calorie snacks fed to children to promote "healthy" dietary habits, and meal skipping to avoid obesity, have been associated with poor growth and weight gain (Pugliese et al 1983, 1987, Lifshitz et al 1987, Lifshitz & Moses 1988).

CLINICAL INTERVENTION

"Fast" foods, convenience foods, and prepackaged high-energy snacks are a permanent part of our children's lifestyle and diet. Manufacturers of these products are offering convenient drive-through windows, 24-hour service, and creative decor; they advertise aggressively, airing television commercials and other advertisements amounting to billions of dollars. In addition, fast-food chains are opening up new markets in suburbs, department stores, schools, parks, industry cafeterias, hospitals, and military installations. At the same time, the types of fast foods and convenience foods available are being modified to meet the goals for human nutrition. For example, salad bars are increasingly common, primarily because of consumer demand. New offerings of low-salt items, "lite" (low-calorie) items, and smaller portions indicate greater nutrition awareness. Also, vending machines are offering dried fruits, nuts, and whole wheat crackers next to the usual selections of candy bars. By including a variety of other foods and making wise choices, children can avoid excess amounts of fat, cholesterol, and sodium and still enjoy the convenience, variety, and flavor of fast food. Table 15–3 lists some general

Table 15–3. Better Choices in the Real World of Fast Food and "Junk" Food.

ITEM	TYPICAL CHOICE	BETTER CHOICE
Pizza	Toppings of extra cheese, sausage, pepperoni, meat	Toppings of peppers, mushrooms, onions, or just low-fat mozzarella cheese
Cheeseburger/ Hamburger	"Big Mac"; double or ¼-lb hamburger, "Whopper"; added cheese, extra sauce; "Jumbo Burger"	Plain, regular hamburger; skip the extra meat, cheese and sauces; choose lean roast beef if available
Potatoes	Baked potatoes with sour cream, butter, cheese, bacon; french fries; home fries	Baked potato without high-calorie toppings; salad with vegetables and a small amount of dressing
Deep fried foods	Fried fish fillet; fried chicken; breaded veal	Avoid these items or remove breading before eating
Breakfast breads	Croissants; donuts; danish	English muffins; whole wheat toast with cinnamon; margarine and small amount of sugar if necessary
Drinks	Milkshakes, soda, punch	Low-fat milk; juices

suggestions on how this can be accomplished. Most studies show appropriate nutritional status for adolescents despite their current food preferences and eating styles (Kovar 1985). Bon appetit!

Independent of the nutritional status and weight of the patient, snacks and sugary foods may produce more dental caries. It has been shown that nonabsorbable sweeteners such as sorbitol and xylitol do not appear to cause dental caries. Indeed, they may even be helpful in counteracting the adverse influences by stimulating salivary flow when chewed after a potential cariogenic snack, such as sticky caramels. Therefore, children and adolescents with active schedules who may not be able to brush their teeth after a snack may benefit from sugarless chewing gum, a habit that doesn't always please parents and teachers (Jensen 1986).

When providing nutritional counseling to a family with special dietary practices or health beliefs, or when caring for an infant or a toddler from such a family, it is important to remember that it is very difficult to change these beliefs or the types of foods they eat (Trahms 1981). Often, one must work within the belief structure and food patterns of the family to ensure that the child is receiving adequate nutrition to support normal growth and development. If the dietary practices are detrimental to the health of the child, efforts must be made to educate the family and modify their attitudes and behaviors regarding diet and nutrition. The family must be seen and counseled more than once, and an accepting and nonjudgmental approach is usually most successful in facilitating change (Truesdell & Acosta 1985).

With infants and children following a vegetarian diet, energy may often be limited. The bulky nature of fruits and vegetables tends to result in satiety before the child's energy needs are met. Therefore, vegan children should be permitted to eat frequently throughout the day so that adequate calories and nutrients can be consumed. Emphasis on nuts, nut butters, avocados, and dried fruit spreads can add calories to the diet. While nut butters can be given to the toddler or preschool child, whole nuts may be dangerous as they may lodge in the child's throat and cause choking. Avocados are an excellent source of calories as well as of copper, potassium, and riboflavin, and can be pureed for infants. Dried fruit purees made from uncooked dried fruit and fruit juice can be substituted for jelly and jams to increase calories and the iron content of infants' or toddlers' diets.

To ensure adequate protein quantity and quality, plant products must complement one another to reach a balance of all the essential amino acids. The traditional combination of foods that provide the essential amino acids are (1) grains and legumes, (2) grains and a small amount of milk, and (3) seeds and legumes. Meat analogues are made from plant foods such as soy, wheat, or nuts and are designed to look and taste like meat. The vitamin and mineral content of these analogues may vary among the different products, and although they may look like meat, they should be eaten with other plant proteins to complement amino acid intake. Further dietary plans for meeting

Table 15–4. Basic Food Guide for Infants and Children on Lacto-Ovo Diets.

			SERVING SIZE					
FOOD GROUP	**SERVINGS PER DAY**	**FOOD ITEMS**	**Infant 0–½ yr**	**Infant ½–1 yr**	**Toddler 1–3 yr**	**Preschooler 4–6 yr**	**Preadolescent 7–10 yr**	**Adolescent 11–18 yr**
Milk and milk products	4	Infant Formula	¾–1 C	¾–1 C	—	—	—	—
		or						
		Milk	—	—	½–¾ C	¾ C	1 C	1 C
		or						
		Cheese	—	—	¾–1 oz	1 oz	1½ oz	1½ oz
		or						
		Yogurt	—	¾–1 C	½–¾ C	¾ C	1 C	1 C
Eggs	1	Egg	—	½	1	1	1	1½
Plant protein	2 or more	Legumes	—	1–6 T	0–¼ C	½ C	½ C	½–¾ C
		or						
		Meat analogues	—	—	¼–½ oz	¾–1 oz	¾–1 oz	1–1¼ oz
		or						
		Textured vegetable protein (TVP)	—	—	0–⅛ oz	½ oz	½ oz	½–¾ oz
Nuts and seeds	2 or more	Nuts and seeds	—	—	—	¼–½ oz	½ oz	½–¾ oz
		or						
		Nut butters	—	—	¼ T	¾ T	1–1¼ T	1–1½ T
Cereals, breads, and whole grains	4 or more	Whole grain bread	—	—	¼–½ slice	¾–1 slice	1–1½ slices	1½–2 slices
		or						
		Cooked cereal	0–1 T	¼ C	¼ C	¼–½ C	½–¾ C	¾–1 C
		or						
		Dry cereal	—	¼–½ C	½ C	¾ C	¾–1 C	1–1½ C
Fruit and vegetables	4 or more	Juice	0–1 oz	⅛–¼C	¼–½ C	½ C	½–1 C	½–1 C
		or						
		Raw	—	—	½ C	½–1 C	1–1½ C	1–1½ C
		or						
		Cooked	1–1½ T	1–2 T	¼–½ C	½ C	½–¾ C	½–¾ C

Fats, oils and sweets: The amount of these foods that should be included in the diet depends on the individual's calorie needs.

Table 15–5. Basic Food Guide for Infants and Children on Vegan Diets.

FOOD GROUP	SERVINGS PER DAY	FOOD ITEMS	SERVING SIZE: Infant 0–½ yr	Infant ½–1 yr	Toddler 1–3 yr	Preschooler 4–6 yr	Preadolescent 7–10 yr	Adolescent 11–18 yr
Fortified soy Milk	4	Isomil or Prosobee or Soyalac or Nursoy	½–¾ C	¾–1 C	¾ C	¾ C	1 C	1 C
Plant protein	2 or more	Legumes	—	1–6 T	¼–½ C	½–¾ C	¾–1 C	½–¾ C
		or Meat analogues	—	—	½–¾ oz	¾–1 oz	1 oz	¾–1 oz
		or Textured vegetable protein (TVP)	—	—	⅛–¼ oz	½ oz	¾ oz	½–¾ oz
Nuts and seeds	2 or more	Nuts and seeds	—	—	—	¼–½ oz	½ oz	½–¾ oz
		or Nut butters	—	—	¼ T	¾ T	1–1¼ T	1–1½ T
Cereals, breads, and whole grains	4 or more	Whole grain bread	—	¼–½ slice	½–1 slice	¾–1 slice	1–1½ slices	1½–2 slices
		or Cooked cereal	0–1 T	¼ C	¼–½ C	½ C	½–1 C	¾–1 C
		or Dry cereal	—	—	½–¾ C	¾ C	¾–1 C	¾–1 C
Fruit and vegetables	4 or more	Juice	0–1 oz	¼ C	¼–½ C	½ C	½–1 C	½–1 C
		or Raw	—	—	½ C	½–1 C	1–1½ C	1–1½ C
		or Cooked	0–1½ T	2 T	¼–½ C	½ C	½–¾ C	½–¾ C
Brewer's yeast	1		—	—	1 T	1 T	1 T	1 T
Molasses	1		—	—	1 T	1–2 T	1–2 T	1–2 T

Fats and sweets: The amount of these foods to be included in the diet depends on the individual's caloric requirements.

Table 15–6. Vegetarian Sources of Critical Nutrients.

NUTRIENT	SOURCE
Calcium	Dairy products, dark leafy greens, fortified soy milk, legumes, peanuts, almonds, and seeds.
Iron	Legumes, dark leafy greens, torula yeast, dried fruits, whole and enriched grains, blackstrap molasses, consuming food that contains vitamin C (citrus fruits, peppers, tomatoes) with any iron-rich food.
Zinc	Eggs, cheese, milk, legumes, nuts, wheat germ, and whole grains.
Riboflavin	Dairy products, eggs, whole and enriched grains (if eaten daily), brewer's yeast, dark leafy greens, legumes.
Vitamin B_{12}	Dairy products, eggs, nutritional yeast, foods fortified with B_{12}, fermented soy products, supplements.
Vitamin D	Fortified milk, fortified soy milk, exposure of skin to sunshine.

the nutrient needs of infants and children following lacto-ovo diets and vegan diets are shown in Tables 15–4 and 15–5, respectively. To overcome some of the nutritional deficiencies seen in vegan diets care must be taken to emphasize foods that are good sources of calcium, iron, zinc, riboflavin, vitamin B_{12}, and vitamin D (Table 15–6).

We do not provide the reader with much advice on how to deal with behavioral feeding problems or how to get children to eat appropriately. These subjects have been addressed by other authors (Satter 1987), and pertain to areas well beyond children's nutrition. It should, however, be remembered that fussy eaters are not born, they're made. Children's eating habits may reflect needs other than nutrition. The rational recommendation is to eat regularly without skipping meals and to feed children a variety of foods and allow them to savor them fully.

REFERENCES

American Academy of Pediatrics Committee on Nutrition. Pediatric nutrition handbook 2nd ed. Elk Grove Village, IL: American Academy of Pediatrics, 1985:53–65.

American Dietetic Association. Position paper on the vegetarian approach to eating. J Am Diet Assoc 1980; 77:61–69.

Arnon SS. Infant botulism. Ann Rev Med 1980; 31:541–560.

Casey V, Dwyer JT. Premenstrual syndrome: Theories and evidence. Nutr Today 1987; 22:4–12.

Cooper CR. Herbal remedies. Hosp Form 1982; 17:1387–1392.

Dwyer JT. Health aspects of vegetarian diets. Am J Clin Nutr 1988; 48:712–738.

Dwyer JT, Dietz WH, Andrews EM, Suskind RM. Nutritional status of vegetarian children. Am J Clin Nutr 1982; 35:204–216.

Eosinophilia myalgia Syndrome—New Mexico. News report. JAMA 1989; 82:3116.

Evans MD, Cronin FJ. Diets of school-age children and teenagers. Family Economic Review US Department of Agriculture 1986; July:14–21.
Fulton JR, Hutton CW, Stitt KR. Preschool vegetarian children. J Am Diet Assoc 1980; 76:360–365.
Gazella JG, Pinto JT. Herbs: Use and abuse. Current concepts and perspectives in nutrition. New York: New York Hospital–Cornell Medical Center, Memorial Sloan–Kettering Cancer Center 1987; 6(2):1–20.
Hendrickse RG. Kwashiorkor and alflatoxins. J Pediatr Gastroenterol Nutr 1988; 7:633–636.
Herbert V. In Barrett and Knight, eds. The health robbers. Philadelphia: George F. Stickley Co., 1976.
Higgenbottom MC, Sweetman L, Nyhan WL. A syndrome of methylmalonic aciduria, homocystinuria, megaloblastic anemia, and neurologic abnormalities in a vitamin B_{12}-deficient breast-fed infant of a strict vegetarian. New Engl J Med 1978; 299:317–323.
Hofferth SL, Phillips DA. Child care in the United States 1970–1995. J Marriage Fam 1987; 49:559–571.
Jensen ME. Responses of interproximal plaque pH to snack foods and effect of chewing sorbitol-containing gum. J Am Dent Assoc 1986; 113:262–266.
Kaufman MR, Siek T. Is "natural" always healthy? J School Health 1980; 50:322–325.
Kaulter DA, Lilly T, Solomon HM, Lynt RK. *Clostridium botulinum* spores in infant foods: A survey. J Food Protect 1982; 45:1028–1029.
Kovar MG. Use of medications and vitamin-mineral supplements by children and youths. Pub Health Rep 1985; 100:470–473.
Larkin T. Herbs are often more toxic than magical. FDA Consumer 1983; 17:5–11.
Lifshitz F. No such thing as junk food. Pediatrics 1989; 84:A86.
Lifshitz F, Moses N. Nutritional dwarfing: Growth, dieting, and fear of obesity. Am Coll Nutr 1988; 7:366–367.
Lifshitz F, Moses N, Cervantes C, et al. Nutritional dwarfing in adolescents. Sem Adolesc Med 1987; 3:255–266.
Maloney MJ, McGuire J, Daniels SR, Specker B. Dieting behavior and eating attitudes in children. Pediatrics 1989; 84:482.
Mercurio KC, Betim PA. Effects of fiber type and level on mineral excretion, transit time and intestinal histology. J Food Sci 1981; 46:1462–1463, 1477.
Mindura TF, Snowden S, Wood RM, Arnon SS. Isolation of *Clostridium botulinum* from honey. J Clin Microbiol 1979; 9:282–283.
Mitchell RE. Herbal medicine. Virg Med 1984; III:753–756.
Morgan KJ, Goungetas B. What is America eating? Proceedings of a Symposium. Food and Nutrition Board, Commission on Life Sciences. Washington, D.C.: National Academy of Sciences, 1986:91–125.
Moses N, Banilivy M, Lifshitz F. Fear of obesity among adolescent females. Pediatrics 1989; 83:393–398.
O'Connell JM, Dibley MJ, Sierra J, Wallace B, Marks JS, Yip R. Growth of vegetarian children. The farm study. Pediatrics 1989; 84:475–481.
Ohsawa G. Zen macrobiotics. Los Angeles: Ignoramus Press, 1965.
Parsons JS. Contaminated herbal tea as a potential source of chronic arsenic poisoning. N Carolina Med J 1981; 42:38–39.

Price C, Brown J. Growth in the health and natural foods industry. USDA Economic Research Service, National Economics Division, Washington, D.C., May 1984.

Pugliese MT, Lifshitz F, Grad G, et al. Fear of obesity: A cause of short stature and delayed puberty. N Engl J Med 1983; 309:513–518.

Pugliese MT, Weyman-Daum M, Moses N, Lifshitz F. Parental health beliefs as a cause of nonorganic failure to thrive. Pediatrics 1987; 80:175–182.

Reinhold JG, Faradji B, Abadi P, Ismail-Beigi F. Decreased absorption of calcium, magnesium, zinc, and phosphorus by humans due to increased fiber and phosphorus consumption as wheat bread. J Nutr 1976; 106:493–503.

Sanders TAB. Growth and development of British vegan children. Am J Clin Nutr 1988; 48:822–825.

Sanders TAB, Purves R. An anthropometric and dietary assessment of the nutritional status of vegan preschool children. J Hum Nutr 1981; 35:349–357.

Satter E. How to get your kid to eat . . . but not too much. Palo Alto. CA: Bull Publishing Co., 1987.

Shull MW, Reed RB, Valadian I, Palombo R, Thorne H, Dwyer JT. Velocities of growth in vegetarian preschool children. Pediatrics 1977; 60:410–417.

Trahms CM. Vegetarianism as a way of life. In Worthington-Roberts B, ed. Contemporary developments in nutrition. St. Louis: C.V. Mosby, 1981.

Truesdell DD, Acosta PB. Feeding the vegan infant and child. J Am Diet Assoc 1985; 85:837–840.

Vyhmeister IB. Vegetarian diets: Issues and concerns. Nutrition and the M.D. 1984; 10:1–3.

Young EA, Sims O, Bingham C, Brennan EH. Fast foods update: Nutrient analysis. Ross Laboratories Publication Dietetic Currents 1986; 13(6).

Zeman FJ, Ney DM. Applications of clinical nutrition. Englewood Cliffs, NJ: Prentice Hall, 1988.

Zmora E, Gorodischer R, Bar-Ziv J. Multiple nutritional deficiencies in infants from a strict vegetarian community. Am J Dis Child 1979; 133:141–144.

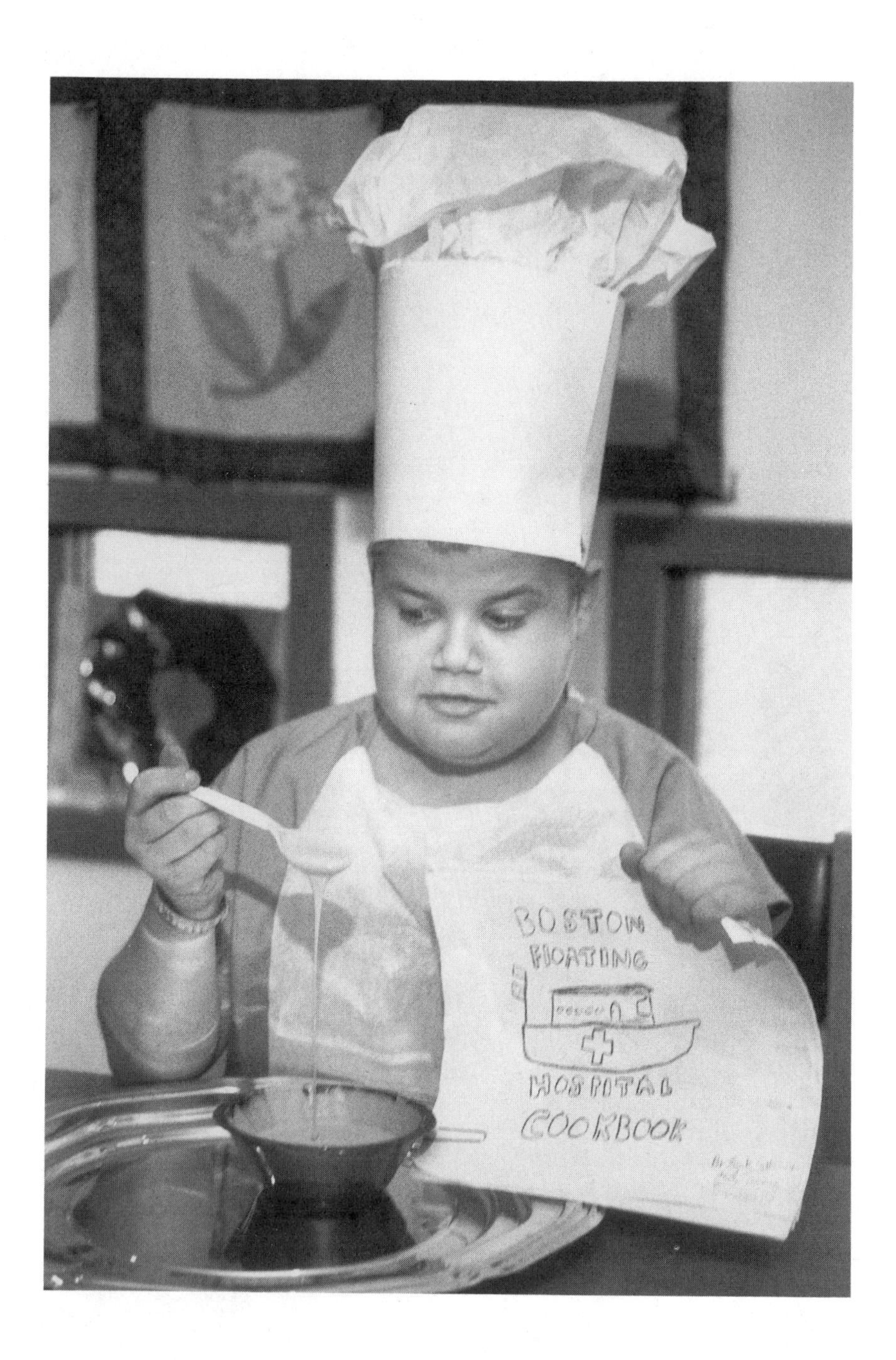
BOSTON
FLOATING
HOSPITAL
COOKBOOK

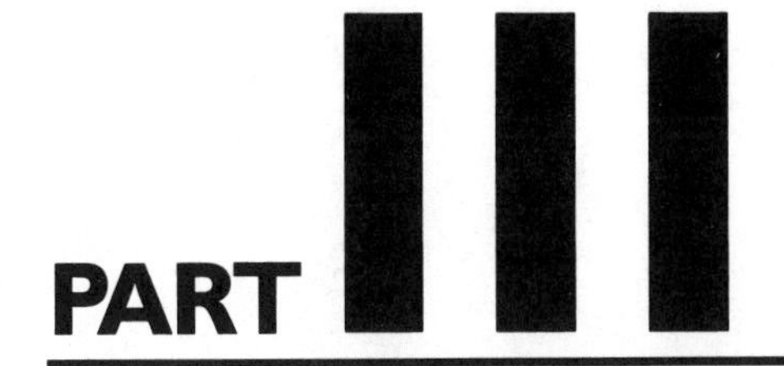

PART III

Nutrition for Special Needs

16

Failure to Thrive

She was not going to let her son become "junk food–dependent." Throughout pregnancy and during breastfeeding she was very careful in selecting her meals and avoiding "junk food." She worried about too much fat, too many sweets, too much salt, and too much cholesterol. When Paul was being weaned, she prepared baby food from "natural" products to avoid "junk"—fat and sugar. Later on she gave him only skim milk and snacks that were "healthy," like fresh vegetables bought from an organic farm. She was so happy that Paul was developing such good eating habits. He didn't even like "junk," and she thought all was wonderful. No wonder she got very upset when her doctor referred her to a specialist because her son had not gained weight in 9 months.

Failure to thrive (FTT) is a common problem in infants less than 1 year of age, accounting for 1 to 5 percent of pediatric tertiary hospital admissions (Powell, Low & Speers 1987). A larger number of FTT infants are managed as outpatients by doctors throughout the country (Mitchell, Gorrell & Greenberg 1980). Failure to thrive, a term usually restricted to infants who fail to grow well, is a sign or symptom, not a diagnosis or a disease state. The causes of FTT are many, and determining the specific etiology can be time-consuming, expensive, and frustrating. Use of the term FTT usually implies that the cause is not immediately apparent.

Physiologically, all FTT infants have alterations due to malnutrition, but the causes of FTT can be categorized as organic or nonorganic. Nonorganic failure to thrive (NOFTT) is a subtype of FTT; it accounts for the majority of FTT infants, although the percentage varies from institution to institution. Nonorganic FTT does not imply a specific etiology, but merely suggests that the cause is primarily external to the infant.

Although FTT is defined as malnutrition resulting in poor growth, NOFTT is more than a growth problem; it is a syndrome consisting of a low rate of weight and/or length gain, delayed development, abnormal behavior, and distorted caretaker–infant interaction (Barbero & Shaheen 1967). In contrast, an infant who has a specific disease that leads to FTT is said to have organic failure to thrive (OFTT) (Rosenn, Loeb & Jura 1980). Examples of organic causes include various congenital syndromes, central nervous system damage, malabsorption and/or diarrhea, chronic "hidden" infection, anemia, heart diseases, renal failure, acidosis of any cause, and endocrine diseases. The problem of OFTT resulting from many disease states is discussed in other chapters of this book that describe the particular illness. Thus, this chapter will focus only on the NOFTT infant.

WHO HAS FTT?

The major clinical presentation of FTT infants is deteriorating growth. Such infants have alterations in the rate of weight gain or they may even exhibit weight loss (Fig. 16–1). Their linear growth may also be affected, but body weight is usually more severely affected than length, especially in infants less than 1 year of age. The more wasted infants have thin chests, wasted buttocks, and prominent abdomens with hanging skin folds under the arms. These features of wasting do not clinically differentiate between NOFTT or OFTT. It should be remembered that weight deficit for length is not always present nor necessary for the diagnosis of FTT and malnutrition (see Chapters 10 and 17).

Although lack of weight gain is the most common presenting complaint of FTT, there may be other common problems that complicate the diagnosis of this illness. For example, these infants may also present with intermittent vomiting, diarrhea, and frequent upper respiratory tract infections (Barbero & Shaheen 1967). Any of these problems could lead to OFTT and therefore need to be investigated. Similarly, NOFTT patients may have associated organic disorders such as a small heart defect, but these medical concerns are not the direct cause of FTT.

A deprived social background and inappropriate nutritional intake are compatible with a nonorganic cause of poor weight gain (Bithoney & Newberger 1987), but such findings may not be forthcoming during the initial examination (Powell 1988, 1990). Proof of a nonorganic etiology is established only by ruling out the many potential disease states that can lead to FTT, and by nutritional rehabilitation, which should induce catch-up growth and weight gain. This important response criterion can be demonstrated in the majority of NOFTT patients even when treatment is initiated prior to certainty of the correct diagnosis (Ellerstein & Ostrov 1985).

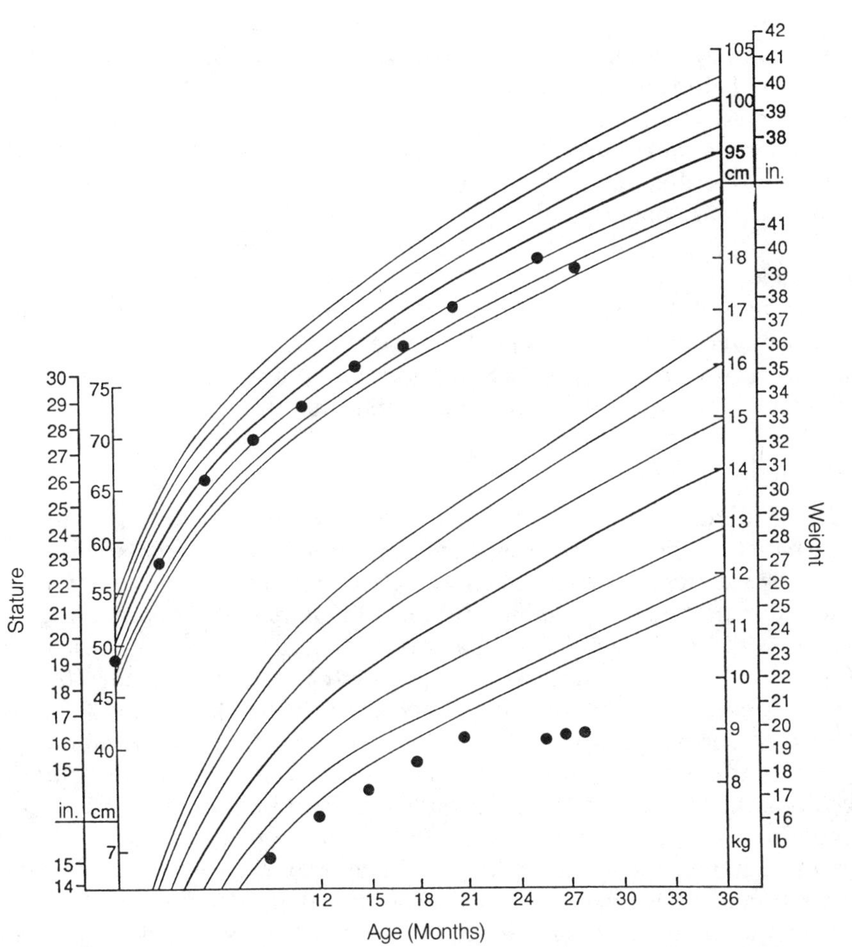

Figure 16–1. A 27-month-old girl failed to thrive since age 21 months. Notice that her body weight failed to progress satisfactorily since age 9 months, when it deviated from the fifth percentile. Prior to that she was gaining weight on the 25th percentile (not shown). However, she failed to gain any weight since age 21 months. In contrast, her length progressed on the 25th percentile, until the last 3 months when it also ceased increasing.

NOURISHMENT OR NURTURING—WHAT IS THE PROBLEM?

Inadequate food intake for age is the most common cause of NOFTT; affected children usually show signs of mild to moderate malnutrition. When malnutrition is severe, an organic problem may be associated with or be the cause of FTT. NOFTT babies do not have evidence of any abnormal losses or abnormal metabolism.

However, assuming decreased caloric intake as the cause of inappropriate weight gain, the question becomes, why are insufficient amounts of food consumed by babies with NOFTT? Although food may be in short supply in some homes, unavailability is not the usual problem in the United States. Are these infants simply not offered enough? Do the infants fail to signal hunger or satiety? Do they have a poor appetite or refuse food? Do the infants not ingest or retain enough food?

FTT babies prove that there is much more to nourishment than the ingestion of food. In most instances, NOFTT results from nurturing practices that are lacking and thus lead to inadequate nourishment. These nurturing factors include maternal attitudes and beliefs, infant behavior, and/or an adverse social and psychologic environment. In addition, nutritional factors per se may also play a part aggravating the feeding behavior and contributing to FTT.

Maternal Attitudes and Beliefs

We have identified parents who deliberately restricted nutrition to their infants based on health practices currently in vogue and recommended for adults by the medical community (Pugliese et al 1987). The following is a description of the dietary habits and nutritional intake of Adam, a 2½-year-old boy with NOFTT who had not gained weight in 9 months. The chronicity of the poor weight gain had affected his length as well: it had fallen from the 25th percentile to below the 5th percentile. At the first interview, Adam was 17 percent underweight for length. His growth chart was similar to the growth of the FTT child shown in Figure 16–1. The specialist promptly noticed that Adam was not ingesting sufficient food for growth. Adam was offered three meals daily with limited snacks between meals. Food was restricted in the home because the parents were concerned that their children ate too much and were obese. Notwithstanding that Adam was not "big," the parents wanted to avoid bad habits and wished to prevent him from becoming obese like his siblings. Adam's dietary intake was as follows:

MENU 1

Breakfast
¾ cup Rice Krispies with ½ cup whole milk
¾ cup apple juice diluted with ¾ cup water

Snack
1 bread stick
½ cup apple juice diluted with ½ cup water

Lunch
¼ regular hamburger with bun
¼ serving french fries
½ cup apple juice diluted with ½ cup water

Dinner
1 pancake with 1 tsp. margarine
¾ cup apple juice diluted with ¾ cup water
¼ cup ice cream

Adam's diet was restricted by his parents, who offered him diluted juice instead of whole milk to limit his caloric intake. He drank as much as 16 ounces of watered-down apple juice each day. Only small portion sizes were given at mealtimes, and there was no opportunity to make up between meals.

Given this diet, Adam's calorie intake was only 84 percent of recommended requirements for normal growth and development (Fig. 16–2A). In addition, he was not eating adequate amounts of protein for his age, and many nutrient intakes were inadequate (Fig. 16–2B). These included vitamin D, vitamin E, vitamin C, calcium, phosphorus, iron, magnesium, zinc, and copper. In fact, Adam had iron deficiency as defined by low iron stores (ferritin levels) but was not yet anemic.

Advice was given to Adam's parents to liberalize his diet. Specific recommendations were to increase his intake of whole milk to 3 cups daily while offering him 1 cup of full-strength juice each day. High-calorie snacks were planned and provided between his meals on a regular basis. However, despite the efforts of the nutritionist and endocrinologist, the mother was resistant to make these changes. Much discussion regarding appropriate nutrition for children was required before the mother conceded to these modifications. These changes were introduced slowly and Adam demonstrated catch-up weight gain. The nutrient quality of his diet also greatly improved. Regardless of these positive changes, the mother continues to worry about him becoming obese, although he is now thriving.

Another example of misguided maternal beliefs that may lead to FTT is the prevalent concern with "junk food." Parents want their children to ingest an appropriate diet and to avoid potentially harmful diets. Thus, products such as apple juice are frequently preferred by parents for feeding their infants. These "natural" juices are used instead of sweets and/or cakes without realizing that excess juice intake may be harmful even though juice itself is not considered "junk food" (see Chapter 15). Excess juice intake may suppress appetite and substitute for other more nourishing drinks, such as milk. The end result may be an unbalanced diet. We have seen children who fail to thrive because juice is given by their parents without any concern since it is not "junk." In Figure 16–3 a well-fed, well-nourished child is shown ingesting 100 percent natural apple juice and a piece of chocolate cake. Which one of these two choices is worse from a nutritional point of view? Both are needed by normal children to provide for their nutrient needs, but any one of them in excess may lead to a "junky diet" (Lifshitz 1989) and failure to thrive.

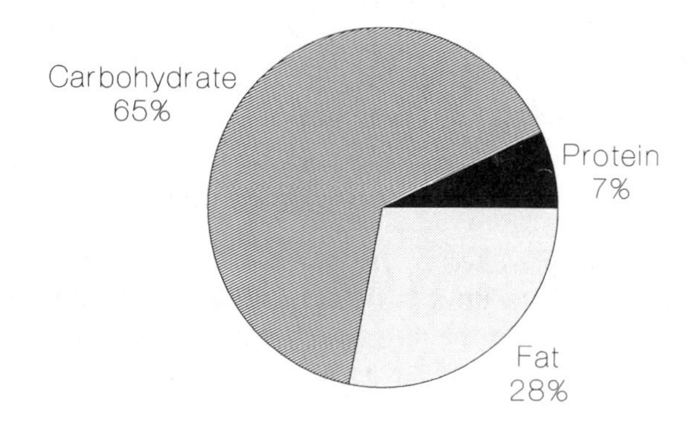

A

Vitamin D 25
Vitamin E 31
Vitamin C 58
Vitamin B12 45
Calcium 36
Phosphorus 40
Iron 36
Magnesium 42
Zinc 21
Copper 19

0 20 40 60 80 100
% R.D.A.

B

■ < 66% RDA

Figure 16–2. **A.** Caloric distribution of Adam's menu. The dietary intake of this 2½-year-old boy with FTT is described in detail in the text (see Menu 1). The parents of this patient subscribed to the idea that restricting excess food in childhood would set up healthier nutritional patterns for their child and prevent him from becoming obese. However, the diet resulted in failure to thrive due to insufficient calories and protein for growth. **B.** Inappropriate nutrient intakes in Adam's menu. Only those micronutrients that were consumed in quantities less than two thirds of the RDAs for a 2½-year-old boy are shown. This FTT patient demonstrated biochemical evidence of iron deficiency.

Infant Behaviors

NOFTT may also result from more complicated problems that are more difficult to determine. For example, NOFTT infants often have delayed motor, language, and social development (Barbero & Shaheen 1967). Many authors have reported a variety of "feeding difficulties" as a cause of decreased nutri-

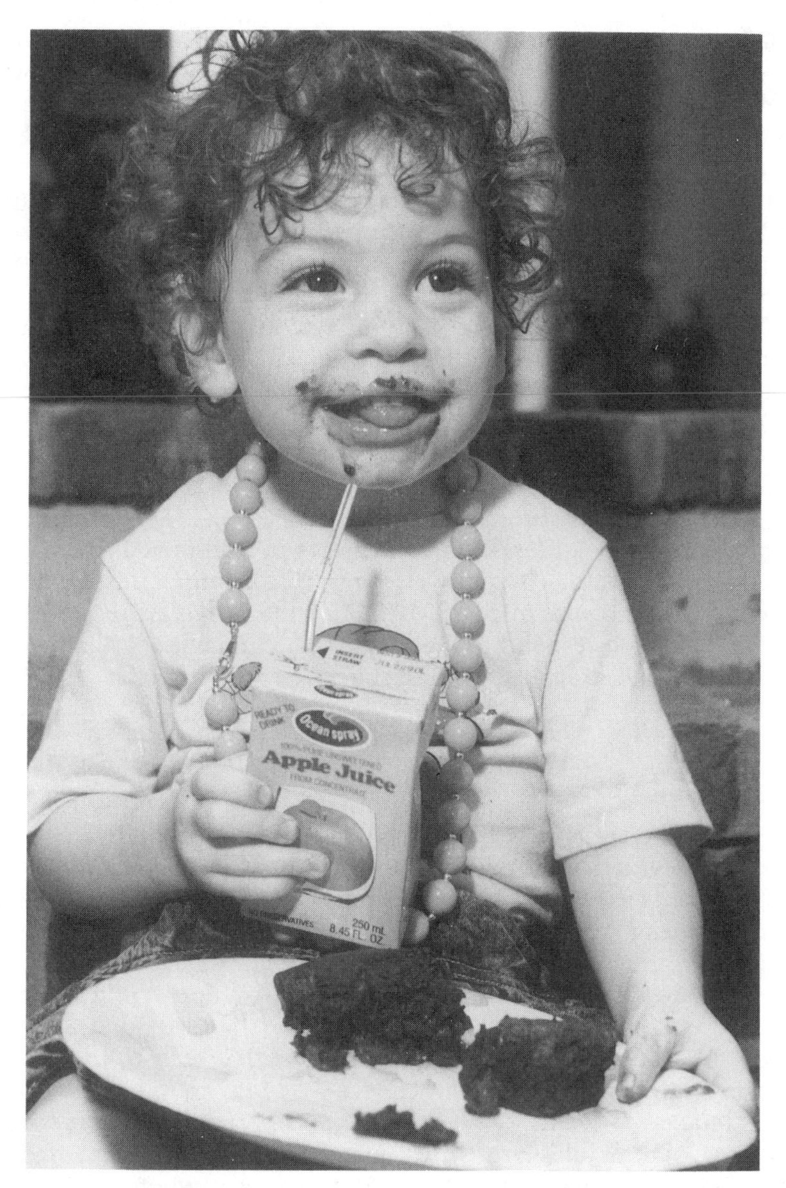

Figure 16–3. Which of the two foods is most appropriate for children—apple juice or chocolate cake?

ent intake in NOFTT infants (Pollitt & Eichler 1976). Also, NOFTT caused by food refusal was reported in infants 16 to 27 months of age who had "abnormal behavior and development" with an inappropriate attachment to their mothers (Chatoor & Egan 1983). Such children may exhibit unusual behaviors, such as wide-eyed stare and gaze avoidance. The infants often clench their fists, do not cuddle, and may actually push away from the caregiver (Powell & Low 1983, Powell, Low & Speers 1987). Obsessive hand and thumb sucking and rumination are less frequently seen abnormal behaviors. These behaviors by themselves may contribute to poor weight gain.

Although apathy and decreased motor activity are recognized behaviors in malnourished infants, many of the abnormal behaviors of NOFTT patients are not attributable to malnutrition alone. These babies are generally not severely malnourished yet they demonstrate more frequent and more intense abnormal behaviors than other infants of equivalent nutritional status (Powell, Low & Speers 1987). These behavioral abnormalities could lead to poor nutritional habits through different mechanisms. For example, they could discourage social interaction, which may be interpreted by the mother as a personal rejection. Alternatively, if the infant demands feeding, the mother may not recognize hunger signals. Or if the signals are recognized, she may be less likely to respond to them because of the infant's apathy and/or her frustration at dealing with an unresponsive baby.

Adverse Social and Psychologic Environment

In the past, reports of NOFTT occurring within the home were rare and usually associated with marked psychopathology in the mother. In 1957 the first case of NOFTT developing at home was reported in which maternal psychopathology was not present (Coleman & Provence 1957). Since then, signs and symptoms of most cases of NOFTT infants brought for medical care in the United States develop in the mother's presence in an apparently appropriate home environment.

There may be problems with the caretaker that lead to an abnormal mother–infant interaction, resulting in NOFTT. Many mothers of NOFTT infants are depressed (Evans, Reinhart & Succop 1972) or come from lower socioeconomic groups and are under multiple stresses (Casey, Bradley & Wortham 1984, Altemeier et al 1985, Bithoney & Newberger 1987). Even mothers from higher socioeconomic groups may not have the emotional strength or motivation to interpret or respond to the needs of the infant. Mothers are often engaged in work outside the home and there may not be an appropriate caretaker to provide the babies' nurturing needs. It is known that NOFTT mothers engage less often in mutual gaze with their babies and interact less with their infants (Berkowitz & Senter 1987). The quantity and quality of social and emotional stimulation may be decreased even before there is clinical evidence of FTT (Pollitt 1975). A positive change in behavior and interactions between the mother and the baby usually follows weight gain (Rosenn, Loeb & Jura 1980, Goldstein & Field 1985). Tactile stimulation seems to be very important for weight gain in little babies (Field et al 1986).

When infants are not nurtured properly they fail to thrive; if severely deprived they may die (Gardner 1972). The need for a fertile, loving environment for the baby has been known for centuries. History relates that King Frederick II of Sicily was interested in learning the innate language of humans and, consequently, he isolated infants to learn what language they would speak spontaneously. These children allegedly died because of lack of communication and attention. Obviously, King Frederick's experiment was unsuccessful, but he did discover that human interaction has a very important role in proper childhood development. At The Johns Hopkins Institution, James Knox described the deaths of infants in Baltimore foundling homes in the year 1915 that were also due to inadequate nurturing (Bakwin 1942).

A classic example of the role of love and attention on the growth of children was reported by Widdowson in 1951. There were two German orphanages that served equivalent diets but were run by women of different personalities. The first matron was unpleasant and domineering and rendered no tender loving care. The infants in the other institution were under the tutelage of a woman who was kind and loved the children for whom she was responsible. The children of the latter orphanage grew better than the children in the first institution (Fig. 16–4). Furthermore, when the supervisors of the orphanages traded workplaces the reverse occurred. Children in the first orphanage who had not grown normally began to grow rapidly when given loving attention. The reverse occurred in the second orphanage, presumably as a result of the absence of attention. These observations demonstrated how important loving compassion and attention are for normal growth in infancy. Since social stimulation was discovered to be an important prevention of FTT, institutions began to attend to social stimulation and the disorder virtually disappeared from institutions.

We must examine more closely the many possible psychologic circumstances that may lead to poor food intake and NOFTT in our current psychosocial structure among apparently well-educated families. To elicit information regarding the psychosocial circumstances of the home may require the expertise of social workers and psychologists. The treatment of NOFTT is a complicated process unless the family is studied in detail. When the social and psychologic environments are not influenced, the FTT child may not improve. There is evidence that up to one third of NOFTT babies fail to catch up in weight despite the best efforts of the family and the physician (Powell 1988, 1990).

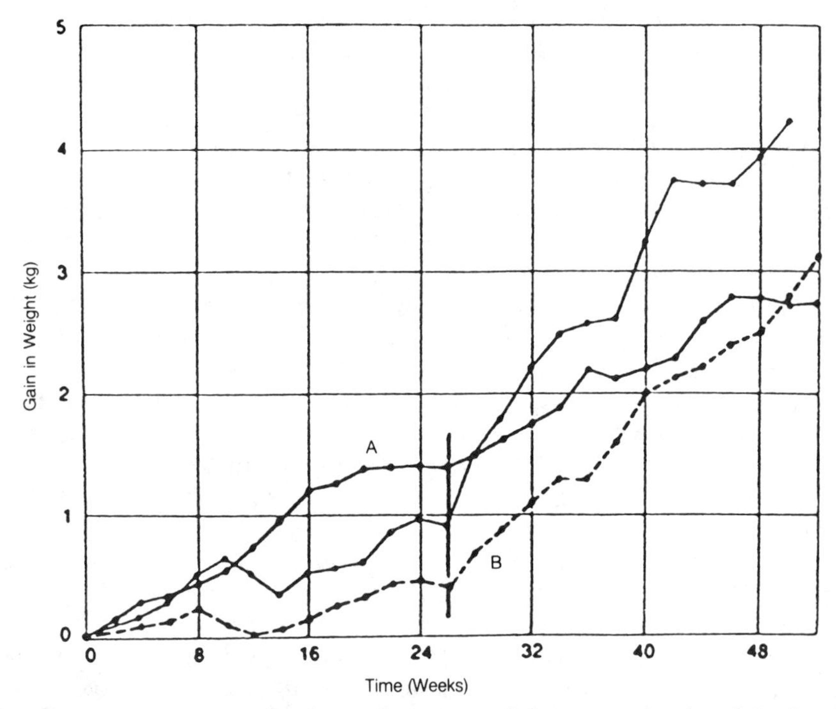

Figure 16–4. For 6 months the orphans in each home received nothing but basic rations, yet the children in Orphanage A, supervised by a kindly matron, gained more weight than most of those in Orphanage B, whose matron was a stern disciplinarian. An exception was a group of favorites of the stern matron at B; they did better than their companions. After 6 months the matron at B was transferred to A and brought her favorites with her. Simultaneously the children at A were given extra rations, whereas the children at B remained on the same basic diet. (The transition is indicated by a vertical line.) Relieved of the stern matron's discipline, the children at B began to show a sharp increase in weight; those at A showed a weight gain that averaged somewhat less than during the preceding 6 months in spite of the larger ration. Again, matron's favorites were an exception: their gain was the greatest of any.

Modified from Gardner LI. Deprivation dwarfism. Sci Am 1972; 76–82.

Nutritional Factors

The syndrome of NOFTT probably results from multiple interacting factors. Both inadequate nutrition (nature) and decreased and/or distorted social stimulation (nurture) contribute to the poor weight gain, delayed development, and abnormal behavior seen in these infants. Furthermore, nutritional deficits, once they occur, may compound the problem regardless of the primary cause that lead to FTT. Iron deficiency during infancy has been associated with anorexia, irritability, and lack of interest in surroundings (Oski 1982). Similarly, zinc deficiency may compound the course of FTT babies (Walravens, Hambidge & Koepfer 1989), and excess lead ingestion may complicate their clinical picture even before the lead blood levels reach a toxic concentration (Bithoney 1986). NOFTT infants were shown to have blood lead levels in a range formerly thought to be safe (15–20 mg/dL) (De la Brude & Choate 1972, Needleham et al 1979). Malnutrition with mild iron and zinc deficiency and increased lead levels are therefore potentially related to the developmental disability of NOFTT babies and thereby lead to a negative social interaction with poor nurturing.

Prompt recognition and treatment of these nutritional abnormalities may ameliorate some of the behavioral, cognitive, and interactive deficits observed in NOFTT infants and therefore facilitate their rehabilitation.

WHAT IS THE OUTCOME OF NOFTT?

The baby who has NOFTT should not be ignored as long-term consequences may occur even when the malnutrition appears to be mild (Oates et al 1985). Quite often the growth and development of infants with NOFTT remains abnormal on long-term follow-up. In one study the weight and length remained below the third percentile in as many as 22 to 26 percent of such patients (Shaheen et al 1968), whereas in another study as many as 42 percent of NOFTT infants continued to have abnormal growth (Glaser et al 1968). Even after 3 to 6 years of follow-up FTT patients were lighter but not necessarily shorter than other children (Mitchell et al 1980). These differences in growth continued even 14 years after the diagnosis and initiation of treatment (Oates, Peacock & Forrest 1985).

NOFTT infants may remain developmentally delayed in spite of improved weight gain. In a study by Singer (1986) NOFTT infants manifested persistent intellectual delays at 3-year follow-up despite maintenance of weight gains achieved during early intervention and treatment. In another study children were significantly behind in language development, reading age, and verbal intelligence even after 13 years of follow-up (Oates & Yu 1971). They also scored lower than the comparison group on a social maturity rating.

Although delayed development is often attributed to early malnutrition, continued exposure to an adverse environment probably plays a major role. The exact role of the mildly elevated lead levels seen in NOFTT babies remains to be determined (De la Brude & Choate 1972 & 1975, Needleham et al 1979). These data therefore suggest that the diagnosis of NOFTT is not without consequences and should always be considered important. Although organic disease may not be present, the NOFTT infant needs intense nutritional rehabilitation, stimulation programs, and the opportunity for a home and social environment conducive to emotional and physical growth.

CLINICAL INTERVENTION

All infants require careful monitoring of body weight and length and head measurements as part of routine baby care. Plotting these measurements on the growth charts will detect abnormalities in the growth of the infants. Crossing more than one major channel of growth (percentile), or the loss of 10 percent of an infant's body weight, is evidence of FTT. In such cases the nutritional intake must be investigated. If weight gain does not occur soon after giving advice to the mother about feedings, the baby needs to be evaluated more intensely. Usually these patients are admitted to the hospital to rule out any possible organic alteration leading to FTT, and simultaneously they receive appropriate nutritional intake to induce weight gain. However, sometimes weight gain does not occur in the first few days in the hospital, particularly while the babies are being studied with tests and X-rays that interfere with feedings. Also, even infants who have OFTT may gain weight in the hospital when appropriate nutrition is given (Ellerstein & Ostrov 1985).

In assessing a FTT child, a careful nutritional evaluation needs to be performed that includes dietary records, feeding patterns, and an assessment of all fluids given (Table 16–1). Often the diet record suggests that the child is receiving adequate calories for weight and length but not for age. This level of intake allows the infant to maintain current weight but does not provide sufficient nutrients for growth. Sometimes the dietary intake is adequate in calories but is deficient in specific nutrients, such as iron or zinc. Often the caregiver has fostered inappropriate eating habits by offering juices instead of milk, or candy as a means of appeasement instead of as a dessert that follows a good meal. At times, feeding difficulties lead to "power struggles" with a loss in nutrient intake for the child and a loss in the parents' nurturing ability.

Medical conditions may contribute to a child's poor appetite. Iron deficiency even without anemia may be a factor (Oski 1982), and zinc deficiency without hypozincemia may be another (Walravens, Hambidge & Koepfer 1989). Also, recurrent respiratory infections, which are common in the malnourished child, may alter the child's appetite. Dentition may make eating difficult or painful. Other conditions such as a mild brain injury (cerebral palsy) may lead to swallowing or sucking problems. The depressed child may appear sad and withdrawn and lose his or her appetite. Sometimes the "poor eaters" described by parents actually bolt down food offered in the hospital or doctor's office; in these cases, withholding of food at home should be considered. Food restriction may be due to health beliefs (Pugliese et al 1987), neglect, or psychologic problems (Blizzard 1990). NOFTT associated with

Table 16–1. Guide for Nutritional History of FTT in Infants and Children.

1. Problems During Infancy
   - Colic ______
   - Diarrhea ______
   - Vomiting ______
   - Spitting ______
2. Feedings During Infancy
   - a. Breastfeeding
     - Schedule ______
     - Supplemental bottle/formula type ______
   - b. Formula type ______ Amount purchased per week ______
     - Schedule of feedings: No. of feedings per day ______
       - Amount per feeding ______
       - Time required per feeding ______
       - Nipple used ______
   - c. Weaned to cup ______ (months)
     - Weaned to glass ______ (months)
     - Straw ______ Plastic ______ Paper ______
3. Vitamin Supplementation ______
4. Eating
   - a. Timing and sequence of feedings offered

	Normal
Strained pureed ______	(3–6 months)
cereals ______	
fruits ______	
vegetables ______	
meats ______	
desserts ______	
Junior ______	(5–6 months)
Ground/mashed ______	(8–10 months)
Chopped fine ______	(10–12 months)
Regular ______	(12+ months)

   - b. Behaviors

Finger foods: small ______ large ______	(9 months)
spoon grasp ______	(10–12 months)
plate-to-mouth ______	(15 months)
independent scooping ______	(12–18 months)
mature grasp ______	(2 years)
fork (spear) ______	(3 years)
knife (spreading) ______	(2½–3 years)
cutting ______	(4–5 years)

5. Positioning During Feeding
   - a. Held: yes ______ no ______ how ______
   - b. Chair
     - lap ______
     - infant seat ______
     - car seat ______
     - high chair ______
     - regular chair ______
     - other ______

Table 16–1. Guide for Nutritional History of FTT in Infants and Children. *(cont.)*

c. Child's position during feeding
   upright ____________
   reclined (angle) ____________
   prone ____________
   supine ____________

6. Time for Meals (minutes)
   30 ________ (normal) 30–45 ________ 45–60 ________ 60+ ________
   Number of meals per day ____________

7. Behavior During Meals
   cooperative ________ uncooperative ________
   attentive ________ inattentive ________
   happy ________ trying ________
   eats with family ________ alone ________

8. Difficulties During Meals
   Drooling? amount ________ asymmetry ________
   Tongue thrusting? Frequency ____________
   Gagging/choking? ____________
   Aspiration pneumonia ____________
   Diagnosis by ____________
   Swallowing difficulties? ____________
   Mouth closure? ____________
   Biting? ____________
   Chewing? ____________
   a. Texture ____________
      Temperature ____________
      Spoon ____________

9. Allergies and/or Intolerances (Yes/No)
   a. List foods: ____________
   ____
   b. List problems that result: ____________
   ____

10. Appetite (Describe)
   ____

11. Food Preferences
   ____
   ____

12. Food Dislikes
   ____
   ____

13. a. Parents' Feelings about Mealtime
   ____
   b. Parents' Dietary Habits ____________
   Follow Diet for 1. Obesity ________ 2. Cholesterol/Low Fat ________ 3. Other ________
   c. Parents wishes for child's weight ____________(amount)
      I wish he/she would eat ____________
      Amount ____________
      Type of foods ____________
   d. Parents concerns with food intake for child ____________
      worried about? obesity ________ cholesterol/fat ________ "junk" ________
      other ____________
   e. Parents concerns with consequences for child ____________

breastfeeding (Hill & Bowie 1983) or food allergies may also occur (see Chapters 12 and 20).

Vomiting in FTT babies is usually mild to moderate and may actually be a sign of rumination disorder. When vomiting occurs esophageal reflux may also be present. It is difficult to determine the precise role of this alteration in the FTT infant. X-rays or other studies may demonstrate esophageal reflux in a large proportion of malnourished infants, which may be of little clinical consequence to the child. In most instances, as the child gains weight, vomiting gradually ceases and the "reflux" and rumination disorder gradually improve. At times, giving feedings thickened with rice cereal and keeping the child upright after feedings may help in this transitional period. When the vomiting is forceful and severe enough to induce weight loss and electrolyte imbalances, or if it is associated with bloody vomitus, then anatomic alterations in the esophagus may be significant as the cause of FTT. In these circumstances medical treatment is needed and surgical repair may be considered. Jejunal feedings should be attempted to improve the nutritional status of these patients (Chapter 28) prior to any surgical intervention, to induce nutritional recovery and improvement in the reflux and to reduce surgical risk.

The diagnosis of NOFTT always demands a very careful history, physical examination, and laboratory assessment to rule out organic disease and/or demonstrate that abnormal clinical or laboratory findings do not solely account for the poor weight gain. At the same time, potential problems with dietary restrictions, atypical maternal and/or infant behavior, or psychologic manifestations require investigation. However, confirmation of the diagnosis of NOFTT is always based on a positive growth and behavioral response to treatment.

Therefore, initial and repeated anthropometric measurements and behavioral evaluations must be obtained with great care to confirm growth and behavioral change. The importance of accurate body-weight measurements cannot be overemphasized. Often, babies are admitted to the hospital and weighed just to find out a few days later that no one can be sure if weight gain occurred due to inaccurate measurements. For infants of about 6 months of age, a weight gain of 1½ ounces per day (45 g) (three times the usual weight gain in this age group) can be considered catch-up growth. Growth may be so fast that the skull sutures split as rapid brain growth exceeds growth of the skull (Pearl, Finkelstein & Berman 1972). There should also be improvement in developmental status and a decrease in abnormal behaviors; the baby may even start smiling!

No specific laboratory tests confirm NOFTT. However, laboratory evaluation is necessary to evaluate the presence and degree of biochemical complications of malnutrition, and to rule out suspected organic disease. The laboratory evaluation of the nutritional status needs to be comprehensive to assess for deficiencies that are not overt (Table 16–2). For example, iron deficiency may be present without anemia.

Table 16–2. Guide for Biochemical Parameters to Be Measured in Patients with FTT.

Parameter	Purpose
CBC with reticulocyte count Serum iron, TIBC Ferritin	Anemias; iron-deficiency
Sedimentation rate	Inflammation/infection
SMAC Transferrin Retinol binding protein Prealbumin Somatomedin C* Urine for creatinine**	Protein malnutrition Fluid balance
Urine for minerals** Serum mineral, vitamin levels	Special nutrient deficiencies
Antigliadin antibodies	Screening test for celiac disease
T_3, T_4, and TSH	Thyroid function test
Venous blood gases with urine pH	Kidney dysfunction; renal tubular acidosis
Serum lead levels	Toxicities

*Usually inaccurate for young children. **24-hour collection is preferable

Initial treatment of malnutrition is most easily accomplished through feeding the young infant formula of about 140 calories per kilogram of body weight per day. Feeding formula alone allows for easy calculation of caloric intake and estimation of losses through vomiting. Nurses or trained therapists should feed the infant initially to allow identification of a feeding problem, and to ensure that intake will be adequate. Tube feedings are rarely indicated except in cases of severe malnutrition and of failure to induce weight gain in the hospital (see Chapter 27).

Observation of mother–infant feeding and nonfeeding interaction is a necessary part of the evaluation. For example, does the mother relax the infant yet gently encourage feeding? Or does she passively feed the infant in a disinterested fashion? In nonfeeding interactions, does she offer a warm and pleasant smile and voice? Does she socially reward the infant for its responses?

Once the infant no longer has a problem with feeding and adequate intake has been achieved, the mother may again feed the infant under observation. Presumably, by this time rapport has been established with the mother, maternal stresses identified, and some social intervention has begun. Education of the mother concerning the infant's nutritional needs is an essential part of therapy, but development and behavioral treatment is also necessary (Powell 1988, 1990). This comprehensive treatment is best accomplished through a team, usually consisting of a physician, nurse, nutritionist, social worker, and developmental therapist.

Continued treatment after discharge from the hospital is necessary and the infant should be followed at regular intervals for a long time. Growth, development, and social behavior must be carefully and continually monitored. Vitamin and mineral deficiencies may become evident only after the baby starts growing and gaining weight. Catch-up growth may be reduced if there is an insufficient positive balance of certain nutrients like iron and zinc. If there is little hope of improvement in the home environment, placement in a foster home may be necessary. All interventions for the treatment of NOFTT must be comprehensive and long-term, and must focus on improving nutrition, mother–infant interaction, and other social and environmental factors if this problem is to be correctly diagnosed, effectively treated, and hopefully prevented.

REFERENCES

Altemeier WA, O'Connor SM, Sherrod KB, Vietze PM. Prospective study of antecedents for nonorganic failure to thrive. J Pediatr 1985; 106:360–365.

Bakwin H. Loneliness in infants. Am J Dis Child 1942; 62:30–40.

Barbero GJ, Shaheen E. Environmental failure to thrive: A clinical view. J Pediatrics 1967; 71:639–644.

Berkowitz CD, Senter SA. Characteristics of mother-infant interactions in nonorganic failure to thrive. J Fam Pract 1987; 25:377–381.

Bithoney WG. Elevated lead levels in children with nonorganic failure to thrive. Pediatrics 1986; 78:891–895.

Bithoney WG, Newberger EH. Child and family attributes of failure to thrive. J Devel Behav Pediatr 1987; 8:32–36.

Blizzard RM. Psychosocial short stature. In Lifshitz F, ed. Pediatric endocrinology: A clinical guide. 2nd ed. New York: Marcel Dekker, 1990.

Casey PH, Bradley R, Wortham B. Social and nonsocial home environments of infants with nonorganic failure to thrive. Pediatrics 1984; 73:348–353.

Chatoor I, Egan J. Nonorganic failure to thrive and dwarfism due to food refusal: A separation disorder. J Am Acad Child Psychiatry 1983; 22:294–301.

Coleman R, Provence S. Environmental retardation (hospitalism) in infants living in families. Pediatrics 1957; 19:285–292.

De la Brude B, Choate MS. Does asymptomatic lead exposure in children have later sequelae? J Pediatr 1972; 81:1088–1091.

De la Brude B, Choate MS. Early asymptomatic lead exposure and development at school age. J Pediatr 1975; 87:638–642.

Ellerstein NS, Ostrov BE. Growth patterns in children hospitalized because of caloric-deprivation failure to thrive. Am J Dis Child 1985; 139:164–166.

Evans SL, Reinhart JB, Succop RA. Failure to thrive. A study of 45 children and their families. J Am Acad Child Psychiatry 1972; 11:440–457.

Field TM, Schanberg SM, Scafidi F, et al. Tactile/kinesthetic stimulation effects on preterm neonates. Pediatrics 1986; 77:654–658.

Gardner LI. Deprivation dwarfism. Sci Am 1972; 76–82.

Glaser HH, Heagarty MC, Bullard DM Jr, Pivchik EC. Physical and psychological development of children with early failure to thrive. J Pediatr 1968; 73:690–698.

Goldstein S, Field T. Affective behavior and weight changes among hospitalized failure-to-thrive infants. Infant Ment Health 1985; 6:187–194.

Hill ID, Bowie MD. Chloride deficiency syndrome due to chloride deficient breast milk. Arch Dis Child 1983; 58:224–226.

Lifshitz F. No such thing as junk food. Pediatrics 1989; 84:A86.

Mitchell WG, Gorrell RW, Greenberg RA. Failure to thrive: A study in a primary care setting, epidemiology and follow-up. Pediatrics 1980; 65:971–977.

Needleham HJ, Gunnoe C, Leviton A, et al. Deficits in psychologic and classroom performance of children with elevated dentine lead levels. N Engl J Med 1979; 300:689–695.

Oates RK, Peacock A, Forrest D. Long-term effects of nonorganic failure to thrive. Pediatrics 1985; 75:36–40.

Oates RK, Yu JS. Children with non-organic failure to thrive, a community problem. Med J Aust 1971; 2:199–203.

Oski FA. Nutritional anemias of infancy. In Lifshitz F, ed. Pediatric nutrition. New York: Marcel Dekker, 1982:123–138.

Pearl M, Finkelstein J, Berman MR. Temporary widening of cranial sutures during recovery from failure to thrive. Clin Pediatr 1972; 11:427–430.

Pollitt E. Failure to thrive: Socioeconomic, dietary intake and mother-child interaction data. Fed Proc 1975; 34:1593–1597.

Pollitt E, Eichler A. Behavioral disturbances among failure-to-thrive children. Am J Dis Child 1976; 130:24–29.

Powell GF. Failure to thrive. In Lifshitz F, ed. Pediatric endocrinology: A clinical guide. 2nd ed. New York: Marcel Dekker, 1990.

Powell GF. Nonorganic failure to thrive in infancy: An update on nutrition, behavior, and growth. J Am Coll Nutr 1988; 7:345–354.

Powell GF, Low J. Behavior in nonorganic failure to thrive. J Dev Behav Pediatr 1983; 4:26–33.

Powell GF, Low JF, Speers MA. Behavior as a diagnostic aid in failure to thrive. J Dev Behav Pediatr 1987; 8:18–24.

Pugliese MT, Weyman-Daum M, Moses N, Lifshitz F. Parental health beliefs as a cause of nonorganic failure to thrive. Pediatrics 1987; 80:175–182.

Rosenn DW, Loeb LS, Jura MB. Differentiation of organic from nonorganic failure to thrive syndrome in infancy. Pediatrics 1980; 66:698–704.

Shaheen E, Alexander D, Truskowsky M, Barbero GJ. Failure to thrive—a retrospective profile. Clin Pediatr 1968; 7:255–261.

Singer L. Long-term hospitalization of failure to thrive infants: Developmental outcome at three years. Child Abuse Neglect 1986; 10:479–486.

Walravens PA, Hambidge KM, Koepfer DM. Zinc supplementation in infants with a nutritional pattern of failure to thrive. A double blind controlled study. Pediatrics 1989; 83:532–538.

Widdowson EM. Mental contentment and physical growth. Lancet 1951; 1:1316–1318.

17

Eating Disorders

"The first time I ever took 60 laxatives I got very scared," Amy said. "Several hours after I took them I started having diarrhea, which I expected because I had been taking 30 laxatives every day. But a few hours later I got very nauseous and started vomiting up the remaining food and undigested laxative pills. I was so nauseous that I couldn't keep down any water. Normally during a laxative purge I wouldn't drink any liquid because I wanted to maximize the weight loss from the laxatives. But when I started getting very painful cramps in my calves and feet and when my feet and hands went into spasms I even tried drinking some orange juice, something I hadn't done in about 10 years because of the calories."

"I ended up spending three days in the hospital. When I got to the emergency room they couldn't hear the bottom number of my blood pressure and had trouble finding a vein to put the IV in. I was given activated charcoal to absorb any remaining laxative in my stomach. I remember my first morning there, I was angry when I got weighed and I didn't lose as much weight as I usually did because the IV had replenished some of the liquid I had lost. I wanted the IV taken out but the doctor said I needed it."

"I have since gotten just as sick many times, but learned that I feel better in 24 hours or so. While I'm feeling my worst I'll vow I'll never do it again. I sometimes even read diet books while I am on the toilet, planning the diet I would start tomorrow so I wouldn't binge and have to purge anymore. I get physically sick when I just see the color pink of the brand of laxatives that has made me so ill."

In the early 1980s, articles in the medical literature reported that bulimia and anorexia nervosa affected as many as 5 to 15 percent of adolescent girls and young women (Pope et al 1984a, b). In other studies the estimated prevalence of bulimia among young women was as high as 22 percent (Leichner et al 1986) and the maladaptive behaviors associated with bulimia nervosa and anorexia nervosa seemed to appear at a younger age than previously expected (Johnson et al 1982, Pyle et al 1983). Eating disorders were considered to be even more common among dancers, modeling students, jockeys, wrestlers, gymnasts, actors, and actresses. Many articles in newspapers and magazines, as well as books devoted to the topic, described rampant epidemics of eating disorders, often implying that dangerous binging and purging behavior was commonly involved.

Prompted by the media alarms and lured by prospects of large profits, an entire industry has grown with numerous outpatient clinics and inpatient facilities to treat bulimia as well as other eating disorders. "In the last two years, we've seen an increase in the number of special facilities that advertise and basically convince people that they have an eating disorder problem," said Lawrence Goelman, president of Cost Care Inc., a company in Huntington Beach, California that reviews claims for medical insurance companies (Miller 1988). Many people are now treated for bulimia and other eating disorders at such outpatient clinics, but national data on the numbers of these patients or the costs incurred by insurance companies, third party payers, and HMOs for their care are difficult to obtain.

EATING DISORDERS AND INAPPROPRIATE EATING BEHAVIORS

Bulimia Nervosa and Anorexia Nervosa

There appears to be a spectrum of eating disorders and inappropriate eating behaviors that afflict schoolaged children, with the most extreme conditions being bulimia and anorexia nervosa. The American Psychiatric Association defines bulimia nervosa as eating binges at least twice a week followed by purging either by self-induced vomiting, strict dieting or fasting, vigorous exercise to prevent weight gain, or use of laxatives or diuretics (Diagnostic and Statistical Manual of Mental Disorders 1987). Anorexia nervosa is a refusal to maintain body weight over a minimal normal weight for age and height. Patients with anorexia nervosa usually have weight loss of 15 percent of their usual body weight, and have an intense fear of becoming obese, even when underweight. They feel fat despite being emaciated and therefore have a distorted body image. Patients with bulimia nervosa and anorexia nervosa often have psychologic disturbances. Anxiety and depression usually develop by the time they seek help, and 5 percent of patients with bulimia nervosa will have attempted suicide. Bulimia nervosa develops in approximately 50 percent of patients with anorexia nervosa, often as a means to control their weight and eating (Herzog & Copeland 1988).

Researchers using a rigorous definition of eating disorders have found that bulimia nervosa and anorexia nervosa are rare, even among college women, a group considered to be very susceptible (Scholte & Stunkard 1987). The first national study found that only 1 percent of all college women had bulimia, and only 0.2 percent of college men had this problem. The group with the greatest prevalence, 2.2 percent, was undergraduate women living in group housing on campus (Drewnowki, Yee & Drahn 1988). The precise incidence of anorexia nervosa has not been clearly determined, with figures ranging from 1 to 10 patients per 100,000 people (Willi & Grossman 1983, Pope et al 1984a, b). The prevalence data for these two severe eating disorders are even lower in children since these problems usually manifest after childhood.

Both psychologic and biologic factors appear to play a part in the development of severe eating disorders. The patient with bulimia and/or anorexia nervosa is usually anxious, lonely, and frustrated, and often reports abnormal appetite and/or difficulty in feeling satieted (Agras 1987, Garner & Garfinkel 1985). It has been shown that in patients with bulimia nervosa there is a blunted meal-induced secretion of the satiety hormone cholecystokinin (Geracioti & Liddle 1988), suggesting a role for biologic factors in inducing satiety and limiting food intake (Hewson et al 1988). In anorexia nervosa other biologic factors have also been implicated, such as high cortisol levels (Smith, Bledsoe & Chhetri 1975, Doerr et al 1984). Eventually, self starvation or binging and purging become habitual. Binging and purging typically begins in the midst of an attempt to lose weight and alternates with periods of food restriction. These cycles of intermittent starvation may play a role in triggering binge eating even among normal men who volunteer for self-starvation (Keys et al 1950).

Atypical Eating Disorders

When the criteria for diagnosis of anorexia nervosa or bulimia nervosa, as established by the American Psychiatric Association, cannot be met, the patients are considered to have atypical eating disorders. Various types of purging behavior, such as self-induced vomiting and use of laxatives and diuretics, are among these types of atypical eating disorders (Killen et al 1986). Additionally, there are many other inappropriate eating behaviors and attitudes among adolescents (Fig. 17–1). Teenagers are often dissatisfied with their body weight and appearance (Feldman, Feldman & Goodman 1988), and have unhealthy approaches toward weight reduction such as fad diets or compulsive exercising (Dwyer et al 1969, Storz & Greene 1983, Yates, Leehey & Shisslak 1983) (see Chapter 14).

In contrast to patients with true anorexia nervosa, patients with atypical eating disorders do not have distorted conceptions about their body image. They usually know they are thin and they want to remain slim and trim (Lifshitz 1985, Lifshitz et al 1987). It is not known whether the presence of a mild

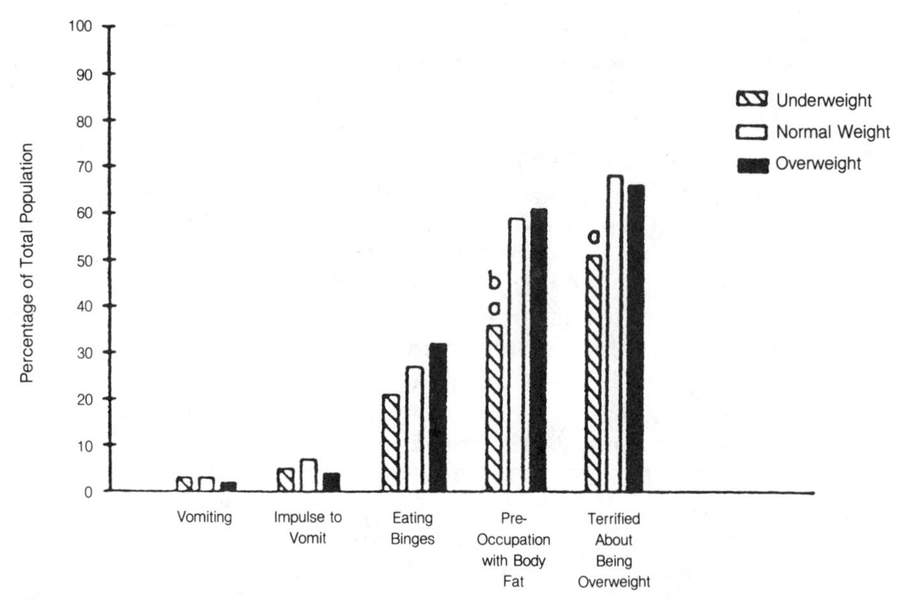

Figure 17–1. The proportion of inappropriate eating attitudes such as fear of obesity and maladaptive eating behaviors among 326 high-school girls varies according to their body weights. Significant differences ($P<0.05$) from normal weight (a) and the overweight group (b) as determined by chi-square test of independence.

From Moses N, Banilivy MM, Lifshitz F. Fear of obesity among adolescent girls. Pediatrics 1989; 83:393–398. Copyright 1989. Reprinted by permission of Pediatrics.

eating disorder could be the beginning of what will develop into true bulimia or anorexia nervosa. Nor is it known whether the fear of becoming obese and associated dieting practices are milder manifestations of anorexia nervosa or bulimia nervosa or represent totally different problems and types of eating disorders (Bruch 1977, Lucas 1986).

A variety of atypical eating disorders that result in poor growth and delayed sexual development has been described during childhood and adolescence (Davis et al 1978, Smith 1980, Button & Whitehouse 1981, Pugliese et al 1983, Lifshitz et al 1987) (Fig. 17–2). One such syndrome, fear of obesity, was defined as self-induced malnutrition due to an exaggerated concern about becoming fat. By skipping meals and avoiding high-calorie foods such as sweets and pastries, these children consumed hypocaloric diets and failed to gain weight and grow. Another group of patients had fears of the consequences of high serum cholesterol levels. They ate low-fat, low-cholesterol diets that were nutritionally inadequate and therefore they failed to grow (Lifshitz & Moses 1989). Even babies whose mothers had fears of allowing their children to become obese or junk food–dependent or to develop atherosclero-

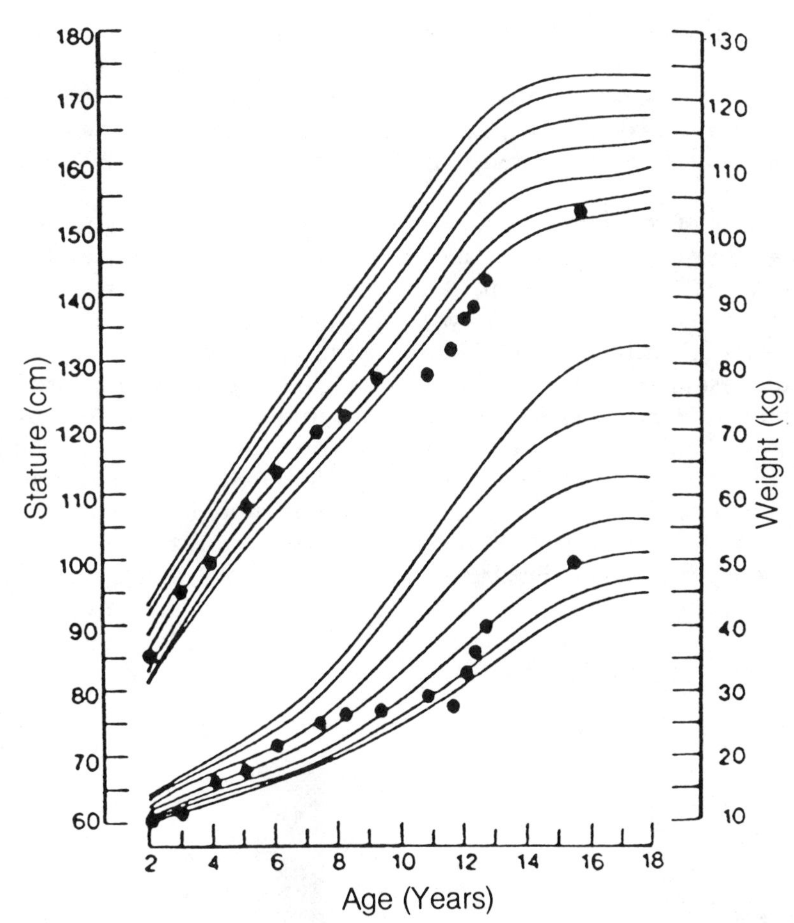

Figure 17–2. Nutritional dwarfing in a patient with an atypical eating disorder. The heights and weights of the patient throughout life are plotted in standard growth charts. Data were provided by the parents, school, and referring physician. This patient was consuming an inappropriate diet due to an atypical eating disorder NOS. An appropriate nutritional intake was initiated at age 12 years. This was associated with catch-up growth and sexual development. Height is represented in the upper panel and weight in the lower one.

From Lifshitz L, Moses N. Nutritional dwarfing: Growth, dieting and fear of obesity. J Am Coll Nutr 1988; 7:367–376. Copyright © 1988.

sis failed to thrive. As a consequence of these fears and health beliefs, the mothers fed them insufficient amounts and types of food to allow for normal growth (Pugliese et al 1987).

Unlike children with bulimia nervosa and anorexia nervosa, the children with these atypical eating disorders were younger and did not have other associated psychologic disturbances. However, growth retardation and delayed sexual development may also occur in patients with anorexia nervosa when the disease starts early in life before growth is completed (Root & Powers 1983). In contrast, patients with bulimia nervosa may appear generally well-nourished and often maintain a normal body weight for their height.

The fear of obesity and inappropriate eating behaviors and attitudes appear to be pervasive among children in the United States (Moses, Banilivy & Lifshitz 1989, Maloney et al 1989). A survey of 325 adolescent females revealed an exaggerated concern with obesity and frequent dieting practices regardless of their body weight (Moses, Banilivy & Lifshitz 1989). Over one third of the students were on diets to lose weight at the time of the survey, and two thirds of them had tried to lose weight in the recent past. Worst of all, dieting was taking place among students who were of normal weight and even among those who were underweight (Fig. 17–3). In contrast, only one half of those who were overweight were on diets to reduce their weight. In another study, which reviewed the growth records of 1017 high-school students from a similar middle-class socioeconomic status, a high incidence of

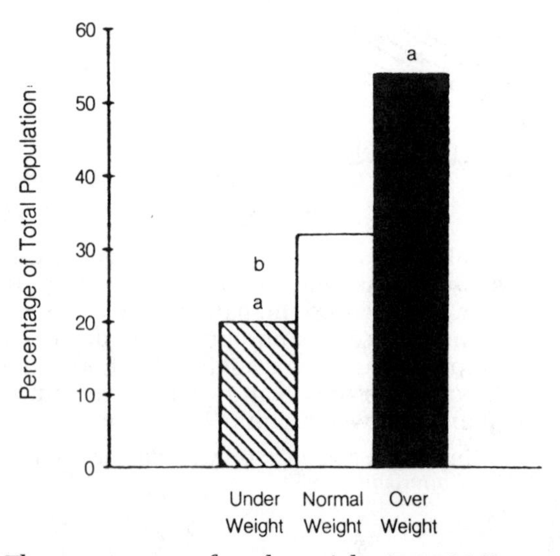

Figure 17–3. The percentage of underweight (n = 118), normal-weight (n = 152), and overweight (n = 152) adolescent girls who were dieting at the time of the survey. Significant differences ($P<0.05$) from normal-weight group (a) and from the overweight group (b) as determined by chi-square test of independence.
From Moses N, Banilivy MM, Lifshitz F. Fear of obesity among adolescent girls. Pediatrics 1989; 83:393–398. Copyright 1989. Reprinted by permission of Pediatrics.

low-weight students was reported. Over 25 percent of these students were below 90 percent of their ideal body weight for height, and 1.8 percent exhibited linear growth retardation associated with poor weight gain (Pugliese, Recker & Lifshitz 1988). These data may reflect the frequent concerns about body weight and the fears of becoming fat among our youth. However, these reports do not necessarily indicate that these students were afflicted with severe eating disorders.

The reasons for the apparent high prevalence of inappropriate eating behaviors and various kinds of atypical eating disorders among adolescents remain unclear. The social and cultural established ideal of thinness has often been blamed (Crisp 1980, Garner et al 1980, Schwartz, Thompson & Johnson 1982, Andersen 1984), and perhaps it is this influence that has resulted in a fertile environment for the development of many types of eating disorders and inappropriate eating behaviors.

When children are afflicted with an eating disorder, the results can be life-threatening. Any self-starvation type of disorder, whether it be true anorexia nervosa or a less severe atypical eating disorder (e.g., fear of obesity), may lead to severe medical and nutritional consequences (Fig. 17–4). Inadequate intake may lead to poor growth and delayed sexual development (Pugliese et al 1983, Lifshitz et al 1987). There may also be other long-term consequences of malnutrition, such as thinning of the bones (osteoporosis), menstrual irregularities, and even infertility later in life (Comerci 1988). With binging and purging behaviors, there may be electrolyte disturbances due to frequent vomiting and/or excessive laxative use. Also, there may be other medical complications in addition to the biochemical imbalances, such as dental enamel erosion, acute gastric dilation that may lead to rupture of the stomach, irritation and inflammation of the lining of the esophogus (esophagitis), enlargement of the salivary glands, and a general susceptibility to infections due to malnutrition (Mitchell et al 1987).

Other Eating Disorders

Two other eating disorders that may afflict children are pica and rumination. Pica, which means abnormal or perverted appetite, is most commonly seen in situations of inadequate maternal care (Eisenberg 1968). It has been suggested that iron-deficiency anemia and zinc deficits may be contributory factors leading to this abnormal eating behavior (Gutelius et al 1962, Hambidge & Silverman 1973). The pathologic significance of pica lies in its unhygienic or socially unattractive aspects of eating unusual things such as dirt. It may also be a health hazard if ingested substances are toxic, such as paint chips containing lead. The life-threatening aspect of pica can be minimized if environmental toxins are removed, but the ubiquity of such substances makes external control difficult. The physician and health care provider should

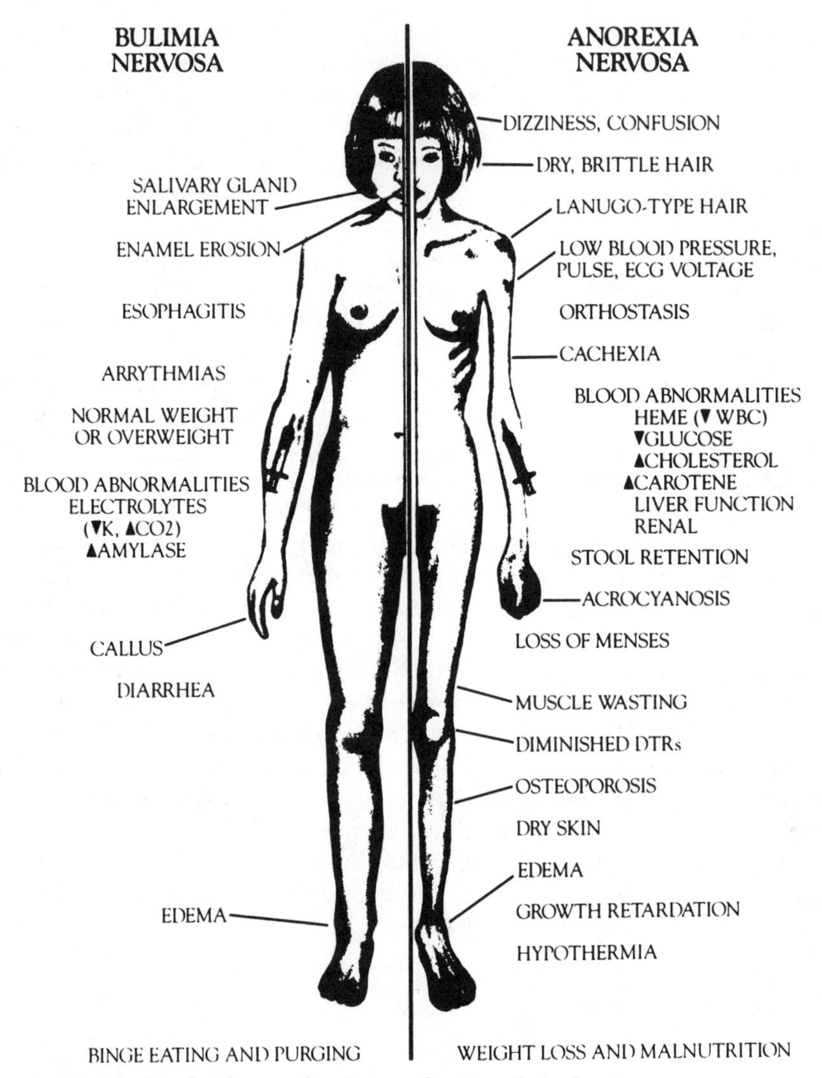

Figure 17–4. Medical complications of eating disorders.

From Kreipe RE, Comerci GE. Assessment of weight loss in adolescents. Columbus, OH: Ross Laboratories, August 1988. Copyright © 1988 Ross Laboratories. Reprinted by permission of Ross Laboratories, Columbus, OH 43216.

search for psychologic as well as physiologic reasons for the perverted appetite and attempt to remedy the lack of supervision that allows the child access to dangerous substances.

Rumination is a syndrome in which the child will return previously swallowed food to the mouth either to be spit out or to be rechewed and reswallowed. Unlike vomiting, rumination is not an unpleasant experience for the child. On the contrary, it is usually associated with feelings of gratification. Rumination has been found to occur more frequently among children with developmental disabilities but it may also be a symptom of a psychologic problem such as a disturbed mother–child interaction. Like vomiting, rumination can lead to electrolyte imbalances, tooth decay, esophagitis, and malnutrition.

Eating Behaviors

There are different types of behaviors in children that lead to "eating problems." Examples of some typical feeding problems among children include refusing to try new foods, "not being hungry," or demanding the same food over and over again. However, these are usually not true eating disorders. The feeding behavior of the child should be viewed calmly and taken in the right perspective as such practices often do not lead to any nutritional alteration. Although the behavior may be bothersome there is little reason to worry about it as long as the child eats sufficiently to gain weight and to grow along the same channels in the growth chart (see Chapter 10). Books are available on the subject of feeding problems and how to get children to eat (e.g., Satter 1987). However, it should be remembered that fussy eaters aren't born, they're made! And they're usually made by parents who can't learn to accept their children's changing food habits.

An important thing to remember is that it is normal for children to sometimes show a real slow-down in their desire for food. This may occur on a given day or even for prolonged periods. For example, when the growth of the child slows down after 1 year of age, less food is required and the appetite decreases. The reverse is also true; adolescents during their growth spurt need enormous quantities of food and they eat a large supply of high-energy products to keep up with the growth demands and activity.

Parents who deprive children of a variety of foods or go to extremes in keeping children away from snacks may set the stage for food obsession and "cheating." In contrast, a mother who uses pressure to get her child to eat can cause more problems once the main battleground becomes the kitchen table and the weapon food. Teasing or using tricks to get food into the child's mouth can result in real resistance and eating difficulties later in life. Another good way to create a fussy eater is to feed them sweets between meals. That curbs the appetite for more nourishing foods, ensuring that the child will pick and fuss at mealtime.

DIETARY INTAKE

Poor nutritional practices are prevalent in all patients with eating disorders. The type and severity of the disorder may determine the dietary selection and the type of nutritional deficiencies found. Also, the stage of the disease will be an important modifier of the type of diet ingested. For example, patients with anorexia nervosa may eat small amounts of special types of foods and may not vomit while they are underweight but when they gain weight, they may begin purging by vomiting or abusing laxatives. Also, patients with bulimia may binge or fast at different stages of their illness. Similarly, patients with other atypical eating disorders may have food-consumption patterns that resemble those of the more severe anorexia nervosa or bulimia nervosa patients or they may eat diets that appear to be in line with the current dietary guidelines recommended for the general population (see Chapters 9 and 25).

Patients with anorexia nervosa have dietary patterns and intakes that are highly variable. Although some eat a balanced diet that includes all the basic food groups, they tend to eat irregularly, skip meals, or severely restrict calories during a meal. The great majority of them fast and select a nutrient-poor diet. Often, they may have capricious choices, such as a vegetarian meal pattern or avoidance of selected food items such as red meat or sweets and desserts. They often exclude carbohydrate (so called carbohydrate-phobia) but at times they gorge on the "forbidden" sweet foods. Anorectic patients are often willing to eat vegetables, lettuce, fresh fruit, cheese, and sometimes eggs to avoid carbohydrates and are often disgusted by milk and meat. Food-intake records of such patients show that they ingest an average of about 1000 calories per day. In these diets, carbohydrates typically provide only 33 percent of the total calories, fats 49 percent, and protein 18 percent. However, other studies have shown that anorectics ate less fat than the average population (Beumont et al 1981).

Bulimic patients may ingest enormous quantities of food during a binge. It has been estimated that they may consume up to 20,000 calories during an eating binge, involving up to 7 pounds of food, chiefly bread, cakes, chocolates, yogurt, cottage cheese, ice cream, doughnuts, soft drinks, cookies, and popcorn. Other estimates are on the order of 3000 to 5000 calories consumed within 1 hour (Johnson et al 1982, Mitchell & Laine 1985). A "sample binge," described by one patient, may be 12 muffins, 1 (12-oz) package of chocolate cookies, 1 pound of chicken salad, *and* 1 coffee cake. The binge may last several hours, with periodic vomiting. Another binge may be 2 packages of Rice-a-Roni, 2 loaves of bread (eaten while waiting for the rice to cook), *and* 8 pieces of fried chicken. After the last of the food is vomited, 120 laxatives are taken. A "small" binge may be 2 or 3 muffins washed down with diet soda to make the vomiting easier. Sometimes the anorectic patient may start out eating a "good" meal, like fish and a vegetable, but suddenly she doesn't feel satisfied so she eats a few slices of bread, some crackers, maybe a big salad. After the first slice of bread, she would get an urge to vomit because it's more than she was "supposed" to have.

In extreme cases these patients may have up to 10 binges per day with-

foods high in fat, with moderate carbohydrate and low protein contents (Mitchell et al 1987, Mitchell & Laine 1985). Virtually all eating binges are immediately followed by purging. In contrast, when these patients are not binging they tend to eat such foods as salads and diet soft drinks (Mitchell & Laine 1985). Even bulimic women will not overeat certain "bad" or "fattening" foods unless they plan in advance to purge afterwards.

The type of food and its taste may also have a role in binge-eating behaviors. Bulimic patients often eat too quickly during a binge to taste anything (Abraham & Beumont 1982). However, all patients feel that the taste and texture of food is important, at least at the beginning of the binge. Often the choices are soft, milky, fluid foods that have a high caloric density, satisfaction, and satiety (Mitchell & Laine 1985).

Overconsumption of foods containing fat and sugar is not restricted to patients with severe eating disorders. College students who binge also make inappropriate food choices (Leon et al 1985). They may select pastries, breads, cookies, and so called "junk food" choices, including salted snacks like pretzels or potato chips, and they often skip meals and eat irregularly (Lacey, Stanley & Crutchfield 1977).

In one study, patients with nutritional dwarfing due to atypical eating disorders had similar food preferences and eating habits as patients in whom a specific fear or health belief was identified (Lifshitz & Moses 1988). Generally, all these patients avoided "junk food" and fatty foods and reduced their intake of red meat, eggs, and shellfish. They ingested limited dairy products; any intake of dairy products was usually of the low-fat variety, such as skim milk instead of whole milk. These patients preferred high-fiber products and low-calorie foods such as vegetables and dietetic sodas. The eating patterns of all patients had many similarities, including small meals and frequent meal skipping. Usually they had no breakfast and ingested a small lunch. Dinner was the only substantive meal that was eaten with the family. They had few if any snacks and when they "indulged," it was on a raw vegetable such as broccoli. These patients rarely consumed high-energy snacks such as pastry or candy. The patients' families generally supported these eating habits. Both patient and family had similar food preferences and eating patterns. The families skipped or hurried through a meager breakfast and ran out to their daily activities. Dinner, a "healthy meal" without excess fat or "junk," was usually rapidly put together, typically when the working parents returned home in the evening.

These patients with atypical eating disorders generally ingested an insufficient amount of calories for age, usually about two thirds of their normal daily caloric requirements (Fig. 17–5) (Lifshitz & Moses 1988). The fat intake of these patients generally did not exceed 33 percent of the total calorie intake. This quantity of fat in the diet was comparable to the amount of fat recommended for a prudent diet and was usually lower than the prevailing

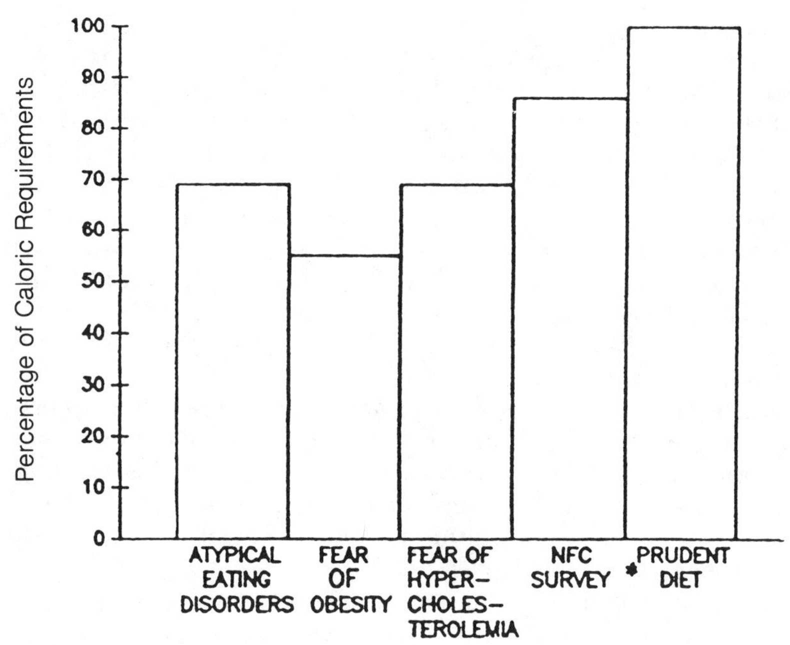

Figure 17–5. Caloric intake of patients with various eating disorders.

*Nationwide Food Consumption Survey 1977–78 (ages 9–18 years). Preliminary Report No. 2, September, 1980.

From Lifshitz F, Moses N. Nutritional dwarfing: Growth, dieting and fear of obesity. J Am Coll Nutr 1988; 7:367–376. Copyright 1988. Reprinted by permission of John Wiley & Sons, Inc.

quantity ingested by the population at large. Patients who feared the consequences of hypercholesterolemia ingested an even lower amount of calories derived from fat, with an average of 24 percent of calories contributed by fat (Lifshitz & Moses 1989).

The low-calorie, low-fat diets, designed largely by eliminating primary foods such as dairy products, meat, and eggs, were deficient in essential nutrients. To consume sufficient calories and minerals without red meat or eggs, large amounts of grains and cereals need to be ingested. However, these were not consumed by the patients studied (Lifshitz & Moses 1988). Without an increased intake of complex carbohydrates and with the traditional American food choices, levels of energy and essential minerals were insufficient in patients with nutritional dwarfing. The intakes of zinc and iron were the most markedly diminished. The intake of other major essential minerals, such as magnesium and calcium, were also below the Recommended Dietary Allowances. The lower the dietary fat content, the lower the quantity of essential minerals in the diet. Indeed, when the fat content of the diet provided less than 25 percent of the calories, the intake of iron and zinc were below 30 and 40 percent, respectively, of the RDA. Growth failure and delayed puberty are well-known complications of inappropriate intake of minerals such as zinc (Prasad 1988).

CLINICAL INTERVENTION

Physicians and health care providers must be aware of the prevailing attitudes and the very frequent inappropriate eating behaviors among children in our population (Moses, Banilivy & Lifshitz 1989, Maloney et al 1989). These attitudes and behaviors may be associated with many medical problems including poor growth and delayed sexual development as well as with many other serious complications (Mitchell et al 1987). It is sometimes difficult to distinguish among the athlete or dancer whose training leads to a low body weight (see Chapter 14), the adolescent who diets to avoid obesity, and the person with an eating disorder. As long as our society equates a thin shape with self-worth, adolescents will diet, engage in inappropriate eating behaviors, become malnourished, and thus fail to grow. The medical and physical histories, the body-weight deficit, the pattern of weight gain or loss, the presence of special nutritional deficits, the eating patterns, and the body image must all be taken into consideration before an eating disorder is considered (Tables 17–1 and 17–2). Often, the diagnosis may not be clear even after psychiatric and psychologic assessments. Many persons will not reveal their inappropriate eating behaviors and must be given support, time, and encouragement before they talk about it. Patients with severe eating disorders will refuse to gain weight even when a physician recommends it. In contrast, patients with atypical eating disorders or misguided health beliefs may object to do so at first, fearing that the added weight will impede their performance or appearance, but will gain weight if necessary.

It should be kept in mind that the general outcome of a patient with an eating disorder is at best guarded. The reported mortality rate may be as high as 18 percent among those with severe eating disorders (Comerci 1988). Death may result from starvation and its complications (e.g., bronchopneumonia and other infections, renal and cardiac failure, electrolyte disturbances) or from suicide. Death from suicide and electrolyte imbalances is more frequent in patients who vomit. Therefore, in any child who does not gain weight or who ceases to grow, an eating disorder and/or an inappropriate health belief that distorts the dietary intake must be considered. In such cases appropriate measures should be taken for accurate medical, psychologic, and nutritional assessments and for prompt treatment, which must involve all aspects of the disease (Health and Public Policy Committee 1986, Comerci 1988).

Table 17–1. Eating Attitudes Test.*

Please place an (X) under the column which applies best to each of the numbered statements. All of the results will be *strictly* confidential. Most of the questions directly relate to food or eating, although other types of questions have been included. Please answer each question carefully. Thank you.

	ALWAYS	VERY OFTEN	OFTEN	SOMETIMES	RARELY	NEVER
1. Am terrified about being overweight.	( )	( )	( )	( )	( )	( )
2. Avoid eating when I am hungry.	( )	( )	( )	( )	( )	( )
3. Find myself preoccupied with food.	( )	( )	( )	( )	( )	( )
4. Have gone on eating binges where I feel that I may not be able to stop.	( )	( )	( )	( )	( )	( )
5. Cut my food into small pieces.	( )	( )	( )	( )	( )	( )
6. Aware of the calorie content of foods I eat.	( )	( )	( )	( )	( )	( )
7. Particularly avoid foods with high carbohydrate content (e.g., bread, potatoes, rice, etc.).	( )	( )	( )	( )	( )	( )
8. Feel that others would prefer if I ate more.	( )	( )	( )	( )	( )	( )
9. Vomit after I have eaten.	( )	( )	( )	( )	( )	( )
10. Feel extremely guilty after eating.	( )	( )	( )	( )	( )	( )
11. Am preoccupied with a desire to be thinner.	( )	( )	( )	( )	( )	( )
12. Think about burning up calories when I exercise.	( )	( )	( )	( )	( )	( )

13.	Other people think that I am too thin.	( )	( )	( )	( )	( )	( )
14.	Am preoccupied with the thought of having fat on my body.	( )	( )	( )	( )	( )	( )
15.	Take longer than others to eat my meals.	( )	( )	( )	( )	( )	( )
16.	Avoid foods with sugar in them.	( )	( )	( )	( )	( )	( )
17.	Eat diet foods.	( )	( )	( )	( )	( )	( )
18.	Feel that food controls my life.	( )	( )	( )	( )	( )	( )
19.	Display self-control around food.	( )	( )	( )	( )	( )	( )
20.	Feel that others pressure me to eat.	( )	( )	( )	( )	( )	( )
21.	Give too much time and thought to food.	( )	( )	( )	( )	( )	( )
22.	Feel uncomfortable after eating sweets.	( )	( )	( )	( )	( )	( )
23.	Engage in dieting behavior.	( )	( )	( )	( )	( )	( )
24.	Like my stomach to be empty.	( )	( )	( )	( )	( )	( )
25.	Enjoy trying new rich foods.	( )	( )	( )	( )	( )	( )
26.	Have the impulse to vomit after meals.	( )	( )	( )	( )	( )	( )

*Scores are derived as follows: A mark on "always" yields 3 points, "very often" 2 points, "often" 1 point; and others 0 points. The only exception is No. 25, which is reversed scoring. Any patient scoring above 20 may have a severe eating disorder.

From Garner DM, Olmstead MP, Bohr Y, Garfinkel PE. The Eating Attitudes Test: Psychometric features & clinical correlates. Psychol Med 1982; 12:871–878. Reprinted by permission of Cambridge University Press.

Table 17–2. Children's Eating Attitudes Test.*

Please place an (X) under the word which best applies to the statements below.
Sample item: I like to eat vegetables.

	ALWAYS	VERY OFTEN	OFTEN	SOMETIMES	RARELY	NEVER
1. I am scared about being overweight.	( )	( )	( )	( )	( )	( )
2. I stay away from eating when I am hungry.	( )	( )	( )	( )	( )	( )
3. I think about food a lot of the time.	( )	( )	( )	( )	( )	( )
4. I have gone on eating binges where I feel that I might not be able to stop.	( )	( )	( )	( )	( )	( )
5. I cut my food into small pieces.	( )	( )	( )	( )	( )	( )
6. I am aware of the energy (calorie) content in foods that I eat.	( )	( )	( )	( )	( )	( )
7. I try to stay away from foods such as breads, potatoes and rice.	( )	( )	( )	( )	( )	( )
8. I feel that others would like me to eat more.	( )	( )	( )	( )	( )	( )
9. I vomit after I have eaten.	( )	( )	( )	( )	( )	( )
10. I feel very guilty after eating.	( )	( )	( )	( )	( )	( )
11. I think a lot about wanting to be thinner.	( )	( )	( )	( )	( )	( )
12. I think about burning up energy (calories) when I exercise.	( )	( )	( )	( )	( )	( )

13. Other people think I am too thin.	( )	( )	( )	( )	( )	( )
14. I think a lot about having fat on my body.	( )	( )	( )	( )	( )	( )
15. I take longer than others to eat my meals.	( )	( )	( )	( )	( )	( )
16. I stay away from foods with sugar in them.	( )	( )	( )	( )	( )	( )
17. I eat diet foods.	( )	( )	( )	( )	( )	( )
18. I think that food controls my life.	( )	( )	( )	( )	( )	( )
19. I can show self-control around food.	( )	( )	( )	( )	( )	( )
20. I feel that others pressure me to eat.	( )	( )	( )	( )	( )	( )
21. I give too much time and thought to food.	( )	( )	( )	( )	( )	( )
22. I feel uncomfortable after eating sweets.	( )	( )	( )	( )	( )	( )
23. I have been dieting.	( )	( )	( )	( )	( )	( )
24. I like my stomach to be empty.	( )	( )	( )	( )	( )	( )
25. I enjoy trying new rich foods.	( )	( )	( )	( )	( )	( )
26. I have the urge to vomit after eating.	( )	( )	( )	( )	( )	( )

*This table is similar to Table 17–1. However, it was devised for children.

From Maloney MJ, McGuire J, Daniels SR, Specker B. Dieting behavior and eating attitudes in children. Pediatrics 1989; 84:482–487. Copyright 1989. Reprinted by permission of Pediatrics.

Patients with severe eating disorders need the combined management of physicians and mental health professionals who are trained to deal with these disorders. Anorectic patients may need to be hospitalized if they are severely malnourished, fail to gain weight, continue to exercise compulsively, or face a particularly life threatening event. Patients with bulimia or other eating disorders who are not severely malnourished may not need to be hospitalized except in the relatively rare instance when they lose complete control over their eating, or they have engaged in excessive purging leading to electrolyte imbalances. In all instances a combined approach of nutritional and psychologic rehabilitation must always be undertaken simultaneously (DoCouto et al 1989).

Nutritional rehabilitation should be a key component of the treatment of these patients (Andersen 1984, Rock & Yager 1987) (Tables 17–3 and 17–4). A good nutritional status must be achieved before the patient can benefit from psychotherapy (Provenzale 1983, Garfinkel & Garner 1984, Rees 1984). Precise, clear nutritional goals must always be agreed upon by the team, and these must be enforced with parents and patients. We recommend the use of a written contract that spells out the goals for weight and dietary intake agreed upon by the patient, the family, and the medical professionals. The patient and family must sign and keep the contract to avoid manipulations and to have clear goals of the treatment and nutritional rehabilitation.

It is important to individualize the diets of these patients and to keep in mind that anorexia nervosa and bulimia nervosa are often found together in the same patient. For children with atypical eating disorders specific nutritional guidance and support are needed to reassure them that an appropriate

Table 17–3. Principles of Nutrition Intervention in Anorexia Nervosa.

1. Increase calorie intake slowly, beginning with 10 to 20 percent of calories above those needed to maintain body weight (usually 800–1200 kcal/d).
2. Prescribe well-balanced diets, with some individual variations according to patient preferences (e.g., vegetarian).
3. Correct any possible vitamin or mineral deficits.
4. Enhance elimination with dietary fiber from grain sources.
5. Reduce sensations of bloating with small, frequent feedings.
6. In behavioral programs, link rewards to caloric intake, not weight gain.
7. Reduce satiety sensations with cold or room temperature foods and with finger foods (e.g., snacks).
8. Provide interactive nutritional counseling as an ongoing process.
9. Reduce excessive caffeine intake.
10. Use liquid supplements when the patient cannot achieve desired intake with solid food and weight gain is not achieved.
11. Provide parenteral nutritional support only in severe cachectic states unresponsive to usual nutritional rehabilitation.

Adapted from Rock CL, Yager J. Nutrition and eating disorders: A primer for clinicians. Int J Eating Disord 1987; 6:276.

Table 17–4. Diet Recommendations to Aid Bulimic Patients.

1. Avoid finger foods; plan meals with foods that require the use of utensils.
2. Increase meal satiety by including warm foods, rather than cold or room temperature foods.
3. Include vegetables, salad, and/or fruit at a meal, to prolong the meal duration; choose whole-grain and high-fiber breads and cereals.
4. Prescribe well-balanced meals, both to increase satiety and to increase the variety of foods eaten.
5. Use foods that are naturally divided into portions, such as potatoes (rather than rice or pasta); 4- and 8-oz containers of yogurt, ice cream, or cottage cheese; precut steak or chicken parts; and frozen dinners and entrees.
6. Include foods containing adequate amounts of complex carbohydrates (which promote meal satiety) and fat (which slows gastric emptying and further enhances the feeling of "fullness").
7. Eat meals and snacks sitting down.
8. Plan meals and snacks, and keep a food diary by recording food prior to eating.
9. Avoid excess carbonated drinks.

Adapted from Rock CL, Yager J. Nutrition and eating disorders: A primer for clinicians. Int J Eating Disord 1987; 6:276.

diet is being ingested without inducing problems that they fear. For example, if a child is afraid of obesity and has nutritional dwarfing, assurance that growth will occur without inducing excess weight gain is very important. In some patients, other phobias or concerns need to be addressed by the nutritionist as well as by the psychiatrist to meet success.

The nutritional rehabilitation of the malnourished patient requires special considerations to induce recovery without endangering the patient's health. It must be kept in mind that patients with eating disorders usually have had a chronic malnourished state to which they have become adapted. Thus, rapid refeeding may induce dangerous changes that could lead to death (Weinseir & Krumdieck 1980) or to other biochemical problems such as a severe drop in serum phosphorus levels (Cummings, Farquhar & Bouchier 1987) or serum zinc concentrations (Lifshitz & Nishi 1980). These alterations may not be evident before weight gain. There may be other problems associated with treatment; for example, the patient may begin vomiting when forced to eat and/or may deteriorate psychologically. When exercise is restricted there may also be decreased bone calcification independent of the dietary intake of calcium. Thus, the treatment needs to be carefully planned and orchestrated to avoid producing more harm than good.

In general, the best approach to nutritional rehabilitation is the least restrictive one that results in weight gain (Neuman & Halvorson 1983). The patient first needs to stop weight loss, followed by weight maintenance, before encouraging a gradual increase in weight through normal self-feeding (Pemberton & Gastineau 1981). The calorie requirements necessary for weight gain in patients with anorexia nervosa vary considerably (Dempsey et al 1984). Initially, a 10 to 20 percent increase above the amount of calories needed to maintain the weight of the patient will suffice for a slow weight gain. Because of the starvation or semistarvation that most of these patients have experienced, a decline in basal energy requirements has taken place. The use of a calculated basal caloric requirements from tables derived from the normal population (see Chapter 9) will therefore overestimate the needs for the undernourished patient.

Even among inpatients, physical activity is the major contributor to calorie need (Kaye et al 1988). In this study, the mean amount of energy that was necessary for a 1-kilogram weight gain was 8301 calories, but individual needs varied from 4561 to 12,723 calories, with the most active patients requiring the greatest caloric intake. The increased physical activity may thus explain the resistance to weight gain commonly noted in anorectic patients. Minimizing activity when weight gain is being sought may greatly decrease the hospitalization time. However, the effect of inactivity on bone density and body composition must also be considered. Patients may gain fat and/or retain fluid rapidly without necessarily getting better nourished by increasing lean body mass.

Enteral or parenteral nutrition for the rehabilitation of patients with eating disorders may be used when oral feedings fail. These nutrition methods are associated with increased morbidity (see Chapters 27 to 29) and they do not provide long-term benefit to patients with severe eating disorders (Bruch 1977, Andersen 1983). Regardless of the method used to achieve nutritional recovery it must be kept in mind that to tolerate weight gain these patients need strong psychotherapeutic support (Neuman & Halvorson 1983, Maloney & Klykylo 1983, Andersen 1984).

The goals of nutritional rehabilitation must be set in accordance with the patient's problem. In children with nutritional dwarfing there may be no body-weight deficit for height, only failure to grow (Lifshitz et al 1987). Thus, these patients' weight goals should be based on attaining the weight that will allow normal growth. In conditions in which body-weight losses occur, nutritional recovery goals need to be set to restore the deficits to allow normal physiologic functioning of the patient.

Many physicians aim to restore the patient's weight to at least 95 percent of ideal body weight (Andersen 1984). However, it should be kept in mind that normal physiologic function can be achieved even when mild malnutrition persists and body weight is not at an ideal level. This includes recovery of all physical and mental components associated with severe malnutrition (Provenzale 1983, Andersen 1983). However, normal menstruation may not occur even when body-weight deficits are fully restored. Moreover, without appropriate psychotherapeutic support the patient may not "tolerate" the weight gain. Thus, individualized supportive guidance is necessary to make adjustments as therapy proceeds. Other aspects of the nutritional status of the patient need to be maintained regardless of body weight. For example, when mineral or vitamin deficiencies occur, these problems must be promptly treated. Long-term follow-up is necessary in most instances since patients with eating disorders usually continue having eating difficulties and/or other psychologic impairments (Schwartz & Thompson 1981).

There is no single therapeutic approach that has emerged as the treatment of choice for eating disorders. A consensus seems to be emerging that optimal management involves combined approaches including nutritional rehabilitation, psychotherapy, behavior modification, family therapy, and, at times, psychotropic medications. In general, treatments tend to be long-term with an uncertain prognosis. Means to prevent eating disorders are unknown. It is hoped, however, that by teaching children and young persons the importance of nutrition and setting examples for an appropriate way to achieve and to maintain a normal body weight, the incidence of eating disorders will decrease and appropriate eating behaviors will develop.

REFERENCES

Abraham SF, Beumont PJV. How patients describe bulimia or binge eating. Psychol Med 1982; 12:625–635.

Agras WS. Eating Disorders. New York: Pergamon Press, 1987.

Andersen AE. In Paige DM, ed. Manual of clinical nutrition. Pleasantville, NJ: Nutrition Publications, 1983:26.1–26.16.

Andersen AE. Anorexia nervosa and bulimia: Biological, psychological, and sociocultural aspects. In Galler JR, ed. Nutrition and behavior. New York: Plenum Press, 1984:305–338.

Beumont PJV, Chambers TL, Rouse L, Abraham SF. The diet composition and nutritional knowledge of patients with anorexia nervosa. J Hum Nutr 1981; 35:265–273.

Bruch H. Psychological antecedents of anorexia nervosa. In Vigersky RA, ed. Anorexia nervosa. New York: Raven Press, 1977:1–10.

Button EJ, Whitehouse A. Subclinical anorexia nervosa. Psychol Med 1981; 11:509–516.

Comerci GD. Eating disorders in adolescents. Pediatr Rev 1988; 10:1–11.

Crisp AH. Anorexia nervosa: Let me be. New York: Grune & Stratton, 1980.

Cummings AD, Farquhar JR, Bouchier IAD. Refeeding hypophosphataemia in anorexia nervosa and alcoholism. Br Med J 1987; 295:490–491.

Davis R, Apley J, Fill F, et al. Diet and retarded growth. Br Med J 1978; 1:539–542.

Dempsey DT, Crosby LO, Pertschuk MJ, Feurer ID, Buzby GP, Mullen JL. Weight gain and nutritional efficacy in anorexia nervosa. Am J Clin Nutr 1984; 39:236–242.

Diagnostic and Statistical Manual of Mental Disorders. 3rd Ed rev. Washington, D.C.: American Psychiatric Association, 1987.

Doerr P, Fichter M, Pirke KM, et al. Relationship between weight gain and hypothalamic pituitary adrenal function in patients with anorexia nervosa. J Steroid Biochem 1984; 13:529–537.

DoCouto C, Reiff D, Stewart E, Lampson-Reiff K. Position of the American Dietetic Association: Nutrition intervention in the treatment of anorexia nervosa and bulimia nervosa—technical support paper. J Am Diet Assoc 1988; 88:68–71.

Drewnowki A, Yee DK, Drahn DO. Bulimia in college women: Incidence and recovery rates. Am J Psychiatry 1988; 145:753–755.

Dwyer JT, Feldman JJ, Seltzer C, Mayer J. Adolescent attitudes toward weight and appearance. J Nutr Ed 1969; 1:14–19.

Eisenberg L. Psychological considerations. In Cook RE, ed. The biologic basis of pediatric practice. New York: McGraw-Hill, 1968:1574–1583.

Feldman W, Feldman E, Goodman JT. Culture versus biology: Children's attitudes toward thinness and fatness. Pediatrics 1988; 81:190–194.

Garfinkel PE, Garner DM. In White PL, Selvey N, eds. Malnutrition determinants and consequences. New York: Alan R. Liss, 1984:305–314.

Garner DM, Garfinkel PE, eds. Handbook of psychotherapy for anorexia nervosa and bulimia. New York: Guilford, 1985.

Garner DM, Garfinkel PE, Schwartz D, Thompson M. Cultural expectations of thinness in women. Psychol Rep 1980; 47:483–491.

Geracioti TD Jr, Liddle RA. Impaired cholecystokinin secretion in bulimia nervosa. N Engl J Med 1988; 319:683–688.

Gutelius M, Millican F, Layman E, Cogen GJ, Dublin C. Treatment of pica with iron given intramuscularity. Pediatrics 1962; 29:1018–1023.

Hambidge KM, Silverman A. Pica with rapid improvement after dietary zinc supplementation. Arch Dis Child 1973; 48:567–568.

Health and Public Policy Committee, American College of Physicians. Position paper. Eating disorders: Anorexia nervosa and bulimia. Ann Int Med 1986; 105:790–794.

Herzog DB, Copeland PM. Bulimia nervosa—psyche and satiety. N Engl J Med 1988; 319:716–718.

Hewson G, Leighton GE, Hill RG, Hughes J. The cholecystokinin receptor antagonist L364,718 increases food intake in the rat by attenuation of the action of endogenous cholecystokinin. Br J Pharmacol 1988; 93:79–84.

Johnson C, Stuckey M, Lewis L, et al. Bulimia: A descriptive survey of 316 cases. Int J Eating Disord 1982; 2:3–16.

Kaye WH, Gwirtsman HE, Obarzanek E, George DT. Relative importance of caloric intake needed to gain weight and level of physical activity in anorexia nervosa. Am J Clin Nutr 1988; 42:989–994.

Keys A, Brozek J, Henschel A, Mickelson O, Taylor HL. The biology of human starvation. Minneapolis: University of Minnesota Press, 1950:846–847.

Killen JD, Taylor B, Telch MJ, et al. Self-induced vomiting and laxative and diuretic use among teenagers: Precursors of the binge-purge syndrome? JAMA 1986; 255:1447–1449.

Lacey JH, Stanley PA, Crutchfield SM. Sucrose sensitivity in anorexia nervosa. J Psychosom Res 1977; 21:17–21.

Leichner P, Arnett J, Rallo JS, et al. An epidemiologic study of maladaptive eating attitudes in a Canadian school age population. Int J Eating Disord 1986; 5:969–982.

Leon GK, Carroll K, Chemyk B, Finn S. Binge-eating and associated habit patterns within college student and identified bulimic populations. Int J Eating Disord 1985; 4:43–57.

Lifshitz F. Nutrition and growth. In Paige DM, ed. Clinical nutrition. Nutrition and growth supplement. St. Louis: C.V. Mosby, 1985; 4:40–47.

Lifshitz F, Moses N. Growth failure—a complication of hypercholesterolemia treatment. Am J Dis Child 1989; 143:537–542.

Lifshitz F, Moses N. Nutritional dwarfing: Growth, dieting, and fear of obesity. J Am Coll Nutr 1988; 7:367–376.

Lifshitz F, Moses N, Cervantes C, et al. Nutritional dwarfing in adolescents. Sem Adolesc Med 1987; 3:255–266.

Lifshitz F, Nishi Y. Mineral deficiencies during growth. In Anast C, DeLuca H, eds. Pediatric disease related to calcium. New York: Elsevier North-Holland, 1980:305–322.

Lucas AR. Anorexia nervosa: Historical background and biopsychosocial determinants. Sem Adolesc Med 1986; 2:1–9.

Maloney MJ, Klykylo WM. An overview of anorexia nervosa, bulimia, and obesity in children and adolescents. J Am Acad Child Psychiatry 1983; 22:99–107.

Maloney MJ, McGuire J, Daniels SR, Specker B. Dieting behavior and eating attitudes in children. Pediatrics 1989; 84:482–487.

Miller D. Dangerous eating disorder may be a false alarm. New York Times, Health Section, August 25, 1988.

Mitchell JE, Laine DC. Monitored binge-eating behavior in patients with bulimia. Int J Eating Disord 1985; 4:177–183.

Mitchell JE, Seim HC, Colon E, Pomeroy C. Medical complications and medical management of bulimia. Ann Int Med 1987; 107:71–77.

Moses N, Banilivy M, Lifshitz F. Fear of obesity among adolescent females. Pediatrics 1989; 83:393–398.

Neuman PA, Halvorson PA. Anorexia nervosa and bulimia: A handbook for counselors and therapists. New York: Van Nostrand Reinhold, 1983.

Pemberton CM, Gastineau CF, eds. Mayo Clinic diet manual: A handbook of dietary practices. 5th ed. Philadelphia: W.B. Saunders, 1981:114–117.

Pope HG Jr, Hudson JI, Yurgelun-Todd D. Prevalence of anorexia nervosa and bulimia in three student populations. Int J Eating Disord 1984a; 3:45–51.

Pope HG Jr, Hudson JI, Yurgelun-Todd D. Anorexia nervosa and bulimia among 300 women shoppers. Am J Psychiatry 1984b; 141:292–294.

Prasad AS. Zinc in growth and development and spectrum of human zinc deficiency. J Am Coll Nutr 1988; 7:377–384.

Provenzale JM. Anorexia nervosa—thinness as illness. Postgrad Med 1983; 74:83–89.

Pugliese MT, Lifshitz F, Grad G, et al. Fear of obesity: A cause of short stature and delayed puberty. N Engl J Med 1983; 309:513–518.

Pugliese M, Recker B, Lifshitz F. A survey to determine the prevalence of abnor-

mal growth patterns in adolescence. J Adolesc Health Care 1988; 9:181–187.
Pugliese MT, Weyman-Daum M, Moses N, Lifshitz F. Parental health beliefs as a cause of non-organic failure to thrive. Pediatrics 1987; 80:175–182.
Pyle RL, Mitchell JR, Eckert ED, et al. The incidence of bulimia in freshman college students. Int J Eating Disord 1983; 2:75–85.
Rees JM. In Mahan LK, Rees JM, eds. Nutrition in adolescence. St.Louis: Times Mirror/Mosby College Publishing, 1984:104–137.
Rock CL, Yager J. Nutrition and eating disorders: A primer for clinicians. Int J Eating Disord 1987; 6:267–280.
Root AN, Powers DS. Anorexia nervosa presenting as growth retardation in adolescence. J Adolesc Health Care 1983; 4:25–30.
Satter E. How to get your kid to eat . . . but not too much. Palo Alto, CA: Bull Publishing Company, 1987.
Scholte DE, Stunkard AJ. Bulimia vs. bulimic behaviors on a college campus. JAMA 1987; 258:1213–1215.
Schwartz DM, Thompson MG. Do anorectics get well?: Current research and future needs. Am J Psychiatry 1981; 138:319–323.
Schwartz DM, Thompson MG, Johnson CL. Anorexia nervosa and bulimia: The sociocultural context. Int J Eating Disord 1982; 1:20–26.
Smith NJ. Excessive weight loss and food aversion in athletes simulating anorexia nervosa. Pediatrics 1980; 66:139–142.
Smith SR, Bledsoe T, Chhetri MK. Cortisol metabolism and the pituitary-adrenal axis in adults with protein calorie malnutrition. J Clin Endocrin Metab 1975; 40:43–52.
Storz NS, Greene WH. Body weight, body image, and perception of fad diets in adolescent girls. J Nutr Ed 1983; 15:15–18.
Weinseir RL, Krumdieck CL. Death resulting from overzealous total parenteral nutrition: The refeeding syndrome revisited. Am J Clin Nutr 1980; 34:393–399.
Willi J, Grossman S. Epidemiology of anorexia nervosa in a defined region in Switzerland. Am J Psychiatry 1983; 140:564–567.
Yates A, Leehey K, Shisslak CM. Running—an analogue of anorexia? N Engl J Med 1983; 308:251–255.

18

Obesity*

Paul, an 8-year-old boy who weighed 120 pounds, came to see his pediatrician for his annual medical examination. Paul's father mentioned his concern regarding his son's recent weight gain and lack of interest in socializing or making new friends. Since early childhood, Paul had tended to be slightly chubby but in the past 2 years, after the family relocated from Maine to New York, Paul's weight increased by 20 pounds! The pediatrician agreed that this was a very important concern and recommended that intervention begin right away. She referred the family to a pediatric obesity program.

An evaluation there revealed that Paul was physically inactive: he spent most of his day watching television, playing computer games, and consuming many high-fat, high-calorie snacks such as ice cream, potato chips, and chocolate. Paul was started on a supervised exercise program in conjunction with a food plan that fit into the family lifestyle. He also joined a tennis league, which met twice a week, and bought a stationary bike so he could exercise at home. Initially it was hard for Paul to make all these changes, but compromises were made. Paul was allowed to watch television and see all his favorite programs as long as he would do so while riding his stationary bicycle. He was also allowed to eat a limited amount of his favorite foods at meal times, but not while watching television. As a result of all his efforts, and by following his nutrition and exercise program, Paul decreased his weight by 15 pounds. He also made new friends in his neighborhood through participation in recreational sports. Paul was no longer embarrassed about his appearance and did not miss his friends from Maine as much as he had before.

*With the help and contributions of Marie Fasano, M.S., R.D.

WHO IS OBESE?

Obesity implies the presence of excess body fat in an amount sufficient to endanger health. However, many people may feel "fat," as the social concepts of obesity and beauty have changed over time. Currently, many children desire an ideal weight that is 10 pounds less than what is considered ideal for their age and height (Moses, Banilivy & Lifshitz 1989). Body weight, the parameter most commonly used to determine obesity, fails to distinguish accurately between being overweight and being overfat. Some individuals may indeed have a larger than average body weight that is actually composed of lean tissue (muscle) as opposed to excessive fat. This can occur in athletes, for instance, who may have reduced fat stores in conjunction with a generously developed musculature. The reverse may also be true for a relatively underweight person who lacks adequate muscle and has a large percentage of body fat. While not overweight per se, this individual is clinically obese and has excess body fat for weight.

However, in most instances, obesity is characterized by excess body weight; thus, most studies and observations that have examined overweight people have most likely assessed people who were obese. Body weight is usually evaluated by comparing the actual body weight of a person with standard weight tables that provide an ideal or desirable weight range based upon height and sex. A body weight in excess of 20 percent over the ideal is indicative of obesity. Tables such as those published by the Metropolitan Life Insurance Company base norms for body weight on the adult size of one's body frame. Yet, frame size is an ill-defined concept with no universally accepted measure for determination. In addition, these tables are based on the supposition that bigger-framed people should be fatter, an assumption that clearly is not accurate. These tables further err by not using age as a variable, thereby eliminating appropriate adjustments for different stages of the life cycle.

For children, age-specific growth charts (National Center for Health Statistics 1977) facilitate a more accurate evaluation of a child's weight since they are based on age, sex, and channels of growth representative of many children in the United States. Additionally, these charts allow the practitioner to view the current weight in light of the child's previous growth patterns and therefore determine the presence of obesity more accurately (see Chapter 10).

The importance of this concept is illustrated by the growth charts of three adolescents shown in Figures 18–1, 18–2, and 18–3. Here, the differences between normal weight, constitutional overweight, and true obesity are demonstrated by the different patterns seen in the height and weight growth curves of each of these three children. These growth charts are from three 14-year-old boys. Each came to see the doctor because of concerns about his body weight; all three weighed 158 lbs (72 kg). Figure 18–1 shows the height and weight of Gary, a child with normal growth who was big but was not

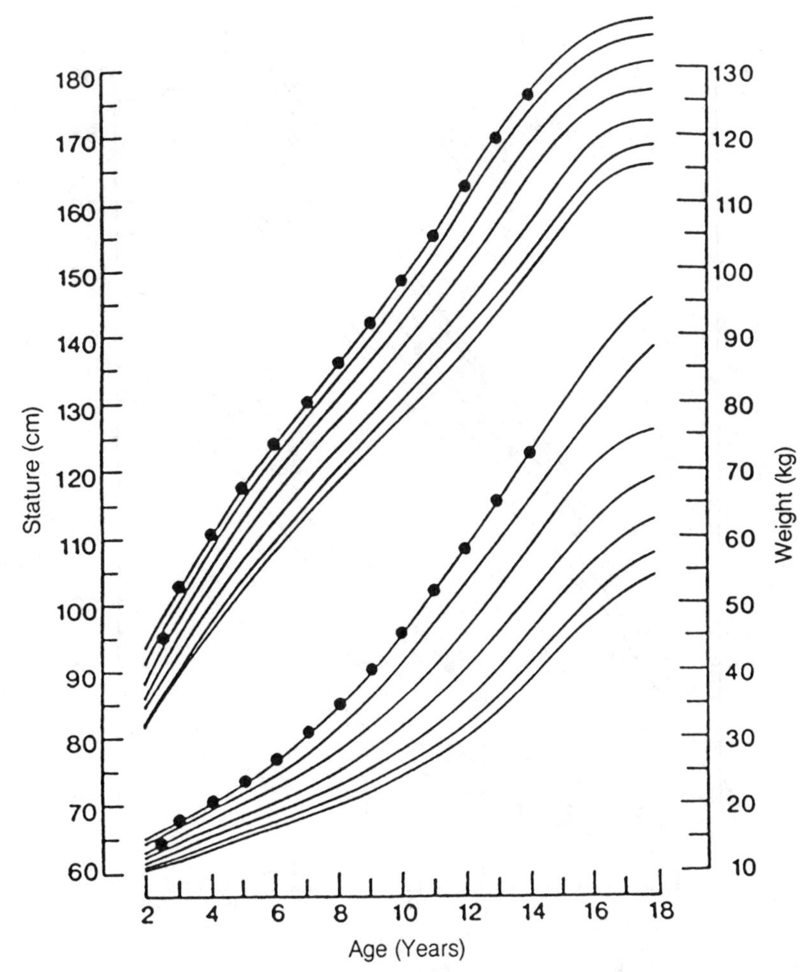

Figure 18–1. Normal growth–tall stature. Normal growth characterized by weight that is proportional to height. This patient is not overweight.

overweight. In his case, the height and the weight were proportional and the pattern of body weight and height advancement consistently followed the 95th percentile for age. Therefore, this patient is tall and does not appear to be obese. Further evaluation of body composition would be necessary (see Chapter 10) in order to determine if Gary had excess body fat; this information cannot be derived from the growth chart data.

Figure 18–2 depicts Jack's growth pattern, which is characteristic of a child who has what we call constitutional overweight. In Jack's case, there is a discrepancy between the body weight and the height. While his growth has remained constant, the weight has progressed along a higher channel than

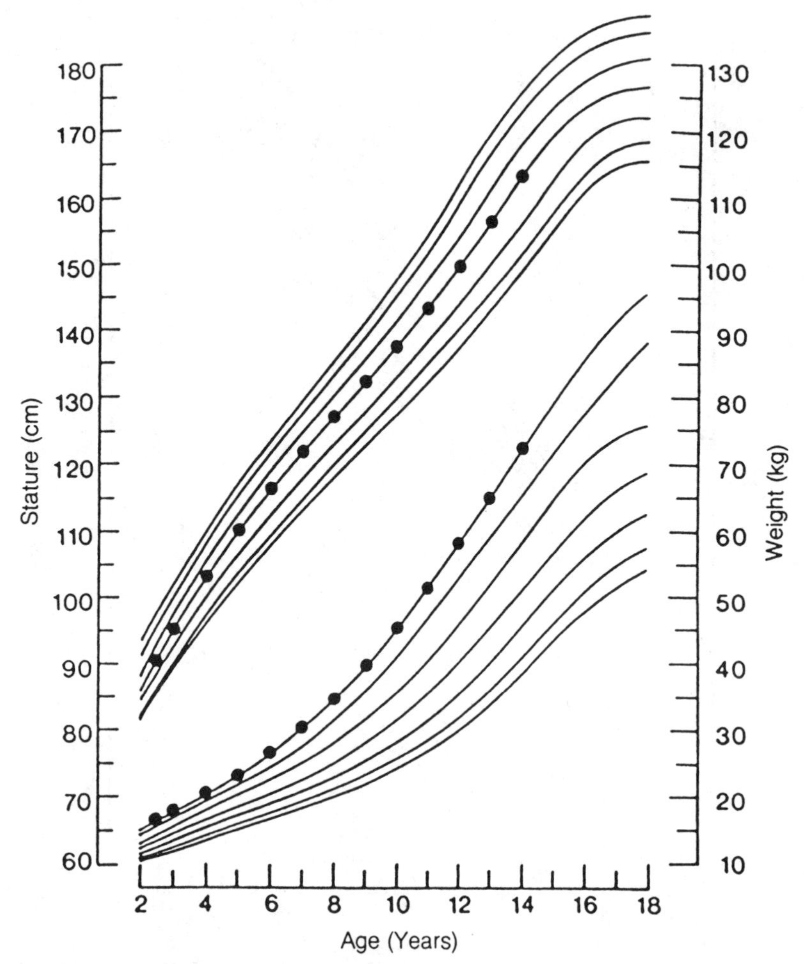

Figure 18–2. Constitutional overweight. Weight is not proportional to height, although both have consistently followed the same channels of growth. This represents a stable pattern of growth with a moderate degree of overweight since height is on a considerably lower channel than weight.

the height. This pattern has characterized Jack's growth since age 2; there have been no deviations from this rate of growth. Even though the patient has excess body weight for height, he has had the same proportion of body weight excess for his stature since early life. This growth chart also provides information regarding the amount of excess body weight for height, thereby implying a possible degree of obesity. Jack has a body weight excess for height of 44 percent; thus, he would be considered moderately obese. If the

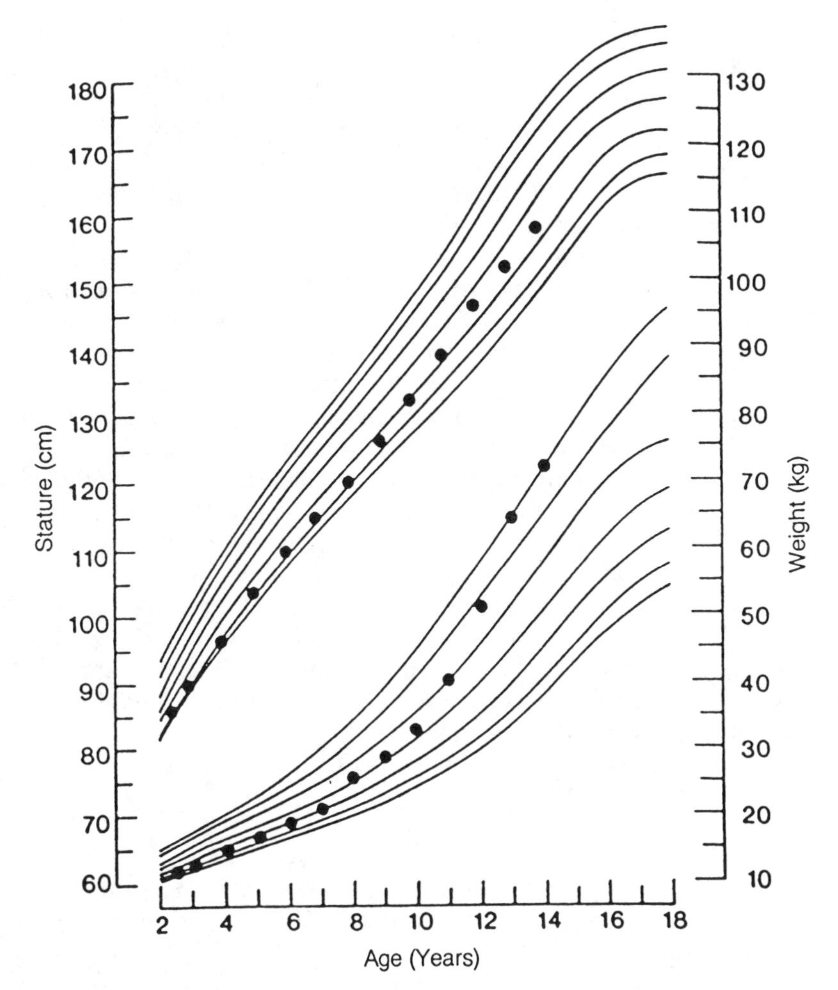

Figure 18–3. Obesity. Weight is progressing upward, crossing over three major percentile channels while height remains fairly stable. This pattern represents a state of true obesity characterized by a disturbing growth pattern. If it continues unabated it may lead to morbid obesity.

body weight excess had been more than 80 percent he would have been considered severely obese.

Gil's growth, on the other hand, demonstrates a clear deviation from a normal growth pattern (see Fig. 18–3). Gil's weight has crossed percentiles, going from the 5th percentile at age 2 to the 95th percentile by age 14. In contrast, height has advanced along similar channels throughout his life, with a mild increase in the last few years. The rate of weight gain has been excessive and represents true obesity with excess weight over height getting progressively worse. Gil's body weight excess for height was 64 percent, which would indicate a moderate degree of obesity, as was found in Jack (see Fig. 18–2) but Gil's progressing weight problem is indeed more serious.

Notice that in each of these clinical cases, the boys were the same weight by age 14. Yet, historical differences in their patterns of height and weight advancement characterize three distinct categories of patients. These boys have very unique appearances, body compositions, and health risks, which necessitate different goals of treatment and modes of intervention. Unfortunately, most studies describing childhood and adult obesity do not consider the pattern of growth and weight gain. Statements are made regarding the rising prevalence of obesity in this country, which may be affecting one in five children (Gortmaker et al 1987), as well as other problems associated with excess body weight without accounting for the rates of weight gain.

We evaluated the growth patterns of over 1000 high-school students and found that excess body weight for height was found in over one third of the students; a similar prevalence was detected for students with body weight deficits for height. Indeed, only a minority of students has a proportional weight for height (Pugliese, Recker & Lifshitz 1988). Nonetheless, most of the students maintained their growth and weight gain patterns along the same percentiles throughout adolescence, and those with excess weight for height had growth records similar to the pattern of constitutional overweight shown in Figure 18–2. Only less than 1 percent of the students had growth patterns of true obesity like that shown in Figure 18–3.

Body Mass Index

Body mass index (BMI) is one of the practical clinical measures that can be used to evaluate for the presence of excess body fat. The calculation for BMI is made as follows:

$$\frac{\text{weight (kg)}}{\text{height}^2\text{ (m)}}$$

The BMI value derived from the calculation allows the individual to be classified as normal (BMI 20–24.9) or obese in different degrees (grade I, BMI 25–29.9; grade II, BMI 30–40; and grade III, >40 BMI).

This BMI system of classification of obesity is important because it has been found that the risk for medical problems of obese patients increases at BMI levels above 25 (Pi-Sunyer 1988). According to the National Center for Health Statistics' Health and Nutrition examination survey (NHANES II 1977), individuals with a BMI exceeding 27 have a markedly increased risk for developing high blood pressure (hypertension), high cholesterol (hypercholesterolemia), and diabetes mellitus. In contrast, when the BMI index is less than 25, there is no apparent physical effect of obesity on the individual although there may be social problems and concerns with body appearance.

It should be kept in mind that BMI was devised to assess obesity in adults, not children. The calculation for BMI is based on facts that assume a stable height, which obviously is not the case in children. For this and for other technical reasons many investigators prefer to evaluate children's obesity based on body weight excess for height (growth charts) and not solely on BMIs. BMIs in overweight children are often inaccurate and the levels for determining obesity are lower than those reported above for adults (Rolland-Cachera et al 1982). Children's 90th percentile for BMI is usually below 22 up to age 10 years and below 27 up to age 16 years.

The BMIs of the three boys previously described facilitates further assessment of their physical states and helps clarify their diagnosis. Gary (see Fig. 18–1), representing a normal growth pattern, has a BMI of 22, the 90th percentile for age and no obesity. Jack (see Fig. 18–2), with constitutional overweight, is moderately obese; his BMI is 27, grade 1 obesity—a mild disorder from a clinical perspective with few health risks, although it is a difficult social problem for a young boy. Gil (see Fig. 18–3), however, is classified as having grade II obesity with a BMI of 30—a more serious imbalance between height and weight with worrisome associated health risks.

Fat Stores

The assessment of fat stores of a child is further accomplished with the use of specific tools for evaluation of body composition. This process allows the practitioner to view an individual's total weight in relation to its actual composition of lean and fat stores. Evaluation of body composition can be accomplished with simple clinical tools such as caliper measurement of skinfolds, or more scientific and accurate measurements such as underwater weighing, electrical conductivity, and total body potassium (see Chapter 10).

Skinfold measurements are popularly referred to as the "pinch test"; it is done by grasping the skin at the side of the waist and measuring the fold; "if more than an inch it's time to lose weight." However, it is often difficult to measure skinfolds, particularly in obese individuals, even when the clinician is experienced in obtaining them. Nonetheless, experienced people can get accurate estimates of the degree and prevalence of obesity in children with these measurements (Gortmaker et al 1987).

Where Is the Fat?

Obesity should also be considered in terms of the location of excess fat deposits. Studies suggest that excess fat in the waist, flank, and abdomen are more detrimental to health than excess fat in the hips or legs (Bjorntorp 1988). It seems that there are important physiologic and pathologic differences in "apple versus pear" appearances among obese people. An excess of body fat in the abdomen is more often associated with the presence of glucose intolerance than when the fat is principally located in the hips or legs (Piers, Struve & Muller 1988). Therefore, the location of the fat sites is a critical element in the evaluation of obesity. Fortunately, fat in the abdomen, which may be the worst for health, is more easily lost with diet and exercise than fat located in the hips and thigh areas.

WHO IS AT RISK?

Many factors have a role in determining who is at risk for becoming obese. Genetic endowment, food intake, and energy expenditure seem to be the most important factors that lead to the development of obesity.

Studies have clearly demonstrated that when obesity begins in childhood it is very likely that it will persist into adulthood. The longer children remain obese, the more likely they are to become obese adults. In one study, 14 percent of obese infants became obese adults, compared with only 6 percent of normal-weight infants (Charney et al 1976). These data show a slightly increased chance that the obese infant will remain obese, but it also points out that most chubby infants *will not* be obese for life. In contrast, 41 percent of 7-year-old overweight children will become obese adults, whereas only 11 percent of their normal-weight counterparts may be obese adults (Stark et al 1981). In general, if childhood obesity is not corrected prior to age 12, the odds for becoming an obese adult are 4:1. If the obesity persists through adolescence, these odds rise to 28:1 (Stunkard & Burt 1967).

There is a strong familial pattern for obesity (Fig. 18–4). The children of obese parents are frequently obese too (Garn & Clark 1976). Boys and girls with two lean parents were the leanest, as compared with boys and girls with two obese parents, who tended to be the fattest. Hence, children of obese parents can be expected to be significantly fatter at all ages than the children of lean parents. By age 17, the children of obese parents are actually three times fatter than the children of lean parents.

A landmark study, involving over 7000 adoptees, lends additional evidence of the genetic role in obesity (Stunkard et al 1986). This report found that weights of the adoptees strongly correlated with the weights of their biologic parents but were not related to the weights of their adoptive parents, even when the children had lived with their adoptive parents since early life. Interestingly, not only the presence and the degree of obesity are genetically determined, but the location and deposition of excess fat is also familial. Figures 18–5 and 18–6 show the differences in the development of subcutaneous fat among fraternal (dizygotic) and identical (monozygotic) twins. The monozygotic pairs display striking similarity in the amount and location of subcu-

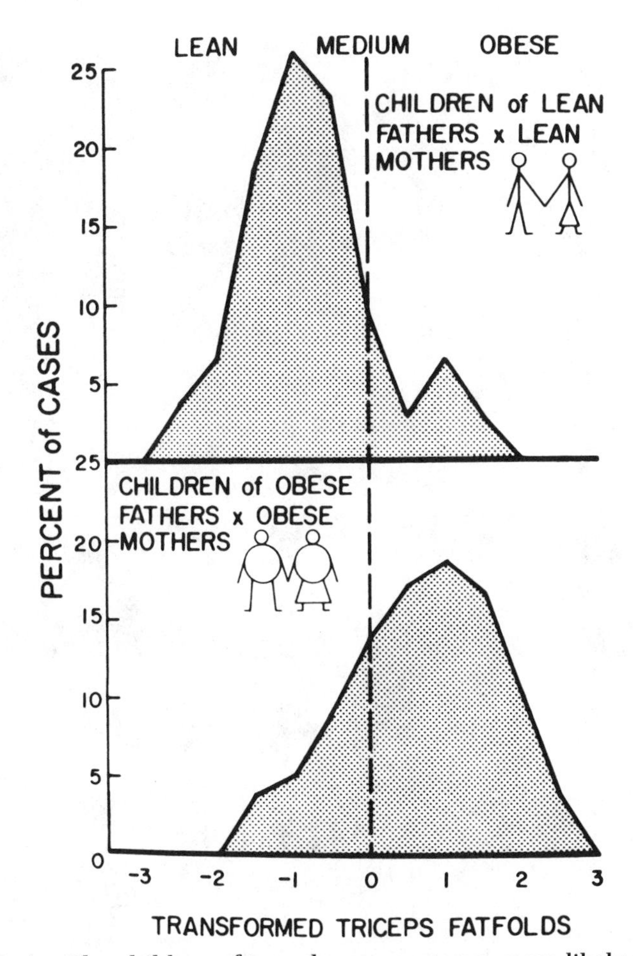

Figure 18–4. The children of two obese parents are more likely to become obese than the offspring of two lean parents.

From Garn SM, Clark DC. Trends in fatness and origins of obesity. Pediatrics 1976; 57:443–456. Copyright 1976. Reprinted by permission of Pediatrics.

taneous fat, whereas the dizygotic pairs, as a group, are characterized by greater differences in total weight, fat deposition, and body shape.

Recent observations have demonstrated that low 24-hour metabolic rates may run in families and that members of these family groups are more likely to develop obesity. Adults from a Southwestern population with a high incidence of obesity were shown to have 24-hour metabolic rates slightly below average (70 calories less per day—the number of calories in 1 slice of bread). The study demonstrated that these individuals had a 60 percent probability

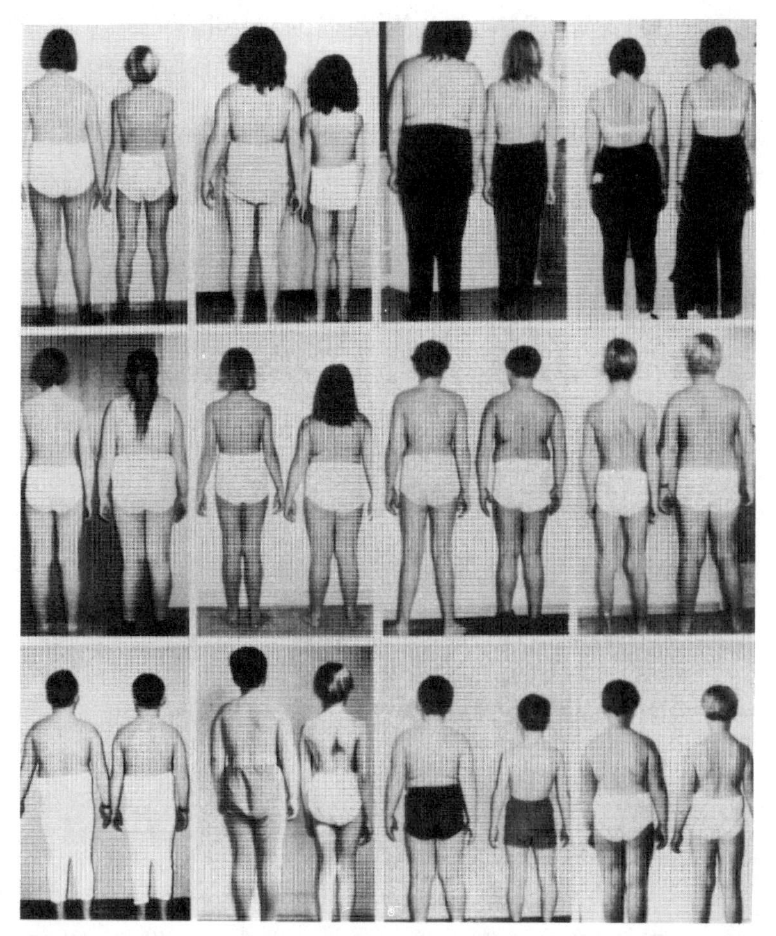

Figure 18–5. Dizygotic twins with dissimilar patterns of body-fat distribution within each set.

From Borjeson M. The aetiology of obesity in children. Acta Paediatr Scand 1976; 65:279-287.

of gaining 10 pounds within a 20-month period (Ravussin, Lillioja & Knowler 1988). In another study 50 percent of infants born to obese mothers were also shown to have lower rates of energy expenditure (Roberts et al 1988). These children advanced to over the 90th percentile of weight for length by 1 year of age. The deficient energy expenditure in both of these studies was not, however, enough to account for the entire amount of excess fat deposition in the subjects. The authors concluded that while the genetic inheritance of a metabolic predisposition to develop obesity played a strong

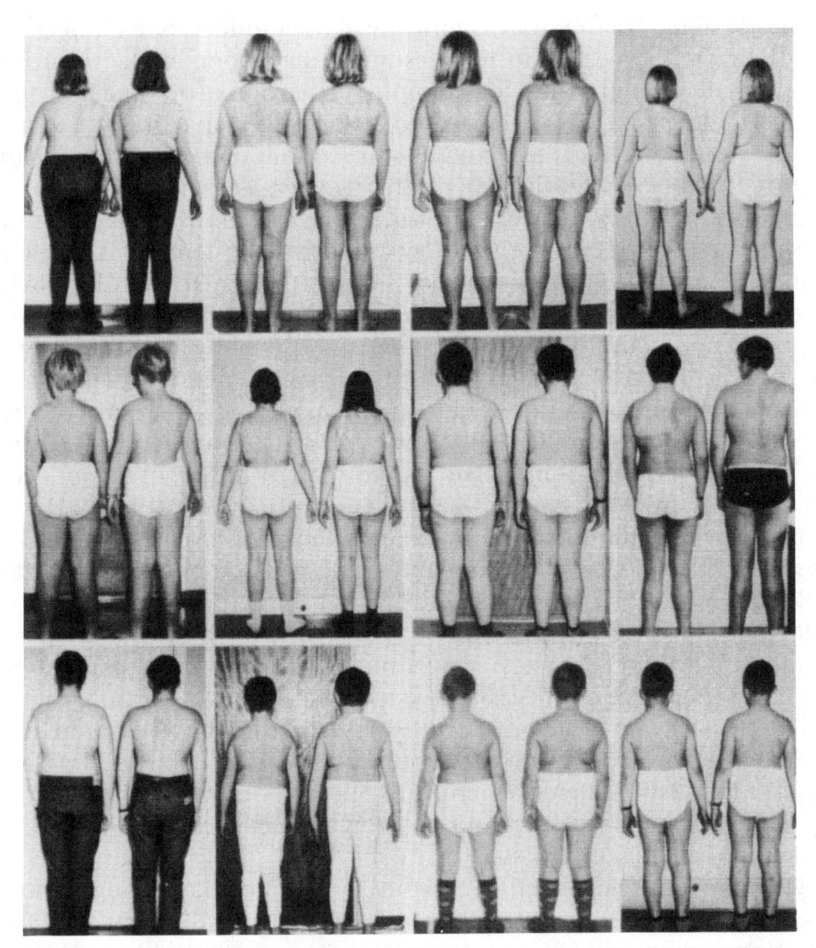

Figure 18–6. Monozygotic twins with similar patterns of body-fat distribution within each set.

From Borjeson M. The aetiology of obesity in children. Acta Paediatr Scand 1976; 65:279-287.

role in the weight gain, other external factors not included in these studies, such as food intake and exercise, also play a significant role.

It is often wondered whether obese children eat excessive amounts of food. They obviously must consume more calories than the amount they expend in order for weight gain to occur, but the amount eaten might not necessarily be "large." As mentioned above, as little as 70 extra calories per day of a positive balance will result in a substantial weight gain over time. The type of food ingested may also vary in obese children, who tend to eat more fat and saturated fat and more calorically dense products (see Chapters 9 and 15). Therefore, it is easier to underestimate the caloric intake of such diets since a small amount of fat—for example, 1 teaspoon of oil—may account for enough calories to tip the balance and result in weight gain.

However, many years ago studies showed that obese children might not eat more than their lean counterparts (Dwyer, Feldman & Mayer 1967, Huenemann 1972). Moreover, even when they consume relatively fewer calories they may remain obese. We now know that this food intake/weight aberration occurs when adaptation to dieting has taken place, resulting in lower energy requirements. For example, after repeated attempts to lose weight (yo-yo syndrome), body composition changes and there is less lean body mass and more fat deposition. This results in decreased metabolic demands and therefore in fewer calories needed to maintain weight. The results of a recent investigation (Epstein et al 1989) show that changes in percent overweight that result from increases in height and no changes in weight do not decrease metabolic rate.

The type and amount of energy expenditures may also be different among obese individuals. Obese children and adults have often been characterized as slow or lazy. Objective studies carried out in the past showed that obese children are less active (Rose & Mayer 1968). Films of obese children performing physical activity also show slower movements, but measurements of energy expenditure are not necessarily decreased since it takes more calories to move a heavier body (Bullen, Reed & Mayer 1964). However, there may be marked differences in spontaneous physical activity while resting among obese individuals. Differences of up to 500 calories per day in energy expended as a result of spontaneous physical activity such as fidgeting may be measured (Ravussin et al 1986).

Sedentary lifestyles of children in the United States have an important role in reducing energy expenditures. Since children spend an average of 25 hours per week watching television it is not surprising that television viewing has been shown to be directly related to the prevalence of obesity. Studies with adolescents have found that with each hour spent viewing television, the prevalence of obesity increases by 2 percent (Gortmaker & Dietz 1987). After following children through the 1970 and 1975 HANES surveys, child-obesity experts determined that "next to prior obesity, television viewing is the strongest predictor of subsequent obesity." They also agree that a dose effect exists, which may be explained by the fact that children tend to consume food while watching television. Their choices tend to reflect foods advertised in commercials—not typical calorie-wise selections for the most part. Moreover, nearly everyone seen on television is thin, yet characters on prime-time television eat an average of eight times per hour! The messages that children receive while viewing television are clearly inconsistent with reality.

There are environmental factors that increase the risk for development of obesity (Dietz & Gortmaker 1984). The likelihood of obesity increases among children of divorced parents (DiNatale et al 1978). The highest prevalence of the disease occurs in single-child families and declines with increasing family size (Ravelli & Belmont 1979). Birth order also appears to play a role; the oldest and youngest child in a family are more likely to become overweight than the intermediate siblings. The physical environment may also play a role in the origin of childhood obesity. According to the National Health Examination Survey, the highest prevalence occurs in the Northeastern United States, followed by the Midwest, South, and West. Likewise, the prevalence of obesity is greater in urban areas than in less-populated regions of the country.

Finally, there may be medical or physiologic conditions that lead to obesity in children. For example, there are very rare genetic diseases in which obesity is an important part of the problem (e.g., Prader-Willi syndrome or central nervous system tumors). Endocrine or glandular alterations are often thought to be the cause of obesity, although this is rarely the case. As a rule, a child who is overweight but who is growing in height and following his or her usual growth channel is not suffering any glandular deficiency (like hypothyroidism) or excess (like hypercorticism [Cushing's syndrome]). Patients with these diseases may be overweight but usually do not grow well in height and, therefore, are short and fat. When an overweight child is not short, endocrine diseases rarely need to be considered as the cause of the obesity.

Among the psychologic reasons for becoming obese, depression should be mentioned. Excess weight gain may be associated with situational depression, as in Paul's case when he gained 20 pounds after he moved from Maine to New York. Divorce and other family problems, or even going away to college, are situations associated with excess weight gain. However, most frequently there are no psychologic causes for becoming obese; rather, there are many psychosocial consequences that overweight children have to face and that may add to their general problems revolving around body weight (see below).

Health Risks

Excess body weight has been associated with increased morbidity and mortality by most investigators (Rimm & White 1980), including the Framingham Study (Garrison & Castelli 1985), the Build and Blood Pressure Study (1959), and the American Cancer Society Study. Obesity has been associated with an increased frequency and severity of many disorders that result in shorter life spans and/or in decreased health (Table 18–1). The Framingham Study showed that each 10 percent weight gain in males resulted in an average 6.6 mm Hg rise in systolic blood pressure, a 2 milligrams per deciliter rise in fasting blood sugar, and an 11 milligrams per deciliter rise in blood insulin levels. In addition evidence suggests that obesity that occurs earlier in life (20–40

Table 18–1. Health Risks Associated with Obesity.

Hypertension
Coronary heart disease
Diabetes mellitus
Atherosclerosis
Thrombophlebitis
Respiratory disease
Gallbladder disease
Osteoarthritis
Ovarian dysfunction
Cancer
Toxemia in pregnancy

years) has a greater influence on cardiovascular disease than late-onset obesity. A high BMI was also found to be associated with heart attacks, sudden death, and angina (coronary insufficiency) (Garrison & Castelli 1985).

For years the search has been on to understand fully the metabolic changes that predispose certain obese individuals to increased morbidity (Keys 1976). The mechanism for the changes in blood pressure and blood sugar levels of overweight persons has been related to the presence of inappropriate insulin action and insulin resistance owing to enlargement of the fat cell (De Fronzo 1980). Weight reduction can reverse many of these metabolic abnormalities in obese individuals; even small amounts of weight loss can rapidly improve the metabolic abnormalities (Fortmann, Haskell & Wood 1988).

Psychologic Risks

The greatest health hazards to the obese child are considered to be psychologic and social. The physical health risks are future problems that the child often does not comprehend, but the loss of self-esteem and discrimination by peers, teachers, and even parents are common problems the obese child encounters daily. Due to their physical size, obese children must contend with many humiliations. In many ways obesity, especially when it reaches morbid proportions, is a physical handicap. For example, obese individuals find it difficult to get in and out of a car or move about in small spaces. Everyday tasks for normal-weight children, such as sitting comfortably in school desks, walking through turnstiles, and playing with the gym class, become frequent sources of frustration and a daily reminder of the fact that they just don't fit in with the rest of the class.

The strong prejudice against the obese cuts across age, sex, race, and socioeconomic status. This contempt for the obese is not surprising given America's preoccupation with thinness, reinforced at every turn by the media, which capitalizes on the theme of "thin is beautiful." As early as age 6, children asked to describe silhouettes of obese youngsters will characterize them as lazy, stupid, ugly, cheats, and liars (Staffieri 1967). When drawings of obese children were combined with drawings of severely disfigured and handicapped children, both children and adults rated the obese figures as representing the least likable person (Richardson et al 1961).

Discrimination is the behavioral enactment of prejudice. Consequently, stigmatization of obese persons occurs in various spheres of social functioning. Obese high-school students applying for acceptance into prestigious colleges were found to have lower acceptance rates than their normal-weight peers of equal academic performance (Canning & Mayer 1966). Not unexpectedly, this discrimination continues into one's adult life as long as the obesity persists. Several reports demonstrate that obese job applicants have a more difficult time obtaining work, and, once employed, may experience discrimination on the job, primarily manifesting itself in earning potential. The authors of one such survey concluded that each pound of extra fat could cost an executive $1,000 a year in decreased earnings (Industry Week 1974).

However, overweight persons on the whole are not significantly more emotionally disturbed than normal-weight persons; those most likely to develop psychopathology specific to their obesity are persons whose weight problem originated in childhood (Stunkard & Burt 1967). These people characteristically view their own bodies as grotesque and loathsome and believe that others view them with hostility and contempt. This disorder is an internalization of parental and peer criticism—not an uncommon occurrence in a society which, despite its increasing prevalence, has found obesity to be unfashionable, unhealthy, and simply "un-American."

WHAT TO DO?

The main rule in medicine when treating a problem is *to do no harm*. This should always be kept in mind when considerations are given to diets and other treatments of obesity. The main goal should be to attain the objective of life-long weight control. Therefore, a realistic goal for body weight needs to be set. For this, it is most important to know the child's pattern of growth and weight gain. In a child like Gary, who is big but tall (shown in Fig. 18–1), dieting for weight reduction is not necessary and could potentially be harmful. In a child like Jack, with constitutional overweight (shown in Fig. 18–2), an adjustment and life-long maintenance of weight has already been achieved. This example illustrates stability regarding weight gain, and any attempt to modify Jack's weight needs to be considered carefully as it may disrupt the balance achieved by this child and create failure and frustrations. In addition, if unrealistic weight loss is attempted the yo-yo effect or growth disturbances may result.

Finally, children like Gil, who had accelerated weight gain over the past 8 years (shown in Fig. 18–3), call for a more aggressive approach to change their pattern of weight gain. This type of patient needs immediate treatment involving all possible avenues to attain the goals, first to stop weight gain, and second to achieve weight loss. The latter must be a slow process for it to be safe and long-lasting. For most of these patients a rate of weight loss of about 1 percent of body weight per week is more than appropriate. Helping the patient to understand that there is no special, quick, or magic remedy for obesity helps to ensure realistic expectations for weight loss.

YO-YO SYNDROME

Recently, research has been shedding light onto the question of "what happens when a person's weight continuously goes up and down?" Answers to this question have led to the realization that the yo-yo syndrome (weight cycling) has a profound effect on physiology and results in negative consequences for the chronic dieter (Ravussin et al 1985).

In essence, repeat dieters learn to cope with dieting. They develop a very efficient metabolism and, in effect, require fewer and fewer calories with each renewed attempt to manage their weight (Hendler, Walesky & Sherwin 1983). In conjunction with a psychologically frustrating situation of failure to control weight, body composition changes during weight cycling. Lean body mass is decreased, and there is an increased fat mass, making the total situation worse than it was before because fat is a relatively metabolically inert tissue. The potential result is a patient who consumes very few calories and yet remains obese. For children, this concept is most important to keep in mind. When a child is not motivated or when he or she is forced to diet, weight may be lost just to be regained soon afterwards. When a parent or doctor forces a diet upon a child, it may ultimately result in a more difficult weight-control problem in the future.

Cycle dieters also may be increasing their risk for heart disease more than if excess weight remained at a stable level. Dieting leads to fat mobilization and during the regaining phase fat deposition in the arteries occurs. The regained weight is more likely to appear on the upper body where it is potentially more harmful (Bjorntorp 1988) and associated with a higher incidence of heart disease and more glucose intolerance (Piers, Strove & Muller 1988).

Strategies to avoid weight cycling should be considered at the beginning of a child's weight-reduction program. As summarized by one expert in the field: "Success lies in the journey, not the destination" (Dalton 1988). When a child is ready to undertake a weight-reduction program, it should represent a serious determination of all involved to produce a successful outcome. There is no magic diet that can accomplish weight loss, there is only a lot of effort.

GROWTH FAILURE

Obese children also have to consider growth in the equation of a weight-loss plan. This concern is unique to children, as adults have finished growing. A child who loses weight is in a negative energy balance and, therefore, may not grow in height (Dietz & Hartung 1985). Obese children who are "motivated" and lose weight may be the ones who exhibit "stunting" of growth. Of course, if the weight loss efforts do not persist for a sufficient time or if they fail, the lack of growth would not be noticed. Dieting during periods of rapid growth, such as infancy or adolescence, results in a higher risk of interfering with height advancement than when dieting occurs during periods of slow growth.

Obese children, in general, are above-average in height for their age and sex. They have a faster rate of growth and reach puberty earlier than non-obese children. Therefore, some physicians tolerate a slowing down of the growth rate during treatment of obesity. This decrease has been reported to bring children more in line with the heights of their parents (Epstein et al 1987). However, the final height may be slightly less than that of their non-obese peers (Merrit 1982). If a child's height velocity slows too drastically, the individual should be reevaluated, and a new program, perhaps with different short-term goals (e.g., decreased rate of weight loss or weight maintenance) should be considered to allow for growth to take place. In some cases it may be sufficient for a child to cease gaining weight and allow the height to catch up with his or her present weight. However, children, like adults, want immediate results with quick gratification, and thus the above plan is often not acceptable.

For the above-mentioned concern with growth during weight reduction, accurate height measurements in managing children with obesity are as important as weight records. They should always be plotted in the growth charts to observe the changes occurring in both height and weight during treatment. Dieting and weight reduction can only be considered successful if there is a normal growth in height proceeding simultaneously with weight loss.

CLINICAL INTERVENTION

It has become increasingly clear that early detection and treatment of obesity should replace the old way of passively waiting for children to outgrow extra pounds. Interventions to induce weight loss must take into account all the factors relating to the development of obesity. Since most of our present knowledge centers on environmental and behavioral factors, these represent the primary areas of intervention for the treatment of obesity. Genetic factors apparently play a very significant part in obesity. This fact can help identify the child who is at risk for obesity and allow treatment to be started early, before obesity reaches extreme proportions and before it is very long-lasting. Both eating and exercise behaviors are imbedded in a web of physiologic, psychologic, social, and cultural influences. Treatment of pediatric obesity must be multifaceted to incorporate sufficiently all the elements necessary for success. Half-hearted attempts to treat obesity lead to failure and frustration and can set the stage for a lifelong struggle with obesity and weight cycling.

Long-term use of medications to suppress the appetite is not indicated in the treatment of obesity. These drugs may help in the beginning of a weight-loss program by suppressing appetite, but the effectiveness of appetite-suppressant drugs appears to decrease with time, and there may be more side effects (Bray & Gray 1988). Therefore, they should not be used in children. Drugs such as bulking agents and nonprescription diet aids such as methylcellulose and other noncaloric bulk materials that inhibit food intake, and pectin, which reduces gastric emptying and increases satiety, have also been used without proof of any long-term benefit (Di Lorenzo et al 1988).

Exercise

Many diets and behavioral treatments of obesity are based on the premise that obese children eat too much. However, it is clear that interventions using diet alone have left a trail of failure and frustration for both the obese patient and the health care practitioners who administer the treatments. Although weight loss may occur with diet alone, reaching the desired weight can be extremely difficult, and even more difficult to maintain. Furthermore, the composition of weight loss on low-calorie regimens constitutes a relatively larger loss of lean body tissue (Newmark & Williamson 1983).

The debate as to whether low activity precedes or results from obesity is likely to continue for years to come. However, it is probably better for the obese child to participate in some form of activity rather than to be sedentary viewing hours of television with advertisements offering an endless variety of calorically dense temptations (Dietz & Gortmaker 1984, 1985).

Physical activity has an enormous effect on human energy expenditure, and the energy cost for most activities is generally greater for heavier people. This is especially relevant for weight-bearing forms of exercise such as walking, where the person must transport the body. Sustained large-muscle activities such as bicycling and swimming can generate metabolic rates six to eight times above the resting level. The importance of exercise is highlighted by the observation that individuals who perform hard physical labor, such as lumberjacks and certain athletes, often consume up to 7000 calories a day, and yet maintain normal weight.

In a recent study an exercise program was proven to be more valuable than dietary treatment in long-term maintenance of weight reduction (Wood et al 1988). Regular aerobic exercise combined with caloric restriction brings about greater reductions in body weight than dieting alone (Hagan et al 1986). However, exercise alone may not decrease body weight in severely obese patients (Bjorntorp 1982). Body fat in these individuals decreases very slowly or not at all with exercise alone. The metabolic effects of exercise resulting in weight reduction pertain to changes in metabolic rates, food intake, and thermogenesis as reviewed elsewhere (Council on Scientific Affairs 1988). These exercise-induced metabolic changes allow the obese patient a greater caloric intake, minimize loss of lean body mass, enhance fat utilization by muscle, and reduce long-term health-risk factors such as hypertension. Long-term conditioning also has multiple psychosocial benefits.

Therefore, no one should attempt to lose weight by diet alone, and obesity treatment should always combine diet with exercise (Epstein et al 1985). However, although physical conditioning by exercise may be helpful, it is not an easy task. An exercise program based on the initial fitness level with a slow progression of intensity, frequency, and duration is necessary to achieve weight control. The reader is referred elsewhere for a discussion of all aspects of formulating exercise prescriptions and programs for children (American College of Sports Medicine 1986). Sustained compliance with exercise is best achieved when the regimen is safe, pleasurable, and adaptable to the child's physical limitations and physical environment.

Diets and Food Management

Many diets and dietary regimens have been used throughout the ages for the treatment of obesity (Weinsier et al 1982). The best diet for overweight children is one of food management: an appropriate reduction in the intake of calories coupled with increased energy expenditure. The diet should provide sufficient calories, fat, and protein to support growth and development and meet the RDAs for vitamins and minerals (see Chapter 9). The caloric restriction should be set at a level that will encourage the mobilization of fat stores, but it should supply energy needs and nutrients necessary for growth. The caloric intake should be based on body size, rate of growth, degree of adiposity, and desired weight and activity level, as well as the likes and dislikes of the child.

As a general rule, moderately overweight children should be placed on a calorie intake and exercise level that will simply prevent further weight advancement or produce a slight weight loss of no more than 1 percent of body weight per week. An example of diet planning is given below.

In the case of Gil (see Fig. 18–3), who weighed 158 pounds (72 kg), weight loss was considered an important goal of treatment. His caloric intake was reported to be 4400 calories per day, or 60 calories per kilogram, which was appropriate to maintain the present weight. However, this was far in excess of his energy requirements for age, which were 2700 calories based on ideal body weight (see Table 9–2, Chapter 9). His usual dietary intake was also high in fat (>40 percent), and he skipped breakfast and lunch and ate a very large dinner. His activity level was low and he spent 6 hours per day watching television.

Utilizing the above-mentioned guidelines, for him to lose 1 percent of his body weight per week he would have to restrict his intake sufficiently to lose 1.5 pounds per week (0.7 kg/wk). This weight loss would result if he ate 750 calories per day less than his usual intake based on the assumption that 3500 calories are needed for every pound of weight loss. Better yet, it would be ideal if he would increase his caloric expenditures with exercise by 200 to 300 calories per day and reduce his caloric intake by 400 to 500 calories per day. Notice that this would allow him to eat a substantial amount during the day—a diet of 3550 calories per day—and still lose weight!

More severe dietary restrictions may lead to loss of lean body mass (Hill et al 1987, Bray & Gray 1988) as well as to nutrient deficiencies and, worst of all, noncompliance. Very-low-calorie diets might set up the groundwork for a lifetime of repeated weight-loss failures. We recognize that patients and parents want immediate rewards and are often very willing and anxious to restrict food intake even more than we recommend during the initial stages of treatment in the hope of achieving quicker results. Sufficient counseling and reassurance might set the goals straight between therapist, patient, and parent for long-lasting results and avoidance of failure and frustration.

It is important to realize that weight loss may not occur every week and that the overall *pattern* of weight change for several weeks should be used to evaluate one's progress. Obese children, especially those who have gone through dieting in the past, may have adjusted to a lower level of dietary consumption while maintaining weight (the yo-yo syndrome). If weight loss does not occur for 2 to 3 weeks, and there is no obvious noncompliance, then a further reduction in the caloric intake or an increase in energy expenditure may be necessary.

Another important immediate goal of nutritional rehabilitation is to modify the diet of the patient in accordance with general principles of good nutrition; that is, to reduce fat to about one third of the calories while increasing complex carbohydrates (see Chapter 9). Gil was managed by increasing vegetables in the diet and substituting other low-calorie snacks for the high-fat foods. Also, the dietary pattern was improved. He was given 3 meals and 2 snacks daily, instead of one large meal. It has long been known that frequent meals are more effective for weight control than a single large meal (Bray 1972, Metzner 1977).

It should be kept in mind that day-to-day variations in caloric intake are characteristic of normal eating patterns and thus they should be permitted as long as the range is within reason. For example, it would be acceptable for Gil, using a 3550-calorie food plan, to have a range of intakes between approximately 3000 and 4000 calories. Along with monitoring the rate of weight loss and growth, the nutrient composition of the diet needs to be evaluated periodically. Special attention should be given to calcium, iron, magnesium, copper, zinc, folacin, and vitamin B_6, as these are the nutrients most likely to be deficient on a reduced intake (USDA 1985).

Finally, it should be noted that discontinuing weight advancement in a patient like Gil does not represent a passive approach to treatment. It may take just as much work and motivation to manage caloric intake and energy expenditure to avoid further weight increases as it would for another patient to lose weight.

Several variations of weight-loss fixes have become popular in attempts to speed up the process of weight reduction (Wadden et al 1983). These modifications include total fasting, very-low-calorie diets, low-carbohydrate diets, protein-sparing diets, and high-protein diets. Table 18–2 presents a summary of many of the diets that are currently in use, with the associated nutrient deficiencies and possible side effects. Despite these negative consequences, their popularity continues to increase (Council of Scientific Affairs 1988). These quick-loss regimens are not appropriate for obese children since they may cause negative nitrogen balance and loss of lean body mass and may affect proper growth and development (Flatt 1973 & 1974). Moreover, none of the quick-fix weight-loss schemes promote healthy eating behaviors for lifelong weight control.

Psychologic/Psychiatric Therapy and Behavior Modification

Psychologic, social, and cultural influences that bear on eating behavior should be addressed as part of a comprehensive strategy to produce behaviors that support weight reduction, maintenance, or both. Psychoanalytic theorists believe that overweight people eat in response to emotional states such as depression. In contrast, behavioral approaches focus primarily on how food cues in the environment trigger overeating. While psychosocial interventions may vary from patient to patient, the important point is to recognize and appreciate that psychologic problems are not usually the cause of obesity.

A landmark report on behavioral control of overeating revealed unprecedented therapeutic success using stimulus-control procedures in the treatment of obesity (Stuart 1967). This led to the development of several behavioral techniques for use in weight-control programs. Some of the techniques included in the programs include (1) self-monitoring of body weight and/or food intake, (2) goal-setting, (3) reward and punishment, (4) aversion therapy, (5) social reinforcement, and (6) stimulus control. Several of these modifications have been found to be effective with children (Epstein 1986, Brownell & Stunkard 1978, Epstein et al 1987).

Positive reinforcement by family and friends, and modifying rate of eat-

Table 18–2. Nutrient Deficiencies and Side Effects Associated with Nutritionally Inadequate Diets.

DIET	POTENTIAL NUTRIENT DEFICIENCIES	POSSIBLE SIDE EFFECTS
Low Carbohydrate		
Air Force Diet	Calcium	Nervousness
Banting Diet	Magnesium	Postural hypotension
Boston Police Diet	Potassium	Ketosis
Brand Name Carbohydrate Diet	B vitamins	Dehydration
Calories Don't Count Diet	Fiber	Hyperlipidemia
Cormillot Thin Forever Diet		
Dr. Atkins Diet Revolution		
Dr. Cooper's Fabulous 14-Day Fructose Diet		
Dr. Stillman's Quick Weight Loss Diet		
Dr. Yudkin's Lose Weight Feel Great Diet		
Drinking Man's Diet		
DuPont Diet		
Fat-Destroyer Foods Diet		
Paul Michael Weight Loss Plan		
Pennington Diet		
Scarsdale Diet		
Ski Team Diet		
Woman Doctor's Diet for Women		
High Carbohydrate		
Best Chance Diet	Calcium	Weakness
Beverly Hills Diet	Iron	Abnormal heart rhythms
Beverly Hills Medical Diet	Zinc	Gastrointestinal symptoms
Carbohydrate Cravers Diet	Sodium	Hair loss
Diet of a Desperate Housewife	Vitamins A, B_{12}, D, E	Kidney stones
Dr. Stillman's Quick Inches Off Diet	Fatty acids	
Hollywood Emergency Diet		
Kempner Rice Diet		
Macrobiotic Rice Diet		
Pritikin Diet		
Protein-Sparing Modified Fast		
Cambridge Diet	Calcium	Death
Last Chance Diet	Copper	Fatigue
Optifast	Magnesium	Gastrointestinal symptoms
Oxford Diet	Potassium	Cold intolerance
University Diet	Protein	Muscle cramps
		Dry skin
		Kidney damage
		Abnormal heart rhythms
Fasting		
	Multiple vitamins and minerals	Nervous and personality disorders
		Bad breath
		Fainting
		Anemia
		Intolerance to cold

Table 18–2. Nutrient Deficiencies and Side Effects Associated with Nutritionally Inadequate Diets. *(cont.)*

DIET	POTENTIAL NUTRIENT DEFICIENCIES	POSSIBLE SIDE EFFECTS
Fasting		
		Metabolic rate decrease Severe headaches Amenorrhea Blurred vision Ulcerated mouth Death

ing, plate size, mealtime distractions, and parental involvement, were found to have a positive outcome on weight loss. Also, time spent viewing television, snack choices, and exercise can be altered through the use of reinforcements for other activities and choices.

Psychosocial interventions for the treatment of childhood obesity are different from all other forms of intervention in that the primary goal is to alter the obese child's habits, not just his or her weight. Although psychologic factors are undoubtedly involved in weight regulation, they interact with one's genetic and physiologic endowment to produce a given physical state. Thus, it seems that treatments that acknowledge all the critical areas related to obesity will need to address several factors. The child belongs to a complex social unit (the family) that has a profound influence on his or her behavior, and psychosocial interventions should include both the child and family.

It should be noted that most areas of behavior modification and of the treatment of obesity have been attempted in children and families who are "motivated" to lose weight and to undergo a treatment program. However, the major problem may be to motivate obese people to initiate and sustain a long-term commitment to weight management. We have found that approximately one half of the patients who seek consultations for obesity join a treatment program (Waldbaum 1982). Those who do not pursue the long-term road have excuses and rationalizations, or may not have the "time, interest, and/or budget." However, even those who do commit themselves to a treatment program may do so, but soon after may drop out or may continue with the program without full compliance.

The Prevention of Obesity

Very few trials have been conducted on the effectiveness of preventive measures of obesity. In the early 1900s, pioneering studies conducted by a pediatrician, Clara Davis, led to the belief that infants would select an appropriate calorie level if supplied with food and left on their own to determine which items and how much they would consume. Several myths have arisen from the misinterpretation of her studies. The most prevalent is the myth that infants and children have the innate ability to select for themselves a balanced, nutritious diet (Story & Brown 1987). In fact, the foods used in those studies were all nutritious, thereby eliminating any possible choice between nutritious and nutritionally weak foods. In addition, Davis pointed out that the mechanism that regulates energy intake was operative only for a diet based on natural foods, and not for processed foods.

In real life the diet from which children make choices has been called a "cafeteria" or "supermarket" diet. With relatively free access to highly palatable choices, the chances for overeating are increased. In fact, obesity occurred among rats given a "cafeteria" diet rather than their usual feed (Sclafani 1980). Thus, free access to highly palatable, nutritionally weak foods may encourage the development of obesity in susceptible individuals.

Children should be encouraged to develop eating habits and exercise patterns that will prevent excessive weight gain. This is especially important for children in high-risk groups, for example, children with obese parents and those who are overweight by the time they start school (Black et al 1983). In some children who may be genetically predisposed to being obese, total caloric intake should be monitored with an emphasis on controlling the percentage of fat calories. Special care should be taken by health care providers to inform the parents of the potential risks and to provide instructions on preventive measures at an early stage.

This early intervention is critical from a treatment standpoint. Initial caloric excess results in enlarged fat cells. Once the fat cells have reached their capacity for size, the actual number of fat cells will begin to increase to provide for excess energy (triglyceride) stores. As an individual moves into this second stage, called "hyperplastic obesity," the condition becomes more refractory to treatment (Buckmanster & Brownell 1988).

The provision of an assortment of nutritious foods will encourage the development of healthy eating habits during childhood and beyond. The available foods should include a variety of fresh or frozen vegetables and legumes; dairy products (low-fat for at-risk children above age 2) (see Chapter 9); fresh fruits and fruit juices; breads (preferably whole grain), pastas, rice, cereals, and other grain products. Children should not be coaxed to eat everything on their plates and should not be expected to like all foods introduced to them. Deciding *how much* food to consume should be the prerogative of the child. Sweets and other nutrient-poor foods should be allowed in limited amounts that will not interfere with the child's consumption of basic foods. Overzealous attempts to avoid "junk food" or to prevent obesity should be discouraged as they may lead to other problems and even failure to thrive (Pugliese et al 1987).

On a larger scale, the schools, the government, and the food industry should support measures that can improve the food habits and exercise patterns of children and adults. Legislation should encourage and standardize a descriptive nutrient label for all packaged foods. Government food programs such as the school lunch program should be based upon the dietary guidelines established by the Surgeon General's Report on Nutrition and Health (U.S. Department of Health and Human Services 1988). The government and local authorities should play a more active role in promoting physical activity through the provision of more community exercise facilities that are affordable to all residents. The government should also regulate commercial slimming organizations and provide standards of treatment to reduce deception and fradulent practices to which obese persons so frequently fall victim. The media should assume a responsible position in regard to idealized concepts of beauty by appropriate programming and feeding messages passed through to children and to society at large. Finally, health insurance companies should assume responsibility in paying for obesity treatment before it leads to more costly long-term complications.

REFERENCES

American College of Sports Medicine: Guidelines for exercise testing and prescription. 3rd ed. Philadelphia: Lea & Febiger, 1986.

Bjorntorp P. Interrelation of physical activity and nutrition in obesity. In White PL, Modeika TD, eds. Diet and exercise: Supervision in health maintenance. Chicago: American Medical Association, 1982:91–98.

Bjorntorp P. Abdominal obesity in the development of non-insulin dependent diabetes mellitus. Diabetes/Metabolism Rev 1988; 4:615–622.

Black Sir D, James WPT, Besser GM. A report of the Royal College of Physicians. J Roy Coll Physicians Lond 1983; 17:5–65.

Borjeson M. The aetiology of obesity in children. Acta Paediatr Scand 1976; 65:279–287.

Bray G. Lipogenesis in human adipose tissue: Some effects of nibbling and gorging. J Clin Invest 1972; 51:537–547.

Bray GA, Gray DS. Treatment of obesity: An overview. Diabetes/Metabolism Rev 1988; 4:655-679.

Brownell KD, Foreyt JP. Handbook of eating disorders: Physiology, psychology, and treatment of obesity, anorexia, and bulimia. New York: Basic Books, 1986.

Brownell KD, Stunkard AJ. Behavioral treatment of obesity in children. Am J Dis Child 1978; 132:403–412.

Buckmanster L, Brownell K. Behavior modification: The state of the art. In Frankle R, Yang M, eds. Obesity and weight control. Rockville, MD: Aspen Systems Corp., 1988.

Build and Blood Pressure Study, 1959. Chicago: Society of Actuaries, 1959.

Bullen BA, Reed RB, Mayer J. Physical activity of obese and non-obese girls appraised by motion picture sampling. J Clin Nutr 1964; 14:211–223.

Canning H, Mayer J. Obesity — its possible effect on college acceptance. N Engl J Med 1966; 275:1172–1174.

Charney E, Goodman HC, McBride M, Lyon B, Pratt R. Childhood antecedents of adult obesity. Do chubby infants become obese adults? N Engl J Med 1976; 295:6–9.

Council of Scientific Affairs. Treatment of obesity in adults. JAMA 1988; 260:2547–2551.

Dalton S. Eating management: A tool for the practitioner. In Frankle R, Yang M, eds. Obesity and weight control. Rockville, MD: Aspen Systems Corp., 1988.

De Fronzo RA. Insulin and renal sodium handling: Clinical implications. In Bjorntorp P, Cairella M, Howard AN, eds. Recent advances in obesity research, III. London: John Libbey, 1980: 37–41.

Dietz WH, Gortmaker SL. Do we fatten our children at the TV set? Television viewing and obesity in children and adolescents. Pediatrics 1985; 75:807–812.

Dietz WH, Gortmaker SL. Factors within the physical environment associated with childhood obesity. Am J Clin Nutr 1984; 39:619–624.

Dietz WH, Hartung R. Changes in height velocity of obese preadolescents during weight reduction. Am J Dis Child 1985; 139:704–708.

Di Lorenzo C, Williams CM, Hajnal F, Valenzuela J. Pectin delays gastric emptying and increases satiety in obese subjects. Gastroenterology 1988; 95:1211–1215.

Di Natale B, Bregani P, Carbone A, et al. Investigations preliminary to devising a programme for prevention of childhood obesity. In Cacciori E, Larun Z, Raiti S, eds. Obesity in childhood. New York: Academic Press, 1978:157.

Dwyer JT, Feldman JJ, Mayer J. Adolescent dieters: Who are they? Physical characteristics, attitudes, and dieting practices of adolescent girls. Am J Clin Nutr 1967; 20:1045–1056.

Epstein LH. Review of behavior treatments for childhood obesity. In Brownell KD, Foreyt JP, eds. Eating disorders. New York: Basic Books Inc., 1986:159–179.

Epstein LH, Rena RW, Cluss P, et al. Resting metabolic rate in lean and obese children: Relationship to parent and child weight and percent overweight change. Am J Clin Nutr 1989; 49:331–336.

Epstein LH, Rena RW, Koeske R, et al. Long-term effects of family-based treatment of childhood obesity. J Consul Clin Psy 1987; 1:91–95.

Epstein LH, Wing RR, Penner BC, et al. Effect of diet and controlled exercise on weight loss in obese children. J Pediatr 1985; 107:358–361.

Fat execs get slimmer paychecks. Industry Week 1974; 180:21, 24.

Flatt JP. The biochemistry of energy expenditure. In Bray G, ed. Recent advances in obesity research. Vol. 2. London, Newman Publishing, 1973:211–228.

Flatt JP, Blackburn GL. The metabolic fuel regulatory system: Implications for protein-sparing therapies during caloric deprivation and disease. Am J Clin Nutr 1974; 27:175–187.

Fortmann SP, Haskell WL, Wood PP. Effects of weight loss in clinic and ambulatory blood pressure in normotensive men. Am J Cardiol 1988; 62:89–93.

Garn SM, Clark DC. Trends in fatness and origins of obesity. Pediatrics 1976; 57:443–456.

Garrison RJ, Castelli WP. Weight and thirty-year mortality of men in the Framingham Study. Ann Intern Med 1985; 103:1006–1009.
Gortmaker SL, Dietz WH, Sobol AM, Wehler CA. Increasing pediatric obesity in the United States. Am J Dis Child 1987; 141:535–540.
Hagan RD, Upton SJ, Wong L, Whittam J. The effects of aerobic conditioning and/ or caloric restriction in overweight men and women. Med Sci Sports Exerc 1986; 18(1):87–94.
Hendler RC, Walesky M, Sherwin RS. Isocaloric sucrose substitution prevents or reverses the diet induced fall in resting metabolic rate. Fourth International Congress on Obesity, New York, 1983:27–36.
Hill JO, Sparling PB, Shields TW, et al. Effects of exercise and food restriction on body composition and metabolic rate in obese women. Am J Clin Nutr 1987; 46:622–630.
Huenemann RL. Food habits of obese and non-obese adolescents. Postgrad Med 1972; 51:99–105.
Keys A. Overweight and the risk of heart attack and sudden death. In Bray GA, ed. Obesity in perspective. Vol. 2. Washington, D.C.: Department of Health, Education and Welfare, 1976: 215–223. NIH Publication No. 75–708.
Merrit RJ. Obesity. Curr Probl Pediatr 1982; 12(11):1–58.
Metzner HL. The relationship between frequency of eating and adiposity in adult men and women in the Tecumseh Community Health Study. Am J Clin Nutr 1977; 30:712–720.
Moses N, Banilivy M, Lifshitz F. Fear of obesity among adolescent females. Pediatrics 1989; 83:393–398.
National Center for Health Statistics, U.S. Department of Health, Education and Welfare. NCHS growth curves for children: Birth to 18 years. Series H, No. 165, DHEW Publication No. (PHS) 78–1650, 1977.
Newark SR, Williamson B. Survey of very-low-calorie weight reduction diets. II. Total fasting, protein-sparing modified fasts, chemically defined diets. Arch Intern Med 1983; 143:1423–1427.
Piers AL, Struve MF, Mueller RA. Body fat distribution and glucose metabolism. J Clin Endocrinol Metab 1988; 67:760–767.
Pi-Sunyer FV. Obesity. In Shils ME, Young VR, eds. Modern nutrition in health and disease. Philadelphia: Lea & Febiger, 1988: 795-816.
Pugliese M, Weyman-Daum M, Moses N, Lifshitz F. Parental health beliefs as a cause of non-organic failure to thrive. Pediatrics 1987; 80:175–182.
Pugliese MT, Recker B, Lifshitz F. A survey to determine the prevalence of abnormal growth patterns in adolescence. J Adolesc Health Care 1988; 9:181–187.
Ravelli GP, Belmont L. Obesity in nineteen-year-old men: Family size and birth order associations. Am J Epidemiol 1979; 109:66–70.
Ravussin E, Lillioja S, Anderson TE, Christin L. Determinants of 24 hour energy expenditure in man: Methods and results using a respiratory chamber. J Clin Invest 1986; 78:1568–1578.
Ravussin E, Lillioja S, Knowler WC. Reduced rate of energy expenditure as a risk factor for body-weight gain. N Engl J Med 1988; 318:467–472.
Ravussin E, Burnand B, Schulz Y, et al. Energy expenditure before and during energy restriction in obese patients. Am J Clin Nutr 1985; 41:753–759.
Richardson SA, Goodman N, Hastorf AH, et al. Cultural uniformity in reaction to

physical disabilities. Am Sociol Rev 1961; 26:241–247.
Rimm AA, White PL. Obesity: Its risks and hazards. In Bray GA, ed. Obesity in America. U.S. Department of Health, Education, and Welfare Publication No. (NIH) 80–359, 1980.
Roberts SB, Savage J, Coward WA, et al. Energy expenditure and intake in infants born to lean and overweight mothers. N Engl J Med 1988; 318:461–466.
Rolland-Cachera MF, Sempe M, Guilloud-Bataille M, Patois E, Pequignot-Guggenbuhl F, Fautrad V. Adiposity indices in children. Am J Clin Nutr 1982; 36: 178–184.
Rose HE, Mayer J. Activity, calorie intake, fat storage, and the energy balance of infants. Pediatrics 1968; 41:18–29.
Sclafani A. Dietary obesity. In Stunkard AJ, ed. Obesity. Philadelphia: W.B. Saunders Co., 1980.
Staffieri JR. A study of social stereotype of body image in children. J Pers Soc Psychol 1967; 7:101–104.
Stark D, Atkins E, Wolff DH, Douglas JWB. Longitudinal study of obesity in the National Survey of Health and Development. Br Med J 1981; 282:12–17.
Story M, Brown JE. Do young children instinctively know what to eat? N Engl J Med 1987; 316:103–105.
Stuart R. Behavioral control of overeating. Behav Res Ther 1967; 5:357–365.
Stunkard A, Mendelsom M. Obesity and the body image. I. Characteristics of disturbances in the body image of some obese persons. Am J Psychiatry 1967a; 123:1296–1300.
Stunkard A, Burt V. Obesity and the body image. II. Age at onset of disturbances in the body. Am J Psychiatry 1967b; 123:1443–1447.
Stunkard A, Sorensen TIA, Hanis C, et al. An adoption study of human obesity. N Engl J Med 1986; 317:193–198.
U.S. Department of Health and Human Services. The Surgeon General's Report on Nutrition and Health, 1988.
USDA, Human Nutrition Service, Nutrition Monitoring Division. Nationwide food consumption survey of food intakes by individuals, women 19–50 years and their children 1–5 years, 1 Day, NFCS, CSFII Report No. 85-1, 1985.
Wadden TA et al. Very low calorie diets: Their efficacy, safety and future. Ann Intern Med 1983; 99:675–684.
Waldbaum R. Childhood obesity: An overview. In Lifshitz F, ed. Pediatric Nutrition. New York: Marcel Dekker, 1982: 273–295.
Weinsier RL, Johnston MH, Doley DM, Bacon JA. Dietary management of obesity evaluation of the time-energy displacement diet in terms of its efficacy and nutritional adequacy for long-term weight control. Br J Nutr 1982; 47:367–369.
Wood PD, Stefanick ML, Dreon DM, et al. Changes in plasma lipids and lipoproteins in overweight men during weight loss through dieting as compared with exercise. N Engl J Med 1988; 319:1173–1179.

19

Diarrhea and Other Gastrointestinal Disorders

The following is an extract of a story published in *Newsweek* (McCabe, *Newsweek*, Dec. 26, 1988).

Nine years ago I had no idea that I would be joining the fraternity of those who have a vital interest in seeing that medical research continues. I was a very pregnant woman in labor. With my husband beside me I gave birth to a 7 pound 1 ounce daughter. It all seemed so easy, but for the next four months she could not gain weight. She was a textbook case of failure to thrive. Finally a hospital test of the salt content in her sweat led to the diagnosis of cystic fibrosis. "Your daughter will not have a long life, but for most of the time, it will be a good life. Her life expectancy is about 13 years, though it could be longer or shorter. As research continues, we're keeping them alive longer," the doctor said.

How has research helped those with CF? Three times a day my daughter uses enzymes from the pancreas of pigs to digest her foods. She takes antibiotics tested on rats before they are tried on humans. As an adult, she will probably develop diabetes and need insulin—a drug developed by research on dogs and rabbits. If she ever needs a heart–lung transplant, one might be possible because of the cows on which surgeons practiced. There is no animal model to help CF research, but now that the CF gene is located, new gene-splicing techniques may create a family of mice afflicted with the disease. Researchers would first learn to cure the mice with drugs, then cautiously try with humans. Come to think of it, it is animal research which has helped my child!

DIARRHEA

Diarrhea is rampant throughout the world. There are approximately 150 million episodes of diarrhea per year in children (Walsh & Warren 1979). Each of the world's 338 million children under the age of 5 years suffers at least two or three episodes of diarrheal illnesses per year. In most of these instances, babies who are otherwise healthy have an uneventful course and recover if proper hydration and dietary treatment are given. However, in the developing world over 7 percent of them die (Walsh & Warren 1979, Synder & Merson 1982, Mason 1986). In other words, each day diarrhea kills 12,600 children before age 5 years. A child living in the poorest areas of the world may have up to 10 episodes of diarrhea per year and diarrhea is associated with over 50 percent of the total deaths (Guerrant et al 1983). Most of these children suffer from infectious diarrhea, whereas in the United States and other developed countries diarrhea is related to many causes (Lifshitz, da Costa Ribeiro & Silverberg 1988) (Fig. 19–1).

Nutrition and Diarrhea

The relationship between nutrition and diarrhea has been apparent since antiquity, when it was recognized that diarrhea could develop after eating and would improve with fasting. There is a clear association between the type of food ingested and the development and outcome of diarrhea (Lifshitz & da Costa Ribeiro 1988) (Fig. 19–2). Contaminated cow's milk fed to babies is the leading cause of diarrhea and its prevalence is highest in the unsanitary conditions associated with poverty. This is due to lack of refrigeration and potable water as well as contamination with flies and poor hygiene. Under these circumstances bottled milk becomes a culture medium for bacteria to grow, multiply, and infect the baby. In contrast, human-milk feeding is the most readily available means to reduce the problems of diarrhea worldwide since it reduces the possibility of contamination of milk and it provides general and local immune factors to prevent infection (see Chapter 12).

Contaminated milk is also a source of diarrhea for older persons, particularly when traveling (traveler's diarrhea [turista]). Infectious diarrhea may also be caused by eating other contaminated foods (Table 19–1). In addition to infections, diarrhea can be induced by other mechanisms by practically everything human beings eat. In this chapter, we describe the intolerances to carbohydrates that produce diarrhea (see below). In Chapter 20, we discuss the food allergies that may also produce diarrhea. In addition, it should be kept in mind that children who are overfed, whether it be formula (see Chapter 13), apple juice (Hyams & Leichter 1985), or even excess fluid, may develop diarrhea (Greene & Ghishan 1983).

Diarrhea is considered to be the most important inducer of malnutrition in the world. Diarrhea and other infections affect the body's economy through a number of mechanisms (Lifshitz 1989). This illness, like many other infections, decreases the appetite. Infants with diarrhea reject most foods, although breast milk is rejected to a lesser extent. The lack of appetite

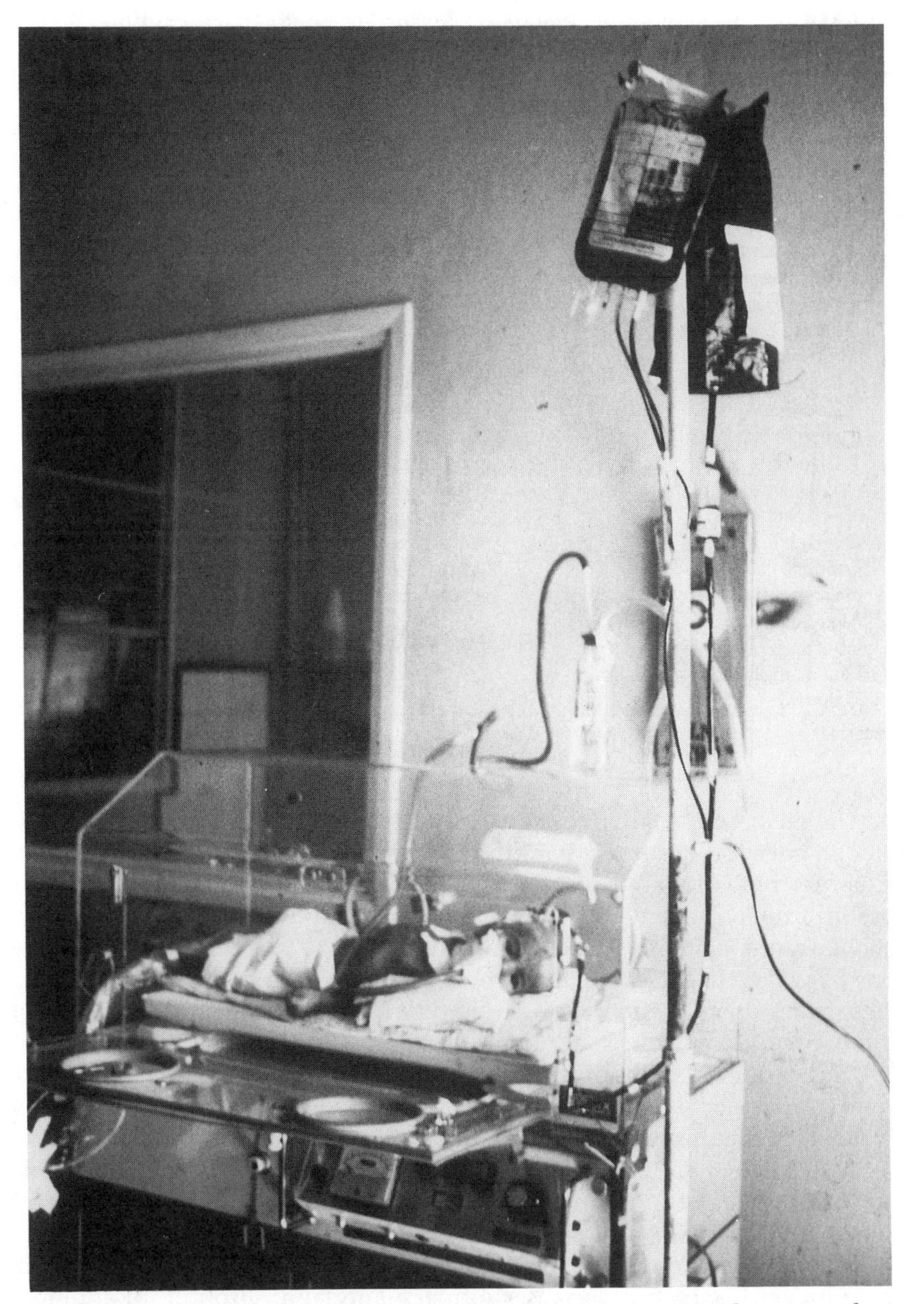

Figure 19–1. An acutely ill infant with severe diarrhea and malnutrition; he is being treated in an intensive-care unit.

Table 19–1. Type of Foods Frequently Associated with Diarrheal Illness.

TYPE OF PROBLEM	USUAL SOURCE OF FOOD
1. Infection	
E. coli (toxigenic)	Restaurant food, milk ("turista")
Salmonella	Eggs, meat, poultry, salads
Norwalk virus	Raw oysters
Vibrio parahaemolyticus	Shrimp, raw fish
Clostridium	Meat or gravy
Yersinia enterocolitica	Seafood, canned meats, ice cream
Aeromonas	Food and water
Protozoan infections	Water, salads
Parasitic infections	Raw fish
2. Toxins/Poisons	
Staphylococcus aureus	Cream-filled pastry
Botulism	Home-processed foods and cans
Scombroid	Tuna and mackerel
Ciguatera	Red snapper
Cadmium poisoning	Food barbecued on refrigerator trays
Solanine	Green sprouts or potatoes
3. Overfeeding	Juice, water, formula
4. Food intolerances	Lactose and other sugars; fat
Malabsorption	Protein
Allergies	
5. Inborn errors of metabolism	All carbohydrate-containing foods.
Glucose/galactose malabsorption	

Modified from Lifshitz F, da Costa Ribeiro H. Diarrheal diseases. In Paige DM, ed. Clinical nutrition. 2nd ed. St. Louis: C.V. Mosby, 1988:447–462.

may be mediated by interleukin I, a hormone released by white blood cells after an infection or some other kind of stress. Thus, the intensity of the anorexia may not correlate with the type or severity of the illness. A child may lose his or her appetite with even mild diarrhea, with anorexia lasting for a few hours or for days or weeks. As much as 20 to 70 percent of food available may be wasted or not eaten during bouts of diarrhea. In addition, when diarrhea strikes there is usually restriction of food intake dictated by medical or popular traditions, beliefs, or taboos to diminish the diarrhea.

The nutritional status of a patient with diarrhea is further altered because there is decreased digestion and intestinal absorption of nutrients (Fig. 19–3). Even when diarrhea is mild, there is sugar (lactose) malabsorption (Kumar et al 1977). Since up to 50 percent of a child's caloric intake is derived from milk sugar, lactose malabsorption secondary to diarrhea accounts for considerable caloric deficit and weight loss. The presence of unabsorbed carbohydrates in the intestinal lumen dilutes bile acid concentrations, which induces protein and nitrogen losses and decreases nitrogen and fat absorption. In addition, there may be loss of cells, plasma, amino acids and other nitrogenous substances, vitamins, and hormones through the stools owing to the intestinal

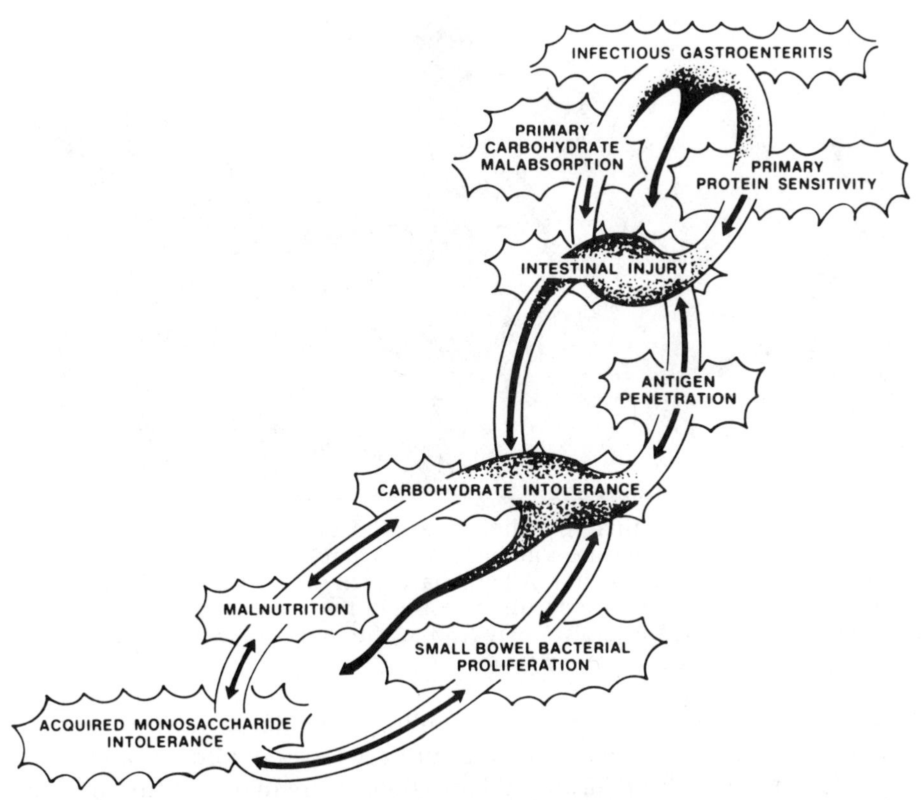

Figure 19–2. Sequence of events leading to chronic diarrhea in infancy. The outcome of an infectious episode of diarrhea often depends on the type of feedings and tolerance for foods fed during the illness. Acquired monosaccharide intolerance denotes an inability to tolerate any feeding including the most simple sugars.

mucosal injury induced by the infection. In the dysentery diarrheas there is also protein-losing enteropathy. Loss of iron from gastrointestinal bleeding may be severe enough to cause anemia and deficiencies of other essential minerals such as magnesium and zinc as well as deficiencies of folic acid and vitamin B_{12}. The use of antibiotics for the treatment of diarrhea may impair intestinal synthesis of vitamin K with resultant hypoprothrombinemia and an increased risk of bleeding problems.

In diarrhea, as in other infections, metabolic alterations occur that have grave negative nutritional implications that are costly and slow to correct (Beisel 1983). These include breakdown of muscle protein; mobilization of white blood cells (leukocytes); sequestration of zinc and iron; and discharge of several hormones, such as insulin, glucagon, vasoactive intestinal polypep-

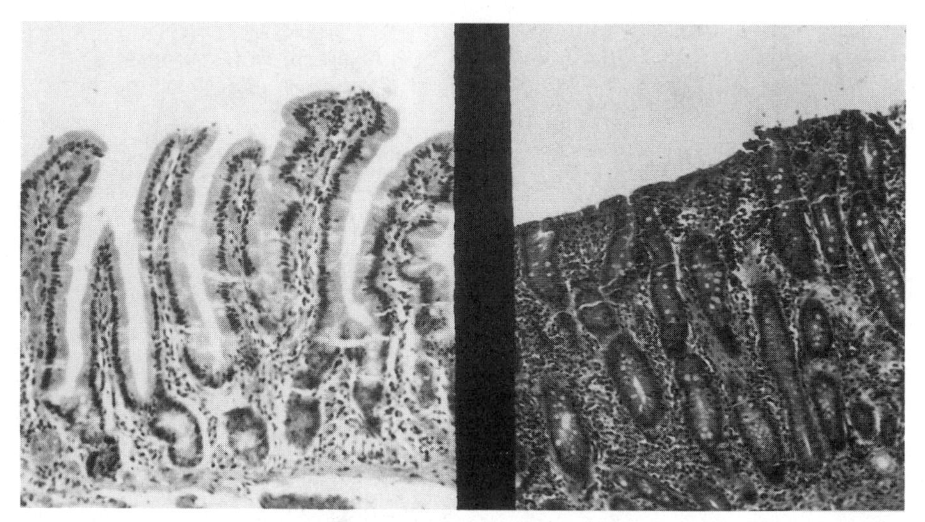

Figure 19–3. The intestinal morphology as seen under a microscope. On the right is a normal small intestine with intact villi where absorption takes place. On the left is a flat intestinal mucosa. All villi have been destroyed; intestinal malabsorption and food intolerance occurs. Intestinal injury due to an infection or to any other destructive mechanism may lead to flattening of the mucosa.

tide (VIP), and other gut hormones (motilin, enteroglucagon, neurotensin). These metabolic alterations account for urinary losses of nitrogen and other essential nutrients. Even during mild infections, there may be nitrogen losses through the urine in amounts ranging from 0.6 to 1.2 grams per kilogram per day. These negative influences rapidly deteriorate the nutritional status of a child with diarrhea. Infants and young children with diarrhea may lose 10 percent or more of their body weight within days.

A child with diarrhea may also develop an allergy to the feedings he or she receives while being sick, whereas the same child without the infection would not have developed such an allergy. Intact dietary proteins pass into the blood owing to intestinal damage as a result of the infections that produce diarrhea. Absorption of intact protein into the circulation may sensitize a susceptible child and induce allergy (see Chapter 20). In addition, there may be carbohydrate intolerances during the illness that are not present when there is no diarrhea (Lifshitz 1980, 1982b, & 1985a). The intestinal malabsorption is often intensified in infants who have diarrhea and lactose intolerance if they are not given dietary therapy.

The presence of continuing dietary intolerances and nutrient losses during diarrhea impair the infant's ability to recover from the initial illness, and the disease may become chronic. These patients may have increased susceptibility to other conditions with spreading infections. Often there are associated ear infections, and at times there may be severe complications, such as necrotizing enterocolitis (NEC). NEC is a life-threatening complication that occurs in infants with diarrhea who have lactose intolerance while being fed milk formula (Coello-Ramirez, Gutierrez-Topete & Lifshitz 1970). NEC may also result from other intolerances or from elemental, hyperosmolar diets fed to the sick patient (Lifshitz 1982a).

NUTRITIONAL MANAGEMENT OF DIARRHEA

Fast Versus Feast

"Bowel rest" has long been recommended in treating a variety of digestive disorders, particularly diarrhea. During the initial treatment for diarrhea, patients are often fasted for up to several days, or food is restricted for up to several weeks, "to provide bowel rest." However, there are no scientific data to support the restriction of oral intake in persons with diarrhea. Moreover, we now know that fasting can only serve to aggravate the high nutritional risks of this illness. Clinicians have long known that breastfeeding should be sustained during diarrhea, and oral fluids are mandatory to hydrate the patient.

Apart from the undesirable metabolic effects of even brief fasts, withholding oral intake may further alter intestinal absorption. Even with intravenous feedings, there may be depletion of intestinal digestive enzymes, cell mass, gut growth, bile and pancreatic secretions, intestinal blood flow and release of enteric hormones when food is withheld. Feedings may be even more critical in a patient with diarrhea, since the positive physiologic effects of oral ingestion are heightened (Pergolizzi et al 1977). Furthermore, oral feedings have an important role in the formation of stool bulk, which helps to restore bowel function.

Even though feedings increase the stool output and diarrhea, children who are fed recover faster and have higher body weights than children who are fasted. Thus, fasting may only be necessary for patients with diarrhea who have specific complications such as paralytic ileus or NEC. However, in all other patients with diarrhea, feedings should be administered. Oral intake is the preferred way to treat patients with gastroenteritis, even if they are vomiting (Hirschhorn 1980).

Oral Hydration

Oral fluids should be given regardless of the cause or severity of the diarrheal episode or the presence of vomiting. Even the most dehydrated infant can be improved with oral hydration solutions (Table 19–2). Intravenous therapy is best reserved for the patient with circulatory failure or central nervous system damage who cannot take water, salts, and calories by mouth, or when oral therapy fails. The latter usually occurs only with very high stool losses (over 10 mL/kg/hr).

To maintain water and electrolyte balance and to prevent dehydration, oral hydration fluids should be initiated as soon as there is evidence of disease (Fig. 19–4). Oral hydration solutions should be given in sufficient quantities to replace the water and electrolyte losses in the stools. In the presence of dehydration, oral fluids must replace the fluid deficits; this should be rapidly accomplished, within 6 to 8 hours if possible, except when there is hypernatremia (high serum sodium). Fever, which often complicates the course of the illness, may increase the risk of hypernatremia, but neither fever nor high environmental temperatures affect the favorable outcome with oral fluid treatment (Hirschhorn 1980). After the dehydration is corrected, oral feedings should begin.

Milk Feedings

Breastfeeding. The fortunate baby who is being breast-fed should continue receiving human breast milk even when he or she has diarrhea (see Chapter 12). Infants fed human breast milk have a lesser chance of acquiring a diarrheal illness, and when they do, they have milder symptoms (Fig. 19–5). Interestingly, breast-fed babies also have a better lactose tolerance despite the relatively higher lactose content in human milk (approximately 7 percent) as compared with cow's milk (approximately 4 percent) (Okuni et al 1972). Moreover, human milk has immunologic advantages and growth factors that may aid in the recovery from infectious diarrhea.

Milk Formula Feedings. When human-milk feeding is unsuccessful, inappropriate, or stopped early proprietary milk formulas must be used (see Chapter 13). However, there is controversy regarding the type and concentration of milk formula that infants with diarrhea should be fed. The World Health Organization recommends diluted cow's milk. The basis for this recommendation is that most patients with diarrhea will improve while being fed diluted milk, which is less expensive and more readily available throughout the world than infant milk formulas (WHO 1984). In contrast, the American Academy of Pediatrics Committee on Nutrition does not recommend unmodified cow's milk or evaporated milk during the first 6 months of life owing to potential problems such as insidious blood loss in the gastrointestinal tract, and dehydration caused by the high renal solute load of cow's milk, which may be tolerated by normal infants but not by babies with diarrhea who have increased water losses. Because of the lactose and unmodified pro-

Table 19–2. Oral Rehydration Solutions and Commercial Products.

	SODIUM (mEq/L)	POTASSIUM (mEq/L)	CHLORIDE (mEq/L)	CARBOHYDRATE (gm/L)	
WHO recommendations*	90	20	80	Glucose	20
Pedialyte	45	20	35	Glucose	25
Pedialyte RS	75	20	65	Glucose	25
Gatorade	23	3	17	Glucose and sucrose	59
Ricelyte	50	25	45	Rice syrup solids	30
Hydra-Lyte	84	10	0	Glucose and sucrose	24
Cherry Koolaid†	2	0.25	7.5	Sucrose	109
Strawberry Jello†	12.5	0.20	0	Sucrose	152
Ginger ale	3.5	0.1		Sucrose and corn syrup	90
Morot's carrot syrup‡	7	35	50	Sucrose, glucose, and fructose	43
Beef broth (bouillon)	170.4	13.7	—	Sucrose	10.5
Apple juice	1.7	2.6	—	Monosaccharides (fructose, sucrose, sorbitol)	125
Tea	1.0	6.8	—	—	—
Cola	6.4	1.2	—	Sucrose	100
7-up	10	NA§	—	Sucrose	100

*Sack RB: Am J Clin Nutr 31:2251–2257, 1978.
†Scanlon JW: Clin Pediatr 9:508–509, 1970.
‡Lenze in Pediatrie. Ed. E. Rossi.
§NA: Not available.

Modified from Lifshitz F, da Costa Ribeiro H. Diarrheal diseases. In Paige DM, ed. Clinical nutrition. 2nd ed. St. Louis: C.V. Mosby, 1988:447–462.

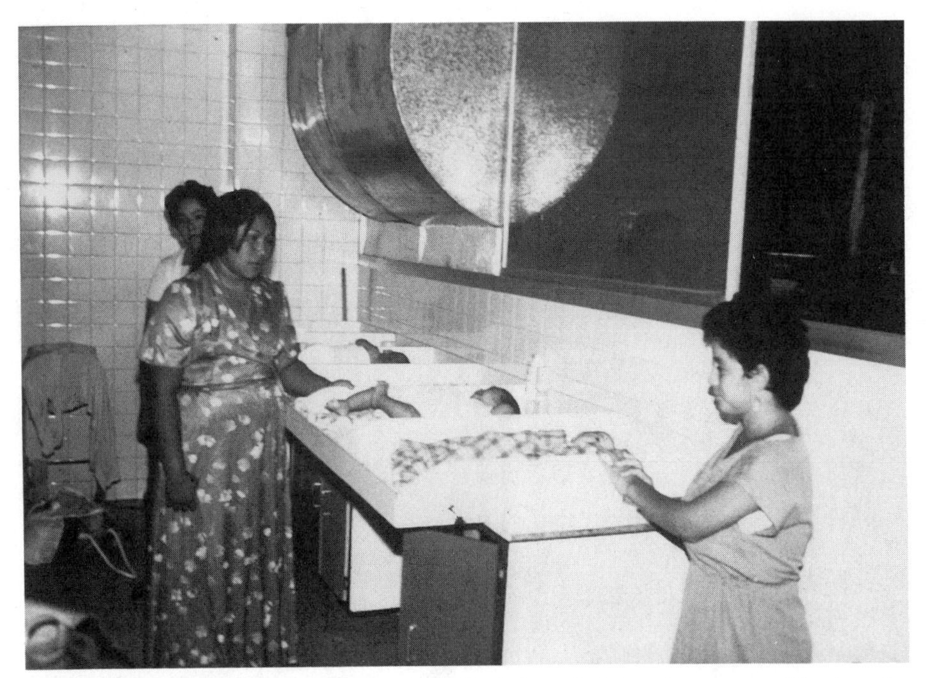

Figure 19–4. An oral hydration unit in a hospital in Monterrey, Mexico. Infants are treated and sent home with oral hydration solutions. The usual stay in this outpatient unit is less than a day. Once the baby is hydrated the danger of diarrhea is usually over.

tein in cow's milk, which are potential sources of intolerance and allergy (Lifshitz 1982b), lactose-free formulas are recommended as the initial feeding for children with severe diarrhea (Barness 1979). In prospective controlled studies we demonstrated that dilute cow's milk was detrimental whereas a lactose free glucose polymer, casein and medium chain fat formula (Portagen®) was best for infants with acute diarrhea (Lifshitz et al 1991). However, for infants with chronic diarrhea a formula with protein hydrolysates was required (Lifshitz et al 1990).

In the United States, special proprietary lactose-free formulas have been prescribed by physicians for the past several years for the treatment of infants with diarrhea, and the incidence of chronic diarrhea following gastroenteritis has declined (Lifshitz 1985b). The most severe forms of the disease—intractable-protracted diarrhea or monosaccharide intolerance (Lifshitz, Coello-Ramirez & Gutierrez-Topete 1970)—are now rarely seen. The reduced prevalence and severity of the diarrhea following infections was also achieved in Europe (Editorial 1987). However, in less developed countries, special formulas are not readily available and cow's-milk feedings are given to the sick infants, leading to chronic diarrhea, malnutrition, and more severe dietary intolerances (Fagundes-Neto, Viaro & Lifshitz 1985, Lifshitz et al 1990). Spe-

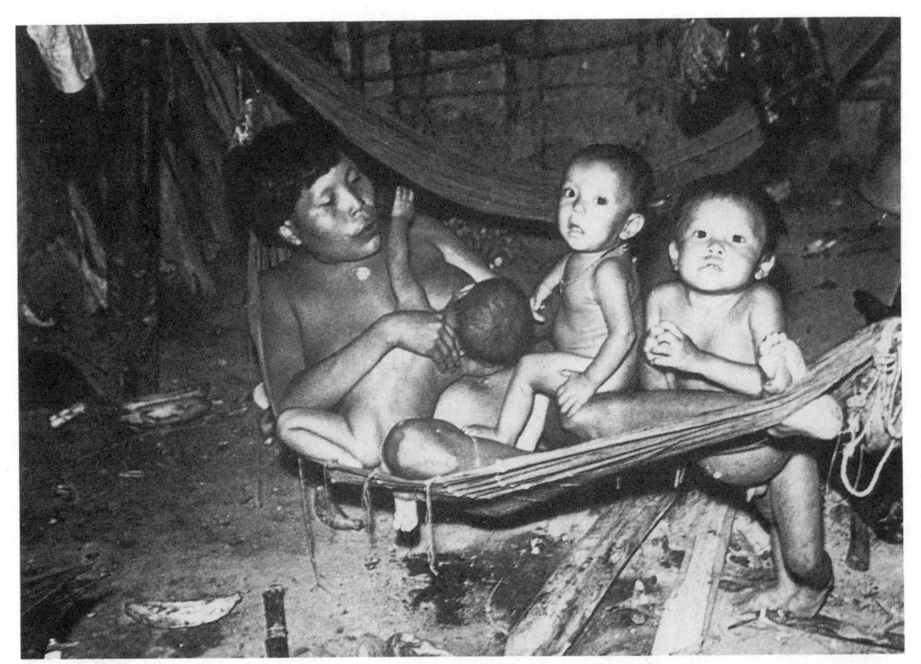

Figure 19–5. Breastfeeding among Indians in the Xingu National Park in the region Amazone river/jungle in Brazil. Courtesy of Dr. Ulysses Fegundo-Neto.

cial formulas are needed to control the diarrhea; they are not to be used for prolonged periods. Dietary intolerances may subside within a few days or may last for a few weeks after the improvement of diarrhea, with complete disappearance after the child grows older. Therefore, once the diarrhea and body weight improve, these infants should be tested to determine whether they have overcome their intolerances and can be upgraded to a conventional milk formula.

Many formulas are available that have been developed for infants with diarrheal disorders (see Chapter 13). These special formulas provide all known nutrients required by the infant at levels similar to those of breast milk, but with specific modifications needed to meet the needs of the sick infant (Lifshitz 1985b). When a physician prescribes a formula for the treatment of a baby with diarrhea most likely the infant will receive a formula that has modified carbohydrate, protein and fat contents (see Chapter 13). Therefore, some of the observed benefits of these formulas may be due to a variety of factors since one formula may effectively treat lactose, protein, and fat intolerance.

Milk formulas derived from soybean or other sources (chicken, lamb, and even frog) instead of cow's milk have been utilized in the treatment of children with diarrhea (Lifshitz 1982b, 1985b). These formulas are often considered to be "hypoallergenic." This is a misconception, since they merely contain a protein source other than cow's milk, which may also induce protein intolerance in susceptible patients (see Chapters 13 and 20). Also available are formulas containing protein hydrolysates instead of whole protein. However, recommending protein hydrolysates as a substitute for cow's-milk protein in all infants with diarrhea is unjustified. The majority of patients with severe diarrhea improve on a formula with casein as the protein source (Lifshitz et al 1971a) and little or no advantage is obtained by using casein hydrolysate for the treatment of such patients (Graham et al 1973, MacLean et al 1980). However, protein hydrolysates may be indicated for patients with chronic diarrhea or for those with specific protein intolerances (see Chapter 20) (Lifshitz 1985b, Fagundes-Neto, Viaro & Lifshitz 1985, Lifshitz et al 1990). Low-fat formulas have no role in the treatment of diarrhea, since the fecal energy loss caused by the fat malabsorption of diarrhea (steatorrhea) is transient, whereas a low-fat intake may lead to chronic persistent diarrhea and malnutrition (Cohen 1979).

How Much to Feed? The quantity of formula fed to an infant with diarrhea should be related to the evolution of the disease. Initially, feedings should be limited to provide maintenance energy requirements (75 kcal/kg/d). Thereafter, the formula intake may be gradually increased if the infant tolerates the feedings and the diarrhea is mild to moderate (stool losses of 30–50 g/kg/d). During this time the fluid balance needs to be maintained by fluids and electrolytes given intravenously or orally, in addition to the formula feedings. Improved consistency of the stools, not the number of diarrheal episodes, should be used to determine advancement in the dietary intake. The number of stools can be misleading, and this alone should not be used as a guide in formula changes. An excessive volume of fluids fed or a rapid advancement of formula intake may also exacerbate diarrhea. This is not an infrequent problem, as babies with diarrhea tend to overeat or drink in excess once the anorexia is improved (Greene & Ghishan 1983). With improvement of the diarrhea the amount of feedings should gradually be increased while the hydration solution is simultaneously decreased until full caloric supply is given to the baby (±110 kcal/kg/d).

The concentration of the formula feedings is also important. Many doctors use a diluted milk formula to treat patients with diarrhea. However, we recommend small amounts of undiluted formula feedings since proprietary formulas contain the right amount of water (1 kcal/1.5 mL of formula) while maintaining the patient's fluid balance with added electrolyte solutions (see Table 19–2). More concentrated formulas or the addition of extra sugar into the formula should be avoided until the diarrhea is controlled, even if the patient is underweight. It is unrealistic to expect improvement in nutrition until the diarrhea is improved. Furthermore, the increased osmolality of the formula due to the added sugar may contribute to prolongation of diarrhea and to other complications such as carbohydrate intolerance or NEC (Lifshitz 1982a).

What About Intravenous Nutrition? In malnourished patients peripheral intravenous nutrient supplements can be a useful early adjunct. Very sick infants may benefit from intravenous glucose, amino acids, and fat when diarrhea is expected to be prolonged and when oral feedings cannot be sustained (see Chapter 28). However, it is difficult to justify a central venous line for total parenteral alimentation if maintenance energy requirements can be provided by peripheral vein and/or oral intake. Generalized infection (sepsis) is a major complication and a potential cause of death in patients with infectious diarrhea given central lines for intravenous nutrition. The use of total intravenous nutrition for infants with diarrhea should be reserved for the infrequent patient who fails enteral nutritional rehabilitation due to intolerances to all foods (Lifshitz, Coello-Ramirez & Gutierrez-Topete 1970, Lifshitz 1985b). Fortunately, constant nasogastric administration of a modified milk formula is usually well tolerated by most infants (see Chapter 27). Such enteral feedings may facilitate the initial stages of the treatment of very malnourished patients, particularly during the anorectic phase of the illness and while they have severe diarrhea (Green et al 1975). However, feedings by mouth at regular intervals should be given once the patient recovers.

Dietary Intake

In older infants and children with diarrheal disease, milk formulas must be supplemented by other foods. All too often, simple foods such as broth, gruel, dry toast, apples, bananas, and tea are prescribed, without regard for the energy needs or likes of the patient. In some areas it has been popular to prescribe a "BRATT" diet (bananas, rice, applesauce, toast, and tea) to treat diarrhea. The usual portion of the BRATT diet provides about 1300 calories for an adult—with 317 grams of carbohydrate, 15 grams of protein, and 3 grams of fat. This is hardly a normal intake and may have detrimental consequences for infants and young children. Furthermore, the diet is low in energy, nitrogen, and fat but high in carbohydrate. It also contains caffeine (75–150 mg/cup of tea), which may perpetuate diarrhea and malnutrition. Nevertheless, it has been advocated on the basis of improvement in the stool consistency because of its high pectin content. Three apples per day yield approximately 2.8 grams of pectin, and three bananas about 3.3 grams. However, the cosmetic improvement of the stools should in no way be interpreted as improvement of the disease!

A low-residue diet is often advocated to decrease the frequency and volume of stools, whereas bran is used to increase stool bulk and help restore motility. Dietary fiber also protects the intestines from the strain of defecation, and this may be important in dysenteric diarrhea when small-volume stools are excreted. The use of 25 to 36 grams of bran per day may decrease the symptoms of cramping and bowel discomfort (Brodribb & Humphreys 1976), although nondigestible bran fiber may cause more flatulence and abdominal distention because of methane gas production.

Once the anorectic phase of the illness improves, a nutritious, well-balanced diet that contains easily digestible components is recommended and should be given in accordance with the needs, likes, and tolerances of the patient. Dietary restriction may have more disadvantages than the intake of a normal diet in patients who do not have specific food intolerances. To avoid deficiencies, the diet should provide adequate amounts of all nutrients.

When presented with a patient with chronic diarrhea, a few nutritional recommendations should be implemented before embarking on an expensive and time-consuming evaluation of an otherwise healthy young child. The following steps should be taken:

1. Restrict apple juice intake and observe the effect.
2. Check fluid intake; it should not exceed 120 milliliters per kilogram per day.
3. Children should not be placed on low-calorie diets to treat chronic diarrhea. Fat intake, if low, should be increased to a level in accordance with age and body weight.

CHRONIC INFLAMMATORY BOWEL DISEASE

Chronic inflammatory bowel disease (CIBD) may affect primarily the small bowel (Crohn's disease) or it may involve the large bowel (ulcerative colitis) (Daum 1988). CIBD may present with a variety of clinical problems including abdominal pain and chronic diarrhea, or it may present with short stature and growth slow down without any other sign or symptom (Kanof, Lake & Bayless 1988). Growth retardation occurs in response to decreased nutrient availability (Motil et al 1982).

It is recognized that the most important problem in CIBD patients is their impaired nutrition. Malnutrition in CIBD results primarily from the lack of appetite (anorexia) and the early satiety or discomfort that accompanies eating. These children decrease the volume and frequency of meals, and they are often described as "picky eaters" by their parents. However, the discomfort that accompanies eating is so subtle that it may not be of concern to either the child or the parent. The total daily calorie intake of CIBD patients usually is appropriate to maintain their weight but is insufficient to allow for normal growth (Kanof, Lake & Bayless 1988). When it is less than requirements for height, weight loss can be substantial (Kirschner 1988).

In addition to poor nutrient intake there may be other alterations that affect the nutritional status of CIBD patients, including impaired nutrient absorption and enhanced water losses through the stools (Kirschner 1988). Iron deficiency may result if blood is lost through the stools and resulting anemia will contribute to the patient's anorexia (Dallman 1982). They may also have other mineral deficiencies, such as magnesium and zinc (Nishi et al 1980, LaSala et al 1985), owing to increased losses of these minerals through the stools and/or reduced absorption (Stumiolo et al 1980). Low serum zinc levels may precede any other biochemical alteration in CIBD (Lifshitz & Nishi 1980).

Nutrition rehabilitation is essential for the treatment of CIBD patients. Treatment may reverse the growth retardation and may even improve the disease itself (Kirschner 1988). Treatment of the nutritional deficits is necessary to start the healing process. For example, if there is iron deficiency, therapeutic doses of iron are needed to replenish the patient's iron stores. The provision of all the necessary nutrients for growth should be attempted throughout the treatment of these patients. When the energy and protein intake of CIBD patients is increased to 60 to 70 calories per kilogram per day and 1.6 to 1.8 grams per kilogram per day, respectively, the patient's growth velocity improves (Kirschner 1988). The main problem is how to achieve these levels of nutrient intake in children with CIBD, since they refuse to eat. Nutritional support has been successfully achieved by a variety of methods (Fig. 19–6). Long-term total parenteral or enteral nutrition at home and even intermittent elemental enteral feedings given for 1 month every 4 months have been shown to be sufficient to allow tripling of the growth rate and improvement of the disease (Belli et al 1988). Some doctors combine low-dose or alternate-day steroid treatment and nutrition supplementation with enteral feedings to prolong the remission of the disease (Whittington, Barnes & Bayless 1977). Surgery for the correction of the growth problem in Crohn's disease should be contemplated only when appropriate nutritional therapy fails.

INTESTINAL PARASITES

Although parasitic infections resulting in diarrhea or intestinal malabsorption are uncommon in the United States, these infections are very prevalent throughout the world (Wittner 1980). Parasites often inhabit the intestinal tract of children, particularly in rural communities in the tropics, and they may affect the child's nutritional status (Stephenson 1980). Parasites are usually removed in food processing or are killed by cooking or freezing. However, eating raw or inadequately cooked food carries the risk of acquiring several types of worms and parasitic infections. Now that sushi and sashimi are popular in the United States, infections acquired from eating raw fish are on the rise (Wittner et al 1989). To avoid parasitic infections, a clean water supply is imperative. If sanitization is questionable, raw foods such as salads should be

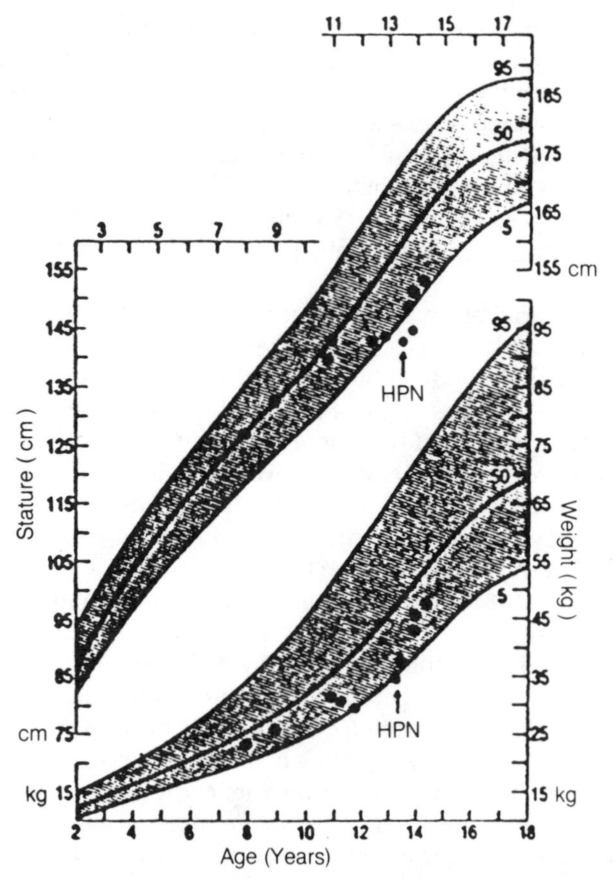

Figure 19–6. The growth pattern of a patient with chronic inflammatory bowel disease. The patient failed to grow and to gain weight before the diagnosis was made. He had essentially no weight gain from age 10 to 13½ years. The patient had a 14-kg (30.8 lb) weight gain and an 11-cm (>4 in.) height increase in 10 months following onset of nocturnal home enteral feedings (HPN).

From Daum F. Pediatric inflammatory bowel disease. In Silverberg M, Daum F, eds. Textbook of pediatric gastroenterology. 2nd ed. Chicago: Year Book, 1988: 392–418.

discouraged. In any case, parasitism should be promptly treated by specific medications.

MALABSORPTION SYNDROMES

Intestinal malabsorption from any cause decreases the total amount of food available to the child and thereby leads to malnutrition. The malabsorption syndrome is characterized by failure to thrive, weight loss, and passage of abnormal stools. A precise diagnosis of the cause of the malabsorption syndrome is essential for proper treatment.

INADEQUATE DIGESTION

Pancreatic Exocrine Insufficiency. Intestinal malabsorption resulting from inadequate digestion due to pancreatic disease is relatively unusual in children. The most common causes of pancreatic insufficiencies are congenital alterations, including exocrine enzyme deficiencies such as amylase, trypsinogen, enterokinase, and lipase deficiencies; the Shwachman–Diamond syndrome; and cystic fibrosis (Kessler & Lebenthal 1988). At times, the pancreas may be affected by viral illnesses or trauma leading to pancreatitis, thereby inducing inadequate pancreatic secretion.

In the newborn, pancreatic insufficiency occurs as a normal developmental event. However, most infants fed an appropriate diet for age gain weight and grow normally. The presence of alternative digestive pathways such as salivary digestion usually compensates for the relative immaturity of pancreatic function. However, if the "system is overloaded," as with overfeeding or earlier introduction of supplements, malabsorption may ensue (Kessler & Lebenthal 1988).

When there is pancreatic insufficiency, oral administration of pancreatic enzymes may be used. There are several products available for pancreatic enzyme replacement, but they have an unpleasant odor and taste. Generally, they are fed at the beginning of the meal to ensure intake, or they are added to the food. (To minimize decomposition, the pancreatic replacement product should not be combined with hot foods or allowed to sit for a long time before eating.) These pancreatic enzyme preparations may be given along with sodium bicarbonate (0.2 g/kg/d) to avoid deactivation by a low pH and to improve enzyme activity. The required dosage of pancreatic enzymes varies from patient to patient depending on the character of the stools and the decrease in their frequency and on the overall improvement of the malabsorption and nutritional state of the patient. Infants usually require 1/4 to 1/2 teaspoon with each feeding; children from 5 to 10 years of age require two to four tablets per meal. Overdosage of pancreatic extracts induces constipation.

Dietary adjustments to facilitate the absorption of food may not be as critical when appropriate enzyme replacement therapy is given. However, restriction of poorly digested foods and liberalization of foods that may not require pancreatic juices for digestion is advisable. For example, when there is amylase deficiency the diet may be limited in complex starches and may be supplemented with glucose polymers (Hodge et al 1983). The same is true for fat intake in conditions of lipase deficiency. In these patients long-chain fats may be replaced in the diet with medium-chain fats. For patients with protein enzyme digestive deficiencies, such as trypsinogen or enterokinase deficiencies, protein hydrolysates are useful. Inadequate digestion may result from combined alterations in pancreatic function, and multiple etiologic factors must be addressed. Patients with pancreatic exocrine insufficiency and bone marrow failure (Shwachman–Diamond syndrome) may require additional blood transfusions and corticosteroid therapy.

Cystic Fibrosis. Cystic fibrosis (CF) is a generalized disease of exocrine glands that leads to secretion of unusually thick mucus. Children with CF show abnormally high sweat sodium and chloride levels, which result from failure of salt reabsorption in sweat gland ducts, and suffer from (1) chronic obstructive lung disease and recurrent and persistent infections leading to respiratory failure and death, (2) exocrine pancreatic insufficiency with fat malabsorption (steatorrhea) as well as malabsorption of many other nutrients, (3) intestinal obstruction (meconium ileus), (4) cirrhosis of the liver, and (5) infertility, especially in males.

Recent studies suggest that insufficient caloric intake may be a long-term complication of CF and a major determinant in the malnutrition and growth failure seen in these patients (Fig. 19–7). Most patients report energy and protein intakes of 80 to 100 percent of the RDA for age, and there may be as much as a 50 percent energy deficit (Hubbard & Mangrum 1982, Bell, Durie & Forstner 1984, Chase, Long & Lavin 1979). This is in contrast with the popular belief that characterizes CF patients as having voracious appetites. Recurrent infections, debilitation, fatigue, and psychologic depression contribute to the anorexia seen in these patients.

Malnutrition in CF may contribute to the morbidity and mortality of these patients (Gerson, Swan & Walker 1987). A marked difference in survival age among CF patients has been attributed to their nutritional status (Kraemer et al 1978). Growth and well-being can also be enhanced in the short term by nutritional rehabilitation. Better pulmonary function of CF patients has been associated with better fat absorption (Gaskin et al 1982), and respiratory muscle strength in CF patients is also improved by nutritional rehabilitation (Mansell et al 1984). However, critical evaluation provides little evidence for the value of aggressive nutritional support in improving the long-term pulmonary disease of CF patients.

Many patients with CF require nutritional support, or supplemental calories beyond usual food intake, to reduce the risk of growth failure and, it is hoped, to improve health status and extend survival (Editorial 1986, Gerson, Swan & Walker 1987). In attempting to maintain adequate caloric intake, many patients with CF find that they need more calories than they can consume. In fact, the actual energy requirements of the child with CF are estimated at 130 to 150 percent of the RDA for age (Hubbard & Mangrum 1982). CF patients also have a higher incidence of gastroesophogeal reflux (Scott, O'Loughlin & Gall 1985) and often, despite pancreatic enzyme replacement,

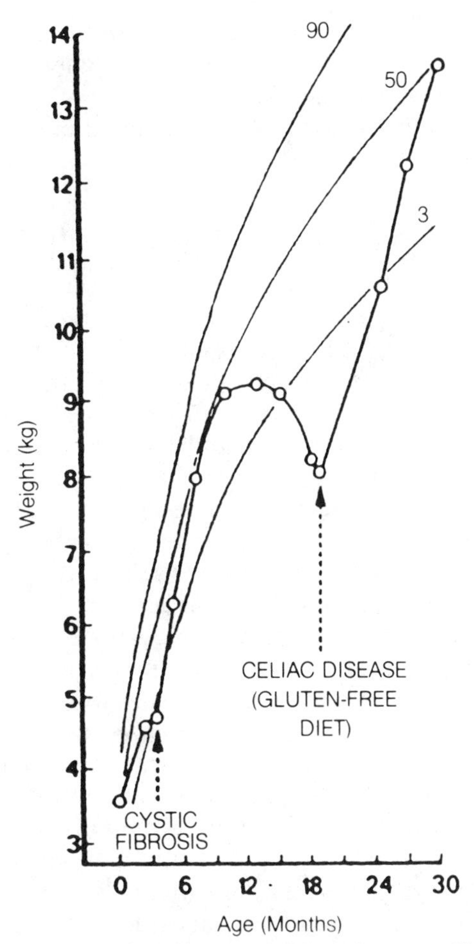

Figure 19–7. The growth pattern of a child with cystic fibrosis and celiac disease. This particular combination of diseases is infrequent but it serves to illustrate the point that weight gain and even weight loss will occur if appropriate digestion and absorption are not present.

From Kelly DG, Grand RJ. Growth failure in intestinal diarrhea. In Lifshitz F, ed. Clinical disorders in pediatric gastroenterology and nutrition. New York: Marcel Dekker, 1980: 349–370.

they have persistent fat malabsorption. These factors further interfere with the child's ability to consume adequate nutrition. Moreover, these patients usually ingest a diet with a relatively lower fat content (about 32 percent of the total energy) despite the presence of fat malabsorption (Lloyd-Still, Smith & Wessel 1989). This is of concern since it has been suggested that patients with CF need a fat intake of 40 percent of total energy intake to prevent burning off dietary essential fatty acids to meet energy needs (Pencharz 1983, Bell, Durie & Forstner 1984). In cystic fibrosis, MCT oil might be beneficial to minimize fat losses in the stool. Nutritional rehabilitation of these patients should also include consideration of other nutrients, as in other patients with malabsorption (see below).

Inadequate Intestinal Absorption

Celiac Disease. Celiac disease, or gluten-induced enteropathy, is a hereditary disorder that is considered the most common chronic intestinal disease causing malabsorption in children (Lebenthal & Branshi 1981). These patients usually have stools that are soft, pale, bulky, and offensive in odor. However, celiac disease is relatively rare in the United States, occurring in probably 1 of every 5000 children. In families who carry the trait for celiac disease, the incidence increases to as high as 5.5 percent.

In patients with celiac disease, the ingestion of products that contain wheat (gluten) causes atrophy of the villi of the small intestine (see Fig. 19–3). Childhood celiac disease usually manifests itself between 6 months and 1 year of age when gluten-containing cereals are first introduced (Young & Pringle 1971). The classic symptoms of this disorder include chronic diarrhea, steatorrhea, malnutrition, irritability, apathy, anemia, and anorexia (Lebenthal & Branshi 1981, Lifshitz & Fagundes-Neto 1983). Substantial muscle wasting and generalized muscle weakness may also occur in association with abdominal distention leading to the typical physical appearance of celiac disease. However, nearly one third of the children with celiac disease do not have diarrhea or steatorrhea at the time of presentation. In fact, the clinical presentation may be one of constipation and fecal impaction. Also, these children may have growth failure as their main clinical problem, and they have been considered to have occult celiac disease (Cacciari et al 1983).

The elimination of all gluten-containing foods, pharmaceutical products, and beverages from the diets of children with celiac disease results in complete remission of clinical symptoms in approximately 2 to 3 weeks (Lifshitz & Fagundes-Neto 1983). The child's appetite improves quickly, as does his or her disposition. The stools become less frequent, more well-formed, and less offensive and the patient exhibits catch-up growth.

Strict adherence to a gluten-free diet is essential for the child with celiac disease. Clinical and histologic improvements are a function of the extent to which gluten is restricted (Lifshitz & Fagundes-Neto 1983). Even small amounts of gluten, such as the amount found in one slice of bread (2–3 g of gluten), may thwart regrowth of the damaged villi in the intestine and cause adverse symptomatology. Also, the duration of nutritional therapy in a patient with diagnosed celiac disease should be life-long in order to manage its symptoms and to avoid potentially life-threatening complications (Young & Pringle 1971, McNish 1980, Lebenthal & Branshi 1981).

To eliminate gluten from the diet, wheat, oats, barley, and rye must be omitted. Families must be carefully instructed to read labels and identify processed foods that may contain hidden sources of gluten. For example, malt flavoring and wheat germ are known to contain gluten, whereas hydrolyzed vegetable protein and emulsifiers are items in which the manufacturer should be contacted for clarification of gluten content.

For the recently diagnosed, malnourished child with celiac disease, calories in excess of normal requirements should be provided, emphasizing protein-rich foods. Maldigestion of lactose and sucrose secondary to intestinal enzyme deficiencies is a problem frequently seen in newly diagnosed celiac patients (Lifshitz, Klotz & Holman 1965). However, after a few weeks of strict adherence to a gluten-free regime, lactose- and sucrose-containing foods can be reintroduced into the diet (Lebenthal & Branshi 1981). Initially, dietary fat should be limited to avoid continued steatorrhea (Broitman & Zamcheck 1980); medium-chain triglycerides (MCT) oil may be administered to supplement the child's caloric intake.

Since celiac disease primarily affects the absorptive capacity of the small intestine, there may be some deficiencies of specific nutrients that need to be treated. Anemia secondary to iron (McGuigan & Volwiler 1964), folate, and/or vitamin B_{12} (Broitman & Zamcheck 1980, Lebenthal & Branshi 1981) deficiencies may be present. There may be deficits of fat-soluble vitamins (A, D, E, and K) due to the underlying fat malabsorption present with untreated celiac disease, and there may be excess losses of calcium, magnesium, and electrolytes in the stool in patients with severe diarrhea and fat malabsorption. In all instances these deficiencies need to be corrected.

Overall, once the child is nutritionally rehabilitated and is receiving a gluten-free diet, future treatment relies solely in avoidance of gluten. Even though a gluten-free diet eliminates the four most frequently consumed grains and their products, it can still provide an adequate intake of all macronutrients and micronutrients if a variety of foods are selected (Moses 1988).

Carbohydrate Malabsorption. Carbohydrate malabsorption may lead to carbohydrate intolerance, a syndrome characterized by diarrhea with acid stools and carbohydrates in feces (Lifshitz 1980, 1982b). The mechanisms that induce diarrhea when there is carbohydrate malabsorption are complex, primarily resulting from the osmotic overload and the sugar fermentation of the unabsorbed carbohydrate (Lifshitz 1982a, 1985b, 1988). The elimination of the offending carbohydrate from the diet results in prompt improvement.

Primary Ontogenetic Lactase Deficiency (Hereditary). Most human beings are not able to digest and tolerate lactose-containing foods such as milk after childhood (Kretchmer 1972, Lifshitz 1985a) due to the disappearance as the person gets older of the intestinal enzyme lactase necessary to digest milk sugar. The persistence of lactase activity into adulthood is the exception, which occurs in a minority of the world's population as an adaptive human evolutionary trait of certain ethnic or racial groups (Fig. 19–8). Those few groups of people are thought to be descendants of populations who had been exposed to milk products from domesticated animals from prehistoric times (Simmon 1981).

There may be some advantages to having lactase deficiency. It may be a defense mechanism against enteric infections. It has been postulated that rotavirus, a deadly virus that induces diarrhea, infects only gut epithelium rich in lactase activity (Lifshitz 1982b). Thus, individuals with high intestinal lactase levels may be more susceptible to rotavirus. In contrast, the genetic mutation that induces intestinal lactase production throughout life offers people the advantage of being able to digest lactose and therefore being able to consume milk and enjoy the benefits of a rich source of protein and calcium.

In individuals with ontogenetic lactase deficiency, lactose malabsorption is usually a clinically insignificant problem since these people may drink moderate amounts of milk (1 or 2 glasses per day) without symptoms. It has been considered inappropriate to discourage milk consumption among individuals with primary ontogenetic lactase deficiency solely because of fear of mild intolerance to milk due to lactose malabsorption (Stephenson & Latham

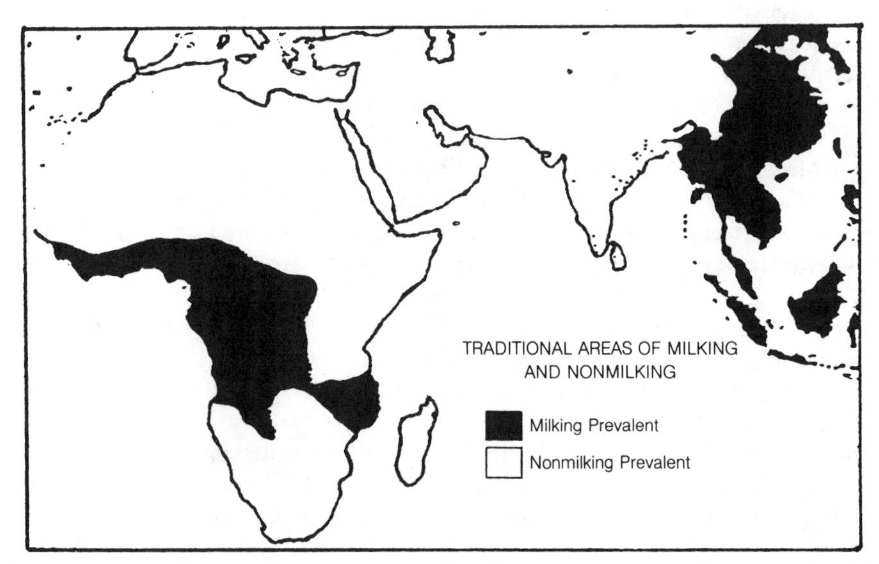

Figure 19–8. The traditional areas of milking and nonmilking in the Old World. The areas of nonmilking habits are also the areas where lactase deficiency and lactose malabsorption are prevalent.

From Simoons FJ. Primary adult lactose intolerance and the milking habit: A problem in biological and cultural interrelations. I. Review of the medical research. AM J Dig Dis 1969; 14:819.

1974). Indeed, most children with ontogenetic lactose malabsorption experience no adverse effects and derive nutritional benefits from moderate milk consumption. This is of importance in locations where inappropriate nutrition is prevalent or when institutional programs provide milk to supplement the diets (e.g., in school lunches).

Lactase deficiency leading to lactose malabsorption is also a normal evolutionary trait in the newborn period, particularly in premature infants. In such babies, good clinical tolerance to lactose-containing formula is usually observed. The amount of lactose in a standard 7.1 percent lactose-containing milk formula, or breast milk, is relatively small. Even if only 22 to 38 percent of the ingested lactose load would be absorbed, such milk feedings are tolerated and these babies gain weight (McLean & Fink 1981). The rapid postnatal rise in lactase activity in the intestine and the scavenger role of colonic bacteria may increase milk tolerance in premature babies. However, the presence of carbohydrate malabsorption may at times trigger metabolic acidosis in such infants (Lifshitz et al 1971b).

Congenital Carbohydrate Malabsorption Syndromes. Carbohydrate intolerance starting soon after birth may occur as a consequence of congenital carbohydrate malabsorption syndromes. This type of carbohydrate malabsorption is seen in patients with rare congenital alterations that involve a single type of carbohydrate, such as lactase deficiency, isomaltase deficiency, or other intolerances (Lifshitz 1985a). Although these are relatively rare disorders, they have an important role in carbohydrate intolerance that may persist for the life of the patient.

In the primary or congenital forms of carbohydrate malabsorption, a prolonged adherence to the dietary regimen is necessary. The offending carbohydrate should be sufficiently restricted from the diet to keep the patient symptom-free and growing at a normal rate. In all instances of congenital intestinal enzyme deficiencies, a gradually increased tolerance of the specific carbohydrate may be observed. The patients may eventually tolerate ordinary diets, but with certain limitations throughout life in regard to their specific intolerance.

Acquired Carbohydrate Malabsorption. Acquired carbohydrate intolerance may occur as a consequence of intestinal damage that results in enzyme deficiencies, or of cellular transport alterations induced by many diseases (Lifshitz 1980, 1982b). Secondary lactase deficiency with lactose intolerance is the most frequent clinical alteration complicating many diseases (Lifshitz 1982b), including infectious diarrhea, celiac disease, surgery, inflammatory processes such as blind loop syndrome, or giardiasis. Systemic alterations may also result in lactase deficiency through a variety of mechanisms, such as primary protein-energy malnutrition, iron deficiency, hypoxia, drugs (birth-control pills), cow's milk and other food allergies, and immunodeficiency disorders (see Fig. 19–2).

There are two clinical conditions that are associated with acquired lactase deficiency even when no alterations in intestinal morphology are demonstrated—alcoholism and osteoporosis (Newcomer et al 1968, Perlow, Baraona & Lieber 1977). Chronic alcoholics, even without malnutrition, have been found to be lactase-deficient; within 2 weeks of abstinence intestinal lactase activity resumes. Also, there is a strong relationship between osteoporosis and lactase deficiency in women. After ethnic backgrounds are matched, lactase deficiency has been found in 26 percent of osteoporotic women, whereas only 3 percent of those with normal bone appearance are lactase-deficient.

The goal of therapy of a patient with acquired carbohydrate malabsorption is to treat the disease that induces the intolerance to dietary sugars. It is also necessary to eliminate all untolerated carbohydrates. However, the capacity to tolerate dietary sugars rapidly recovers; thus, these dietary restrictions are not necessarily permanent. After the diarrhea improves, these patients may begin to tolerate an increased number of carbohydrates, but lactase is usually the last one to recover (Lifshitz 1982b). Eventually even lactose can be tolerated by patients with acquired intolerances once the primary illness is improved.

CONSTIPATION

In infancy and childhood a complaint of constipation normally follows an observation by the parents that the child is having difficulty passing stools and appears to be in pain. Usually there is a decrease in the frequency of stool and a hardening of its consistency. Often constipation is bothersome but clinically insignificant. However, if constipation is associated with poor weight gain, refusal to eat, or vomiting, appropriate investigation is necessary.

The feeding history is an important component of the initial assessment of a child with constipation. Breast-fed infants normally have soft, easy-to-pass stools. Weaning an infant from breast milk to formula frequently coincides with the onset of constipation. A change in bowel habits may not in itself be an abnormality, and an increase in the total water intake may be all that is necessary to resolve the constipation.

For constipated children, dietary fiber needs to be given in sufficient quantities to induce a stool consistency that is easy to pass. A list of the fiber contents of cereals, breads, crackers, fruits, and vegetables in child-size portions is a helpful tool for parents (Table 19–3). This list should include a written reminder that an adequate fluid intake is essential when extra fiber is given. Children usually accept natural food sources more readily than special products (e.g., raisin bran muffins, fresh fruit, high-pulp juices, whole grain crackers).

Sometimes when a stool is hard to pass children will try to hold it back,

Table 19–3. Dietary Fiber Content of Foods.

FOOD	AMOUNT	FIBER (g)
Breads/cereals		
White rice	1/3 cup	0.5
Whole wheat bread	1 slice	1.3
Whole wheat crackers	6	2.2
Oatmeal	3/4 pkg	2.5
Corn flakes	3/4 cup	2.6
Bran chex	3/4 cup	6.2
Fruits		
Grapes, white	10	0.5
Raisins	1/2 tablespoon	1.0
Banana	1/2 medium	1.5
Apple	1/2 large	2.0
Prunes, dried	2	2.4
Strawberries	1 cup	3.1
Blackberries	3/4 cup	6.7
Meat, milk, eggs	—	0
Vegetables		
Spinach, raw	1 cup	0.2
Cucumber	1/2 cup	1.1
Sweet potatoes, baked	1/2 medium	2.1
Green beans	1/2 cup	2.1
Carrots	1/2 cup	2.4
Broccoli	1/2 cup	3.5

Adapted from Anderson JW. Plant fiber in foods. University of Kentucky Medical Center, 1980.

and constipation can result. The stool becomes impacted, and as it collects, the colon expands to accommodate the mass. With expansion, the colon loses its normal sensitivity to the stimulation that leads to expulsion of contents, and the condition worsens. The child becomes uncomfortable, appetite decreases, and weight gain may slow. Encopresis or fecal soiling may result from chronic constipation.

The first course of therapy for constipated children normally includes cleaning the colon to remove the impacted stool. This can be done with an enema or a cathartic, and is followed by oral mineral-oil therapy. Mineral oil acts as a nonabsorbable lubricant to ease the passage of stool.

Orally administered mineral oil has been associated in the past with interference of the absorption of fat-soluble vitamins but recent investigations did not find an effect on the level of fat-soluble vitamins. However, to ensure good overall vitamin status an appropriate diet should be ingested (see Chapter 9) and if this is not possible multivitamins may be given at some time other than when the mineral oil is given.

The dose of mineral oil is 1 to 5 milliliters per kilogram per day, given in two doses. For example, a child weighing 20 kilograms would receive 1½ tablespoons of mineral oil in the morning and at bedtime. Getting the child to accept mineral oil doses often requires special expertise on the part of the dietitian. There are flavored products that may be more acceptable to some children. If these are not accepted, the dietitian can suggest offering the oil blended with a strong flavored juice (e.g., orange juice, apricot nectar). Mineral oil also can be disguised by mixing it into a fatty food, such as ice cream, for the bedtime dose.

CLINICAL INTERVENTION

In children with diarrhea oral hydration solutions are most important and must be given as soon as liquid stools begin (Fig. 19–9). The diet for children with gastrointestinal disorders should be selected after the specific diagnosis has been established. In all instances an adequate amount of calories to allow normal weight gain and catch-up growth should be provided. In patients with diarrhea and other gastrointestinal disorders emphasis should be given to treating the patient rather than the stools. Increasing stool losses might be associated with an increased food intake, but the increased proportion of nutrients being absorbed might be sufficient to improve the nutritional status of the patient. In well-nourished children most diarrheal syndromes are more a nuisance than a serious illness, and require only relief from cramps and diarrhea. Drugs that may be of help include Lomotil (dysherolylate) and Imodium (loperamide). However, these should not be used if symptoms continue for more than a few days. For those who are sicker and/or have specific infections, the physician may prescribe antibiotics.

Regarding intestinal malabsorption problems, an increasing body of evidence suggests that medium-chain triglycerides as the predominant source of dietary fat is beneficial. Supplemental MCT preparations should be considered for patients with severe malabsorption and malnutrition. The rationale for the use of this agent is that MCTs are easily hydrolyzed even with limited amounts of conjugated bile salts or pancreatic enzymes. In addition, medium-chain fatty acids are more readily taken up by the mucosal cells and are transported into the portal vein. MCTs are available as an oil or as a powder that can be added to food (see Chapter 27). However, MCTs may have side effects, including acidosis and/or high blood levels of medium-chain fatty acids, specifically in patients with impaired hepatic function. Additionally, MCT therapy can induce diabetic ketoacidosis in susceptible individuals and may induce gastrointestinal symptoms and diarrhea.

For patients with celiac disease who require a gluten-free diet, details of the gluten content of foodstuffs in specific tables and cookbooks should be consulted (Moses 1988). In general, any food containing wheat, wheat flour, rye, barley, or malt should be eliminated from the diet. Careful efforts should be made to avoid foods that frequently contain concealed "gluten," includ-

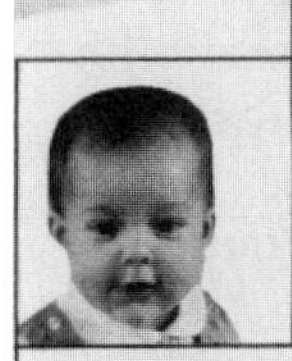

Diarrhea can be dangerous. It drains water and salts from your child. If these are not put back quickly, your child can get dehydrated and may need to be hospitalized. To protect your child follow these steps:

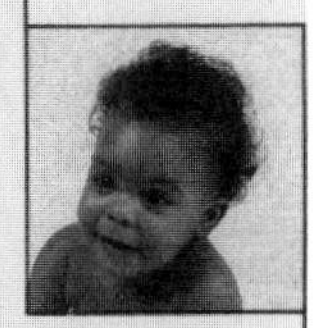

MANAGING DIARRHEA

1. As soon as diarrhea starts, give your child fluids. An oral electrolyte solution is the best fluid to give. This will put the water and salts back into your child's body that are lost with diarrhea.

- You can get these solutions at grocery and drug stores.
- If under 2 years old give ½ cup every hour using a small spoon. Call your doctor or public health clinic.
- If over 2 years old give ½ to 1 cup every hour.
- Keep giving the oral electrolyte solution until the diarrhea stops.
- If your child vomits, continue to give the oral electrolyte solution, using a teaspoon. Give one teaspoon every 2—3 minutes until vomiting stops. Then give regular amount.
- Do not give sugary drinks such as Gatorade, cola drinks or apple juice. They can make your child's diarrhea worse.

NO

Sports Drink · Apple Juice · Soda

These have the WRONG amounts of water, salts and sugar.

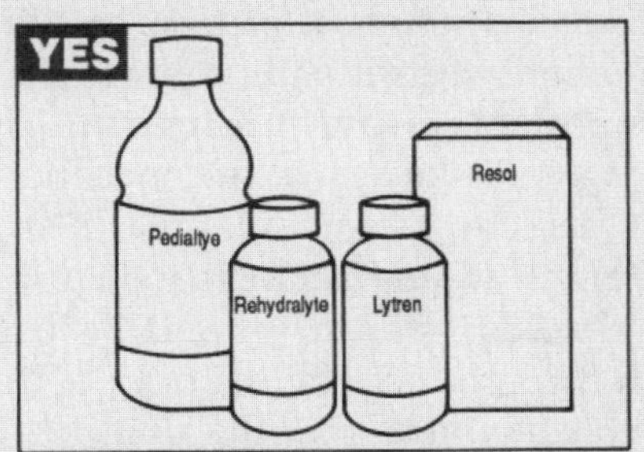

Oral electrolyte solutions have the RIGHT amounts of water, salts and sugar.

2. Continue to feed your child as recommended by your doctor or public health clinic. Food will help your child stay healthy.

- If breast-fed continue to breast feed.
- If on formula continue to give formula.
- If on solid foods continue to give regular diet. Good foods to give include cooked meat, cooked cereal or bananas.

DANGER SIGNS OF DIARRHEA

Your child may need medical help if the diarrhea is more serious than usual. You should call your doctor or public health clinic immediately if:

the diarrhea lasts more than 24 hours,
the diarrhea gets worse,
there are any signs of dehydration:
decreased urination
sunken eyes
no tears when child cries
extreme thirst
unusual drowsiness or fussiness

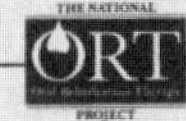

(202) 625-2570

Figure 19–9.
From American Academy of Pediatrics (AAP).

ing meatloaf, canned meat dishes, frankfurters, cold cuts, beer and ale, commercial salad dressings, some commercial ice creams, food prepared with bread, and cracker crumbs. Allowed foods, including rice, soy, potatoes, and cornmeal flour, may be used as "breading" or in stuffing or gravies. Additional information on celiac disease and gluten-free products can be obtained from:

American Celiac Society, Inc.
45 Gifford Avenue
Jersey City, NJ 07304

National Celiac Sprue Society
5 Jeffrey Road
Wayland, MA 01778

The sources of carbohydrates in foods should be considered when there is carbohydrate malabsorption (Weyman-Daum 1988). The common carbohydrates in fruits are fructose, glucose, sucrose, and starch; in vegetables and mature dry legumes, sucrose and starch; in cereal and cereal products, starch and small amounts of sucrose; and in spices and condiments, starch. Syrups and other sweets usually contain glucose, maltose, and polysaccharide dextrins. Honey contains fructose and glucose. Milk and milk products are the major sources of lactose in concentrations varying from 5.8 percent in yogurt to 7 percent in human milk. For individuals who are highly lactose-intolerant, adding lactase to milk prior to ingestion is recommended. Lactase, marketed as Lact-Aid, is available in a liquid form or as tablets to add to milk. With this product, the majority of the lactose is digested and most patients can tolerate milk, deriving all its benefits.

The diagnosis of gastrointestinal disorders occasionally requires a therapeutic trial of nutritional rehabilitation. For example, clinical and biochemical response to a gluten-free diet would help make the diagnosis of celiac disease. Without improvement of the underlying malnutrition and the secondary digestive and absorptive alterations of gastrointestinal diseases, the diagnosis may not be clear. However, the response to therapy should never substitute for a diagnostic work-up.

Patients with gastrointestinal disorders may also require specific replacement therapy to correct the associated vitamin and mineral deficiencies. The possibility of vitamins A, B, E, D, and K deficiencies should be considered. Vitamin B_{12} and folic acid deficits may also be present, and severe potassium and magnesium deficiency may be encountered. Iron deficiency and anemia are also frequent. The treatment of specific deficiencies is shown in Table 19–4.

The intestinal tract is not floating free in outer space; disturbances in other

Table 19–4. Vitamin and Mineral Replacement for Children with Malabsorption Syndromes.

Vitamin A

Water-soluble preparation for fat malabsorption: 10,000 to 20,000 units for daily maintenance, >100,000 units for severe deficiencies.

Vitamin B_6 (Pyridoxine)

Initial dose 2.5 mg/d; if convulsion of unknown cause occurs, give 5 to 10 mg/d.

Vitamin B_{12}

Intramuscular injection must be given; initial dose of 1000 μg followed by 100 to 200 μg given every 1 to 2 months; for the treatment of pernicious anemia, dose may vary from 1000 to 5000 μg depending on condition.

Folic Acid

Initial dose of 10 to 20 mg daily for 7 days to treat anemia, 5 to 10 mg for daily maintenance; if there is diarrhea or inability to take supplement by mouth, parenteral administration of 1 mg/d for 4 to 5 days is needed.

Vitamin K

Water-soluble preparation for fat malabsorption: 2 to 5 mg for daily maintenance.

Vitamin E

Water-soluble preparation for fat malabsorption: 25 to 50 IU for infants; 100 to 200 IU for children.

Vitamin D

For daily maintenance, 400 to 800 IU; may be mixed with MCT oil to improve absorption; water-soluble form available.

Calcium

1. Calcium chloride (27% elemental calcium): 1 to 2 g/d for infants; 2 to 4 g/d for children, not to exceed 5% concentration when given in milk.
2. Calcium lactate (0.3% elemental calcium): 0.5 g/kg/d to be given in divided doses.
3. Calcium gluconate (9% elemental calcium): 3 to 6 g/d for infants; 6 to 10 g/d for children to be given in divided doses not exceeding 10% concentration in solution.

Iron

Oral ferrous sulfate

Iron dextran parenteral preparations given when malabsorption dictates oral nutrient supplementation; dose: wt (kg) $\times$ (13.5 $-$ Hgb (g%)) $\times$ 2.5 = mg of elemental iron needed to be given in divided doses.

Magnesium

For treatment of hypomagnesemia, magnesium can be given parenterally, either intravenously or intramuscularly, 3 mEq/kg/d, not to exceed 60 mEq/d.

1. Magnesium sulfate: 50% solution provides 4 mEq/mL
2. Magnesium chloride: 4 g provides 40 mEq
3. Magnesium citrate: 6 g provides 40 mEq

Oral dose: 2 to 3 mEq/kg/d; dose should be increased gradually to avoid diarrhea.

organ systems have intestinal repercussions, and diarrhea and gastrointestinal disorders may affect other parts of the body. Even the benign belching and burping, or feeling bloated and distended, are troublesome, and passing gas can be embarrassing. The food one eats has a bearing on the welfare of the patient and the symptoms of the gastrointestinal disease.

REFERENCES

Barness LA, ed. Pediatric nutrition handbook. Evanston, IL: American Academy of Pediatrics, 1979.

Beisel WR. Metabolic effects of infection. Progr Food Nutr Sci 1983; 8:43–75.

Bell L, Durie P, Forstner GG. What do children with cystic fibrosis eat? J Pediatr Gastroenterol Nutr 1984; 3(Suppl):137–146.

Belli DC, Seldman E, Bouthillier L, et al. Chronic intermittent elemental diet improves growth failure in children with Crohn's diseases. Gastroenterology 1988; 94:603–610.

Brodribb AJM, Humphreys DM. Diverticular disease: three studies. Part I— Relation to other disorders and fiber intake. Part II—Treatment with bran. Part III—Metabolic effect of bran in patients with diverticular disease. Br Med J 1976; 1:424–430.

Broitman SA, Zamcheck N. Nutrition in diseases of the gastrointestinal tract. B. Nutrition in diseases of the intestine. In Goodhart RS, Shils ME, eds. Modern nutrition in health and disease. 6th ed. Philadelphia: Lea & Febiger, 1980; 332–340.

Cacciari E, Salardi S, Lazzari R, et al. Short stature and celiac: A relationship to consider even in patients with no gastrointestinal tract symptoms. J Pediatr 1983; 103:708–711.

Chase HP, Long MA, Lavin MH. Cystic fibrosis and malnutrition. J Pediatr 1979; 95:337–347.

Coello-Ramirez P, Gutierrez-Topete G, Lifshitz F. Pneumatosis intestinalis. Am J Dis Child 1970; 120:3–9.

Cohen SA. Chronic nonspecific diarrhea. Dietary relationship. Pediatrics 1979; 64:402–407.

Dallman PR. Manifestations of iron deficiency. Semin Hematol 1982; 19:19–30.

Daum F. Pediatric inflammatory bowel disease. In Silverberg M, Daum F, eds. Textbook of pediatric gastroenterology. 2nd ed. Chicago: Year Book, 1988: 392–418.

Editorial. Supplementary nutrition in cystic fibrosis. Lancet 1986; 1:249–251.

Editorial. What has happened to carbohydrate intolerance following gastroenteritis? Lancet 1987; 1:23–24.

Fagundes-Neto U, Viaro T, Lifshitz F. Glucose polymer intolerance in infants with diarrhea and disaccharide intolerance. Am J Clin Nutr 1985; 41:228–234.

Gaskin K, Gurwitz D, Durie P, Corey M, Levison H, Forstner G. Improved respiratory prognosis in patients with cystic fibrosis with normal fat absorption. J Pediatr 1982; 100:857–862.

Gerson WT, Swan P, Walker WA. Nutrition support in cystic fibrosis. Nutr Rev 1987; 45:353–360.

Graham GG, et al. Lactose-free medium-chain triglyceride formulas in severe malnutrition. Am J Dis Child 1973; 126:330–335.

Green H, et al. Protracted diarrhea and malnutrition in infancy: Changes in intestinal morphology and disaccharidase activities during treatment with total intravenous nutrition or oral elemental diets. J Pediatr 1975; 87:695–704.

Greene HL, Ghishan FK. Excessive fluid intake as a cause of chronic diarrhea in young children. J Pediatr 1983; 102:836–840.

Guerrant RL, Kirchhoff LV, Shields DS, Natious MK, Leslie J, deSeusa JG. Prospective study of diarrheal illness in northeastern Brazil: Patterns of disease, nutritional impact, etiologies and risk factors. J Infect Dis 1983; 148:986–997.

Hirschhorn N. The treatment of acute diarrhea in children: A historical and physiological perspective. Am J Clin Nutr 1980; 33:637–663.

Hodge C, Lebenthal E, Lee PC, Topper W. Amylase in the saliva and in the gastric aspirates of premature infants: Its potential role in glucose polymer hydrolysis. Pediatr Res 1983; 17:998–1001.

Hubbard VS, Mangrum PJ. Energy intake and nutrition counseling in cystic fibrosis. J Am Diet Assoc 1982; 80:127–131.

Hyams JS, Leichtner AM. Apple juice. An unappreciated cause of chronic diarrhea. Am J Dis Child 1985; 139:503–505.

Kanof ME, Lake AM, Bayless TM. Decreased height velocity in children and adolescents before diagnosis of Crohn's disease. Gastroenterology 1988; 95:1523–1527.

Kessler J, Lebenthal E. The exocrine pancreas. In Silverberg M, Daum F, eds. Textbook of pediatric gastroenterology. Chicago: Year Book, 1988: 362–391.

Kirschner BS. Nutritional consequences of inflammatory bowel disease on growth. J Am Coll Nutr 1988; 7:301–308.

Kraemer R, Rudeberg A, Hadorn B, Rossi E. Relative underweight in cystic fibrosis and its prognostic value. Acta Paediatr Scand 1978; 67:33–37.

Kretchmer N. Lactose and lactase. Sci Am 1972; 227:70–78.

Kumar V, et al. Carbohydrate intolerance associated with acute gastroenteritis. Clin Pediatr 1977; 16:1123–1127.

La Sala MA, Lifshitz F, Silverberg M, Wapnir RA, Carrera D. Magnesium metabolism studies in children with inflammatory disease of the bowel. J Pediatr Gastroenterol Nutr 1985; 4:75–81.

Lebenthal E, Branshi D. Childhood celiac disease—A reappraisal. J Pediatr 1981; 98(5):681–690.

Lifshitz F. Carbohydrate intolerance as a result of inborn errors of carbohydrate absorption. In Wapnir RA, ed. Congenital metabolic diseases. New York: Marcel Dekker: 1985a: 347–351.

Lifshitz F. Interrelationship of diarrhea and infant nutrition. In Lebenthal E, ed. Textbook of gastroenterology and nutrition in infancy. 2nd ed. New York: Raven Press, 1989:657–664.

Lifshitz F. Necrotizing enterocolitis and feedings. In Lifshitz F, ed. Clinical disorders in pediatric nutrition. New York: Marcel Dekker, 1982a:513–530.

Lifshitz F. Nutrition for special needs in infancy. In Nutrition for special needs in infancy. New York: Marcel Dekker, 1985b:1–10.

Lifshitz F. Secondary carbohydrate intolerance in infancy. In Lifshitz F, ed. Clinical disorders in pediatric gastroenterology and nutrition. New York: Marcel Dekker, 1980:327–340.

Lifshitz F, ed. Carbohydrate intolerance in infancy. New York: Marcel Dekker, 1982b.

Lifshitz F, Coello-Ramirez P, Gutierrez-Topete G. Monosaccharide intolerance and hypoglycemia in infants with diarrhea. I. Clinical course of 23 infants. J Pediatr 1970; 77:595–603.

Lifshitz F, Coello-Ramirez P, Gutierrez-Topete G, Cornado-Cornet MC. Carbohydrate intolerance in infants with diarrhea. J Pediatr 1971a; 79:760–767.

Lifshitz F, da Costa Ribeiro H. Diarrheal diseases. In Paige DM, ed. Clinical nutrition. 2nd ed. St. Louis: C.V. Mosby, 1988:447–462.

Lifshitz F, da Costa Ribeiro H, Silverberg M. Childhood infectious diarrhea. In Silverberg M, Daum F, eds. Textbook of pediatric gastroenterology. 2nd ed. New York: Year Book, 1988:284–329.

Lifshitz F, Diaz-Breussen S, Martinez Gorza V, Abdo Bassals F, Diaz DelCastillo E. The influence of disaccharides on the development of systemic acidosis in the premature infant. Pediatr Res 1971b; 5:213–225.

Lifshitz F, Fagundes-Neto U, Castro-Ferreira V, et al. The response to dietary treatment of patients with chronic postinfectious diarrhea and lactose intolerance. Am J Coll Nutr 1990; 9:1–10.

Lifshitz F, Fagundes-Neto U. The malabsorption syndrome. In Silverberg M, ed. Advanced textbook of pediatric gastroenterology. New Hyde Park, NY: Medical Examination, 1983; 314–320.

Lifshitz F, Klotz A, Holman GH. Intestinal disaccharidase deficiencies in gluten sensitive enteropathy. Am J Dis Child 1965; 10:47–57.

Lifshitz F, Nishi Y. Mineral deficiencies during growth. In Anast C, DeLuca H, eds. Pediatric diseases related to calcium. New York: Elsevier North-Holland, 1980:305–321.

Lifshitz F, Fagundes Neto U, Garcia Olivo CA, Cordano A, Friedman S. Refeeding of infants with acute diarrheal disease. J Pediat (in press).

Lifshitz F, Fagundes Neto U, Castro Ferreira V, Cordano A, da Costa Ribeiro H. The response to dietary treatment of patients with chronic post infectious diarrhea and lactose intolerance. J Am Coll Nutr 1990; 9:231–240.

Lloyd-Still JD, Smith AE, Wessel HU. Fat intake is low in cystic fibrosis despite unrestricted dietary practices. JPEN 1989; 13:296–298.

MacLean WC, et al. Nutritional management of chronic diarrhea and malnutrition: Primary reliance on oral feeding. J Pediatr 1980; 97:316–322.

Mansell AL, Andersen JC, Muttart CR, et al. Short-term pulmonary effects of total parenteral nutrition in children with cystic fibrosis. J Pediatr 1984; 104:700–705.

Mason JO. Enteric disease and health for all: A public health perspective. Pediatr Infect Dis 1986; 5:57–60.

McGuigan JE, Volwiler W. Celiac sprue: Malabsorption of iron in the absence of steatorrhea. Gastroenterology 1964; 47:635–641.

McLean WC Jr, Fink BB. Lactose digestion by premature infants: Hydrogen breath test results versus estimates of energy loss. In Paige DM, Paige TM, eds. Lactose digestion: Clinical and nutritional implications. Baltimore, MD:

Johns Hopkins University Press, 1981:203–213.
McNish AS. Coeliac disease: Duration of gluten-free diet. Arch Dis Child 1980; 55:110–111.
Motil KJ, Grand RJ, Maletskos CJ, Young VR. The effect of disease, drug and diet on whole body protein metabolism in adolescents with Crohn's disease and growth failure. J Pediatr 1982; 101:345–351.
Moses NS. Gluten-free diets. In Chiaramonte LT, Schneider AT, Lifshitz F, eds. Food allergy. A practical approach to diagnoses and management. New York: Marcel Dekker, 1988:421–433.
Newcomer AD, Hodgson SF, McGill DB, Thomas PJ. Lactase deficiency: Prevalence in osteoporosis. Ann Intern Med 1968; 89:218–220.
Nishi Y, Lifshitz F, Bayne MA, Daum F, Silverberg M, Aiges H. Zinc status and its relation to growth retardation in children with chronic inflammatory bowel disease. Am J Clin Nutr 1980; 33:2613–2621.
Okuni M, et al. Studies on reducing sugars in stools of acute infantile diarrhea, with special reference to differences between breast fed and artificially fed babies. Tohoku J Exp Med 1972; 107:395–402.
Pencharz PB. Energy intakes and low fat diets in children with cystic fibrosis. J Pediatr Gastroenterol Nutr 1983; 2:400–402.
Pergolizzi R, Lifshitz F, Teichberg S, Wapnir RA. Interaction between dietary carbohydrates and intestinal disaccharidase in experimental diarrhea. Am J Clin Nutr 1977; 30:482–489.
Perlow W, Baraona L, Lieber CS. Symptomatic intestinal disaccharidase deficiency in alcoholics. Gastroenterology 1977; 72:680–684.
Scott RB, O'Loughlin EV, Gall DG. Gastroesophageal reflux in patients with cystic fibrosis. J Pediatr 1985; 106:223–227.
Simmon FJ. Geographic patterns of primary adult lactose malabsorption: A further interpretation of evidence for the Old World. In Paige DM, Bayless TM, eds. Lactose digestion—Clinical and nutritional implications. Baltimore, MD: Johns Hopkins University Press, 1981:23–48.
Stephenson LS. Nutritional and economic implications of soil-transmitted helminths with special reference to ascariasis. In Lifshitz F, ed. Clinical disorders in pediatric gastroenterology and nutrition. New York: Marcel Dekker, 1980:391–409.
Stephenson LS, Latham MC. Lactose intolerance and milk consumption: The relation of tolerance to symptoms. Am J Clin Nutr 1974; 27:296–303.
Stumiolo GC, Molokhia MM, Shields R, Turnberg LA. Zinc absorption in Crohn's disease. Gut 1980; 21:387–391.
Synder JP, Merson MN. The magnitude of the global problem of acute diarrheal disease: A review of surveillance data. Bull WHO 1982; 60:605.
Walsh JA, Warren RS. Selective primary health care: An interim strategy for disease control in developing countries. N Engl J Med 1979; 301:967–974.
Whittington PF, Barnes V, Bayless TM. Medical management of Crohn's disease in adolescence. Gastroenterology 1977; 72:1338–1344.
Wittner M. Protozoan diarrheas: Dientamoebiasis and Giardiasis. In Lifshitz F, ed. Clinical disorders in pediatric gastroenterology and nutrition. New York: Marcel Dekker, 1980:315–323.
Wittner M, Turner JW, Jacquette G, Ash LR, Salgo MP, Tanowitz HB.

Eustrongylidiasis—A parasitic infection acquired by eating sushi. N Engl J Med 1989; 320:1124–1143.
World Health Organization. Control of diarrheal diseases. A manual for the treatment of acute diarrhea. Geneva: World Health Organization, 1984, Rev. 1.
Young W, Pringle EM. 110 children with coeliac disease, 1950–1969. Arch Dis Child 1971; 46:421–436.
Weyman-Daum M. Milk-free, lactose-free, and lactose-restricted diets. In Chiaramonte LT, Schneider AT, Lifshitz F, eds. Food allergy. New York: Marcel Dekker, 1988:401–420.

20

Food Allergies and Intolerances

Allison, a 3-year-old girl, and Sara, her 1-month-old sister, were sent to the pediatric nutrition specialist because of severe "food intolerances." Allison had a life-long history of intolerance to most foods. At birth, when started on a regular cow's milk–based infant formula, she had persistent "cramps" and was therefore switched to soy formula at 1½ weeks of age, without improvement. Only diluted infant formula was "somewhat tolerated" until 10 months of age. Solid foods were introduced around 3½ months, but Allison was "allergic" to most foods. Only natural yogurt, small amounts of butter, green beans, and onions "could be tolerated." When Allison's sister Sara was born, the mother started her on a "hypoallergenic formula" as a "precautionary measure." However, Sara's mother insisted that even with this formula, Sara was developing "allergic symptoms" similar to her sister's problem, and she refused to introduce any new foods into her diet. As a consequence of the restrictive nature of the children's diets, they both failed to thrive.

"What food is to one, to others is bitter poison" (Titus Lucretius Carus 55 BC). The terms "food allergies" and "intolerances" refer to a wide variety of disorders. These, along with the terms "adverse reaction" or "sensitivity to food," are generally used to describe any abnormal physiologic response to an ingested food. Food allergies or intolerances vary in the mechanisms that lead to the adverse reaction and therefore should be clearly identified. True food allergy or hypersensitivity is an immunologically mediated reaction. A food allergy is usually caused by the body's immune system reacting to certain foods, food additives, or food contaminants (allergens). When the child is exposed to an allergen the patient identifies the "invasion" by producing antibodies that elicit the allergic response. Such immunologically mediated reactions may produce a variety of clinical problems (Iyngkaran & Abdin 1982). For example, wheat sensitivity may produce celiac disease in some patients (see Chapter 19), but only nonspecific symptoms of food allergy in other children. To complicate matters further, food allergy may induce a very acute dangerous reaction (anaphylaxis) only under special conditions. For example, the ingestion of food antigen may trigger a reaction during exercise, whereas no problem results when the same food is ingested at other times (Buchbinder et al 1983).

Food intolerance is a reaction that occurs in the absence of classic allergic phenomena. In other words, there is no immunologically mediated reaction leading to the abnormal response to a food or food product. Food intolerance may result as a consequence of many different mechanisms and types of reactions.

The so-called anaphylactoid reactions occur when large quantities of histamine are consumed, as in poisoned scombroid fish (tuna or mackerel), mahi-mahi, or Swiss cheese. Food intolerance occurs with the ingestion of food poisons or other products contained in unsafe forms of food. Death may follow ingestion of toxic mushrooms, solanine poisoning can result from the ingestion of green potatoes, excess gas and abdominal discomfort may occur following meals of insufficiently cooked beans, and vitamin A intoxication has been reported from the ingestion of large amounts of chicken liver.

There are many natural pharmacologic agents that may contaminate foods and are capable of inducing food intolerances. For example, vasoactive amines, which are often found in contaminated cheese (tyramine) or chocolate (phenylethylamine), may provoke a variety of problems, yet these foods are safe when they are not contaminated by the toxic agents.

Specific inborn errors of metabolism may also lead to adverse reactions to food (see Chapter 25). These are caused by the ingestion of ordinarily safe foods by individuals who are unable to metabolize specific ingredients or components of the food. For example, many people cannot digest milk sugar (lactose) and therefore they cannot tolerate milk. Lactose intolerance occurs as a normal event in the majority of the healthy world population owing to a high prevalence of genetic lactase deficiency (see Chapter 19). It may also occur in sick individuals with infectious diarrhea due to transient deficiency of the intestinal enzyme lactase (see Chapter 19). In other instances, food intolerances may occur as a result of medications. For example, patients taking monoamine oxidase (MAO) inhibitors for psychologic depression cannot tolerate aged cheeses and certain wines (e.g., Chianti) because of their tyramine content.

Psychologic causes have also been implicated in food intolerances. The reverse is also true; that is, food intolerances have been thought to lead to psychologic problems. Patients seen in allergy clinics with suspected food allergies and/or food intolerances demonstrate a high occurrence of neurotic depression and other neuroses. They also present with personality disorders and may not reproduce their symptoms of food intolerance when tested blindly (Pearson & Keith 1983). Thus, psychogenic reactions commonly are expressed as food intolerances in the general population.

COMMON FOOD ALLERGIES

Approximately 140 foods have been shown to cause immediate allergic reactions in humans (Atkins 1983). The presence or absence of allergy depends on the genetic immune response of the patient (Fig. 20–1). Also, several outside factors may determine whether or not a food will be allergenic, including the way the food was prepared, processed, or stored and the circumstances of ingestion. The methods of processing affect the molecular configuration of the potential allergen and hence its allergenicity. For example, heating cow's milk transforms some of its proteins, thereby lowering its allergenicity (Bahna & Gandhi 1983). The tolerance of some patients to fish, fruit, and vegetables may be improved by cooking or freezing (Hannuksela & Lahti 1977). However, cooking alone is often ineffective in reducing the allergenic activity of food because most major allergens tend to be heat-stable.

Foods from the same biologic family, like the citrus fruits, may contain similar antigens (Table 20–1). Therefore, a person who is allergic to oranges may have an adverse response to other citrus fruits. Additionally, it should be kept in mind that there may be cross reactivity among various foods. Food families in which cross-reactivity has been noted include various milks and milk products (e.g., cow's-milk and soy-milk formulas), citrus fruits, legumes, shellfish, mollusks, and crustaceans (American Academy of Allergy and Immunology 1984). Therefore, children allergic to one member of a food family should be made aware of the potential for problems with other foods even if they are not biologically related. In contrast, some food products within a given species are not necessarily cross-reactive. For example, children allergic to eggs can usually tolerate chicken and other poultry-derived products.

Food allergies manifest themselves in a variety of ways. The most common signs and symptoms of food allergy are listed in Table 20–2. There are many other subjective symptoms that have been blamed on food allergy, including irritability and sleeplessness. However, these are difficult symptoms to evaluate with precision and their association with food allergy cannot be clearly ascertained. For example, although recent evidence suggests that milk allergy may be related to sleep disturbances in infancy (Kahn et al 1988), these data are new and need to be critically reviewed as many children with proven severe

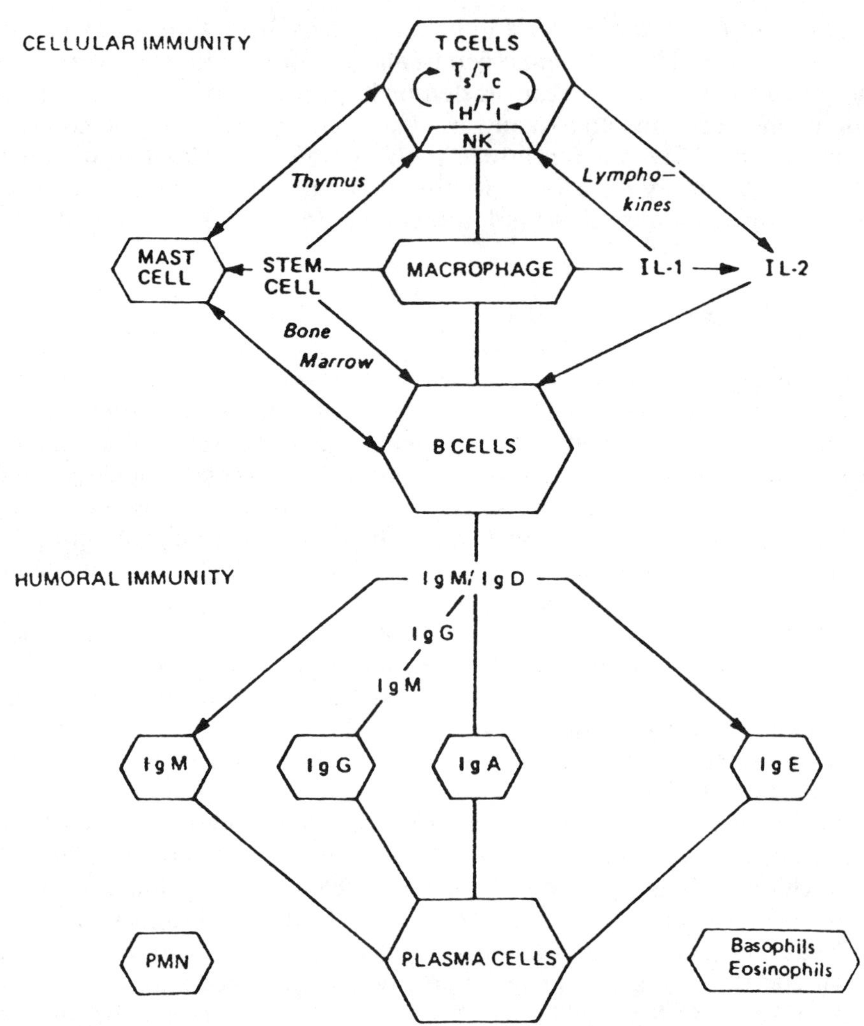

Figure 20–1. Cellular and humoral immune pathways in food sensitivity. T_ST_C = suppressor-cytotoxic T cells, T_HT_I = helper-inducer T cells; IL-1, IL-2 = interleukins; Ig = immunoglobulin; PMN = polymorphonuclear leukocytes.

From Frieri M. IgE/IgA bearing cells in gut lymphoid tissue with special emphasis on food allergy. In Chiaramonte LT, Schneider AT, Lifshitz F, eds. Food allergy. A practical approach to diagnosis and management. New York: Marcel Dekker; 1988:45–70.

Table 20–1. Foods Commonly Implicated in Food Allergies.

VEGETABLES							
Legumes	**Mustard**	**Parsley**	**Potato**	**Grass**	**Lily**	**Laurel**	**Sunflower**
Beans	Broccoli	Anise	Chili	Barley	Asparagus	Avocado	Artichoke
Cocoa bean	Brussels sprouts	Caraway	Eggplant	Corn	Chives	Camphor	Lettuce
Lentil	Cabbage	Carrot	Peppers	Oats	Garlic	Cinnamon	Sunflower
Licorice	Cauliflower	Celery	Potatoes	Rice	Leek		
Peanut	Mustard	Coriander	Tobacco	Rye	Onions		
Peas	Radish	Cumin	Tomato	Wheat			
Soybean	Turnip	Parsley					
Tamarind	Watercress						
FRUITS							**GRAINS**
	Gourd	**Plums**	**Citrus**	**Cashew**	**Nuts**	**Beech**	**Cereals**
	Cantaloupe	Almond	Grapefruit	Cashews	Brazil nut	Beechnut	Wheat
	Cucumber	Apricot	Lemon	Mango	Pecan	Chestnut	Corn
	Honeydew	Cherries	Lime	Pistachio	Walnut	Chincapin nut	
	Melons	Peaches	Mandarin				
	Pumpkin	Persimmon	Orange				
	Squash	Plums	Tangerine				
	Zucchini						
ANIMALS							
	Mammals (meat/milk)	**Birds (meat/egg)**	**Fish**		**Crustaceans**	**Mollusks**	
	Cow	Chicken	Catfish	Salmon	Crab	Abalone	
	Goat	Duck	Cod	Sardine	Crayfish	Clams	
	Pig	Goose	Flounder	Snapper	Lobster	Mussels	
	Rabbit	Hen	Halibut	Trout	Prawn	Oysters	
	Sheep	Turkey	Mackerel	Tuna	Shrimp	Scallops	

From Rao YAK, Bahna SL. Dietary management of food allergies. In Chiaramonte LT, Schneider AT, Lifshitz F, eds. Food allergy. A practical approach to diagnosis and management. New York: Marcel Dekker, 1988:351–375.

Table 20–2. Common Signs and Symptoms of Food Allergy.

Respiratory manifestations
—Asthma
—Allergic rhinitis, cough
Skin manifestations
—Urticaria and angioedema
—Dermatitis (eczema)
Gastrointestinal manifestations
—Vomiting
—Diarrhea/constipation
—Abdominal pain
—Colic (infants)
Life-threatening
—Anaphylaxis

food allergies do not exhibit these nonspecific problems. However, any sign or symptom that suggests a possible allergy is worth investigating.

Cow's Milk

Cow's milk is the most common offending agent causing food allergy in infants and small children. The onset of cow's-milk allergy (CMA) usually occurs during infancy, as most babies receive some form of cow's milk during the first year of life (Lebenthal 1975, Bahna 1980). Even babies fed human milk may be exposed to cow's milk passively through breast feedings if their mothers consume cow's milk. Thus, human-milk feedings may also sensitize a very susceptible infant (Jakobsson & Lindberg 1978). The reported prevalence of CMA has been estimated to range from 0.3 to 7.5 percent in children (Jakobsson & Lindberg 1979). A more reasonable prevalence for milk allergy in the general pediatric population in the United States is probably 1 to 3 percent (Bahna & Heiner 1980). However, CMA may be present in up to 30 percent of children with specific allergic problems such as eczema (Bachman & Dees 1957). Often, CMA is confused with lactose intolerance because the latter condition also causes diarrhea and other gastrointestinal (GI) complaints with the ingestion of milk (see Chapter 21).

Infants and small children are exposed to large quantities of cow's milk considering the amount consumed in relation to their small size. Also, they have immature intestinal mucosal barriers that allow the passage of milk-protein allergens into the blood. This may sensitize susceptible babies because they also have immature immune systems (Roberton et al 1982). The most allergic fraction in cow's milk is β-lactoglobulin, which accounts for 10 percent of the protein content in cow's milk. β-lactoglobulin is not present in human milk. Casein is the second most allergic component of cow's milk and contributes as much as 82 percent of the protein content (Bahna & Heiner 1980). In addition, there are over 20 other different types of proteins in cow's milk, each with a potential to induce allergy in susceptible babies.

It should be kept in mind that allergic reactions from milk ingestion may also be caused by foreign substances in the milk rather than by the milk-protein constituents. Such substances may reach the milk either directly from the animal or indirectly during various stages of handling and processing. For example, patients who are highly sensitive to penicillin have had severe reactions after ingesting milk that contained minute quantities of this antibiotic. In the United States the Food and Drug Administration prohibits adding penicillin to milk or selling milk for human consumption from cattle receiving this antibiotic.

The clinical presentation of milk allergy is diverse and may assume any or all of the problems listed in Table 20–2. In addition, GI tract bleeding, both frank and occult, has been associated with milk allergy (Wilson, Lahey & Heiner 1974). Homogenized whole cow's milk has been shown to be more offensive than proprietary cow's-milk formula or heat-treated milk (Fomon et al 1981), and the amount of blood loss in CMA is usually proportional to the amount of milk consumed (Wilson, Lahey & Heiner 1974). The blood loss may go undetected for long periods and result in profound iron-deficiency anemia that does not respond well to iron therapy unless milk is eliminated from the diet.

In some children CMA may present as a form of milk-induced enteropathy that predominantly involves the intestinal lining (mucosa) and results in a profound loss of protein in the stools (Lebenthal et al 1970). This type of protein-losing enteropathy usually presents during infancy or early childhood with malabsorption, growth retardation, anemia, edema, and low serum protein levels (hypoalbuminemia and hypogammaglobulinemia).

In other children, CMA may lead to chronic pulmonary symptoms, with wheezing and clear, watery, or mucoid discharge from the nose (rhinorrhea) along with chronic serous otis media, recurrent upper respiratory infections, and chronic cough (Heiner 1984). Individuals with this condition (Heiner syndrome) usually have failure to thrive, GI disturbances, eosinophilia, iron deficiency, and elevated serum precipitins to cow's-milk proteins. These symptoms of Heiner syndrome will improve within a few days of cessation of milk intake.

Hen's Eggs

Hypersensitivity to hen's eggs has been estimated to occur in about 5 percent of children with allergies. The most allergenic protein in the chicken egg is ovomucoid, which is found only in the egg white. This protein accounts for only 4 percent of the total egg-white proteins (American Academy of Allergy and Immunology 1984). It is heat-stable and, therefore, cooking does not greatly minimize the allergenicity of egg whites. In contrast, the egg-yolk protein contains only minor allergens and is a rich source of high-quality proteins and minerals. Therefore, egg yolks may be used for infants feedings, while egg whites should be avoided (see Chapter 13).

Legumes

The peanut is one of the most potent allergens of all the legumes, capable of eliciting severe, life-threatening reactions (Fries 1982). Sensitivity to peanuts is much more likely to persist into adulthood than are CMA and hen's egg allergies (Bock 1982). Heating the peanut does not appear to reduce its allergenicity; rather, studies have suggested that it may increase its allergic potency (Nordlee et al 1981). Other peanut products, such as flour or flavorings, appear to have as much allergenicity as the pure peanut. However, the oil extract has little or no allergenic activity. In addition, peanuts are dangerous because they may be aspirated into the wind pipe (trachea) instead of being swallowed or they may end up in the ears or nose of young children.

Soybeans are another potential allergen in the legume family. This allergen may be of increased importance in the future because of its frequent use in our food supply as a protein extender or food supplement. In the past, soy-protein milk formulas were considered less allergenic than cow's-milk formulas and were used in the management of CMA in infancy. However, we now know that soy protein is as antigenic as cow's-milk protein (Taitz 1982). As many as one third of infants who are allergic to cow's milk are also allergic to soy-protein formulas (see Chapters 13 and 19). Therefore, using soy-based formulas in the treatment of CMA or diarrhea does not necessarily eliminate the problem and may simply expose the infant to another potential antigen. As with peanut oil, soybean oil is generally nonallergenic (Bush et al 1985).

Fish and Shellfish

Allergy to fish is more common in such countries as Japan and Norway, where per capita consumption of fish is relatively high. Shellfish, which includes mollusks (clams, scallops, oysters, and mussels) and crustaceans (crab, lobster, shrimp, and crawfish), contain potent allergens with cross-reactivity among shellfish. More recently, structural similarities have been found among crustacean allergens and between crustaceans and mollusk allergens. Studies have shown that fish contain both common and species-specific allergens (Aas 1966). The most completely characterized fish allergen is allergen M of the codfish.

Fish allergy usually produces skin rashes (urticaria), choking, angioedema, asthma, or a combination of these symptoms within minutes of fish ingestion. The reaction occurs whether the fish is raw or cooked, indicating that the major allergens of fish are heat-stable. Many fish-sensitive patients also react to inhaled fish emanations (Chiaramonte, Schneider & Lifshitz 1988). Asthma, angioedema, and even anaphylaxis have been reported following inhalation of steam from cooking fish, presumably because of nebulization of the allergen, which is of low molecular weight (Aas 1969).

Wheat and Corn

Wheat and corn are the most common allergens among the cereals. Wheat flour is one of the most complex allergenic foods. It can cause wheat allergy as an ingestant and baker's asthma as an inhalant, and the gluten fraction can cause celiac disease (gluten sensitivity) (see Chapter 21). Also, wheat products have been observed to cause contact dermatitis. The principal protein fractions of wheat are albumin, globulin, gliadin, and glutenin. All four of wheat's protein fractions show major allergenic activity, but wheat allergy, baker's asthma, and gluten sensitivity are each caused by different wheat-protein fractions (Sutton et al 1982).

Corn can be one of the most problematic food allergies to manage because corn products, in the form of meal, starch, or syrup, are used in a wide variety of foods. Processed meats, peanut butter, jam and jelly, cheese, ice cream, cookies, cakes, and candy may all contain corn in one form or another and elicit reactions in a corn-sensitive patient (Chiaramonte, Schneider & Lifshitz 1988).

Food Additive Intolerances

Food additives may also be the cause of food intolerance. Additives are generally classified into one of four broad categories: flavors and flavor enhancers, preservatives and antioxidants, colorings, and texturing agents. Currently there are over 2500 different additives being used, and they are ubiquitous in food (Juhlin 1987). Consequently, it is often quite difficult to diagnose and treat problems resulting from food additives. Unlike classic allergic reactions to foods, the role of the immune system in food-additive sensitivity is unclear. There is evidence of an immune-mediated (IgE) reaction denoting allergy in only a few cases involving sulfiting agents. In most other cases, nonimmunologic mechanisms are most likely to cause the intolerance.

Tartrazine (FD&C yellow no. 5) is used in a wide variety of foods to impart a bright yellow color or other colors, such as maroon, rust, and turquoise. Examples of foods containing this colorant include salad dressing, canned vegetables, frankfurters, catsup, cheese, and butter. Children, who generally consume larger than average quantities of candies, gum, soft drinks, and jellies, ingest up to 150 milligrams daily, most often with good tolerance (Collins-Williams 1985). In some instances, clinical manifestations of tartrazine intolerance are bronchial asthma (Spector, Wangaard & Farr 1979), urticaria, and angioedema (Settipane et al 1976). Several investigators have reported a role of tartrazine in the development of hyperactivity or hyperkinesis in children (Feingold 1975a,b); however, this association remains doubtful (Harley et al 1978).

Although tartrazine has been the food coloring most studied, other azo and non-azo dyes may also cause urticaria and bronchoconstriction (Juhlin 1980). Azo dyes implicated in allergic reactions include amaranth (FD&C red no. 2), bonceau (FD&C red no. 4), and sunset yellow (FD&C yellow no. 6). The non-azo dyes implicated include brilliant blue (FD&C blue no. 1), erythrosin (FD&C red no. 3), and indigotine (FD&C blue no. 2) (Schneider & Codispoti 1988).

Monosodium glutamate (MSG) is a commonly used flavor enhancer. It is often added to many canned, dry packaged, and frozen processed foods such as soups, gravies, and salad dressings, as well as condiments and spices. Chinese foods contain a particularly high amount of MSG, approximately five to 10 times the average amount of other foods. Thus, a food intolerance caused by ingestion of Chinese food is known as the "Chinese restaurant syndrome" (CRS). The most severe asthmatic reactions to MSG have been reported in adults. However, very few reports have focused on MSG intolerance in children, though they may also have symptoms like those associated with CRS in adults. The adverse reaction to MSG is believed to result from an inborn defect in gluatmate transport or metabolism (Asnes 1980), not from an immunologic mechanism.

Sulfites have been added to foods for centuries as antioxidants to inhibit both enzymatic and nonenzymatic browning of foods, to retard oxidation, and to prevent microbial spoilage (Stevenson & Simon 1981). They are also used as sanitizing agents in food containers and fermentation units. The leading food sources of sulfiting agents are dried fruits, salad-bar lettuce, beer and wine, citrus drinks, prepared potato products, avocadoes and guacamole, grape juice, and shrimp. Exposure to a large dose of sulfites is far more likely to occur in restaurants and salad bars, where many foods are treated with sulfites to maintain a fresh appearance. The average daily intake at home is estimated to be 2 to 3 milligrams per day, whereas a single restaurant meal may contain 25 to 100 milligrams. It should be kept in mind that the amount of sulfite may not be as important as the food to which the sulfiting agent is applied. Sulfited lettuce, for example, appears to be particularly provocative because there is nothing in lettuce to react with a sulfiting agent and transform it into a more innocuous substance. Also, sulfite sensitivity may be more common among children than adults (Towns & Mellis 1984), leading to asthma ranging from mild wheezing to severe life-threatening bronchospasm (Wolf & Nicklas 1985).

In addition to food colorings, MSG, and sulfiting agents, other food additives when given in large quantities have been cited as a cause of adverse reactions to food. These substances include (1) benzoic acid and related compounds, such as sodium benzoate and 4-hydroxybenzoic acid used as antimicrobial preservatives in a wide variety of foods such as dressings, jam, licorice, margarine, powdered milk and potatoes and cereals; and (2) the synthetic antioxidants butylated hydroxyanisole (BHA) and butylated hydroxytoluene (BHT), which are widely used in foods containing fats and oils to inhibit these foods from turning rancid and developing an unpleasant odor and taste.

Molds and fungi, which naturally occur in foods, may also provoke intolerances. Although molds are generally regarded as airborne allergens inhalation is not the usual mechanism by which molds and their spores enter the body. Molds and fungi are often ingested with contaminated foods and thus may result in adverse reactions. Fungi are also used in food processing such as ripening agents for certain cheeses (e.g., brie, camembert, roquefort) and in the preparation of alcoholic beverages.

Food spoilage is another source of fungi in foods. Fresh and canned fruits are a fertile environment for mold growth owing to their high sugar and acid content. Meat, baked goods, and, to a lesser degree, vegetables are all susceptible to fungi and mold growth. Dairy products such as butter and cheese may also be contaminated by mold if stored too long. Pasteurization of milk does not kill all fungi spores. Mycotoxins such as aflatoxins are produced by molds and can negatively affect health and lead to malnutrition (see Chapter 26).

NUTRITIONAL CONSIDERATIONS IN FOOD ALLERGIES AND INTOLERANCES

The most important nutritional consideration in food allergy is to avoid the offensive food product while taking special care to ensure that the diet provides all the necessary nutrients for normal growth and development. This is often not easy to achieve. For example, a child who is unable to tolerate milk and consumes an entirely milk-free diet may be deficient in calcium, protein, vitamins A and D, riboflavin, and zinc. Thus, to maximize calcium intake, non–milk-containing calcium-rich foods such as oranges, broccoli, whole wheat breads, eggs, dried fruit, and legumes (peanut butter) should be emphasized in planning an appropriate menu. The other potential nutrient deficits also need to be addressed by encouraging more meat intake for additional protein and zinc, by providing fruits and vegetables for vitamin A, and green leafy vegetables for riboflavin.

An example of an appropriate milk-free diet for a 6-year-old child (20 kg; 44 lb) is shown below.

MENU 1: Milk-Free Diet

Breakfast

½ cup orange juice

1 scrambled egg with 1 tsp. milk-free margarine (parvae)

½ slice whole wheat bread with 1 tsp. jam

Lunch
¾ peanut butter and jelly sandwich
¾ cup apple juice
small box of raisins (1.5 oz)

Snack
½ cup apple juice
1 banana
2 sandwich cookies

Dinner
¾ cup enriched pasta with spaghetti sauce
3 ounces meatballs
½ cup broccoli with 1 tsp. milk-free margarine (parvae)
½ cup salad with oil and vinegar dressing (milk-free)
½ cup apple juice
½ cup canned peaches in light syrup

Snack
½ cup sherbet (milk-free)

This milk-free diet provides a well-balanced diet with adequate calories and protein (Fig. 20–2A). However, calcium, zinc, copper, sodium, vitamin B_{12}, and vitamin D are deficient to meet this growing child's nutrient needs (Fig. 20–2B). Vitamin D is not a big concern since it can be synthesized by the skin from sunshine. In contrast, the vitamins and minerals need to be supplemented to meet recommended requirements (see Chapters 3 and 9).

Let's now assume that in addition to milk this same 6-year-old girl was also allergic to eggs. Her menu might now look as follows:

MENU 2: Milk- and Egg-Free Diet

Breakfast
½ cup orange juice
½ cup oatmeal cooked with ¾ cup soybean milk and 1 tsp. milk-free margarine
½ sliced peach

Lunch
¾ peanut butter and jelly sandwich on whole wheat bread
¾ cup apple juice
small box of raisins (1.5 oz)

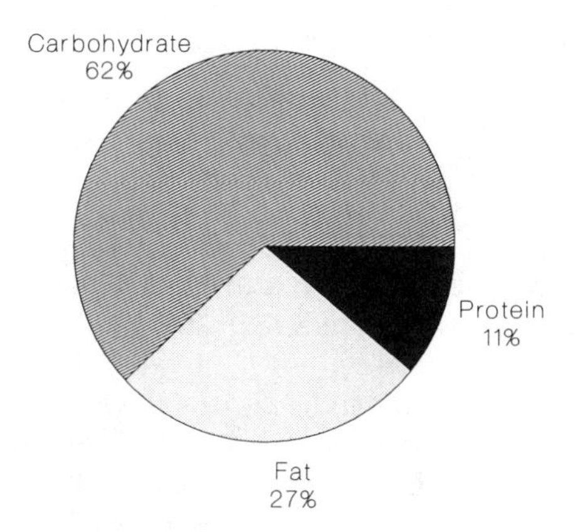

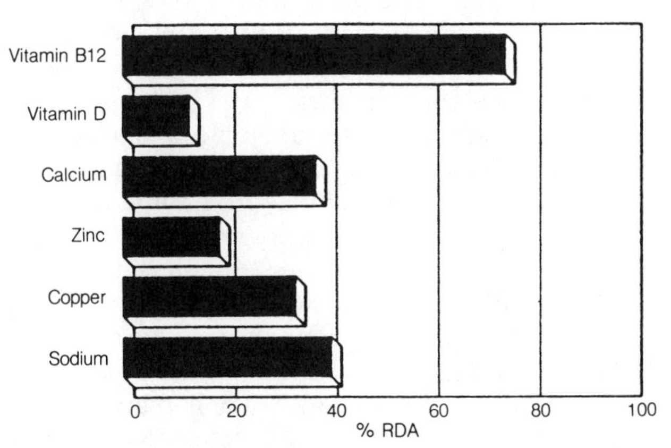

Figure 20–2. A. Caloric Distribution of a Milk-Free Diet. This milk-free diet (Menu 1) provides adequate calories for a 6-year-old girl (80 kcal/kg). **B.** Inappropriate Nutrient Intakes of a Milk-Free Diet. The micronutrients that are deficient (< ⅔ RDA) are shown.

Snack
½ cup apple juice
1 banana
2 sandwich cookies

Dinner
¾ cup enriched pasta with spaghetti sauce
3 ounces meatballs (egg-free)
½ cup broccoli with 1 tsp. milk-free margarine
½ cup salad with oil and vinegar dressing

½ cup apple juice
1 orange

Snack
fruit ice

As with the milk-free diet, the milk- and egg-free menu meets a growing 6-year-old girl's calorie and protein needs (Fig. 20-3A). However, it is deficient in calcium, zinc, copper, sodium, vitamin B_{12}, and vitamin D despite the addition of soybean milk (Fig. 20–3B). Zinc intake is even lower with the elimination of egg, which is an excellent source of this nutrient in the diet and would therefore need to be supplemented. Further elimination of the soybean milk and substitution of the peanut butter sandwich with a tuna fish salad sandwich would make this menu legume-free. This may be needed by those unfortunate patients who cannot tolerate these foods. With a milk-, egg-, and legume-free diet zinc, calcium, and vitamin D would be the main deficiencies while all other nutrient requirements could be met.

It is important to remember that with multiple food allergies the variety of the diet becomes very limited. This may be more dramatic in children who may have limited food preferences and may have some resistance to try new foods. Therefore, a precise diagnosis is necessary to help in planning the nutritional intake of children with food allergies. The previous example of a child who needed a milk-free diet because of milk allergy (an unusual problem in a 6-year-old child) needed supplementation to ensure the intake of calcium and zinc. If the child was lactose-intolerant (a frequent problem in non-white-Anglo-Saxon children), complete avoidance of milk may not have been necessary. Lactose-intolerant patients are often able to ingest milk in small amounts (Stephenson & Latham 1974) or with enzyme predigestion (see Chapter 19).

DIAGNOSIS OF FOOD ALLERGIES AND INTOLERANCES

An accurate diagnosis of food allergies and intolerances is important to avoid unnecessary dietary restrictions. Since there is no single laboratory or immunologic test that confirms food allergies and intolerances, the diagnostic process may be cumbersome (Bock et al 1978). In the past, a suspected food was eliminated and the amelioration of clinical symptoms was sufficient evidence for a diagnosis. This method is inaccurate and may lead to a misdiagnosis, which can result in an unnecessarily prolonged avoidance of a food with the potential for developing nutritional deficiencies or neglect from the underlying undiagnosed disease.

In Table 20–3, a summary evaluation of food allergy is shown. A comprehensive assessment is essential for accurate diagnosis. It should include a de-

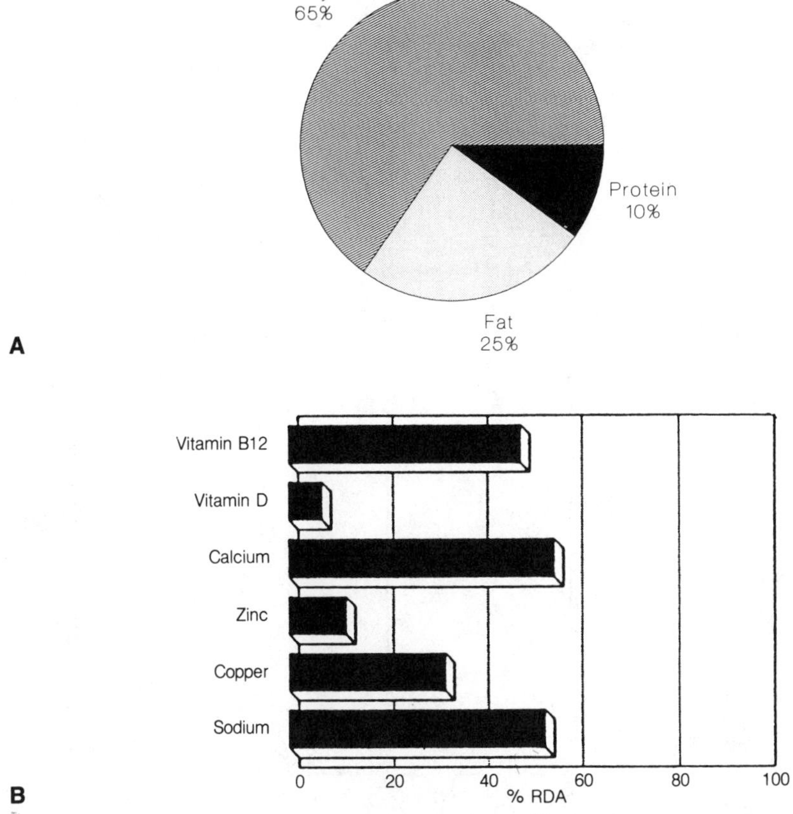

Figure 20–3. **A.** Caloric Distribution of a Milk- and Egg-Free Diet. This milk-free, egg-free diet (Menu 2) provides adequate calories for a 6-year-old girl (82 kcal/kg). **B.** Inappropriate Nutrient Intakes of a Milk- and Egg-Free Diet. The micronutrients that are deficient (< ⅔ RDA) are shown.

tailed evalution of food intake and nutritional status. The time from ingestion of food to onset of symptoms and the quantity and type of food necessary to produce a reaction should be noted. The possibility of an anaphylactic reaction needs to be elicited. A review of restricted and accepted foods provides information on the nutritional adequacy of the patient's diet. When examining a patient with food allergies an experienced physician may be able to detect specific signs that suggest allergic conditions, such as allergic shiners, Morgan–Denne lines, nasal creases, and dermatitis, and distinguish clinically urticaria from other rashes that may not be related to allergic reactions.

Skin testing remains the basic technique used by clinical allergists to assess for food allergies, even though they are of questionable reliability. Much of the

Table 20–3. Summary of Evaluation of Food Allergy.

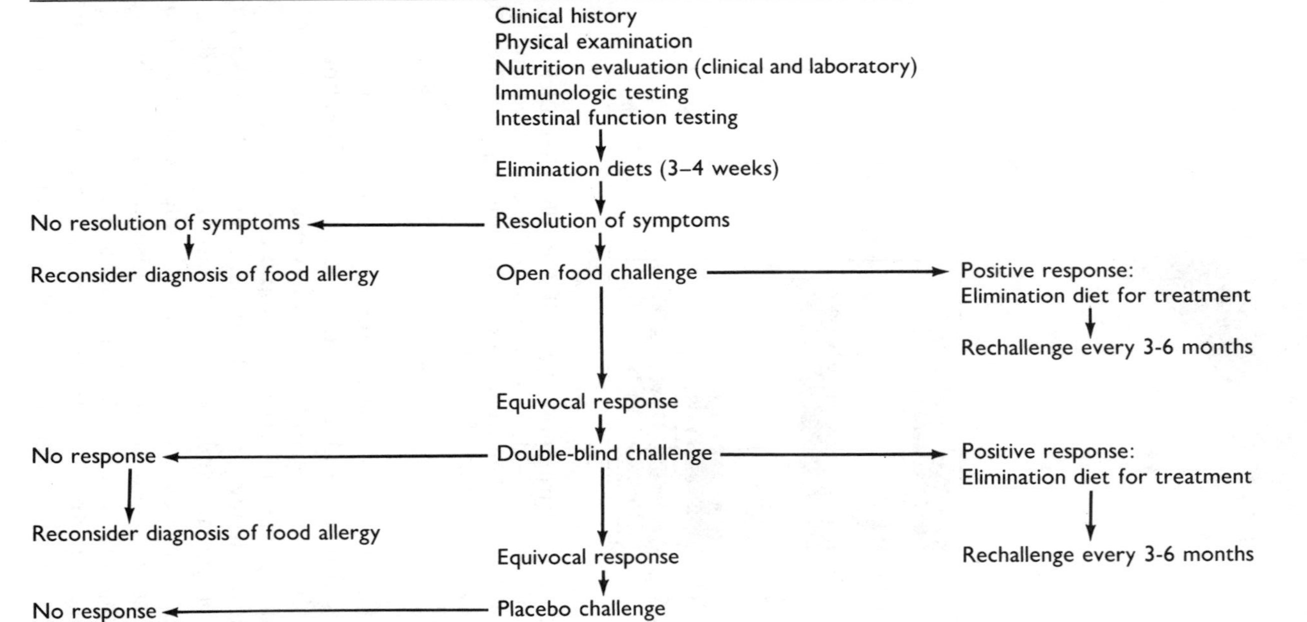

Adapted from Rentschler LA, Moses NS. Protein challenges. In Chiaramonte LT, Schneider AT, Lifshitz F, eds. Food allergy. A practical approach to diagnosis and management. New York: Marcel Dekker, 1988: 465–472.

confusion surrounding food skin tests arises from the lack of verification of the antigenicity of the extracts and from failure to determine objectively the relationship between skin-test results and the clinical reactions following ingestion of the suspected food. In children less than 3 years old, a negative skin test is even less valuable in detecting food sensitivity than in older children.

The radioallergosorbent test (RAST), an in vitro radioimmunoassay to measure circulating immunoglobulin E (IgE), may be useful in selected patients with suspected food allergies. However, it is the current recommendation of the American Academy of Allergy and Immunology that skin testing be used in preference to RAST testing except in very special clinical situations (Chiaramonte, Schneider & Lifshitz 1988), such as severe eczema or other skin conditions. When there is a history or risk of anaphylaxis, RAST must be employed first. Other sophisticated immunologic tests for food allergy include RAST inhibition assay, enzyme-linked immunosorbent assay (ELISA), and gel diffusion techniques. These tests are still in the early stages of development and thus remain only research tools (Chiaramonte, Schneider & Lifshitz 1988).

Often, it is necessary to obtain other laboratory tests to assess possible disorders that may mimic food allergies or to recognize some of the consequences and/or complications of the disease. In patients with diarrhea and other GI complaints the presence of carbohydrate intolerance should be ruled out, as this is often associated with or confused for food allergies. This can be done by determination of sugars and pH of the stools or by a lactose tolerance test and/or breath hydrogen test (see Chapter 19). Also, an assessment of some possible damage induced by the allergy may help establish a diagnosis and/or help plan an appropriate treatment. Intestinal function should be measured (see below), and laboratory data should include an assessment of the nutritional status of the patient (see Chapter 10).

After the medical evaluation is completed, the next step is to eliminate all the foods in the diet that are suspected of causing an adverse reaction. When no particular food(s) can be clearly identified as the culprit the patient may be assessed by an elimination diet study (Table 20–4). This includes exclusive feeding of a hypoallergenic liquid diet such as Vivonex, Criticare HN, Nutramigen, Pregestimil, or Alimentum (see Chapters 13, 19, and 27), or feedings of a standard "nonallergenic" diet.

Once an elimination diet is started it is necessary to continue it for 2 to 4 weeks to assess the patient's response. Daily food records and a symptom diary should be kept and compared with the complaints reported during the initial evaluation. The diagnosis of potential food allergies can be made if symptoms resolve while on the elimination diet, but confirmatory tests are necessary once the patient is symptom-free. For example, a patient with diarrhea due to food allergies needs to show normalization of stools, absence of fecal blood, and disappearance of cells and eosinophils in the stools once the offending food is eliminated. During this time a normal weight gain with adequate ca-

Table 20–4. Elimination Diets.

Elimination Diet 1 (infants 0 to 6 months)*
Hypoallergenic formula
Elimination Diet 2 (6 months to 2 years)†
Hypoallergenic formula
Rice or poi
Pears or bananas
Lamb
Elimination Diet 3 (children 2 years or older)
Beverage: tea (only sugar may be added)
Bread: traditional Ry-Krisp (not seasoned Ry-Krisp)
Cereal: rice, white, brown, wild, puffed, flour
Fats: lamb fat dripping, pure; olive oil, pure
Fruits: all must be thoroughly cooked; nothing added but sugar: apricots, cherries, peaches, cranberries, prunes
Fruit juices: apricot, cranberry, prune
Meat: Lamb
Miscellaneous: ripe olives, pure vanilla extract, gelatin (pure and unflavored), baking soda, tapioca (pure), citric acid (buy from drugstore), cream of tartar
Sweets: sugar (white or brown), sugar syrups (homemade), sugar and water candies (pure or homemade), jams and preserves (homemade from allowed fruits and sugar)
Vegetables: all must be thoroughly cooked, seasoned only with salt and fats allowed; beets: fresh, dried at home, canned, or commercially canned if only salt and/or sugar added

*In special circumstances this may be progressed to elimination diet 2, in a stepwise fashion, adding rice, then pears, and then lamb every 3 to 4 days.
†After 1 month or more on this diet, foods in elimination diet 3 may be added gradually, one at a time.

Adapted from Parathyras AJ, Greenberg L. Diagnostic diets. In Chiaramonte LT, Schneider AT, Lifshitz F, eds. Food allergy. A practical approach to diagnosis and management. New York: Marcel Dekker, 1988:395–399.

loric intake must be demonstrated for 2 to 4 weeks. Lack of improvement of symptoms while receiving the elimination diet would suggest reconsideration of the diagnosis.

A provocative food challenge is the next step in the diagnosis of food allergy since many symptoms may improve independently of dietary manipulations. The age of the subject often determines how the food challenges should proceed. In infants, food challenges are not recommended until the body weight returns to at least the pre-illness level. For the food challenge, the child should ingest a meal that contains the "test" food in the amount normally consumed at one meal that had produced symptoms (Adams & Mahan 1984). Average portions of the test food are consumed for 3 to 4 consecutive days. If the patient remains asymptomatic, the food does not need to be restricted in the diet. When more than one food challenge is necessary to test for several food allergies, the food challenges should be separated by 1 week as a precaution against overlapping symptoms. If life-threatening anaphylactic reactions are possible, the patient should *not* be challenged.

The patient and the family may know they are being challenged (open food challenge) if their cooperation can be elicited. However, double-blind food challenges are indicated if the response to the open food challenge was found to be equivocal or if the patient (or family) has strongly held opinions, nonspecific symptoms, or multiple problems with several foods. For the double-blind food challenge capsules are available that contain the dried form of several foodstuffs (Rentschler & Moses 1988). Also, many of the most common food allergies, such as cow's milk, soybean flour, whole-wheat flour and other grains, dried egg, peanuts and other nuts, can be tested blindly by obtaining, in the grocery store, the dry forms of these foods which are less expensive than the premade capsules. Freeze-dried, powdered foods designed for campers also can be placed into capsules. In young children, the test food can be masked in formula, mashed potatoes, or juice.

The amount of dry food administered as a test dose is governed by the apparent degree of sensitivity. Generally, the test dose of a particular food ranges from as low as 10 milligrams to as much as 2 grams for the initial dose. It is necessary to remember that water has been removed from the dried food when calculating the dose for the challenge. For example, to give a child 2 ounces (61 g) of milk, it is necessary to give 8 grams of dried powdered milk.

Test foods are given before breakfast after a fast of at least 6 hours. After the test challenge, the patient is carefully monitored both clinically and by laboratory testing (see below) for 1 to 4 hours to detect immediate allergic reactions. Asymptomatic patients receive a second test dose of the food being investigated at the end of the first observation period. For the second food challenge, the dose is increased two to ten times the original dose. The challenge observation phase continues with successively larger dosages until the patient consumes the equivalent of a full load of hydrated food. Failure to confirm the adverse reaction to food suggests a misdiagnosis or a psychologic cause for the problem. As many as 60 percent of suspected adverse reactions may fall into this category (Chiaramonte, Schneider & Lifshitz 1988). For blind challenge tests, the food tested and the placebo need to be concealed in the same manner and be given under the same conditions, and the results of the two tests are compared to establish the diagnosis.

Laboratory tests performed during the food challenges may provide objective evidence of clinical and subclinical reactions resulting from a test food. Laboratory criteria for demonstrating a positive reaction to an acute food challenge include (1) an increase in peripheral-blood white-cell count (polymorphonuclear leukocyte count of $>4000\ mm^{-1}$) between that in a blood sample drawn immediately before oral challenge and that in a sample drawn 6 to 8 hours after the challenge; (2) evidence of blood in the stool (usually microscopic); and (3) the induction of leukocytes in Hansel-stained smears of stool mucus and Charcot–Leyden crystals or eosinophilic debris in stool mucus. When a child's symptoms are specifically related to the GI tract, it is useful to perform a D-xylose absorption test and a breath hydrogen test before and after a food challenge. An asymptomatic child receiving an elimination diet who shows normal D-xylose and breath hydrogen tests would rule out primary intestinal diseases. However, after a food challenge with the offending agent, these studies may become abnormal, suggesting intestinal mucosal damage induced by a specific food.

There is a need for frequent administration of food challenges in the first few years of life because of the transient nature of adverse reactions to food in young children. A few food allergies, usually peanut and egg, persist in causing symptoms for a number of years. In contrast, adverse reactions to milk are often promptly "outgrown." Children who have a reaction to a food for several consecutive months should be challenged at 3- to 6-month intervals depending on the severity of the reaction. When it becomes apparent that a food is continuing to cause adverse reactions, the interval can be lengthened to a year or more. However, if the food allergies are limited and specific or if they induce a very severe reaction, the challenge may be delayed, provided there is an appropriate overall dietary intake.

PREVENTION OF FOOD ALLERGY

Recognition of infants at risk of developing allergic disease is the first step toward the prevention of food allergies. Allergy is a multifactorial disease with a strong inherited tendency. However, no genetic marker has yet been identified for its prediction. While the overall prevalence of allergy in young children is 20 percent (Matthew et al 1977), if neither parent has problems with allergies the prevalence is as low as 13 percent (Hamburger 1979). In contrast, if one parent is atopic the prevalence of allergy in the offspring increases to 29 percent, and when both parents are allergic the prevalence of allergy increases to 47 to 100 percent (Hamburger 1980). A family history of allergy is found in 70 percent of babies with cow's-milk intolerance (Jakobsson & Lindberg 1979).

It is now known that an allergic illness results from a complicated interrelationship between the genetic predisposition for allergies and the environmental influences to which a child may be exposed. A fetus may have exposure to food allergens prenatally through placental passage, after birth through breast milk, or in the first few months of life through early solid feedings. Contact with any one of the food allergens at these stages of development may result in food allergy, whereas this would not occur if exposure had taken place later in life. Specific sensitization to such allergens as wheat (Kaufman 1971), milk, egg (Michel et al 1980), and microfilaria (Weil et al 1983) has been documented to occur even before birth. Nevertheless, specific prenatal sensitization to food is a rather infrequent event in human infants (Kjellman & Croner 1984, Hamburger et al 1983). Moreover, modification of maternal diet during late pregnancy in attempts to reduce allergy in atopic families has not proven to be effective (Chiaramonte, Schneider & Lifshitz 1988).

For many years breastfeeding has been considered the best approach to prevent food sensitization and allergic disease in infancy. The relatively low incidence of allergies among breast-fed infants may be due to multiple factors (see Chapter 12), but food intolerances and sensitivities can occur in highly sensitive fully breast-fed infants (Lake, Whitington & Hamilton 1982, Jakobsson & Lindberg 1983). Egg antigen and cow's-milk protein antigens have been identified in maternal breast-milk samples. Maternal ingestion of cow's milk has been shown to cause infantile colic (Jakobsson & Lindberg 1983) and colitis (Lake, Whitington & Hamilton 1982) in highly sensitive exclusively breast-fed infants. The elimination of cow's-milk protein from the maternal diet was an effective treatment for colic in 30 to 40 percent of breast-fed infants.

In contrast, it has been postulated that ingestion of small quantities, or the delayed introduction of food allergens such as cow's milk, could increase later sensitization (Jarrett & Hall 1979). However, a delay of 1 year of cow's-milk ingestion did not increase cow's-milk sensitization either clinically or immunologically in infants of allergic parents following a strict food prophylaxis (avoidance) regimen (Hamburger et al 1983).

Prolonged breastfeeding for at least 6 months of age and/or use of hypoallergenic infant formulas is strongly encouraged in the offspring of documented immunologically atopic parents (Table 20–5). To reduce the potential for food sensitization by passage of allergenic food proteins through breast milk, mothers are often instructed to avoid totally milk, egg, and peanut ingestion during lactation and to take supplemental calcium (1500 mg daily). Avoidance of cow's milk and soy milk, and delayed introduction of solid foods after 6 months of age have also been recommended to reduce the development of food allergies in infancy (Chiaramonte, Schneider & Lifshitz 1988). However, attempts at strict dietary adherence to avoid the development of food allergy is not always effective, perhaps owing to the genetic predisposition and to significant obstacles of avoidance of certain allergens.

Table 20–5. Dietary Avoidance Regimen for Prevention of Food Allergy.

Infant
Prolong breastfeeding (>4 months)
Hypoallergenic infant formula
Delayed solid-food introduction (>6 months)
6–12 months (vegetables, rice, meat, fruit)
12–18 months (milk, wheat, corn, citrus, soy)
24 months (egg)
36 months (peanut, fish)
Mother
Eliminate milk, egg, and peanuts during pregnancy and lactation

Adapted from Zeiger RS. Prevention of food allergy. In Chiaramonte LT, Schneider AT, Lifshitz F, eds. Food allergy. A practical approach to diagnosis and management. New York: Marcel Dekker, 1988: 329–350.

CLINICAL INTERVENTION

The primary treatment for food allergy is the accurate identification and avoidance of the offending allergens. In general, this is a safe and effective approach, although it may not be easy to accomplish, especially if there are multiple food allergies or if the allergen is ubiquitous in the food supply. Children and their families must receive extensive training to learn how to avoid the offending food or food additive. This information may also extend to avoidance of cross-reacting foods in highly sensitive children. The close interaction between a board-certified allergist, nutritionist, and pediatrician is often necessary for the successful management of these patients.

Nutrition education of the allergic child and his or her family should include instruction on food labeling, information regarding eating away from home, and a variety of food alternatives and recipes. Often the degree of compliance of the patient will depend on the completeness of the nutritional guidance that is provided. There are numerous resources to help the professional and the family follow the prescribed diet to manage the food allergies (Chiaramonte, Schneider & Lifshitz 1988).

Nondietary therapy and pharmacologic therapy of food allergy such as sublingual drops and food injections are generally considered ineffective. Certain drug treatments, however, have been useful in certain conditions. For example, antihistamines have been used in the therapy of food allergies known to result in the release of histamine, which causes a wheal, flare, or itch response. These types of drugs may therefore be helpful in the treatment of adverse reactions to foods when the symptoms include urticaria/angioedema, conjunctivitis, and rhinitis (Phanuphak, Shocket & Kohler 1978). Additionally, the use of certain drugs primarily prescribed for ulcer therapy in the treatment of the GI consequences of food reactions has been suggested (Celestin et al 1975).

Sodium cromoglycate, or cromolyn, has been used in inhalation therapy for the treatment of asthma for the past 20 years. More recently, it has been established as a potentially useful drug in the treatment of food allergy (Collins-Williams 1985). Its mechanism of action in the GI tract is inhibition of mediator release from mast cells, thereby reducing gut permeability and decreased absorption of allergens into the bloodstream (Falth-Magnusson et al 1984). However, this treatment is not recommended for all patients with food allergy. Cromolyn is indicated for individuals who cannot eliminate the offending food allergen owing to its ubiquitous nature or who have so many food allergies that they cannot be given adequate nutrition with the necessary restrictive diet. High-dose cromolyn has not yet been shown to be safe for long-term use in infants and children, so it should not be used without proper informed consent and continued monitoring for toxicity.

Other drugs, such as prostaglandin inhibitors for the treatment of gluten-induced enteropathy (celiac disease) and irritable bowel syndrome (Lessof, Anderson & Voulten 1983), theophylline (Caldwell, Sharma & Hurtubise 1978), and a variety of vitamins (Collipp et al 1975, Schacter & Schlesinger 1982) have been suggested in the possible treatment of food intolerances. However, further studies are needed to demonstrate their usefulness, if any. Adrenergics, specifically epinephrine, are an important pharmacologic therapy for anaphylactic reaction to foods. This is a life-saving drug in the event of inadvertent ingestion of an allergenic food in a child with great sensitivity (often to eggs, nuts, peanuts and milk) and should always be kept handy for emergencies.

REFERENCES

Aas K. Antigens and allergens of fish. Int Arch Allergy 1969; 36:152–155.

Aas K. Studies of hypersensitivity to fish. A clinical study. Int Arch Allergy 1966; 29:346–363.

Adams EJ, Mahan LK. Nutritional care in food allergy and food intolerance. In Kraus MV, Mahan LK, eds. Food, nutrition, and diet therapy. 7th ed. Philadelphia: WB Saunders, 1984:644–646.

American Academy of Allergy and Immunology Committee on Adverse Reactions to Food, National Institute of Allergy and Infectious Diseases. Adverse reactions to foods. Washington, D.C.: U.S. Department of Health and Human Services, NIH Publication No. 84-2442, July 1984:7–26.

Asnes RS. Chinese restaurant syndrome in an infant. Clin Pediatr 1980; 19:705–706.

Atkins FM. The basis of immediate hypersensitivity reactions to foods. Nutr Rev 1983; 41:229–234.

Bachman KD, Dees SC. Milk allergy. I. Observations on incidence any symptoms in "well" babies. Pediatrics 1957; 20:393–399.

Bahna SI, Gandhi MD. Milk hypersensitivity. I. Pathogenesis and symptomatology. Ann Allergy 1983; 30:218–223.

Bahna SL, Heiner DC. Allergies in milk. New York: Grune and Stratton, 1980.

Bock SA, Lee WY, Remigio LK, May CD. Studies of hypersensitivity reactions to foods in infants and children. J Allergy Clin Immunol 1978; 62:327–334.

Bock SA. The natural history of food hypersensitivity. J Allergy Clin Immunol 1982; 69:173–177.

Buchbinder EM, Bloch KJ, Moss J, Guiney TE. Food-dependent, exercise-induced anaphylaxis. JAMA 1983; 250:2973–2974.

Bush RK, Taylor SL, Nordlee JA, Busse WW. Soybean oil is not allergenic to soybean-sensitive individuals. J Allergy Clin Immunol 1985; 76:242–245.

Caldwell JH, Sharma HM, Hurtubise PE. Eosinophilic gastroenteritis and extreme allergy: Immunopathological comparison with non-allergic gastrointestinal disease. Gastroenterology 1978; 74:1016.

Celestin LR, Harvey V, Saunders JHB, et al. Treatment of duodenal ulcer by metiamide. A multicentre trial. Lancet 1975; 2:779–781.

Chiaramonte LT, Schneider AT, Lifshitz F, eds. Food allergy. A practical approach to diagnosis and management. New York: Marcel Dekker, 1988.

Collins-Williams C. Clinical spectrum of adverse reactions to tartrazine. J Asthma 1985; 22:139–143.

Collipp PF, Goldzier S, Weiss N, Soleymani Y, Snyder R. Pyridoxine treatment of childhood bronchial asthma. Ann Allergy 1975; 35:93–97.

Falth-Magnusson K, Kjellman N-IM, Magnusson K-E, Sundqvist T. Intestinal permeability in healthy and allergic children before and after sodium cromoglycate treatment assessed with different-sized polyethylene-glycols (PEG 400 and PEG 1000). Clin Allergy 1984; 14:277–286.

Feingold BF. Hyperkinesis and learning disabilities linked to artificial food flavors and colors. Am J Nurse 1975a; 75:797.

Feingold BF. Why your child is hyperactive. New York: Random House, 1975b.

Fomon SJ, Ziegler EE, Nelson SE, Edwards BB. Cow milk feeding in infancy: Gastrointestinal blood loss and iron nutritional status. J Pediatr 1981; 98:540–545.

Fries J. Peanuts: Allergic and other untoward reactions. Ann Allergy 1982; 48:220–226.

Hamburger RN. Development of atopic allergy in children. In Johansson SGO, ed. Diagnosis and treatment of IgE-mediated diseases. Proceedings of the International Allergy Symposium, Uppsala, September 24–26, 1980. Amsterdam: Excerpta Medica, 1980: 30–34.

Hamburger RN. Heredity, IGE and the development of atopic allergy. In Hamburger RN, ed. Allergy unmasked. Noodbridge, NJ: Medical Education Dynamics, 1979:10–19.

Hamburger RN, Heller S, Mellon M, O'Connor RD, Zeiger RS. Current status of the clinical and immunologic consequences of a prototype allergic disease prevention program. Ann Allergy 1983; 51:281–290.

Hannuksela M, Lahti A. Immediate reactions to fruits and vegetable. Contact Dermatitis 1977; 3:79–84.

Harley JP, Ray RS, Tomasi L, et al. Hyperkinesis and food additives: Testing the Feingold hypothesis. Pediatrics 1978; 61:818–828.

Heiner DC. Respiratory diseases and food allergy. Ann Allergy 1984; 53:657–664.

Iyngkaran N, Abdin Z. Intolerance to food proteins. In Lifshitz F, ed. Pediatric nutrition. New York: Marcel Dekker, 1982:449–483.

Jakobsson I, Lindberg T. A prospective study of cow's milk allergy in Swedish infants. Acta Paediatr Scand 1979; 68:853–859.

Jakobsson I, Lindberg T. Cow's milk as a cause of infantile colic in breast-fed infants. Lancet 1978; 2:437–439.

Jakobsson I, Lindberg T. Cow's milk proteins cause infantile colic in breast-fed infants: A double-blind crossover study. Pediatrics 1983; 71:268–271.

Jarrett E, Hall E. Selective suppression of IgE antibody responsiveness by maternal influence. Nature 1979; 280:145–147.

Juhlin L. Incidence of intolerance to food additives. Int J Dermatol 1980; 19:548–551.

Juhlin L. Intolerance to food additives. In Marzulii FN, Maibach HI, eds. Advances in modern toxicology. Vol. 4, Dermatoxicology and pharmacology. New York: John Wiley & Sons, 1987:455.

Kahn A, Francois G, Sottiaux M, et al. Sleep characteristics in milk-intolerant infants. Sleep 1988; 291–297.
Kaufman HS. Allergy in the newborn: Skin test reactions confirmed by the Prausmitz-Kustner test at birth. Clin Allergy 1971; 1:363–367.
Kjellman NI, Croner S. Cord blood IgE determination for allergy prediction—A follow-up to seven years of age in 1,651 children. Ann Allergy 1984; 53:167–171.
Lake AM, Whitington PF, Hamilton SR. Dietary protein-induced colitis in breast-fed infants. J Pediatr 1982; 101:906–910.
Lebenthal E. Cow's milk protein allergy. Pediatr Clin North Am 1975; 22:827–833.
Lebenthal E, Leon J, Lewitus Z, Matoth Y, Freier S. Gastrointestinal protein loss in allergy to cow's milk beta-lactoglobulin. Isr J Med Sci 1970; 6:506–510.
Lessof MH, Anderson JA, Voulten LJF. Prostaglandins in the pathogenesis of food intolerance. Ann Allergy 1983; 51:249–250.
Matthew DJ, Taylor B, Norman AP, Turner MW, Soothill JF. Prevention of eczema. Lancet 1977; 1:321–324.
Michel FB, Bousquet J, Greillier P, Robinet-Levy M, Coulomb V. Comparison of cord blood immunoglobulin E and maternal allergy for the prediction of atopic disease in infancy. J Allergy Clin Immunol 1980; 65:422–430.
Nordlee JA, Taylor SL, Jones RT, Yunginger JW. Allergenicity of various peanut products as determined by RAST inhibition. J Allergy Clin Immunol 1981; 68:376–382.
Pearson DJ, Keith JB. Diet and illness. Lancet 1983; 1:1259–1261.
Phanuphak P, Shocket A, Kohler PF. Treatment of chronic idiopathic urticaria with combined H_1 and H_2 blockers. Clin Allergy 1978; 8:429–433.
Rentschler LA, Moses NS. Protein challenges. In Chiaramonte LT, Schneider AT, Lifshitz F, eds. Food allergy. A practical approach to diagnosis and management. New York: Marcel Dekker, 1988:465–472.
Roberton DM, Paganelli R, Dinwiddie R, Levinsky RJ. Milk antigen absorption in the preterm and term neonate. Arch Dis Child 1982; 57:369–372.
Schacter EN, Schlesinger A. The attenuation of exercise-induced bronchospasm by ascorbic acid. Ann Allergy 1982; 49:146–150.
Schneider AT, Codispoti AJ. Allergic reactions to food additives. In Chiaramonte LT, Schneider AT, Lifshitz F, eds. Food allergy. A practical approach to diagnosis and management. New York: Marcel Dekker, 1988:117–151.
Settipane GA, Chafee FH, Postman IM, et al. Significance of tartrazine sensitivity in chronic urticaria of unknown etiology. J Allergy Clin Immunol 1976; 57:541–546.
Spector SL, Wangaard CH, Farr RS. Aspirin and concomitant idiosyncracies in adult asthmatic patients. J Allergy Clin Immunol 1979; 64:500–506.
Stephenson LS, Latham MC. Lactose intolerance and milk consumption: The relation of tolerance to symptoms. Am J Clin Nutr 1974; 27:296–303.
Stevenson DD, Simon RA. Sensitivity to ingested metabisulfite in asthmatic subjects. J Allergy Clin Immunol 1981; 68:26–32.
Sutton R, Hill DJ, Baldo BA, Wrigley CW. Immunoglobulin E antibodies to ingested cereal flour components: Studies with sera from subjects with

asthma and eczema. Clin Allergy 1982; 12:63–74.
Taitz LS. Soy feeding in infancy. Arch Dis Child 1982; 57:814–815.
Titus Lucretius Carus. De Rerum Natur, Book 4, 1, 637 (55 BC).
Towns SJ, Mellis CM. Role of acetyl salicylic acid and sodium metabisulfite in chronic childhood asthma. Pediatrics 1984; 73:631–637.
Weil GJ, Hussain R, Kumaraswami V, Tipathy SP, Phillips KS, Olten Sen EA. Prenatal allergic sensitization to helminth antigens in offspring of parasite-infected mothers. J Clin Invest 1983; 71:1124–1129.
Wilson JF, Lahey ME, Heiner DC. Studies on iron metabolism. V. Further observations on cow's milk induced gastrointestinal bleeding in infants with iron-deficiency anemia. J Pediatr 1974; 84:335–344.
Wolf SI, Nicklas RA. Sulfite sensitivity in a seven-year-old child. Ann Allergy 1985; 54:420–423.

21

The Handicapped Child

Cathy entered the world as a very sick baby with severe birth defects. She had eye, ear, and kidney problems as well as a congenital heart defect that required surgery before she was 1 month old. To make matters worse, Cathy was unable to drink enough formula to gain weight because of a slow, weak suck. Tube feedings were started to help Cathy gain weight and grow. However, by 7 months of age, Cathy's mom convinced the doctors to discontinue tube feedings because she thought the tube was irritating Cathy's throat and was not allowing her to learn to suck and swallow normally. This is when Cathy's trouble with nutrition began. No matter how hard the mother tried to feed Cathy, she was not able to eat enough by mouth. Cathy would only take a thickened liquid that her mom would prepare from skim milk, cereal, sugar, oil, and water. Due to a lack of oral motor coordination, she could not take any food from a spoon; she could tolerate only small amounts of bottle feedings given very, very slowly. By 4 years of age, Cathy weighed only 19 pounds and was severely underweight and malnourished.

Many handicapped children with physical and/or neurologic conditions may have difficulties consuming a diet adequate to support normal growth. In these developmentally disabled children, malnutrition can occur quite early in life and may further compromise their already limited neurologic and developmental growth. Inadequate protein and energy intakes in infants and children have been associated with decreased brain growth and inappropriate nerve functioning (Torin & Viteri 1988), and specific mineral deficiencies such as iron may have adverse consequences on mental development and concentration abilities in infants and young children (Pollitt et al 1988). However, these detrimental effects of malnutrition do not seem to lead to prolonged intellectual deficits if nutritional status is improved and proper educational intervention is undertaken (Joos & Pollitt 1987). It is therefore essential to meet the nutritional needs of these handicapped children and to help the families and health professionals who care for these special children identify nutritional problems before they become severe.

Handicapped children are at greater risk than normal children for nutritional problems. These children often have feeding difficulties, which may arise from neuromuscular incompetence as seen in patients with seizure disorders or cerebral palsy. Also, they may have physical deformities such as cleft palate that make feeding a difficult task. Children who are born deaf and blind without any other physical or medical handicap may demonstrate malnutrition and growth failure owing to early feeding difficulties that persist throughout childhood (Thommessen, Riis & Kase 1989). In addition, there may be psychosocial issues for the handicapped child, including inappropriate mother–child interactions during feeding. Unusual feeding behaviors such as eating nonfood items (pica), and tantrums during mealtimes may also interfere with achieving a well-balanced dietary intake.

Handicapped children may have specific medical conditions that alter their nutritional needs. For example, a child with heart disease and recurrent infections with fever has an increased nutrient requirement to cover the increased expenditures owing to the stress of these conditions. Other handicapped children have metabolic disorders such as phenylketonuria (PKU) and food allergies and intolerances that require special restrictive diets, which may further compromise the child's nutritional status (see Chapters 20 and 25). Additionally, medications often used to treat specific problems of a handicapped child may interfere with the child's ability or desire to eat or may negatively interact with some of the nutrients in the diet (Table 21–1).

NUTRITIONAL ASSESSMENT

A comprehensive nutritional assessment should be a component of every handicapped child's health care. The basic features of such an evaluation are reviewed in Chapter 10. However, there are a few specific concerns for handicapped children that require some attention here.

As with all infants and children, monitoring changes in weight and length or height is the key to determining whether a child is receiving adequate nutrition. Although growth retardation is commonly seen in handicapped children, particularly those with central nervous system dysfunction, it is critical to determine whether any nutrition-related causes may be contributing to poor growth. These children should be growing at a constant rate, and any sudden changes in their established growth patterns should alert the health professional to a potential nutrition problem (see Chapter 10).

In some cases physical problems such as scoliosis, contractures, or an in-

Table 21–1. Impact of Drugs on Nutrition.

DRUG	POTENTIAL NUTRITIONAL SIDE EFFECTS
Anticonvulsants	
Phenobarbital	Vitamin-D deficiency
Primidone (Mysoline)	rickets and fractures
Diphenylhydantoin	Folic-acid deficiency
(Dilantine)	macrocytic anemia
Valproic acid	adverse CNS effects
(Depakene)	Gingival hyperplasia
	Transient nausea/vomiting
Stimulants	Anorexia, inadequate intake, weight loss
Antidepressants	
Tricyclic	Gastrointestinal problems
	nausea, vomiting, diarrhea
	Altered appetite and taste acuity
	Thickening of saliva
	dry mouth, increased dental caries
Monoamine oxidase	With tyramine ingestion, headaches, palpitations, or hypertension
Tranquilizers/sedatives	Weight gain
	Altered taste acuity and appetite
Antibiotics	
Tetracycline	Gastrointestinal disturbances, loose stools
	Reduced vitamin-K absorption
	Reduced calcium and iron absorption
Trimethoprim	Folic-acid deficiency
	Increased phenylalanine levels

ability to stand make it impossible to obtain accurate length or height measurements in handicapped children. When accurate heights or lengths cannot be obtained, arm span, sitting height, leg length, and other body-segment measurements must be used as estimates of the child's growth. There are standards available for many of these body-segment measures as they relate to height in normal children (Lifshitz & Cervantes 1990), and the progressive increase over time of a particular body segment may offer evidence of growth in these children.

Growth charts for healthy children are not always appropriate for use in the handicapped child. Special growth charts are available for children with Down syndrome (Cronk et al 1988), Turner's syndrome (Lyon, Preece & Grant 1985), and premature babies (see Chapter 3). Other specific growth charts are available for other conditions (Lifshitz 1990). If a specific growth chart is not available, the child's ideal weight for length or height can be compared with their actual weight to determine the degree of under- or overnutrition.

Frequently, the diagnosis of failure to thrive (FTT) is made in patients who suffered intrauterine growth retardation (IUGR) (see Chapter 11). Because of the concern with their growth they may be subjected to unnecessary diagnostic and therapeutic studies. One such patient was evaluated twice for FTT, and forced feedings were advised and enforced to increase weight gain and growth, to no avail (Fig. 21–1). A cursory examination of the anthropometric measurements of this patient ruled out the diagnosis of FTT. He more than tripled his birth weight by 1 year of age and quadrupled it by 2 years. Similarly, his length remained proportional to weight throughout. FTT cannot be considered when birth weight is tripled within the first year of life, because this rate of growth occurs in normal children. However, when children start with a tremendous size deficit, they may be expected to remain proportionally small thereafter (see Chapter 11).

Although body-composition determinations may be helpful in assessing a child's muscle and fat mass, standards are not available for children with specific handicaps. However, serial body weight and body composition measurements will add more insight into the quality of weight changes and may be more reliable than weight alone as an index of fatness and undernutrition in these children.

The nutritional history of a handicapped child should record the type and amount of food consumed, the physical effort required for feeding, and the time needed to finish a meal. These babies may have a weak, slow suck and work very hard with each meal. Excessive sweating during feeding is an indication of the enormous efforts these small babies make to take nourishment. They may also require a long time to ingest small amounts, and many calories they receive are "used up" by the effort of feeding. The type and extent of feeding assistance required, oral–motor control, posture, and caretaker–child interaction are all important observations to make during a feeding assessment.

Although the benefits of medications in the treatment of certain problems seen in children with developmental disabilities cannot be denied, their adverse nutritional consequences should not be ignored (see Table 21–1). Some of these medications may directly cause nutritional deficiencies. For example, certain anticonvulsant drugs may lead to folic-acid deficiency, but folic acid supplementation may reduce the efficacy of the medication to control seizures (Baylis et al 1971). These medications also interfere with vitamin D metabolism, and children receiving long-term anticonvulsant therapy are at an increased risk for developing rickets (Lifshitz & MacLaren 1983). Handicapped children who are bedridden and are not exposed to sunlight are particularly prone to have low serum calcium (hypocalcemia) and phosphorus (hypophosphatemia) levels. As a consequence, they may have bone thinning (rickets) and frequent fractures, which can be prevented by increased dosages of vitamin D. Other medications may indirectly affect the child's nutrition by causing a loss of appetite, an alteration in taste perception, and gastrointestinal problems such as nausea, vomiting, diarrhea, and malabsorption.

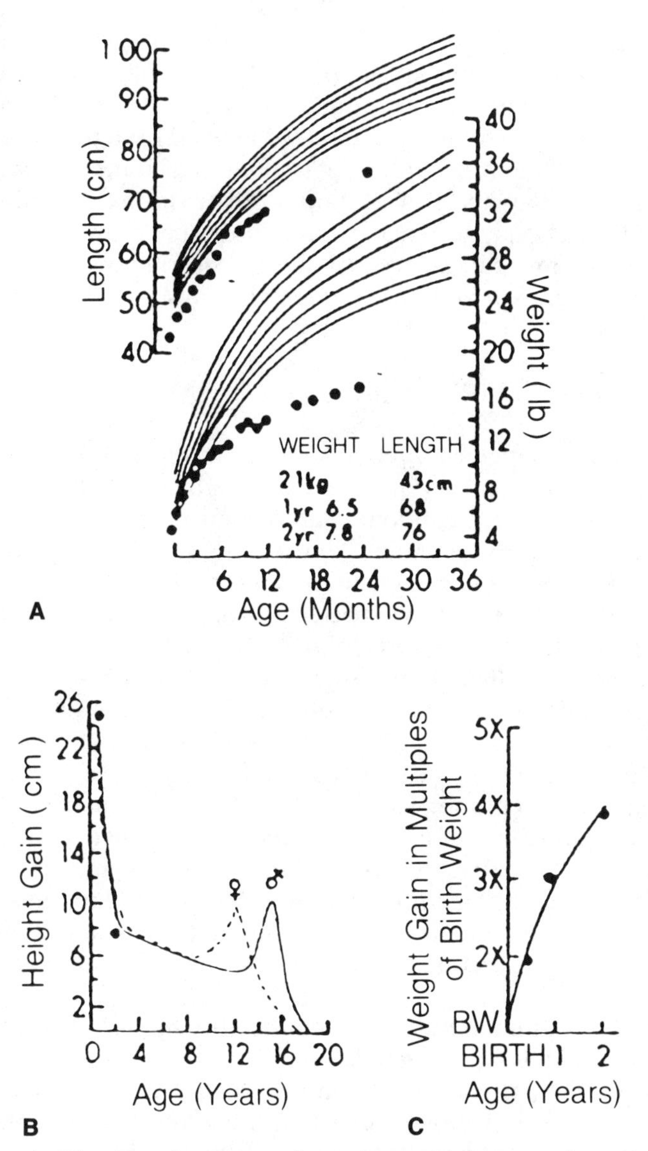

Figure 21–1. A. The growth pattern of a patient with intrauterine growth retardation. B and C. The height and weight velocities plotted against normal standards. Note that this patient did not have FTT despite the apparent fall off in length and weight because he was growing at a normal velocity.

Modified from Lifshitz F, Cervantes C. Short stature. In Lifshitz F, ed. Pediatric endocrinology. New York: Marcel Dekker, 1990:3–42.

The biochemical assessment of the nutritional status is similar for all children including those with handicaps and/or developmental disabilities (see Chapter 10). Since pica, the consumption of nonfood items, is frequently seen in mentally retarded children, serum lead levels should be routinely assessed (Gibson et al 1967) to rule out lead poisoning, which may be associated with developmental delay and FTT (Bithoney 1986, Davis & Svendsgaard 1987). Other specific tests may be needed if the nutritional assessment reveals ingestion of other noxious substances that may be contributing factors to the handicapped child's growth and developmental delays.

NUTRITIONAL NEEDS

Physically handicapped children differ from normal children in the way they grow, their physical activity, and their state of health, thereby affecting their nutritional needs. These children often demonstrate growth retardation and some type of motor dysfunction. They may be stiff (hypertonic) or limp (hypotonic). Therefore, the energy requirements for healthy children, which are based on age and sex given an expected rate of growth and activity, cannot be directly applied to handicapped children. The recommended energy requirements for these children should be based on their height rather than their age. For example, a 4-year-old handicapped girl with a height of only 35.5 inches (90 cm) has the average height of a 2½-year-old. Therefore, the energy needs for this child would be based on the RDAs for energy for a 2½-year-old rather than for her chronologic age of 4 years (see Chapter 9).

There are guidelines of estimated energy requirements for specific developmental disabilities that are based on the child's height (Table 21–2). However, these guidelines may not apply to infants and older adolescents. Any guideline is only an estimate of a child's needs. Growth and weight gain must be monitored to ensure an adequate intake while avoiding undernutrition and/or obesity.

No special vitamin or mineral is required by children with developmental disabilities. The RDAs are generally used as guidelines (Committee on Dietary Allowances 1989). The most common nutrient deficiencies seen in such patients include calcium, iron, and vitamin C (McKibbin, Toselana & Duckworth 1968, Peeles & Lomb 1951, Leamy 1953). Otherwise, these children, like all other children, need to eat a well-balanced, varied diet that provides all the necessary nutrients for health (see Chapter 9).

The use of vitamins in excess of normal requirements has often been advocated in the treatment of children with developmental disabilities (Rimland, Callaway & Dreyfus 1978, Feingold 1975). However, no benefit of such practices has been demonstrated on the intellectual and physical development of the developmentally disabled child (AAP 1981). Vitamin toxicity may result

Table 21–2. Recommended Energy Requirements for Children with Developmental Disabilities.

DEVELOPMENTAL DISABILITY	GUIDE FOR CALORIC INTAKE			
	kcal/kg	kcal/lb	kcal/cm	kcal/in.
Normal				
Infant 0–0.5 year	115	52	—	—
Infant 0.5–1 year	105	48	—	—
Toddler 1–3 years	100	45	14.4	36.6
Preschool 4–6 years	85	39	14.5	36.8
Down Syndrome				
Boys	—	—	16.1	40.9
Girls	—	—	14.3	36.3
Prader–Willi Syndrome				
For maintenance	—	—	10–11	26.7
For weight loss	—	—	8.5	21.6
Spina Bifida				
For weight loss*	—	—	7.0	17.8
Cerebral Palsy				
5–11 years, mild/moderate activity	—	—	13.9	35.3
5–11 years, limited activity	—	—	11.1	28.2

*Generally recommended to be 50 percent of the caloric requirements of a normal child.

from megavitamin therapy, with symptoms of nausea, vomiting, diarrhea, headaches, blurred vision, liver damage (Haslam, Dalby & Rademaker 1984), and many other problems (see Chapter 9). Families with developmentally disabled children are very vulnerable to unconventional and potentially dangerous nutritional claims to help their children. In many cases, these vitamin fallacies offer hope where there is no cure. Adherence to unconventional dietary treatments may divert attention and resources from the more needed psychosocial care and rehabilitation of the handicapped child.

Children with developmental disabilities may not be able to drink enough fluid because of physical deformities or mental deficits. Some children cannot communicate or understand their need to drink to quench thirst, and children who are tube-fed must rely on their caretakers to provide them with sufficient water. The use of concentrated formulas decreases the likelihood that a child's fluid requirements will be met. Excessive fluid losses because of diarrhea, vomiting, or mouth-breathing may require additional fluid to maintain adequate hydration status.

Under normal circumstances general fluid requirements are 1.0 to 1.5 milliliters of water for each calorie consumed. For example, a baby that requires 640 calories a day will need to receive 640 to 960 milliliters of water (2.5–3 cups) a day. The energy and water required can easily be provided by giving the child 32 ounces of milk formula. Infant formulas contain almost 90 percent water (see Chapter 13) and are balanced to provide the appropriate amount of water in relation to the calories supplied. However, when more concentrated formulas are used, or when there are excessive fluid losses, care must be taken to ensure sufficient water intake. Weight loss of greater than 5 percent of body weight, dry mucous membranes, sunken eyeballs with absence of tears, reduced skin turgor, and limited urine output are all signs and symptoms of dehydration (Hochman, Grodin & Crone 1979).

COMMON NUTRITION PROBLEMS

Underweight and Failure to Thrive

It is not uncommon for children with developmental disabilities to have slow growth and be underweight. Although there may be a specific genetic predisposition for some handicapped children to be small, impaired nutrient intake owing to oral–motor dysfunction, increased energy needs, and malabsorption are causes of nutritional FTT in the developmentally disabled child. Specific problems such as gagging, vomiting, and rumination often develop in handicapped children due to inappropriate oral reflexes.

Gagging is a normal oral reflex that prevents food from being swallowed or inhaled into the trachea (windpipe). A strong, overactive gag reflex may interfere with a child's ability to chew and swallow solid foods, whereas a weak gag reflex may lead to aspiration and choking. Gagging may also be a behavioral ploy by children to get attention or express dislike for a given food. An occupational or speech therapist may need to work with the child and the mother to lessen or strengthen the gag reflex.

Rumination, the process of returning already-swallowed food back to the mouth to be rechewed and swallowed, is frequently reported in children with developmental disabilities (Kalisz & Ekvall 1978). As with vomiting, it may lead to dehydration, aspiration pneumonia, gastrointestinal blood loss, and malnutrition. It may also be the cause of dental problems. Rumination may be caused by psychologic disturbances such as inappropriate mother–child interaction or may be a result of an organic problem associated with vomiting and gastrointestinal reflux. Therefore, an interdisciplinary approach including a physician, speech/occupational therapist, psychologist, nutritionist, and dentist is warranted for the care of children with these inappropriate behaviors as well as to care for all patients who fail to thrive (see Chapter 16).

Overweight and Obesity

Developmentally disabled children, especially those with Down syndrome, mental retardation, spina bifida (myelomeningocele), spastic cerebral palsy, and Prader–Willi syndrome are often overweight and may become severely obese. The inability to be physically active appears to be an important part in the etiology of excess weight gain and accumulation of fat. Being overweight makes it even more difficult to care for these children, who depend on the physical support of others.

The recommended treatment of overweight or obesity in handicapped children is similar to the approach taken in normal children (see Chapter 18). However, it is even more difficult for handicapped children to lose weight given the limited ability to exercise and to elicit their cooperation and motivation. Children with Prader–Willi syndrome exhibit an uncontrollable urge to eat excessive amounts of food. Therefore, prevention of obesity must be part of the care of infants and children with this handicap since they are at risk of becoming obese.

In addition to an appropriate dietary intake, children who are unable to do traditional exercises such as running or biking need to incorporate other types of physical activity to help them maintain a normal rate of weight gain. For example, children with spina bifida who cannot use their legs may learn to swim or use a special exercise bicycle with hand pedals. Almost all handicapped and developmentally disabled children are able to exercise in some fashion, and this should be encouraged not only to maintain a balance of energy needs but also as a very good way to improve health and self-worth (see Chapter 14). Olympics and other competitive sports for the handicapped are already a part of our lives!

CLINICAL INTERVENTION

For the handicapped child, timely and appropriate nutritional intervention is essential to limit the deficits imposed by the underlying medical condition and to maximize growth and development. In deciding what course to take for feeding a handicapped child, the medical and nutritional history must be considered. For example, Steven, a 4-month-old baby with Down syndrome and congenital heart disease, had difficulty ingesting adequate nutrition to gain weight and to grow. He had been failing to gain weight since birth, and he weighed only 10 pounds (4.6 kg). Given the seriousness of his heart condition, surgery to repair the problem was needed but it had to be postponed until he gained weight and was in better nutritional health. When Steven was given bottle feedings of a standard infant formula providing 20 calories per ounce, he would tire easily and sweat profusely. It would take him at least an hour to take only 4 ounces of formula, and he was only consuming about 15 ounces a day. Given the underlying medical condition and the increased energy expenditures the estimated caloric requirements for this child were as high as 150 calories per kilogram of body weight. This baby would therefore need to take at least 34 ounces a day of regular infant formula to meet his calorie requirements.

To meet Steven's nutritional needs, increasing the caloric density of the formula might be considered. A more concentrated preparation of the infant formula can be used to provide 24 or even 27 calories per ounce. However, even if the baby were to tolerate this stronger formula with a higher osmotic load, the baby would receive only 405 calories a day (88 kcal/kg body weight) if he was able to take the same 15 ounces as before. This level would still be insufficient to allow him to grow.

Nutritional supplements such as modular carbohydrate or fat supplements used to increase the caloric density of formula were also considered for this baby. Although these products add calories, they do not add protein, vitamins, or minerals. Therefore, their use may dilute the nutritional quality of the formula and result in protein and other nutrient deficiencies (see Chapters 3 and 27). Also, using carbohydrate modular supplements or even adding cereal and fruit as a means of increasing calories may do more harm than good in patients with heart defects or pulmonary disease. The metabolism of carbohydrates is associated with increased carbon dioxide production, and the need to expire excess carbon dioxide may further exacerbate compromised respiratory function.

Therefore, the only reasonable solution for this baby who could not take adequate nutrition by mouth was tube feedings (see Chapter 27). Continuous tube feedings have been shown to improve an infant's ability to tolerate larger amounts of formula without causing heart failure and to improve their absorptive capacity (Vanderhoof et al 1982). Infants with congenital heart defects receiving continuous enteral feedings gain weight and thereby can tolerate an earlier and a safer surgical intervention. A standard infant formula could be fed continuously through a nasogastric tube. It would be prudent to start with the same total volume of 15 to 16 ounces that Steven was able to take by mouth and infuse the formula over a 24-hour period infusion rate of 20 milliliters per hour. The volume of feeding should be gradually increased until the baby gains weight at a rate of 30 grams per day or less if the baby's fluid tolerance is reached earlier. If necessary, the formula may be more concentrated (24–27 kcal/oz) to ensure adequate intake within the fluid restrictions imposed by the heart disease.

Special formulas that are low in sodium may not be necessary for infants with congenital heart defects and FTT. Regular infant formulas contain a relatively low sodium content that mimics breast milk: approximately 230 milligrams (10 mEq) of sodium per liter of formula. A formula lower in sodium, such as Similac PM 60/40, provides only three quarters of the sodium content of regular infant formula and therefore might be insufficient to cover the baby's basal sodium needs of 2 to 3 milliequivalents per 100 calories consumed. In addition, these babies might have increased sodium losses since they are usually given diuretics and other sodium-wasting medications.

Some babies with congenital heart disease may not be able to grow despite the best possible nutritional treatment. The heart defect may be so severe that no matter how hard one tries to provide adequate nutrition, it is impossible to keep up with the increased energy requirements and altered metabolism secondary to the disease, and/or to avoid cardiac failure. The only hope for such babies is to correct their cardiac defect by surgical intervention and to provide aggressive nutritional rehabilitation after the surgery.

Children with developmental disabilities who have feeding problems can be taught to accept food by mouth with proper "feeding" therapy. The use of special feeding utensils, such as thick plastic spoons, special nipples, and adaptive drinking devices, as well as proper postural support of a correctly positioned hand to steady the jaw and specially designed wheelchairs or feeding seats may be necessary (Fig. 21–2 to 21–4). Also, the texture of the diet is very important to handicapped children. Their ability to eat, as well as to enhance the development of oral motor skills, may depend on the type of food given. Some children will never advance from a pureed diet, while others may accept only very soft-textured food. These children often do not accept hard, more textured foods owing to mouth tenderness or simply the refusal to accept any dietary changes.

In a pureed diet, all the foods are blended to a smooth consistency appro-

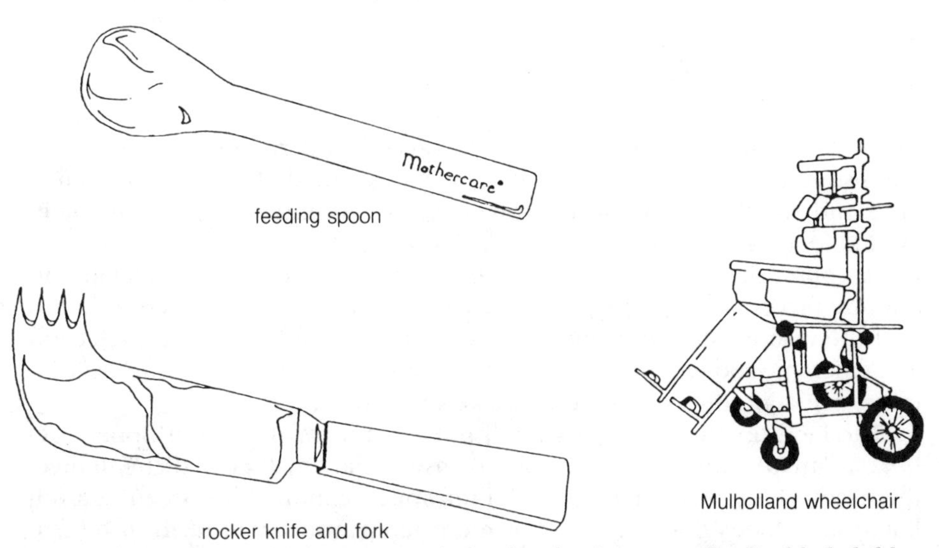

Figure 21–2. Special feeding utensils for the developmentally disabled child.
From Heinrichs E, Rokusek C. Nutrition and feeding for the developmentally disabled. South Dakota State Medical Association, 1985. Developed by South Dakota University Affiliated Facility Center for the Developmentally Disabled, and South Dakota Department of Education and Cultural Affairs Child and Adult Nutrition Services.

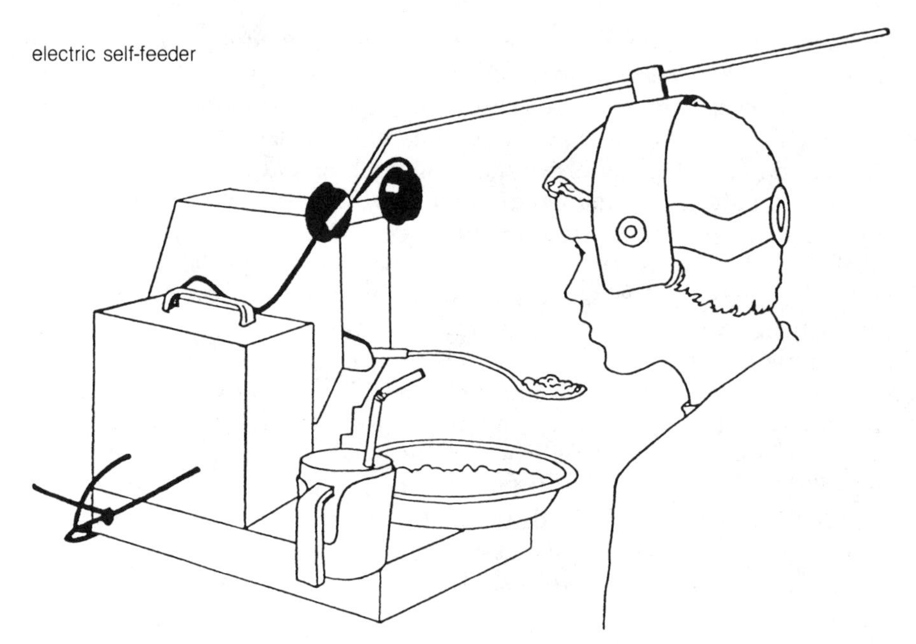

Figure 21–3. Special feeding utensils for the developmentally disabled child. From Heinrichs E, Rokusek C. Nutrition and feeding for the developmentally disabled. South Dakota State Medical Association, 1985. Developed by South Dakota University Affiliated Facility Center for the Developmentally Disabled, and South Dakota Department of Education and Cultural Affairs Child and Adult Nutrition Services.

priate for a child who cannot chew or swallow properly. However, different foods should not be blended together. Each food should have its own unique taste and smell and should be appetizing. A ground diet contains finely ground foods as well as soft fruits and vegetables that are easy to chew; this diet is appropriate for a child who cannot chew but can swallow. Soft foods in bite-size pieces are appropriate for the child with more advanced oral motor skills. New foods should be introduced gradually to avoid complete rejection of a different food texture. Foods that are sweet such as cookies and fruit increase saliva production and may make swallowing easier.

The food texture of a diet should not interfere with its nutritional adequacy. Careful planning is necessary to ensure that any type of diet will meet the needs of a growing child. For handicapped children who require a full liquid diet, foods that are liquid at room temperature will need to be fed. Some variability in consistency may be included depending on the feeding skills of the child. For example, blended meat in broth may be included if the child is able to control swallowing of slightly thickened feedings.

The following is an example of a full liquid diet for a 3-year-old handicapped girl who weighs 28½ pounds (13 kg).

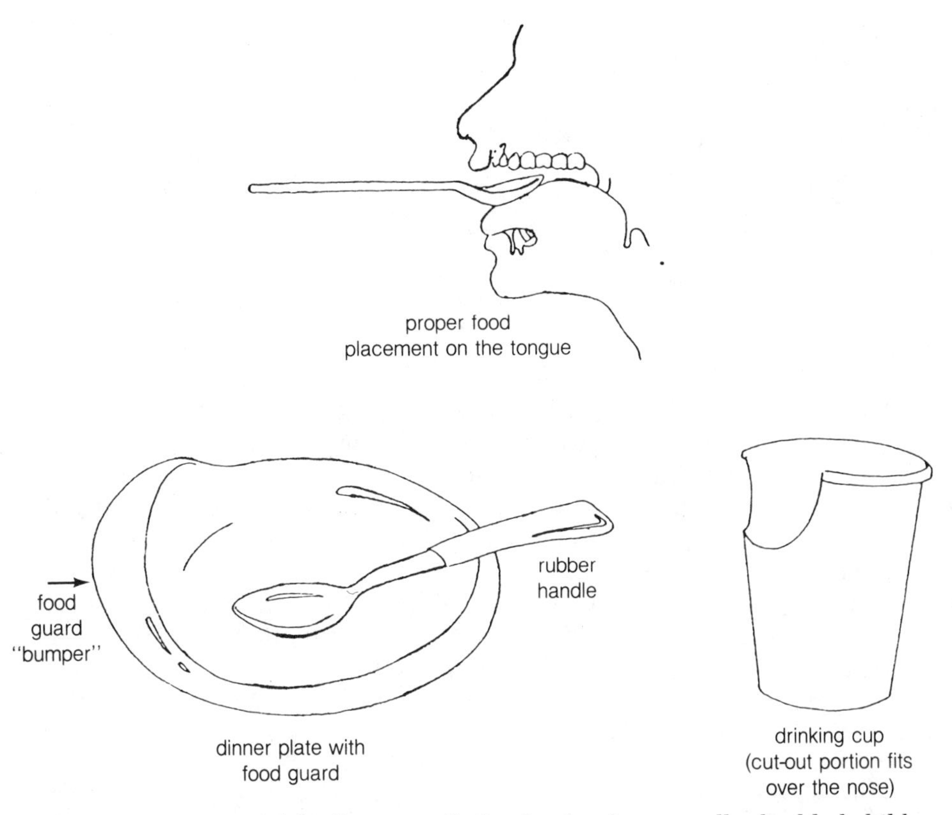

Figure 21–4. Special feeding utensils for the developmentally disabled child.
From Heinrichs E, Rokusek C. Nutrition and feeding for the developmentally disabled. South Dakota State Medical Association, 1985. Developed by South Dakota University Affiliated Facility Center for the Developmentally Disabled, and South Dakota Department of Education and Cultural Affairs Child and Adult Nutrition Services.

MENU 1

Breakfast
½ cup refined cooked cereal (Cream of Wheat, rice, or farina)
½ cup orange juice
½ cup whole milk
½ tsp. margarine

Snack
½ cup eggnog

Lunch
½ cup cream of vegetable soup
½ cup whole milk
½ cup pureed fruit

Snack
½ cup milkshake with instant breakfast powder

Dinner
½ cup cream of potato soup
½ cup blended beef in broth
½ cup whole milk

Snack
½ cup cooked, strained cereal
½ tsp. margarine
½ cup juice

This full liquid diet designed for Jane meets all of her nutritional needs with the exception of zinc. However, some children with severe feeding difficulties may not be able to tolerate eggs or blended red meats, which are excellent sources of iron, zinc, and vitamin B_{12}. In such cases, the handicapped child might benefit from a nutritionally complete formula designed as a meal replacement (see Chapter 27). Small, frequent feedings are recommended with a full liquid diet to ensure that the child takes enough fluid without becoming too full at each meal. Overfeeding may lead to problems with gastrointestinal reflux, vomiting, and eventually obesity.

If the patient's feeding skills are more advanced, progression to a soft diet with greater food texture is indicated. A typical menu of a soft, "lumpy" diet that is appropriate for a 5-year-old child who is learning to chew but who can swallow foods is given below.

MENU 2

Breakfast
½ cup unsweetened cereal
½ cup whole milk
½ ripe banana
½ cup orange juice

Snack
2 white crackers without seeds
1 tsp. cream cheese
1 tablespoon raisin puree (2 tablespoons raisins with juice)
½ cup apple juice

Lunch
1 ounce finely ground meat stewed in broth
½ cup tender, well-cooked carrots and peas
½ cup whole milk
½ cup plain custard

Snack
canned peaches without skin
½ cup whole milk

Dinner
½ cup well-cooked vegetable soup
½ cup macaroni with tomato sauce (may be blended with sauce to avoid stickiness)
grated cheese
½ cup whole milk

Snack
½ cup plain ice cream

This menu provides foods that can be swallowed without chewing so that choking is minimized. It is relatively high in sodium (2152 mg) and low in zinc and copper, primarily owing to the commercially prepared soups and gravies; homemade products with limited added salt can be substituted for these ready-to-use products if controlled sodium intake is required. As with any diet a variety of foods helps to ensure nutritional adequacy.

Handicapped children require special attention in accordance with their specific problems to ensure that their nutritional intake is adequate. The complete nutritional arsenal, ranging from tube feedings, to liquid diets, to pureed food, to regular, well-balanced diets needs to be used to feed infants and children with developmental disabilities at various stages of their lives. If the major concern is FTT, the infant and child should be managed according to the guidelines discussed in Chapter 18. On the other hand, overweight children with developmental disabilities may require more specific interventional strategies than typically applied for overweight children without handicaps. As always, the goal is nutritional health!

REFERENCES

American Academy of Pediatrics. Policy Statement: Megavitamins and mental retardation. Elk Grove Village, IL: American Academy of Pediatrics, August, 1981.

Baylis EM, Crowley JM, Preece JM, Sylvester PE, Marks V. Influence of folic acid on blood-phenytoin levels. Lancet 1971; 1:62–64.

Bithoney WG. Elevated lead levels in children with nonorganic failure to thrive. Pediatrics 1986; 78:891–895.

Brown JE, Davis E, Flemming PL. Nutritional assessment of children with cerebral palsy in the Lakeville Sanatorium. Am J Public Health 1953; 43:1310–1317.

Committee on Dietary Allowances, Food and Nutrition Board, National Research

Council. Recommended dietary allowances. 10th ed. Washington, D.C.: National Academy of Sciences, 1989.
Cronk C, Crocker AC, Pueschel SM, et al. Growth charts for children with Down Syndrome: 1 month to 18 years of age. Pediatrics 1988; 81:102–110.
Davis JM, Svendsgaard DJ. Lead and child development. Nature 1987; 329:297–300.
Feingold BF. Why your child is hyperactive. New York: Random House, 1975.
Gibson SLM, Lam CN, McCrae WM, et al. Blood lead levels in normal and mentally deficient children. Arch Dis Child 1967; 42:573–578.
Haslam RHA, Dalby JT, Rademaker AW. Effects of megavitamin therapy on children with attention deficit disorders. Pediatrics 1984; 74:103–111.
Hochman HI, Grodin MA, Crone RK. Dehydration, diabetic ketoacidosis, and shock in the pediatric patient. Pediatr Clin North Am 1979; 26:803–826.
Joos SK, Pollitt E. Nutritional status and behavior. In Grand RJ, Sutphen JL, Dietz WH, eds. Pediatric nutrition: Theory and practice. Boston: Butterworth, 1987:307–312.
Kalisz K, Ekvall S. Rumination. In Pediatric nutrition in developmental disorders. Springfield, IL: Charles C. Thomas, 1978.
Leamy CM. A study of the food intakes of a group of children with cerebal palsy in the Lakeville Sanatorium. Am J Public Health 1953; 43:1310–1317.
Lifshitz F, Cervantes C. Short stature. In Lifshitz F, ed. Pediatric endocrinology. New York: Marcel Dekker, 1990:3–42.
Lifshitz F, MacLaren NK. Vitamin D dependent rickets in institutionalized mentally retarded children receiving long term anticonvulsant therapy. J Pediatr 1983; 83:612–620.
Lifshitz F. Pediatric endocrinology. New York: Marcel Dekker, 1990:983–1051.
Lyon AJ, Preece MA, Grant DB. Growth curve for girls with Turner syndrome. Arch Dis Child 1985; 60:932–935.
McKibbin B, Toselana PA, Duckworth T. Abnormalities in vitamin C metabolism in spina bifida. Dev Med Child Neurol 1968; 15 (Suppl): 55–57.
Peeles S, Lomb MW. Comments on the dietary practices of cerebral palsied children. J Am Diet Assoc 1951; 27:870.
Pollitt E, Saco-Pollitt C, Leibel RL, Viteri FE. Iron deficiency and behavioral development in infants and preschool children. Am J Clin Nutr 1988; 43:555–565.
Rimland B, Callaway E, Dreyfus P. The effect of high doses of vitamin B_6 upon autistic children: A double-blind cross-over study. Am J Psychiatry 1978; 135:472–475.
Thommessen M, Riis G, Kase BF. Nutrition and growth retardation in 10 children with congenital deaf-blindness. J Am Diet Assoc 1989; 89:69–73.
Torin B, Viteri FE. Protein-energy malnutrition. In Shils ME, Young VR, eds. Modern nutrition in health and disease. Philadelphia: Lea & Febiger, 1988:746–773.
Vanderhoof JA, Hofschire RJ, Baluff MA, et al. Continuous enteral feedings. An important adjunct to the management of complex congenital heart disease. Am J Dis Child 1982; 136:825–827.

22

Diabetes Mellitus

When Dr. Morton Ryder, a 1918 graduate of Cornell University Medical College, journeyed to Toronto in June 1922 to see Dr. Frederick Banting, the survival of Ryder's diabetic nephew was much in doubt. This young boy had developed diabetes mellitus 2 years earlier and was expected to die soon. Weighing only 26 pounds, 5-year-old Teddy Ryder had been kept alive by the only known treatment for diabetes: a near-starvation diet consisting of jellies, washed-bran cookies, and cabbage. After his first meal of this extremely restrictive diet in the hospital Teddy commented, "Mama, they don't know how to feed little boys here." Years later he would recall, "They'd give you cabbage; they'd cook this stuff three times, they'd throw out the juice and with it most of the flavor. So you had this sort of colorless, tasteless roughage, and I guess you thought you'd eaten after you finished it." Luckily, in February 1922 a newspaper report from Toronto broke the electrifying news of the insulin experiments of Drs. Banting and Best. Dr. Ryder worked quickly to obtain insulin for his nephew. Teddy's life began again and he was able to eat what he liked! Today, thanks to his uncle's intervention, Ted Ryder lives comfortably in his West Hartford apartment, having taken insulin longer than anyone else in the world. He is 71 years old (Wardner 1988).

The day-to-day management of patients with diabetes mellitus is very demanding despite the great advances made since the discovery of insulin. We now know that there are different types of diabetes mellitus. The two major forms are the juvenile form, more appropriately known as insulin-dependent diabetes mellitus (type I, IDDM), which results from insulin deficiency, and the adult form, non–insulin-dependent (type II, NIDDM). The symptoms are similar; patients with diabetes may complain of the 3 Ps—polydipsia (severe thirst), polyuria (excess urine), and polyphagia (excess eating), which result from either a lack of insulin (type I) or an inability of insulin to exert its action despite excess levels (type II). Either of the two types of diabetes can occur at any age, but type I is more frequent in children. Even today the long-term outlook of many patients with diabetes is bleak despite their best efforts and those of their families and physicians. By 20 years' duration of the disease, a great majority of these patients will have developed small-artery disease of vital organs such as the kidneys and eyes and atherosclerosis, and may suffer a premature death.

NUTRITION AS A CAUSE OF OR RISK FACTOR FOR DIABETES MELLITUS

It was long suspected that nutrition played a major part in the development of diabetes mellitus. Populations in countries who "Westernized" their diet and lifestyle also coincidentally "Westernized" the incidence of diabetes mellitus. This was observed in Japan after World War II and in Israel among the new Eastern immigrants settling in a Westernized Israeli culture, as well as among aboriginal populations (Cohen, Teitelbaum & Saliternik 1972, Wicking et al 1981). Under these circumstances up to a tenfold increase in the risk of developing diabetes mellitus occurred (West 1974a, Wicking et al 1981).

Obesity is the major link between nutrition and the increased risk of developing diabetes mellitus. We have known for many years that the greater the degree and the longer the duration of the adiposity, the higher the risk in susceptible individuals of developing the disease (West & Kalbfleich 1971). However, it is not known whether an excess caloric intake or the type of dietary carbohydrate or fat triggers the development of the disease. An increased incidence of diabetes seems to parallel increased sugar consumption (Cohen, Teitelbaum & Saliternick 1972, West 1974a). However, greater sugar consumption is often associated with high-fat and high-calorie intake, as well as with lifestyle changes such as decreased exercise. Older studies in human beings suggest that sugar and fat may not be important contributing factors to the incidence of diabetes apart from their effects on the level of caloric consumption and effects on the amount of fat in the body (West & Kalbfleich 1971, West 1972, 1974a, 1974b). However, experimental animal studies demonstrated that refined sugars by themselves might increase the risk of developing diabetes mellitus (Cohen, Teitelbaum & Saliternik 1972). Other nutritional factors that may be associated with the increased risk of developing IDDM include high-protein feedings (Elliot & Martin 1984), food additives (Helgason & Jonasson 1981), and low-fiber diets (Trowell 1974). It has also been reported that a large number of diabetic children were never breast-fed (Borch-Johnsen 1984), and/or were fed soy-protein formula in infancy (Fort et al 1986). However, the amount of food and the total caloric intake remain the most important factors for increasing the risk of developing diabetes mellitus. A reduction in the amount of food consumption without any other dietary changes reduces the incidence of diabetes dramatically (Gerritsen et al 1974).

Specific nutritional deficiencies may also have a role in the development of diabetes mellitus (Table 22–1). Vitamin and mineral deficiencies, such as zinc, chromium, manganese, copper, magnesium, or vitamin B_6, may lead to high blood glucose levels (Kirchgessner, Roth & Weigand 1976). Vitamin E- and selenium-deficient diets have also been shown to increase the susceptibility to diabetes by decreasing the antioxidant, protective state of the organism. Under these conditions the organism becomes susceptible to injury by free radicals, which may lead to pancreatic beta-cell damage and insulin deficiency (Slonim et al 1983, Beherns et al 1986). Vitamin C deficiency has also been implicated in diabetes mellitus by enhancing platelet aggregation, leading to an increased tendency to blood clotting (Pecoraro & Chen 1987).

Although specific nutrient deficiencies may result in impaired glucose tolerance, their role in clinical diabetes is less certain. The micronutrient status in diabetic patients varies greatly (Mooradian & Morley 1987) and their serum vitamin and mineral levels may be low, normal, or high as compared with nondiabetic matched peers. These serum levels may also vary in accordance with many different clinical factors, such as degree of sugar excretion in the urine, duration of the illness, and/or dietary intake.

Table 22–1. Micronutrient Status of Type I Diabetic Patients.

MICRONUTRIENT	USUAL LEVELS IN BLOOD*
Trace elements	
Zinc (Zn)	↓
Calcium (Ca)	↓
Magnesium (Mg)	↓
Manganese (Mn)	↓
Copper (Cu)	↓ or NL
Iron (Fe)	NL
Chromium (Cr)	↑
Selenium (Se)	↑
Vitamins	
1,24-Dihydroxycholecalciferol	↓
B_6	NL or ↓
B_{12}	NL or ↓
C	NL or ↓
Thiamin	NL
A	?
E	↑

*↓ = decreased; ↑ = increased; NL =normal; ? = unknown.

Modified from Mooradian AD, Morley JE: Micronutrient status in diabetes mellitus. Am J Clin Nutr 1987; 45:877–895.

In addition, the role of vitamin and mineral therapy on the evolution of the disease itself remains unclear. For example, zinc and chromium deficiency may diminish insulin secretion and reduce insulin effectiveness. Therapeutic doses of chromium but not zinc improves both of these factors. Serum magnesium concentrations in diabetic patients are usually reduced, but replacement therapy is difficult and without evident benefit. Supplementation with vitamin C has not been proven useful since it does not prevent the increased tendency to form blood clots in diabetic patients. On the other hand, nicotinamide supplements are believed to slow the destruction of pancreatic beta cells in newly diagnosed diabetics, thereby extending the "honeymoon phase" of the disease (Vague et al 1985).

NUTRITION AND THE COMPLICATIONS OF DIABETES MELLITUS

Short-Term Complications

Nutrition has a very important role in the acute complications of diabetes. What the patient eats directly affects blood sugar levels. Other factors influencing blood sugar levels include the time between insulin injection and food intake, the type of insulin, and the number and timing of meals and snacks. For example, an individual with diabetes who ingests an overload of sugar may develop high blood sugar (hyperglycemia), which then requires more insulin treatment. The blood glucose level may then fall to a low level, which requires ingestion of sugar. A possible vicious cycle, leading to poor control, may ensue. Dietary factors have also been implicated in other metabolic consequences of diabetes, such as ketosis. The presence of by-products of fat metabolism—ketones—in the blood occurs when fat is used for energy because glucose is unavailable to the cells (West 1974a, Helgason & Jonasson 1981). Sometimes one of the ketones, acetone, will appear in the urine of a diabetic individual following intake of a high-fat meal.

Nutritional management, not insulin alone, is necessary for diabetic patients. For example, Pete, $5^{10}/_{12}$ years of age, received insulin twice daily. This was considered insufficient since he had high blood sugar levels and high sugar excretion in the urine. He also showed a high level of glucose bound to hemoglobin (glycosylated hemoglobin), which is indicative of long-term poor control. Despite increased dosages of insulin, Pete continued to excrete large quantities of glucose in his urine and demonstrated high fasting blood glucose levels, yet he gained 13 pounds of weight (6 kg) in 12 months (Fig. 22–1). Patients who are not receiving sufficient insulin are in negative nitrogen balance and will not gain weight. A patient such as Pete, who is gaining excessive weight, is not lacking insulin; hence he must be overeating. Indeed,

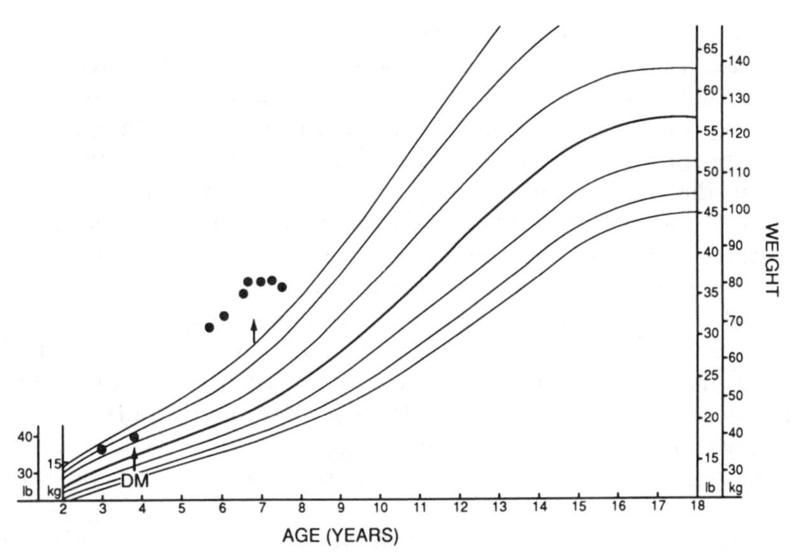

Figure 22–1. Overeating in IDDM. This child developed diabetes mellitus (DM) at age $3^{10}/_{12}$ years. He was treated with insulin twice daily in increasing dosages yet he had poor control of the disease. He had a very high blood sugar level and constantly excreted excess sugar in the urine. Additionally, his glucose-bound hemoglobin (glycosylated hemoglobin) was high, which indicated long-term poor control. When a nutritionist intervened and dietary and exercise changes were made (↑), he ceased gaining weight and his diabetes control improved.

a look at his weight chart clearly shows that he became obese after age $3^{10}/_{12}$ years when he was diagnosed as having diabetes mellitus. He was afraid of insulin reactions and was overeating. When changes in the basic dietary intake and caloric expenditures were made, there was an improvement in the control of the disease and he ceased gaining excess weight.

Long-Term Complications

The long-term complications of diabetes have long been related to nutritional intake (West 1972, West 1974a). For example, diabetics in Japan have less gangrene and coronary artery disease than diabetics in Western countries. Diabetics among the Navajo Indians in America, the African Nigerians, and the Pacific populations also have a lower incidence of hardening of the small blood vessels of vital organs than do other populations with this disease (West 1972, West 1974a). This finding may be related to the nutrition habits of these groups of patients; that is, their lower intake of animal fats. However, genetic factors that immunologically alter the pancreatic beta cell may be critical in determining the effect of the environmental input (diet) on the expression of the disease and/or its complications (Zimmet 1979).

Coronary Artery Disease. Coronary artery disease is the second leading cause of death for individuals who have had IDDM for more than 30 years (National Diabetes Advisory Board 1985). The number of cardiovascular deaths is reportedly 11 times greater in these patients than in age- and sex-matched peers (dorman et al 1984). Also, one third of all non–insulin-dependent diabetic individuals die of coronary artery disease. Of the risk factors for coronary artery disease, serum cholesterol and other fats in the blood are the most responsive to dietary intervention. Epidemologic surveys and dietary intervention trials provide strong evidence that dietary fat and cholesterol restriction can exert favorable influences on plasma lipid levels (Hoeg & Brewer 1987). Appropriate treatment of diabetes mellitus, which includes dietary management and exercise, is clearly associated with prompt improvement in plasma very-low-density lipoprotein (VLDL) and low-density lipoprotein (LDL) concentrations (the "bad" type of cholesterols) and increased high-density lipoproteins (HDL) (the "good" type of cholesterol).

Renal Disease. Renal disease poses an even more imminent threat to individuals with IDDM than coronary artery disease. Renal disease accounts for one half of all deaths in IDDM, and end-stage renal disease is the primary cause of death in diabetic children between 15 and 30 years (Dorman et al 1984). Traditionally, diabetic dietary recommendations have emphasized a low-carbohydrate, low-fat, high-protein diet. However, excessive protein ingestion may play a role in the loss of kidney function owing to an increase in renal blood flow, which results in an increased glomerular filtration rate and structural changes (Laouri et al 1982). It appears that high protein intake may increase the work load of the kidney; protein restriction could restore appropriate glomerular filtration load before structural changes have advanced to overt nephropathy (see Chapter 23). Thus, it seems prudent to maintain protein intake at recommended levels for growing children and to avoid excess protein intakes.

NUTRITION IN THE MANAGEMENT OF DIABETES MELLITUS

To develop a rational approach to the treatment of diabetes with appropriate dietary objectives and strategies, one must understand the human nutrition needs of the normal population and of children at different stages of life (see Chapter 9). We now know that diabetic patients should follow the same standards for human nutrition as the normal population (ADA 1987, Nuttail 1980). The concept of the "diabetic diet" or "exchange diets" can be replaced by appropriate food selections and eating patterns that conform to general nutritional recommendations. However, IDDM individuals need to eat more regularly than others to minimize blood glucose variations and to provide calories at the time of maximum insulin action in order to ensure efficient energy utilization (Fig. 22–2). Nutritional adjustments are important during periods of illness and other stresses. Decisions regarding food intake in IDDM patients should be individualized, depending upon blood and/or urine glucose monitoring, lifestyle, physical activity, type of insulin, and time and site of insulin administration. Timing of snacks may change with use of different types of insulin as they have different peak effects and duration of action (Lifshitz & Fort 1984).

In adult diabetic patients who do not require insulin treatment, a reduction of body fat by dietary restriction of calories and increased exercise are most important (Strefa, Boyko & Rabkin 1981). Return to normal glucose tolerance is possible but uncommon in these patients, primarily because of the difficulties in weight reduction and weight maintenance. However, even a small amount of weight loss may help control the diabetes and alleviate the need for oral medications.

Most young individuals with diabetes require insulin for treatment and, thus, calorie restrictions are usually not needed. Often during periods of catch-up growth, for example, following recovery from various illnesses or ketoacidosis, the required caloric intake can be enormous. Caloric requirements should be dictated by age, sex, and activity as well as by individual variability to provide for normal growth and development. Individual appetites are usually the best indicators of calorie needs and can be the sole determinant of total dietary intake unless excessive or inadequate weight gain is occurring.

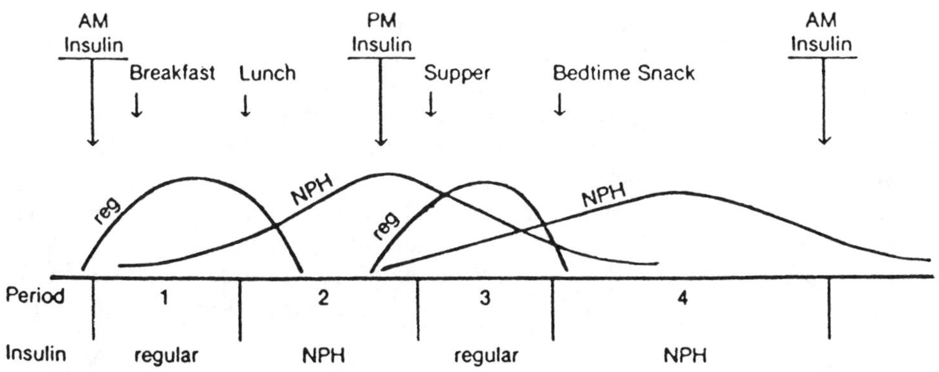

Figure 22–2. The timing and action of two different types of insulin. The consumption of meals at regular intervals in relation to the insulin shots is essential to maintain appropriate blood sugar levels and to ensure adequate control of the disease and nutrition of the patient.

From Chase PH. Understanding insulin dependent diabetes. 6th ed. Denver: The Guild of the Children's Diabetes Foundation at Denver, 1988.

Carbohydrate restriction has not been recommended in IDDM for many years (West 1973a) because insulin requirements are related more to total fuel supply than to the amount of carbohydrate ingested. When carbohydrate is restricted, the diet is too high in fat, cholesterol, and protein, which may contribute to the higher incidence of coronary heart disease and atherosclerosis. Thus, the amount of carbohydrate in the diet should be liberalized and individualized, ideally up to 55 to 60 percent of total calories, but refined sugars should be reduced in the diet of diabetics, as for all healthy human beings.

Glycemic Index

For years the dietary recommendations for diabetics were based on the belief that all carbohydrate foods act in predictable ways—namely, that complex carbohydrates such as starches cause a lower rise in blood glucose than simple, rapidly absorbed carbohydrates such as sugar. Recently, investigators have attempted to classify individual foods by the extent to which they raise blood glucose values. This is called the "glycemic index," which was developed by measuring the response of blood glucose to 50 grams of carbohydrate portions of common foods and assigning each food a relative value (Jenkins et al 1984).

The insulin dose given to IDDM patients was found to be the main factor in the glycemic response to mixed meals containing various types of carbohydrate (Weyman-Daum et al 1987). When a proper adjustment of the insulin dose is made, the type of carbohydrate in a mixed meal does not appear to have significant effects on blood glucose levels in children with longstanding IDDM (Fig. 22–3 and 22–4). The idea that a judicious selection of carbohydrate-containing foods can effectively control blood sugar levels captured the imagination of many physicians and health care professionals. The movement toward accepting a "glycemic index" in the selection of foods gathered momentum rapidly. However, the Council of the American Diabetes Association concluded that current evidence does not permit a precise appraisal of the clinical utility of the glycemic index (ADA 1986). On the other hand, there are data indicating that the diet has an important impact on insulin requirements, but that when insulin requirements are met normal blood glucose levels (euglycemia) prevail regardless of the type of food consumed (Vlachokosta et al 1988). To date, there is no evidence that the clinical course of diabetes is improved by the long-term intake of foods with a low glycemic index.

Fiber

An increase in dietary fiber has been associated with lower plasma glucose levels in patients with diabetes. Unrefined soluble fiber—that is, fiber primarily from fruits and vegetables—is most effective in decreasing the plasma glu-

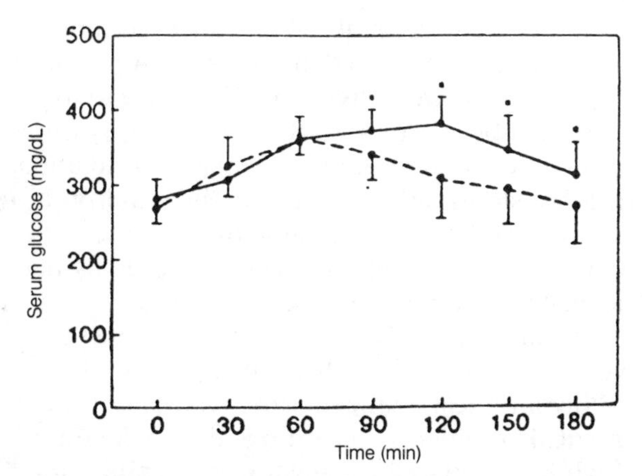

Figure 22–3. The glycemic response after a high-glycemic (solid line) and a low-glycemic (broken line) breakfast when no adjustment of insulin was made. Data are mean ±SEM. * = a significant difference between groups ($P<0.05$) at that time point by post-hoc t test.

Data from Weyman-Daum M, Fort P, Recker B, Lifshitz F. Glycemic response in children with insulin dependent diabetes mellitus after high or low glycemic index breakfast. Am J Clin Nutr 1987; 46:798–803.

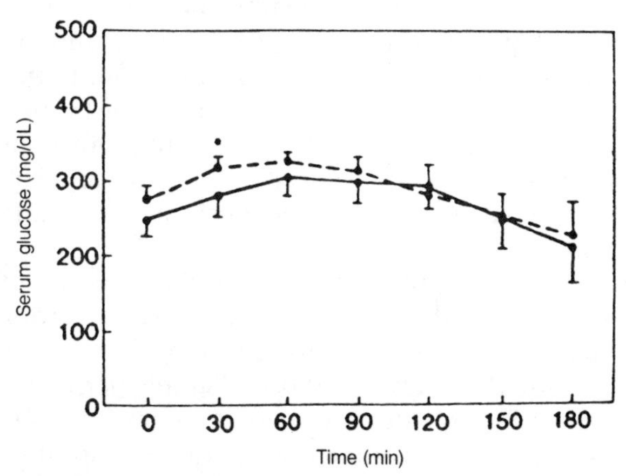

Figure 22–4. The glycemic response after a high-glycemic (solid line) and a low-glycemic (broken line) breakfast when insulin dose was adjusted for grams of carbohydrate. Data are mean ±SEM. * = a significant difference between groups ($P<0.05$) at that time point by post-hoc t test.

Data from Weyman-Daum M, Fort P, Recker B, Lifshitz F. Glycemic response in children with insulin dependent diabetes mellitus after high or low glycemic index breakfast. Am J Clin Nutr 1987; 46:798–803.

cose response to meals (Jenkins et al 1977). However, long-term benefits of increased dietary fiber have not been demonstrated. A recent study indicated that increasing dietary fiber two to five times did not lead to improvement in diabetic control (Hollembeck, Coulston & Reaven 1986). Moreover, a significant increase in the fiber content of the diet may lead to abdominal cramping, discomfort, loose stools, and excess gas. The child on a high-fiber diet may be easily satiated and may not be able to consume a diet adequate for growth. Due to the interference with absorption caused by high-fiber intake, it is also possible that patients following high-fiber diets would require supplements of calcium or trace minerals. Careful attention must be paid also to the insulin dose given to patients who embark on high-fiber diets, because hypoglycemia can follow a radical change in fiber content of the diet. There are also many practical problems regarding the palatability of a high-carbohydrate, high-fiber, low-refined-sugar diet in children.

DIETARY GUIDELINES

An ideal diet for diabetic individuals should provide adequate energy to attain and/or maintain optimum weight and growth. The diet should be high in unrefined carbohydrate, with foods such as fruits, vegetables, milk, and grains. Inclusion of added refined carbohydrates should be limited to no more than 10 percent of the total calories. However, consideration of the psychosocial needs of children should be made, allowing them to eat sweets in moderation, to develop a more appropriate self-image, and to adjust to their disease. This consideration may be especially important in the earlier stages of the disease when radical dietary changes may not be needed. Exercise offers an excellent opportunity for a balance with the consumption of refined carbohydrate. Exercise will decrease insulin resistance and subsequently increase glucose uptake, allowing for greater consumption of simple sugars (Bogardus et al 1984).

Fat should be limited to 30 percent of the total calorie intake, with no more than 10 percent of total calories coming from animal sources (saturated fat). The cholesterol content should not be more than 150 milligrams per 1000 calories, or should not exceed 300 milligrams per day. Protein in the American diet generally provides up to 20 percent of the total calories. At present, it seems prudent to recommend that the protein in the diet be limited to no more than 15 percent of the total calories. However, levels as low as the RDA for sex and age may be more acceptable for diabetic patients. Protein intake should also be modified in children with diabetic nephropathy, who may need even less than 8 percent of protein in their diets. The diet should also supply vitamins and minerals to avoid deficiencies (Levine 1987).

In the following example we present the dietary intake of Johnny, a 6-

year-old boy who weighed 46 pounds (21 kg) and was 45.7 inches (116 cm) tall before and after he became diabetic. Menu 1 shows his ordinary food intake before he became diabetic.

MENU 1

Breakfast
1 cup orange juice (8 oz)
2 slices toast with butter (2 tsp.)

Lunch
1 cup whole milk
1 sandwich with 1 slice cheese and lettuce
pretzels
carrot sticks

Snack
none

Dinner
1 hamburger (3 oz) with bun
½ cup of broccoli with tsp. butter
8 ounces orange juice

Snack
1 cup whole milk
4 creme-filled sandwich cookies

This dietary intake was typical and included the usual food selections that many American children like. However, he was ingesting a diet that is now considered less than desirable for all healthy children. The meal provided all the calories he needed for his age (1710 kcal) but was high in fat (38.4 percent), especially saturated fatty acids, with 208 milligrams of cholesterol, and was low in carbohydrate (46.7 percent). Also, it was inadequate in essential minerals and vitamins; for example, it provided less than 50 percent of the RDA for zinc and copper.

In contrast, when he became diabetic, a diet was recommended which included all the foods he liked, yet this diet was considered even better and healthier than his previous intake. Menu 2 shows his recommended food intake after he became diabetic.

MENU 2

Breakfast
½ cup orange juice
¾ cup Rice Krispies

½ cup whole milk
1 slice toast with 1 tsp. margarine

Lunch
peanut butter and jelly sandwich
carrot and celery sticks
small bag pretzels
½ cup apple juice

Snack
¾ cup whole milk
2 sandwich creme-filled cookies

Dinner
1 hamburger (3 oz) lean meat
½ cup rice with 1 tsp. margarine
½ cup broccoli with 1 tsp. margarine
8 ounces orange juice

Snack
¾ cup whole milk
2 slices cinnamon bread with 1 tsp. margarine

Notice that the recommended dietary changes provided a food intake that was more in accordance with the recommendations and goals for human nutrition needs without sacrificing any of the likes of the child.

This dietary intake is improved in regards to fat content (31.9 percent of calories) and a more equal distribution of saturated, polyunsaturated, and monounsaturated fatty acids. Also, there are more calories derived from carbohydrates (53.2 percent) and the cholesterol intake was reduced to 115 milligrams per day! It also provides more zinc and iron (100 percent). This improved diet went beyond improving Johnny's intake; his whole family also changed the way they ate!

The most difficult aspect of this dietary advice is persuading dietitians, physicians, and allied health personnel that a liberal normal dietary intake with a high proportion of complex carbohydrates is not bad for individuals with diabetes. In many instances this may require changing the health beliefs and dietary practices of the family and community, since the patient may find that such a regimen will require him or her to eat more starches than do family or friends. In surveys of the dietary intake of children with diabetes treated in our center, most patients underreport their total caloric and carbohydrate intake (Marks et al 1981, Alemzadeh et al 1989). It is possible that our population continues to cling to the old belief that the diabetic diet should be low in carbohydrates, despite being instructed otherwise.

For years we have known that the majority of individuals with diabetes do not follow, on a long-term basis, appropriate dietary recommendations (West 1973a). There are also problems in the formulation and implementation of diet prescriptions (West 1975), and limitations in methods of educating patients. Therefore, more effective ways to assess dietary intakes and to educate diabetic patients must be developed.

No special dietetic foods or sweeteners are recommended for diabetic children. These products are not necessary. They cost much more than ordinary foods without offering significant advantages (see Chapter 8). Moreover, the use of artificial sweeteners and special dietetic products may give the individual or family a false perception of treating the diabetes, when, in fact, the most beneficial diet is one derived from a variety of ordinary food. Awareness of the relationship between food composition and diabetes control is the key. Avoidance of sugar per se is not a panacea.

CLINICAL INTERVENTION

The ultimate goal in nutrition education and counseling is to promote behavioral changes. For this to occur, a phased plan of nutrition counseling is important. The key components of such a plan include the initial or "survival" phase and the in-depth or counseling phase. The American Diabetes Association recommends that in the initial phase, a simplified, individual meal plan and an introduction to the basics of meal planning with a variety of ordinary foods be made. This can be achieved through two or three 45-minute sessions after diagnosis and one to three 45-minute follow-up sessions with the family in the first 2 to 3 months after diagnosis.

During the second in-depth and continuing phase, the person with diabetes and his or her family learn how to make decisions about food selection and diabetes control. The approach must be realistic and provide as much flexibility as possible in accordance with general nutrition goals. Educational tools should also be appropriate for the individual, taking into account age and educational level. Because the in-depth phase requires continuing education and counseling, the American Diabetes Association has recommended that children and adolescents with diabetes be seen by a nutritionist at least every 6 months, preferably every 3 months.

Whenever possible, a team approach to education and counseling should be used that focuses on the person with diabetes and includes family members and "significant others" as integral parts of the education program. A team of professionals should consist of a pediatric endocrinologist, clinical nurse specialist, nutritionist, exercise physiologist, social worker, and psychologist.

It is evident that nutrition and diabetes are intimately interrelated. A better understanding of this association may not only help reduce the risk and causes of diabetes, but may also ameliorate some of the complications of the disease and improve its management. However, further studies are needed to help bring about the changes in eating patterns for the improved health of the population as a whole, as well as of specific groups such as diabetic individuals, to prevent degenerative diseases (National Dairy Council 1977). We are experts at getting facts and outlining goals; we are far less successful in implementation and follow-through, largely because of the relative crudity of our motivational techniques.

A better understanding of specific nutritional needs in diabetes is needed; for example, we are only beginning to explore the essential mineral needs in diabetics, particularly during growth. Low serum magnesium levels are frequently encountered in diabetics, especially in those who are poorly controlled. Glycosuria (glucose in the urine) is accompanied by marked urinary losses of magnesium and other minerals essential for normal health. Deficiency of these ions have been implicated in many of the complications of diabetes mellitus and other degenerative disease (Fort 1982, Seelig 1982). Indeed, this may be an area where nutritional requirements in diabetics may be different from those of normal populations, particularly since no perfect control of the diabetes can be achieved with standard therapy methods (Lifshitz & Fort 1984). Therefore, further research must be done on nutrition and diabetes. Meanwhile, patients should be counseled to follow the general principles of healthy diets, eat a variety of foods, and follow the nutrition goals recommended for the population at large. Nutrition, as important as it is in the control of IDDM, is only one of three important components for the therapy of these patients. Insulin and exercise are also necessary for the successful management of the disease. What the patient eats needs to be very closely bound to the type, dosages, and timing of insulin administration and to the patient's activity. The interaction of these three components is the key to successful patient management.

REFERENCES

Alemzadeh R, Goldberg T, Fort P, Recker B, Lifshitz F. The validity of 24-hour dietary recalls in children with insulin-dependent diabetes mellitus (IDDM): Reported dietary intakes in patients with IDDM. J Am Coll Nutr 1989; 8:450 (abstract).

American Diabetes Association Position Statement. Nutritional recommendations and principles for individuals with diabetes mellitus, 1986. Diabetes Care 1987; 10:126–132.

American Diabetes Association Position Statement. Glycemic effects of carbohydrates: A different perspective. Diabetes Care 1986; 9:641–647.

Behrens WA, Scott WS, Madere R, Trick K, Hanna K. Effect of dietary vitamin E on the vitamin E status in the BB rat during development and after the onset of diabetes. Ann Nutr Metab 1986; 30:157–165.

Bogardus C, Ravussin E, Robbins DC, Wolfe RR, Horton ES, Ethan AH. Effects of physical training and diet therapy in carbohydrate metabolism in patients with glucose intolerance and non insulin dependent diabetes mellitus. Journal 1984; 53:311–318.

Borch-Johnsen K. Relationship between breast feeding and incidence rates of insulin dependent diabetes mellitus. Lancet 1984; 2:1083–1086.

Cohen AM, Teitelbaum A, Saliternik R. Genetics and diet as factors in development of diabetes mellitus. Metabolism 1972; 21:235–240.

Dorman JJ, Laporte RE, Kuller LH, et al. The Pittsburg Insulin Dependent Diabetes Mellitus (IDDM) Morbidity and Mortality Study: Mortality results. Diabetes 1984; 32:274.

Elliot RB, Martin JM. Dietary protein: A trigger of insulin dependent diabetes in the BB rat? Diabetologia 1984; 26:297–299.

Fort P. Magnesium and diabetes mellitus. In Lifshitz F, ed. Pediatric nutrition, infant feedings, deficiencies, diseases. New York: Marcel Dekker, 1982:223–240.

Fort P, Lanes R, Dahlem S, et al. Breast feeding and insulin dependent diabetes mellitus in children. J Am Coll Nutr 1986; 5:435–441.

Gerritsen GC, Blanks MC, Miller RL, Dulin WE. Effect of diet limitation on the development of diabetes in prediabetic Chinese hamsters. Diabetologia 1974; 10:559–565.

Helgason T, Jonasson MR. Evidence for a food additive as a cause of ketosis-prone diabetes. Lancet 1981; 2:716–722.

Hoeg JM, Brewer HB. Definition and management of hyperlipoproteinemia. J Am Coll Nutr 1987; 6:157–163.

Hollembeck CB, Coulston AM, Reaven GM. To what extent does increased dietary fiber improve glucose and lipid metabolism in patients with noninsulin-dependent diabetes mellitus (NIDDM)? Am J Clin Nutr 1986; 43:16–24.

Jenkins DJA, Leeds AR, Gassull MA, Cochet B, Alberti GMM. Decrease in post-prandial insulin and glucose concentrations by guar and pectin. Ann Intern Med 1977; 86:20–23.

Jenkins DJA, Wolever TMS, Jenkins AL, Josse RG, Wong GS. The glycemic response to carbohydrate foods. Lancet 1984; 2:388–391.

Kirchgessner M, Roth HP, Weigand E. Biochemical changes in zinc deficiency. In Prasad AS, ed. Trace elements in human health and disease. Vol. I. New York: Academic Press, 1976:189–225.

Laouri D, Kleinkneckt C, Gubler MC, Ravet U, Broyer M. Importance of proteins in the deterioration of remnant kidneys, independent of other nutrients. Inter J Pediatr Nephrol 1982; 3:263–269.

Levine SE. Renal failure: Diabetic nephropathy. In Powers MA, ed. Handbook of diabetes nutritional management. Rockville, MD: Aspen Systems Corp., 1987:378–397.

Lifshitz F, Fort P. Common problems in the management of children with insulin dependent diabetes mellitus. In Lifshitz F, ed. Common pediatric disorders. New York: Marcel Dekker, 1984:3–23.

Marks ML, Lifshitz F, Fort P, et al. Dietary intakes of juvenile diabetics. Diabetes 1981; 30:284 (abstract).

Mooradian AD, Morley JE. Micronutrient status in diabetes mellitus. Am J Clin Nutr 1987; 45:877–895.

National Dairy Council. Statement on Dietary Goals for the U.S., July 20, 1977. Select Committee on Nutrition and Human Needs, U.S. Senate, Dietary Goals for the U.S.—Supplemental Views. Nov., 1977:703–708.

National Diabetes Advisory Board. Diabetes in America. HNS, PHS, NIH. 1985 Publication No 85-1468, Aug.

Nuttail FQ. Dietary recommendations for individuals with diabetes mellitus, 1979: Summary of report from the Food and Nutrition Committee of the American Diabetes Association. Am J Clin Nutr 1980; 33:1311–1312.

Pecoraro RE, Chen MS. Ascorbic acid metabolism in diabetes mellitus. In Burns JJ, Rivers JM, Machlin LW, eds. Third Conference on Vitamin C, Part IV: Health and disease. Vol. 498. New York: New York Academy of Sciences 1987:248–258.

Seelig MS. Nutritional roots of combined system disorders. In Lifshitz F, ed. Pediatric nutrition, infant feedings, deficiencies, diseases. New York: Marcel Dekker, 1982:327–351.

Slonim AE, Surber ML, Page DL, Sharp RA, Burr IM. Modification of chemically induced diabetes in rats by vitamin E: Supplementation minimizes and depletion enhances development of diabetes. J Clin Invest 1983; 71:1282–1288.

Strefa D, Boyko E, Rabkin SW. Nutrition therapy in non-insulin dependent diabetes mellitus. Diabetes Care 1981; 4:84.

Trowell H. Diabetes mellitus death rates in England and Wales 1920–1970. Lancet 1974; 2:998–1002.

Vague P, Vialettes B, Lassman-Vague V, Vallo JJ. Nicotinamide may extend remission phase in insulin-dependent diabetes. Lancet 1985; 1:619.

Vlachokosta FV, Piper CM, Gleason R, Kinzel L, Kahn CR. Dietary carbohydrate, a Big Mac, and insulin requirements in Type I diabetes. Diabetes Care 1988; 11:330–336.

Wardner LH. The world's longest insulin patient. Cornell University Medical College Alumni Quarterly 1988; 49:30–34.

West KM. Diabetes in American Indians and other native populations of the world. Diabetes 1974a; 23:841–844.

West KM. Diabetes Mellitus. In Anderson LE, Coursin DB, Schneider HA, eds. Nutritional support of medical practice. New York: Harper & Row, 1975:278–296.

West KM. Diet therapy of diabetes: An analysis of failure. Ann Intern Med 1973a; 79:425–434.

West KM. Epidemiologic evidence linking nutritional factors to the prevalence and manifestations of diabetes. Acta Diabetol Lat 1972; 9 (Suppl):405–429.

West KM. Epidemiology of adiposity. In Vague J, Boyer J, eds. The regulation of the adipose tissue mass. Proceedings of the Fourth Meeting of Endocrinology. Amsterdam: Excerpta Medica, 1973b.

West KM. Is the risk of becoming diabetic affected by sugar consumption? In Hillerbrand SS, ed. Epidemiological observations on 13 populations of Asia and the Western Hemisphere. Proceedings of the Eighth International Sugar Research Symposium, Bethesda, MD, 1974b:33–43.

West KM, Kalbfleich JM. Influence of nutritional factors on prevalence of diabetes. Diabetes 1971; 20:99–108.

Weyman-Daum M, Fort P, Recker B, Lifshitz F. Glycemic response in children with insulin dependent diabetes mellitus after high or low glycemic index breakfast. Am J Clin Nutr 1987; 46:798–803.

Wicking J, Ringrose H, Whitehouse S, Zimmet P. Nutrient intake in a partly Westernized isolated Polynesian population. The Funafuti Survey. Diabetes Care 1981; 4:92–95.

Zimmet P. Epidemiology of diabetes and its microvascular manifestations in Pacific populations: The medical effects of social progress. Diabetes Care 1979; 2:144–153.

23

Renal Disease

Roy's first day in school was very difficult and upsetting. He was teased by his classmates who called him "shortie." Even the teacher did not believe he was 7 years old. She thought that he was in the wrong class and wanted to send him back to kindergarten. Indeed, he had not grown since age 3, and he looked very young for his age. However, his mom felt he was just a small kid. On the advice of the teacher, he was seen by a pediatric endocrinologist who detected severe renal disease as the cause of his poor growth and short stature. He was born with valves that blocked the urine flow and produced back-up pressure, which ultimately resulted in kidney damage and renal failure.

Chronic renal failure (CRF) may develop either rapidly or slowly, over periods varying from months to decades. Owing to the large reserve capacity of the kidneys, patients with CRF may remain relatively symptom-free until their renal function is significantly decreased. Therefore, patients are often unaware of the existence of renal disease until it is quite advanced, as in Roy's case.

It has long been appreciated that the nutritional status of CRF patients is altered and that the dietary intake of these patients requires modification. In the past, the only treatment was the restriction of protein and salt (sodium), and sometimes potassium. This dietary treatment impressively reduced nitrogenous waste products as measured by lower blood urea nitrogen (BUN) levels. Today's dietary care of patients with renal disease is more complicated. Since the CRF patient's condition changes with time, the nutrition specialist must also be able to alter the care to meet the patient's changing needs. Dietary modifications vary greatly depending on the medications and on the type of treatment given to clear the waste products out of the blood—namely, hemodialysis, peritoneal dialysis, or renal transplantation (Broyer et al 1983).

WHAT HAPPENS WHEN THERE IS KIDNEY FAILURE?

The clinical findings of the child with renal disease reflect the decreased function of the failing kidney and the toxic effects of the excessive accumulation in the blood of nitrogenous waste products (uremia). Different stages of renal insufficiency have been arbitrarily defined by the amount of glomerular filtration rate (GFR) present (Table 23–1) (Colburn 1984). When a patient has a GFR of less than 10 milliliters per minute he or she is considered to have end-stage renal disease (ESRD). As a result of the inability to regulate the biochemical milieu, children with renal disease usually fail to grow (Rizzoni et al 1986, Polinsky et al 1987), and short stature occurs in 50 percent of these children (Chantler & Holliday 1973). Also, they may develop other complications such as high blood pressure (hypertension), acidosis, and malnutrition.

Several factors contribute to malnutrition in the uremic child. Renal disease leads to poor appetite and to an inability to distinguish flavors and aromas (Anonymous 1981, Mahajan et al 1983). Therefore, these patients lose their interest and taste for food and have a marked decrease in nutrient intake. The alterations in food consumption contribute to the decreased height, weight, and lean body mass of children with renal disease (El-Bishti et al 1981).

In addition, the small amount of food consumed is not properly utilized since the metabolic processes are altered by the uremia. Alterations in glucose and insulin metabolism (hypoglycemia), high serum lipid levels (hyperlipidemia), abnormal plasma amino acid patterns, low serum protein (hypoproteinemia), high potassium (hyperkalemia), low calcium (hypocalcemia) and high serum phosphate (hyperphosphotemia) occur in uremic patients. The metabolic alterations of renal disease also lead to an impaired ability to maintain acid/base balance with bicarbonate and electrolyte wastage and resultant acidosis. In addition, there is bone softening (rickets in children and osteomalacia in adults) which is incapacitating for the patient as it causes bone pain and contributes to growth retardation. The diseased kidneys are unable to produce the final active product of vitamin D (1,25-

Table 23–1. Different Stages of Renal Insufficiency.

STAGE	PERCENT OF NORMAL RENAL FUNCTION
Normal*	100
Mild	40–80
Moderate	20–40
Severe	<20

*Normal renal function is measured as 80 to 120 milliliters of fluid filtered by the kidney per minute (GRF).

Adapted from Colburn JW. General concepts and management of chronic renal failure. In Bricker NS, Kirschenbaum MA, eds. The kidney: Diagnosis and management. New York: John Wiley, 1984.

dihydroxy cholecalciferol) which creates actual or relative vitamin D deficiency and higher levels of parathyroid hormone leading to bone osteodystrophy.

The treatment for renal disease may further stress the metabolic homeostasis of patients with CRF. For example, low protein diets which may be used to adjust the degree of uremia of the patient may in itself contribute to malnutrition by exacerbating negative nitrogen balance. Also, the large doses of steroids often given for the treatment of renal failure may lead to increased urinary losses of nitrogen, calcium and other nutrients. Dialysis treatment leads to increased amino acid and mineral losses (Dworkin et al 1987). On the other hand, there may also be toxic effects of medications. For example, aluminum hydroxide, which is given to decrease the high phosphate levels of these patients might result in anemia and bone disease due to aluminum toxicity (Swartz et al 1987).

NUTRITIONAL REQUIREMENTS

Energy

Energy requirements for uremic children may be different from those of normal healthy children. Children with CRF usually ingest less than 80 percent of the Recommended Dietary Allowance (RDA) and they have a reduced growth velocity (Simmons et al 1971). However, even when they ingest 100 percent of their energy requirement they fail to grow at normal rates (Rizzoni, Basso & Setari 1984, Betts, Magrath & White 1977). In all cases of renal disease, sufficient energy must be provided to reverse the negative nitrogen balance and to improve the uremia (Martin 1980). As a general rule, energy needs are higher as the renal insufficiency worsens as indicated by a decline in the GRF. Also, the disease process that caused CRF increases the metabolic requirements of the child. For example, in acute renal insufficiency there may be hypercatabolism due to inflammation or infection.

Protein

Many of the metabolic changes of CRF patients are responsive to modification of the protein intake. Acidosis and nitrogen and phosphate retention are some of the problems for which limited protein intake is recommended. However, when protein intake is decreased, care must be taken to avoid protein malnutrition. It is generally advised that children with renal disease who are not being dialyzed receive protein intakes that approximate the RDA (Committee on Dietary Allowances 1989). These range from 0.8 to 2.2 grams per kilogram of body weight depending on the age of the child (see Chapter 9). This dietary intake represents a reduction of protein intake for most children living in the United States, who usually ingest enough protein to provide for 15 percent or more of the calories consumed. However, the patient with renal disease who loses excess protein through the urine may have to increase the protein intake. Although proteinuria may exceed 30 grams per day in rare instances, the usual average daily urinary losses incurred by patients with nephrotic syndrome are only about 8 to 9 grams, the amount of protein in one egg. Thus, it is very easy to replace losses and maintain the protein balance in these patients by simple dietary means.

Protein losses through dialysis treatment must be considered in the estimation of the nutritional needs of the CRF patient (Baum et al 1982, Salusky, Kopple & Fine 1983, Broyer et al 1983). With peritoneal dialysis, protein losses are more marked and inversely proportional to body weight (Blumenkranz et al 1981, Giordano, DeSanto & Capodiacasa 1981, Wassner & Corcoran 1984). In children these losses have been measured at 9 to 15 grams per treatment (McVicar 1982). Loss of protein with peritoneal dialysis is 2.5 to 4 grams per kilogram for an infant, 3 grams per kilogram for a toddler, 2.5 grams per kilogram during childhood and 1.5 grams per kilogram in adolescence (Wilkens 1986). However, precise protein requirements for these children remain unclear, but protein intakes as high as 3.5 to 4.0 grams per kilogram per day with energy intake above 75 percent of the RDA have been recommended (DeSanto et al 1981, Warren & Conley 1983, Wassner & Corcoran 1984). In CRF children on hemodialysis, there is a concern that increasing the protein intake would necessitate additional hemodialysis. However, this has not been demonstrated; rather, these children probably require relatively normal protein-energy ratios and little if any protein restriction if energy intakes are maintained (Grupe, Harmon & Spinozzi 1983).

High biological value protein such as egg, milk, and meat should be incorporated into the CRF child's diet, whereas the use of supplements of essential amino acids to promote positive nitrogen balance in these children is controversial. The acutely uremic and catabolic child may not be able to synthesize nonessential amino acids from essential amino acids. Also, certain nonessential amino acids, such as histidine and arginine, may become "conditionally essential" in renal disease. Thus, all amino acids are needed for the CRF patient, and the best source of amino acids is high-quality protein from food, not supplements, which may lead to an imbalanced amino acid profile and compromised endogenous protein synthesis.

The use of ketoacid analogues to achieve positive nitrogen balance has met with mixed reviews. While some studies demonstrate that CRF patients can convert these nitrogen-free analogues into amino acids (Bergstrom et al 1978) other investigations have shown no benefit and even noted such problems as elevated serum calcium and retinol concentrations (Burns et al 1978). Furthermore, experience with the use of ketoanalogues of essential amino acids for children is even more limited (Giordano 1980, Giordano et al 1978).

Carbohydrates and Fat

Requirements for carbohydrate and fat intakes for CRF patients do not differ from the recommendations for healthy children. However, if protein intake is to be somewhat limited, the proportion of carbohydrates need to be increased (to 60 percent of the caloric intake). Specifically, simple sugars and sweets should be reduced in the diet while complex carbohydrates and starches increased (see Chapter 9).

The fat intake of the CRF patient should not exceed 30 percent of the total calories consumed. At about 50 percent loss of renal function, hypertriglyceridemia often ensues (Frank et al 1977). In uremia, the liver increases production of triglycerides because of abnormalities in the enzymes needed for lipid clearance (Cramp, Tickner & Beale 1977, Bagdade, Yee & Wilson 1978). Moreover, hemodialysis does not improve the child's hyperlipidemia. Thus, the distribution of calories as well as the type of carbohydrate and fat in the diet have to be balanced in accordance with current guidelines for meeting human nutrition needs (see Chapter 9). Fat intake may need to be restricted below 30 percent to help lower blood triglyceride levels.

Fluid

The fluid needs of patients with renal disease vary widely. In patients who lose their renal concentrating ability and have increased urine losses (polyuria), water intake requirements may be as high as 3000 milliliters (over 3 quarts) per day. In contrast, as renal disease becomes progressively more severe with very reduced GFR, it becomes critical to decrease the fluid intake to prevent fluid overload. Thus, in CRF children fluid intake is limited only to the amount needed to cover output and fluid losses, which must include the insensible water lost through the skin. By monitoring weights daily one can identify accumulation or deficits of fluids: each 1000 milliliters (33.3 oz) of retained fluid will mean an increase of 2.2 pounds (1 kg) in weight.

Vitamins and Minerals

Patients with CRF frequently have vitamin and mineral abnormalities even when they have only mild renal insufficiency (Gentile et al 1988). Specifically, there is evidence that these patients have an increased requirement for vitamin B_6 (pyridoxine). In patients with uremia the pyridoxine from food cannot be converted in the body to pyridoxal phosphate because of reduced levels of the cofactor necessary for this reaction and decreased associated enzymatic functioning (Stone, Warnock & Wagner 1975). There may also be symptoms of vitamin B_6 deficiency in uremic patients, including peripheral neuropathy, CNS depression, and diminished immune response. Folic acid may also be deficient in CRF patients owing to the increased binding of this vitamin to protein and/or inactivation by cyanate in uremia (Francis, Thompson & Kromdieck 1977).

Patients being treated with either hemodialysis or peritoneal dialysis lose water-soluble vitamins. Thus, replacement of water-soluble vitamins, including thiamin, riboflavin, niacin, biotin, pantothenic acid, and vitamin B_{12}, should be given in amounts to meet the RDAs. Higher doses of vitamin B_6, folate, and vitamin C may be given if deficiency states exist. However, these preparations should be given after dialysis or the vitamins will be washed out by the dialysate. In contrast, vitamins A and E should not be supplemented as levels of these nutrients may already be elevated in CRF patients, since these fat-soluble vitamins are not removed by dialysis. However, vitamin K supplementation may be warranted for children receiving long-term antibiotic therapy.

The kidney plays a very important regulatory role in mineral homeostasis; thus, CRF patients may be expected to have altered mineral metabolism with or without clinical consequences. The most important mineral alterations seen in renal disease pertain to alterations in phosphate, calcium, and vitamin D (Slatapolsky & Bricker 1973, Portale et al 1984). The dietary phosphorus requirements in CRF (GFR <20 mL/min) are lower than normal. However, it is almost impossible to restrict dietary phosphorus intake sufficiently to control the high serum phosphate levels in CRF patients. Thus, aluminum phosphate–binding antacids are often necessary to decrease the intestinal absorption of phosphorus, thereby helping to prevent hyperphosphatemia, secondary hyperparathyroidism, and renal osteodystrophy. As soon as the serum phosphorus level is below 7 milligrams per deciliter, the aluminum antacid is changed for a calcium carbonate–phosphate binding medication given in sufficient amounts to counteract the amount of phosphorus ingested each day until the levels of this mineral return to normal. Among the foods recognized to have a high phosphorus content are milk, cheese, legumes, and whole-grain foods. However, phosphorus is greatest in cereal, fruits, peanuts, and drinks such as Coca Cola.

The amount of vitamin D and calcium intakes must be increased in CRF patients. The active final product of vitamin D metabolism that is normally produced by the kidney—1,25-dihydroxycholecalciferol—is now commercially available for the prevention and treatment of the bone demineralization that occurs in renal disease. Usually, large quantities of calcium are also needed by CRF patients owing to the alterations in the absorption and metabolism of this mineral. The increased calcium needs of CRF patients can be met only with calcium salt supplements.

The healthy kidney resorbs about 99 percent of the sodium filtered by the glomerulus, adjusting the amount resorbed to the body's need. As renal failure progresses, however, the ability to adapt to changes in sodium intake is lost. Thus, patients who retain sodium require sodium restrictions, while "salt wasters" require added salt. In general, sodium intake should be permitted at a level of 3 milliequivalents per 100 calories (69 mg/100 kcal) unless restriction is required, when 1 milliequivalent per 100 calories (23 mg/100 kcal) or less may be necessary (McVicar 1982). The use of diuretics usually makes it possible to allow more sodium intake in the diet.

The same dichotomy is true for potassium—children with renal disease may have either low or elevated levels of this ion in their blood. Both high and low potassium levels are life-threatening conditions. In general, 2 milliequivalents (78 mg) of potassium for every 100 calories consumed can be given to CRF children who are not retaining potassium. With end-stage renal disease, hyperkalemia occurs due to the inability of the kidney to excrete potassium. For these patients, diet modification to restrict potassium intake may help avoid potassium accumulation in the blood. In the latter case, potassium intake should be limited to 1 milliequivalents per 100 calories (39 mg/100 kcal) or less (McVicar 1982). The use of diuretics usually makes it possible to allow a higher potassium intake.

Iron-deficiency anemia may be present in children with CRF, and oral or parental iron therapy may be used. However, most anemias in renal disease are not related to iron but to a decreased production and survival of red blood cells resulting from the renal disease. Another mineral—zinc—has received some attention as a potential cause of the anorexia in uremic children (Hambridge et al 1972). However, zinc deficiency has not been demonstrated to be an important contributor to the poor eating habits of children with uremia. Although zinc replacement is necessary if a deficiency exists, its effect on appetite may not be dramatic (Condon & Freeman 1970).

There are other minerals which may be altered in patients with CRF as a result of the treatments they are given. For example, low blood selenium levels have been reported in adult patients undergoing either hemodialysis or peritoneal dialysis (Dworkin et al 1987) but no specific clinical abnormality has been associated with this alteration. Therefore, routine supplementation of this mineral may not be warranted. In contrast, magnesium is not dialyzable but it may become deficient because of treatment with diuretics which enhance losses in the urine.

In patients with CRF there is also a concern regarding accumulation of trace minerals like aluminum. This element is contained in phosphate binders and other products used in the treatment of uremia and have been associated with aluminum induced bone disease, microcytic anemia, and encephalopathy (Nathan & Pederson 1980, Andreoli et al 1984, Salusky et al 1984). Thus, other alternative phosphate binders such as calcium carbonate may need to be used (Andreoli et al 1987).

NUTRITIONAL ASSESSMENT

Children with renal insufficiency require close monitoring of their nutritional status. Complete assessments should be undertaken frequently given the constantly changing nature of their disease. These children may be very resistant to nutritional rehabilitation so it is important to identify early signs of nutritional deficits and to provide appropriate intervention before the onset of malnutrition.

Serial weight and height measurements remain an important part of the nutritional assessment for children with renal disease, although they are not always simple to interpret. These children have fluid retention and expanded blood volume which leads to overestimation of lean body mass if absolute weight is used to calculate their energy needs. Thus, ideal body weight for age can be used as a guideline, or weight for height at the 95th percentile if there is fluid accumulation and in conditions of stunting (McVicar 1982). "Dry weight," or the weight at normal hydration, should be used to assess these patients. Dry weight can be obtained when the patient's blood pressure and serum sodium levels are near normal and when edema is not present. For children receiving dialysis, the dry weight is obtained at the end of the dialysis treatment.

It is important to note that the growth failure in children with renal disease may not be simply a consequence of poor nutrition (Powell 1988). Thus, growth may not be an appropriate measure of adequate nutrition in these metabolically abnormal children (Broyer 1982, Arnold, Danford & Holliday 1983). Metabolic acidosis (McSherry 1978), hyperosmolarity; sodium, potassium, and chloride depletion (Buktus, Alfrey & Miller 1974); and low serum phosphorus may all contribute to poor bone growth in children with renal disease. Inhibition of somatomedin, the intermediary substance by which growth hormone acts to induce growth, is also present in uremia. Additionally, many drugs such as steroids, which are often used to treat kidney disease, can also interfere with normal growth in children. Psychosocial dysfunction, hypertension, and anemia may also play a role in the growth failure seen in renal disease.

Estimation of body composition using standard methods, such as triceps skinfold and arm circumferences, may also be misleading in the edematous child. As with weight, measurements may be taken when the patient's fluid status has normalized. More sophisticated techniques, such as bioelectrical impedance, which measures body water to calculate fat weight, may be quite useful in determining hydration status in the short term as well as in assessing body composition (see Chapter 10).

Biochemical parameters typically used to assess nutritional status are poor indicators of malnutrition in patients with CRF. Overhydration can result in abnormally low values of serum proteins such as albumin and transferrin and vitamins and minerals. Urinary excretion of nutrients will also be askew given the underlying renal disease. In many cases, one may have to rely on clinical symptomatology to detect deficiency states or more cumbersome assessments using tissue analysis.

Evaluation for skeletal maturation and radiologic signs of renal bone disease (osteodystrophy) should be performed frequently. Skeletal status can be evaluated by x-ray studies of the knee. The most frequently noted radiologic evidence of osteodystrophy is a general decrease in density of bone tissue and thin cortical shafts reflecting osteoporosis. Rickets or osteomalacia is seen as a mottling of the bone endings (metaphysis).

CLINICAL INTERVENTION

Most nephrologists now believe that children with reduced renal function will remain short for their age despite the best efforts to correct energy malnutrition, renal osteodystrophy, acidosis, salt wasting, and other abnormalities (Powell 1988). Recently there have been successful experimental trials using growth hormone treatment. However, the nutritional status of the CRF child needs to be monitored and maintained as close to optimal as possible. Roy, the 7-year-old boy with CRF, was provided with proper guidance on what to eat to maintain good nutritional status. With treatment, he was able to grow well along the 5th percentile of the standard growth charts although his siblings and parents were taller. This relative good growth occurred despite moderate renal insufficiency and despite the fact that he was slightly underweight for height.

The menu shows Roy's intake on a typical day of a "low-protein, low-salt diet."

MENU

Breakfast
¾ cup sugared corn flakes
½ cup whole milk
1 cup orange flavored drink

Lunch
1 cup grape juice
1 hard boiled egg and 2 tablespoons mayonnaise for egg salad
1 slice white bread
6–8 carrot strips
10 jelly beans

Snack
½ cup whole milk
½ cup sweetened applesauce with ¼ cup nondairy whipped topping

Dinner
⅓ cup pasta with tomato sauce and 1 ounce ground beef
1 cup soda
½ cup sweetened fruit cocktail

Snack
ice popsicle

This diet pattern was recommended by the nutritionist from food exchange lists. Exchange lists for renal disease, which are numerous, distinguish foods according to their protein, sodium, and potassium content, since these are the nutrients that are most carefully monitored.

One of the important features of Roy's diet is that a source of high biological value protein was present at each meal: milk at breakfast and snack, an egg at lunch, and beef at dinner. It is often recommended that 70 to 80 percent of the protein intake comes from high biological value protein and that it is evenly distributed throughout the day. In Roy's case approximately 24 grams of the total 30.7-gram protein intake (78 percent) was contributed by excellent protein sources (Fig. 23–1A).

This diet provided Roy with a caloric intake slightly above the RDAs for a healthy 7-year-old child: 32 calories per pound of body weight (70 kcal/kg). Given Roy's weight deficit for height (2 kg), it is warranted to increase his caloric intake above these general recommendations to promote catch-up gain. This may be accomplished by adding high-calorie foods that are low in protein, such as specially marketed low-protein cookies, breads, and pastas. Commercial formula supplements designed to provide energy sources without adding protein or unacceptable amounts of electrolytes may also be utilized; these include CalPower, Controlyte, Hycal, Moducal, Polycose, Sumacal, and Lipomul (see Chapter 27).

The protein content of Roy's diet is low, contributing only 7 percent of the total calories (see Fig. 23–1A). However, the level of intake is slightly in excess of established protein requirements of 1.0 grams per kilogram of ideal body weight or 20 grams a day. Notice that by substituting regular bread and pasta with the low-protein variety and eliminating ½ cup milk, the protein content of the diet would be approximately 22 grams and thus would more closely meet the established requirements. This additional modification would be necessary if Roy's uremic symptoms persisted at the somewhat higher level of protein intake.

However, there are many nutrient deficiencies present in Roy's diet, including vitamin D, folacin, calcium, magnesium, zinc, and copper (Fig. 23–1B). These vitamins and minerals need to be supplemented. For children with CRF, it is generally recommended that a multivitamin and a vitamin D metabolite be given when the GFR falls below 50 percent of normal functioning (Wilkens 1986). Calcium supplementation should also be provided to

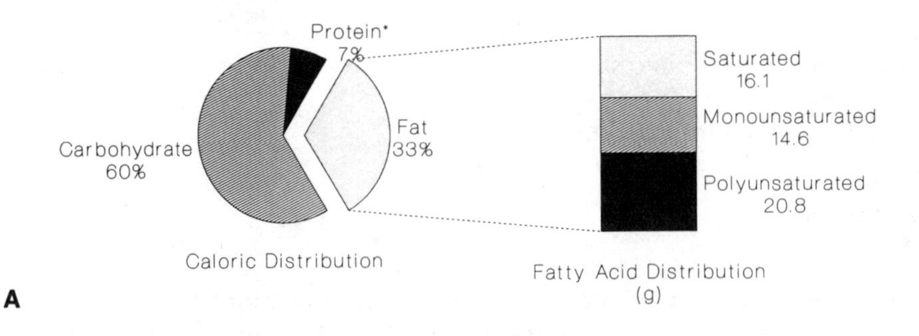

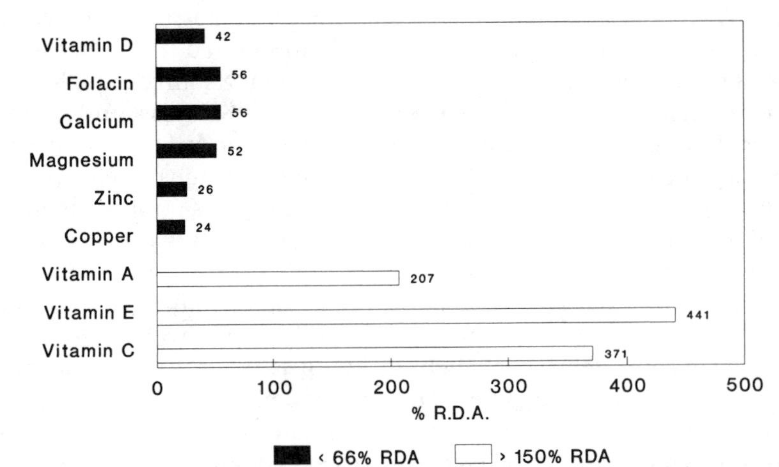

Figure 23–1. **A.** Caloric Distribution of Roy's Menu for Chronic Renal Disease. (Protein is 78 percent high biological value protein.) **B.** Inappropriate Nutrient Intakes in Roy's Menu for Chronic Renal Disease. Percent of RDAs are for a 7-year-old boy.

achieve 800 milligrams per day for children 4 to 10 years of age. Roy's diet alone provided about half of this amount, and an additional 400 milligrams of calcium was needed to meet requirements.

By avoiding foods with added salt or other sodium compounds as well as restricting the use of salt seasoning in cooking, Roy's diet was relatively low in sodium, providing 1520 milligrams (66 mEq) per day, or 3.16 milliequivalents per 100 calories. In Roy's case, this level of sodium was slightly higher than the requirements would dictate. However, as Roy demonstrated a stable weight and normal blood pressure, this level of sodium intake was not considered a problem. For most conservatively managed children with renal failure, sodium intake ranging from 1000 to 2000 milligrams (43–87 mEq) per day is usually appropriate. Sodium restriction below 1000 milligrams (43 mEq) is usually met with poor compliance because food is unpalatable. If such severe restriction is necessary, special tips for the use of alternative seasonings are available (Law 1983, Mayes 1984).

The use of salt substitutes is not always recommended, as many of these products contain potassium in varying amounts (Table 23–2). When renal functioning is severely impaired or in conditions of catabolic illness hyperkalemia (elevated serum potassium levels) will occur if potassium intake is not restricted. In patients with renal acidosis who require a buffer, sodium-free, potassium citrate (Polycitra-K) is recommended.

Similar nutrition intervention must be undertaken for children undergoing dialysis for end-stage renal disease. With dialysis, energy requirements are similar to those established for predialysis treatment, but if a glucose-free dialysate is used, a variable amount of glucose will be lost and must be replaced in the diet. In contrast, peritoneal dialysis, which includes glucose in the dialysate, will contribute to the child's overall energy intake. Also, feelings of nausea during and after dialysis may interfere with a child's ability to consume adequate calories; caloric supplementation may therefore be necessary. Protein intake does not have to be restricted when dialysis is used. Both hemodialysis and peritoneal dialysis promote protein loss, and higher levels of protein intake are required for replacement.

Sodium, potassium, and fluid intake for a child receiving either hemodialysis or intermittent peritoneal dialysis must be restricted. However, for children undergoing continuous ambulatory peritoneal dialysis, these dietary constituents may not have to be restricted unless there is fluid retention and high blood pressure. In fact, supplemental sodium may be necessary if there are excessive losses during dialysis. Vitamins and minerals may be in-

Table 23–2. Potassium Content of Salt Substitutes.

	POTASSIUM	
PRODUCT	**mEq/tsp.**	**mg/tsp.**
Morton's Salt Substitute	70	2730
No Salt (Norcliff Thayer, Inc.)	68	2652
Diamond Crystal	66	2574
Adolph's Salt Substitute	65	2535
Nu-Salt (Sugar Foods Corp.)	55	2145
Featherweight Garlic Salt Substitute	53	2067
Morton's Seasoned Salt Substitute	50	1950
Featherweight K Salt Substitute (Chicago Dietetic Supply, Inc.)	49	1911
Featherweight Seasoned Salt Substitute	43	1677
Adolph's Seasoned Salt Substitute	33	1287
Featherweight Poultry Seasoning	16	624
Featherweight Meat Seasoning	16	624
Featherweight Fish Seasoning	15	585

Adapted from Zeman FJ, Ney DM. Applications of clinical nutrition. Englewood Cliffs, NJ: Prentice Hall, 1988.

creased to replace losses into the dialysate, primarily the water-soluble vitamins described above.

The most important consideration for the child receiving a kidney transplant is to maintain the patient in the best possible nutritional status to facilitate recovery from this major surgical procedure. Protein, sodium, and potassium need not be restricted after the transplanted kidney is functioning well. However, additional calories, protein, vitamins, and minerals may be indicated if the child was malnourished prior to transplantation. The use of steroids and other immunosuppressant drugs, which are used to decrease rejection of the donor kidney, may lead to carbohydrate intolerance. Restric-

Table 23–3. Guidelines for Nutritional Management of Renal Disease in Children.

<table>
<tr><th colspan="2">WITHOUT DIALYSIS</th></tr>
<tr><td colspan="2">— ↑ energy requirements ≥ 100% R.D.A.
↑ carbohydrate intake
→ maintain fat intake ≤ 30% of calories
— ↓ protein intake to R.D.A.
↑ high biological value protein (50–75% total protein intake)
— ?-↑ vitamin B_6 and folacin requirements
↓ phosphorus requirement
↓ intake and include phosphate binders
— ↑ vitamin D requirements
↑ supplement active form of vitamin D
— ↑ calcium requirement
↑ supplement calcium salts
— ↑/↓ sodium and potassium needs depending on urinary losses or retention</td></tr>
<tr><th colspan="2">WITH DIALYSIS</th></tr>
<tr><th>Hemodialysis</th><th>Peritoneal Dialysis</th></tr>
<tr><td>— ↑ energy requirements
replace loss in dialysate</td><td>— ↓ energy intake
consider contribution of glucose in dialysate</td></tr>
<tr><td colspan="2">↑ protein intake (50–65% high biological value)</td></tr>
<tr><td>— ↓ sodium, potassium, and fluid intake</td><td>— IPD: ↓ Na, K, fluid intake
— CAPD: Liberalize intake</td></tr>
<tr><td>— ↓ phosphorus requirement
↓ intake; use phosphate binders</td><td>— Liberalize phosphorus intake with use of phosphate binders</td></tr>
<tr><td colspan="2">↑ calcium intake</td></tr>
<tr><td>— ↑ iron supplementation
anemia secondary to blood loss with dialysate</td><td></td></tr>
<tr><td colspan="2">↑ water-soluble vitamins
↓ vitamin A, magnesium and other nondialyzable trace elements</td></tr>
</table>

IPD = intermittent peritoneal dialysis
CAPD = continuous ambulatory peritoneal dialysis

tion of simple sugars and concentrated sweets may be helpful to control hyperglycemia. Calcium, phosphorus, and vitamin D supplementation may still be required to treat persistent renal osteodystrophy and replace calcium in the bone.

The clinical management of children with CRF is not simple (Table 23–3). However, with appropriate medical and nutritional rehabilitation and conscientious compliance with dietary guidelines, these children can now expect to maintain their health at a sufficient level to enjoy and live productive and satisfying lives. Of current interest is the aim at preventing through dietary means the progression and deterioration of kidney function in patients with chronic renal disease. A "modification of diet in renal disease" (MDRD) is being undertaken to determine whether low-protein, low-phosphorus diets along with strict blood pressure control can slow or even halt the progression of kidney failure. Further information regarding this study and patient eligibility may be obtained by calling (800) 344-DIET. A new report indicates that renal function may be preserved with restriction of dietary protein; this intake was effective in slowing the progression of renal disease (Ihle et al 1989).

REFERENCES

Andreoli SP, Bergstein JM, Sherrard DJ. Aluminum intoxication from aluminum-containing phosphate binders in children with azotemia not undergoing dialysis. N Engl J Med 1984; 310:1079–1084.

Andreoli SP, Dunson JW, Bergstein JM. Calcium carbonate is an effective phosphorus binder in children with chronic renal disease. Am J Kidney Dis 1987; 9:206–210.

Arnold WC, Danford D, Holliday MA. Effects of caloric supplementation on growth in children with uremia. Kidney Int 1983; 24:205–209.

Anonymous. Decreased taste acuity in chronic renal patients. Nutr Rev 1981; 39:207–210.

Bagdade JD, Yee E, Wilson DE. Hyperlipidemia in renal failure: Studies of plasma lipoproteins, hepatic triglyceride production and tissue lipoprotein lipase in a chronically uremic rat model. J Lab Clin Med 1978; 91:176–186.

Baum M, Powell D, Calvin S, et al. Continuous ambulatory peritoneal dialysis in children: Comparison with hemodialysis. N Engl J Med 1982; 307:1537–1542.

Bergstrom J, Ahlberg M, Albestrand A, Furst P. Metabolic studies with keto acids in uremia. Am J Clin Nutr 1978; 31:1761–1766.

Betts PR, Magrath G, White RH. Role of dietary energy supplementation in growth of children with chronic renal insufficiency. Br Med J 1977; 1:416–418.

Blumenkranz MG, Gahl GM, Kopple JD, et al. Protein losses during peritoneal dialysis. Kidney Int 1981; 19:593–602.

Broyer M. Growth in children with renal insufficiency. Pediatr Clin North Am 1982; 29:991–1003.

Broyer M, Niaudet P, Champion G, Jean G, Chopin N, Czernichow P. Nutritional and metabolic studies in children on continuous ambulatory peritoneal dialysis. Kidney Int 1983; 24:S106–S110.

Buktus DE, Alfrey AC, Miller NL. Tissue potassium in chronic dialysis patients. Nephron 1974; 13:314–324.

Burns J, Gresswell E, Ell S, et al. Comparison of the effects of keto acid analogues and essential amino acids on nitrogen homeostasis in uremic patients on moderately protein-restricted diets. Am J Clin Nutr 1978; 31:1767–1775.

Chantler C, Holliday MA. Growth in children with renal disease with particular reference to the effects of calorie malnutrition. Clin Nephrol 1973; 1:230–242.

Colburn JW. General concepts and management of chronic renal failure. In Bricker NS, Kirschenbaum MA, eds. The kidney: Diagnosis and management. New York: John Wiley, 1984.

Committee on Dietary Allowances, Food and Nutrition Board, National Research Council. Recommended dietary allowances. 10th ed. Washington, D.C.: National Academy of Sciences, 1989.

Condon CJ, Freeman RM. Zinc metabolism in renal failure. Ann Intern Med 1970; 73:531–536.

Cramp DG, Tickner TR, Beale DJ. Plasma triglyceride secretion and metabolism in chronic renal failure. Clin Chim Acta 1977; 76:237–241.

DeSanto NG, Capodicasa G, Pluvio M, et al. Protein-energy requirements of children and adolescents on CAPD: Preliminary results of nitrogen balance studies. In Gruskin NB, Norman ME, eds. Pediatric nephrology. Boston: Martinus Nijhoff, 1981:199.

Dworkin B, Weseley S, Rosenthal WS, Schwartz EM, Weiss L. Diminished blood selenium levels in renal failure patients on dialysis: Correlations with nutritional status. Am J Med Sci 1987; 293:6–12.

El-Bishti M, Burke J, Jones W, et al. Body composition in children on regular hemodialysis. Clin Nephrol 1981; 15:53–60.

Francis KT, Thompson RW, Kromdieck CL. Reaction of tetrahydrofolic and cyanate from urea solutions: Formation of an inactive folate derivative. Am J Clin Nutr 1977; 30:2028–2032.

Frank W, Rao TKS, Manis T, Freidman E. Uremic hyperlipoproteinemia: Correlation with residual renal function and duration of maintenance hemodialysis. Trans Am Soc Artif Intern Organs 1977; 23:59–64.

Gentile MG, Manna GM, D'Amico G, et al. Vitamin nutrition in patients with chronic renal failure and dietary manipulation. Contrib Nephrol 1988; 65:43–50.

Giordano C. Amino acids and ketoacids—Advantages and pitfalls. Am J Clin Nutr 1980; 33:1649–1653.

Giordano C, DeSanto NG, Capodiacasa G. Amino acid losses of children on CAPD. Int J Pediatr Nephrol 1981; 2:85–88.

Giordano C, DeSanto NG, DiToro R, et al. The imbalance effect of amino acid and keto acid diet for growth of the uremic infant. In Proceedings of the Seventh International Congress of Nephrology. Basel: Karger, 1978:477.

Grupe WE, Harmon WE, Spinozzi NS. Protein and energy requirements in children receiving chronic hemodialysis. Kidney Int 1983; 25:S6–10.

Hambridge KM, Hambridge G, Jacobs M, Baum JD. Low levels of zinc in hair, anorexia, poor growth and hypogeusia in children. Pediatr Res 1972; 6:868–874.

Ihle BU, Becker GJ, Whitwork JA, Charlwood RD, Kincaid-Smith PS. The effects of protein restriction on the progression of renal insufficiency. N Engl J Med 1989; 321:1773–1777.

Law M, ed. The renal family cookbook. Downsview, Ontario: The Renal Family, Inc., 1983.

Mahajan S, Speck J, Varghese G, et al. Zinc metabolism in nephrotic syndrome. Kidney Int 1983; 23:129.

Martin KJ. Renal disease. In Freitag JJ, Miller LW, eds. Manual of medical therapeutics. 23rd ed. Boston: Little, Brown, 1980.

Mayes K. The sodium-watcher's guide. Santa Barbara, CA: Pennant Books, 1984.

McSherry E. Acidosis and growth in non-uremic renal disease. Kidney Int 1978; 14:349–354.

McVicar MI. Nutritional consequences of kidney disease. In Lifshitz F, ed. Pediatric nutrition: Infant feedings, deficiencies, and diseases. New York: Marcel Dekker, 1982:297–316.

Nathan E, Pederson SE. Dialysis encephalopathy in an non-dialyzed uremic boy treated with aluminum hydroxide orally. Acta Paediatr Scand 1980; 69:793–796.

Polinsky MS, Kaiser BA, Stover JB, et al. Neurologic development of children with severe chronic renal failure from infancy. Pediatr Nephrol 1987; 1:157–165.

Portale AA, Booth BE, Halloran BP, et al. Effect of dietary phosphorus on circulating concentrations of 1,25 dihydroxyvitamin D and immunoreactive parathyroid hormone in children with moderate renal insufficiency. J Clin Invest 1984; 73:1580–1589.

Powell DR. Renal disease and growth retardation. Growth: Genetics and Hormones. New York: McGraw Hill, 1988; 4:1–3.

Rizzoni G, Basso T, Setari M. Growth in children with chronic renal failure on conservative treatment. Kidney Int 1984; 26:52–58.

Rizzoni G, Broyer M, Guest G, et al. Growth retardation in children with chronic renal disease: Scope of the problem. Am J Kidney Dis 1986; 7:256–261.

Salusky IB, Coburn JW, Paunier L, Sherrara DJ, Fine RN. Role of aluminum hydroxide in raising serum aluminum levels in children undergoing continuous ambulatory peritoneal dialysis. J Pediatr 1984; 105:717–720.

Salusky IB, Kopple JD, Fine RN. Continuous ambulatory peritoneal dialysis in pediatric patients. A 20-month experience. Kidney Int 1983; 15:S101–105.

Simmons JM, Wilson CJ, Potter DE, Holliday MA. Relation of calorie deficiency to growth failure in children on hemodialysis and the growth response to calorie supplementation. N Engl J Med 1971; 285:653–656.

Slatapolsky E, Bricker NS. The role of phosphorus restriction in the prevention of secondary hyperparathyroidism in chronic renal disease. Kidney Int 1973; 4:141–145.

Stone WJ, Warnock LG, Wagner C. Vitamin B_6 deficiency in uremia. Am J Clin Nutr 1975; 28:950–957.

Swartz E, Dombrouski J, Burnatowska-Hledin M, Mayor G. Microcytic anemia in dialysis patients: Reversible marker of aluminum toxicity. Am J Kidney Dis 1987; 9:217–223.

Warren S, Conley SB. Nutritional considerations in infants on continuous peritoneal dialysis (CPD). Dial Transplant 1983; 12:263.

Wassner SJ, Corcoran M. Nutritional considerations after the institution of dialysis. In Brodehl J, Ehrich JHH, eds. Pediatric nephrology. Berlin: Springer-Verlag, 1984:92.

Wilkens K, ed. Suggested guidelines for nutrition care of renal patients. Renal Dietitians Practice Group, The American Dietetic Association, 1986.

24

The Cholesterol Concern

Fred just had such a nice 10-year birthday, which was celebrated along with his father's 42nd birthday and had their favorite dessert. But soon after his father had a heart attack and was found to have high cholesterol levels in his blood. Fred's dad was no longer able to eat his favorite dessert and had to avoid many other foods. His heart problems continued, necessitating heart surgery by the time Fred was 14 years old. At that time, Fred was also found to have a high cholesterol level. He was so surprised because he was secretly following the same diet as his father. After all, he didn't want to have clogged arteries by the time he was 40! Moreover, poor Fred had not grown and had not developed like his friends, and the doctors told him that this poor growth was because of his low-fat, low-cholesterol diet. This diet was not giving him all the calories and minerals he needed for growth and sexual maturation.

CHOLESTEROL AWARENESS

The 1980s was the beginning of the age of cholesterol awareness. Nowadays, there is no way of avoiding advice and information regarding cholesterol; it is available to the public by all types of media and health professionals. The cholesterol age first began in 1912 when Anitschkow fed this substance to rabbits and produced hardening of the main blood vessels of the heart (aortic atherosclerosis). Not until the 1970s was cholesterol considered a major risk factor for human coronary artery disease (CAD). However, most physicians ignored this fact unless cholesterol values were extremely high, usually above 300 milligrams per deciliter. In the 1980s the importance of cholesterol values became increasingly recognized by both patients and physicians as many studies showed that lowering cholesterol decreased CAD and rates of heart attacks (myocardial infarction).

The clinical, experimental, and epidemiologic evidence linking dietary animal fat (saturated) to increased serum cholesterol levels and increased risk of CAD is substantial (NIH Consensus Conference 1985). These data provide the basis for the current dietary recommendations made by the National Institute of Health, the American Heart Association, and others to reduce the total amount of saturated fat and cholesterol intake to promote improved health and to reduce the incidence of chronic illness such as heart disease.

The American Heart Association (Weidman et al 1983), the National Institutes of Health Consensus Development Panel (1985), as well as individual medical authorities (Newman et al 1986), believe that atherosclerosis has its roots in childhood and that adherence to a prudent diet from early life will lessen the risks of chronic illness in later life. Lauer and associates found that elevated cholesterol levels during childhood were associated with hypercholesterolemia in adulthood (Lauer, Lee & Clarke 1988). Therefore, for preventive health care, many medical organizations recommend that everybody, including children and adolescents, consume a lower fat and cholesterol diet.

However, the Committee on Nutrition of the American Academy of Pediatrics has worried about potential problems for children who are eating low-fat, low-cholesterol diets (AAP 1986). Low-fat, low-cholesterol diets in our culture usually result from elimination of highly nutritious products such as red meat, eggs, and dairy products without the necessary increase in grains and cereals to provide for a well-balanced diet. In fact, we have recently described children in whom growth failure was associated with unsupervised dietary treatment of high cholesterol levels (Lifshitz & Moses 1989) (Fig. 24–1).

What Is My Cholesterol Level?

We have the technology to recognize and diagnose hypercholesterolemia with great ease, and pediatricians are availing themselves of cholesterol screening methodology with increasing frequency (Nader et al 1987). Everybody is getting a cholesterol measurement! About 100 million blood cholesterol tests were performed in the United States in 1986 at a cost to patients and insurers of between $1.5 billion and $1 trillion dollars (Bogdanich 1987). The serum cholesterol level test is the most commonly performed clinical laboratory procedure. The first thing that many patients ask their doctors to do is to measure their cholesterol; their next question is, what was my cholesterol value last year?

The National Cholesterol Education Program and the Expert Panel on Detection, Evaluation, and Treatment of High Blood Cholesterol in Adults both define total blood cholesterol values of less than 200 milligrams per deciliter

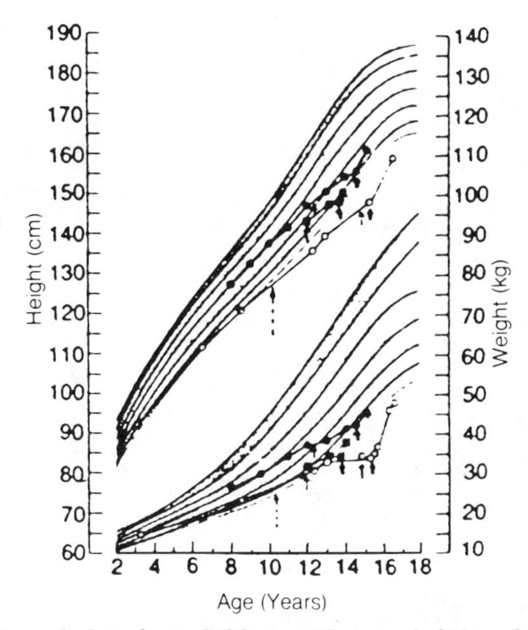

Figure 24–1. Growth data for 3 children with growth failure following the diagnosis of hypercholesterolemia. The extreme growth percentiles shown denote the 5th and 95th percentiles. The diagnosis of hypercholesterolemia and initiation of dietary treatment by the pediatrician are indicated by a thin arrow. In the patient represented by open circles, the dashed arrow represents onset of father's heart problems and dietary restrictions. The thick arrow denotes intervention with appropriate nutritional counseling.

From Lifshitz F, Moses N. Growth failure: A complication of dietary treatment of hypercholesterolemia. Am J Dis Child 1989; 143:537–542.

as desirable, 200 to 239 milligrams per deciliter as borderline, and greater than 240 milligrams per deciliter as high. In children up to age 19 years all levels above 200 milligrams per deciliter are considered high. Values above 170 to 200 milligrams per deciliter are considered borderline, while values below 170 are considered desirable (Fig. 24–2).

Many variables can influence a cholesterol measurement. In a survey of 5000 testing laboratories, it was found that almost one half did not meet the desired goal of being accurate to within 5 percent of the true cholesterol value (Roberts 1987). This study also found significant variability from laboratory to laboratory. A test of a known blood sample with a cholesterol level of 262 milligrams per deciliter was sent to several laboratories throughout the country; their results ranged from 101 to 524 milligrams per deciliter.

Cholesterol values can also be significantly influenced by other factors,

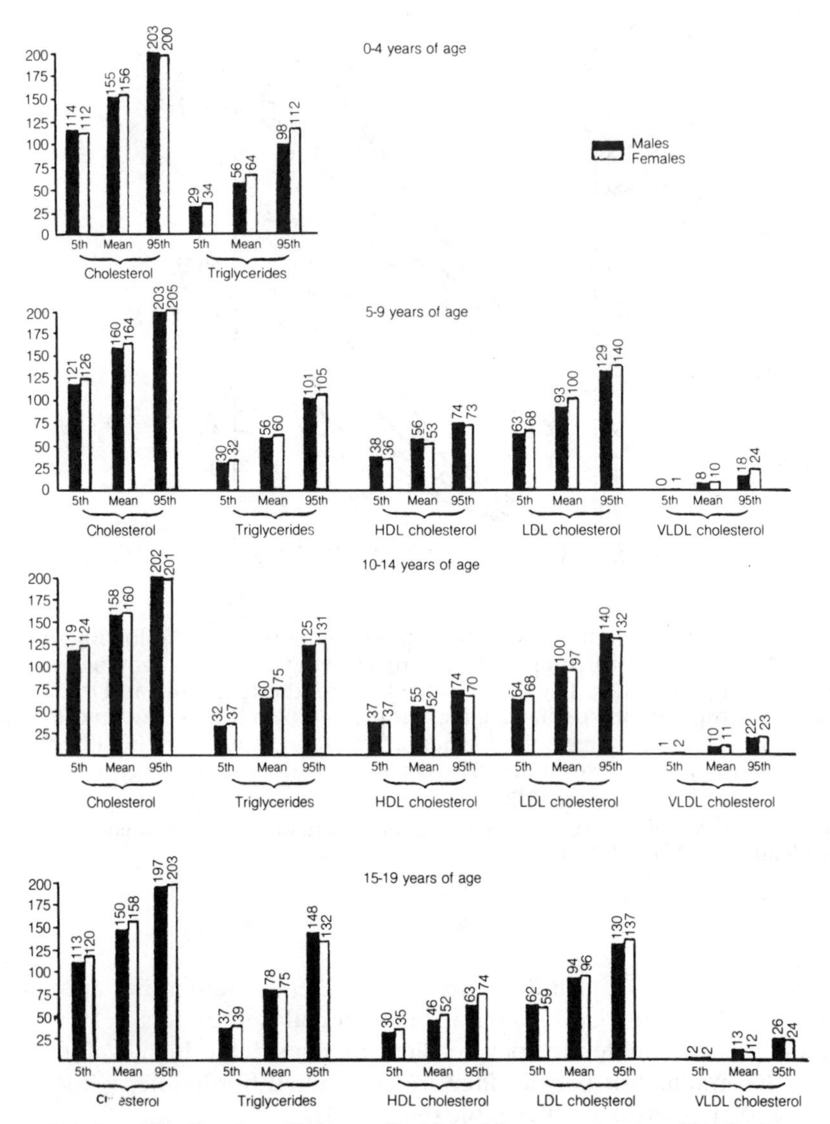

Figure 24–2. Distribution of plasma lipid and lipoproteins (mg/dL) for boys and girls from infancy through adolescence.

Data from Lipid Research Clinics. Population Studies Data Book. Department of Health and Human Services (NIII) 80-1527. Vol 1. The Prevalence Study.

particularly sex and age (Fig. 24–3). Additional factors include whether the patient is standing or sitting, whether the tourniquet has been left on, and what time of day the blood is taken. Another variable for serum cholesterol is time of year. The average cholesterol was 7.4 mg/dl higher in December than in June (Roberts 1987). This effect was not related to diet or weight or to when the last meal was ingested; indeed, serum cholesterol levels do not need to be measured after fasting.

Other factors besides the cholesterol value are important in evaluating a patient's risk of developing atherosclerosis (AAP 1989). Important clinical factors that must be considered are family history of a heart attack and heart disease, particularly in a young person, and the presence of diabetes mellitus, high blood pressure, and obesity. Other significant risk factors include being male, being female on birth-control medication, smoking, and inactivity (Lauer, Lee & Clarke 1988).

In addition, cholesterol levels have to be interpreted in relation to the type of cholesterol found in the blood, not just the level (see Fig. 24–2). The low-density lipoprotein (LDL) accounts for the greatest percentage of cholesterol and it appears to be responsible for depositing fat in the artery walls. For this reason, this type of cholesterol is known as "bad" cholesterol. Another lipro-protein "package" that the body makes is called high-density liproprotein (HDL). HDLs contain the greatest amount of protein and the smallest amount of cholesterol. HDL is believed to take cholesterol away from cells and trans-

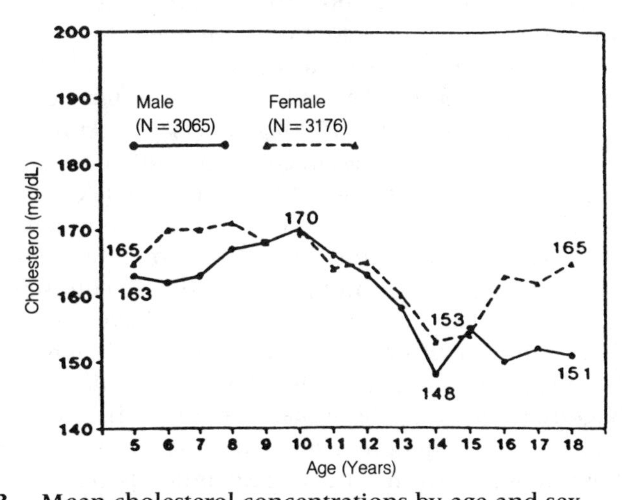

Figure 24–3. Mean cholesterol concentrations by age and sex.

Modified from Resnicow K, Morley-Kotchen J, Wynder E. Plasma cholesterol levels of 6585 children in the United States: Results of the know your body screening in five states. Pediatrics 1989; 84:969-976.

port it back to the liver for processing or removal. Researchers have noted that persons with higher levels of HDL have less heart disease. Thus, HDLs are now known as the "good" cholesterol. Women generally have higher levels of HDL, and this may explain in part why they have fewer heart attacks than men. Higher levels of HDL usually are found in people who exercise regularly, don't smoke, and maintain normal weight. Among young adolescents aged 12 to 14 years, initiation of light or moderate smoking for 1 to 2 years was associated with lower HDL-cholesterol concentrations compared with nonsmoking adolescents (Dwyer et al 1988). Therefore, even short-term smoking at low levels (1 to 39 cigarettes per week) results in an increased risk of cardiovascular disease, and smoking may be worse than the blood cholesterol itself and/or the dietary cholesterol intake.

Should children have their cholesterol checked? The American Academy of Pediatrics recommends that all children in families with high-risk factors should have a cholesterol check, but routine testing for all children is not needed (AAP 1986). The blood cholesterol level is influenced by the foods children eat and by their particular body chemistry, which is inherited just as hair or eye color. Thus, the body's response to a diet is determined by inheritance, as well as by the fat and cholesterol content of that diet. However, two recent studies found that without routine screening of serum cholesterol levels, a large number of children who may be at risk with high blood levels of this fat would not be identified by the presence of family history alone (Garcia & Moore 1989, Griffin et al 1989). These data suggest that for thorough identification of young children with elevated cholesterol levels, mass screening will be necessary, but it does not imply that everyone should be screened at the present time. Two new studies found that universal screening of cholesterol in childhood must be reserved, as there is a high number of children with elevated cholesterol levels on screening who as adults do not meet criteria for intervention (Lauer & Clarke 1990). Universal screening and interventions to lower blood cholesterol levels in children would be expensive and the risks may exceed the benefits of such action (Newman et al 1990). Many other factors must be considered before making this recommendation. Accurate measurements of cholesterol and the LDL fraction must be readily available to the pediatrician, and thorough professional counseling must be implemented for those families who are found to have high levels. When families are left to their own devices, low-fat, low-cholesterol diets may be inappropriate and growth failure or weight loss may result (see Fig. 24–1) following the diagnosis of hypercholesterolemia (Fig. 24–4). Also, the safety and efficacy of dietary and/or long-term drug treatment for hypercholesterolemia for children has not been proven. Until these conditions are met the subject of cholesterol screening will remain controversial, and families without a genetic predisposition should not worry needlessly.

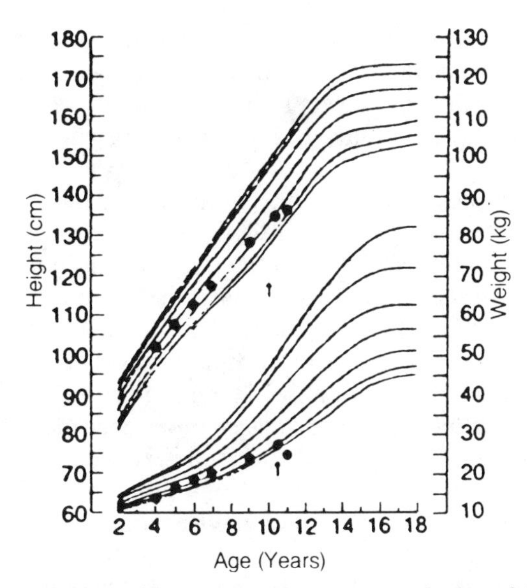

Figure 24–4. Growth data of 1 child with acute weight loss following the diagnosis and treatment (arrow) of hypercholesterolemia of 6.37 mmol/L. (246 mg/L).

Modified from Lifshitz F, Moses N. Growth failure: A complication of dietary treatment of hypercholesterolemia. Am J Dis Child 1989; 143:537-542.

HOW TO LOWER CHOLESTEROL LEVELS

Fat is a major source of calories in the American diet, accounting for up to 40 percent of the total caloric intake and contributing 300 to 500 milligrams of cholesterol each day (see Chapter 9). Epidemiologic surveys, dietary intervention, and many experimental studies have provided strong evidence that if we change our habits to reduce dietary fat intake to about 30 percent of calories, with animal (saturated) fat making up only one third of total fat intake, vegetable (polyunsaturated) fat making up another third, and dietary intake of cholesterol reduced to no more than 300 milligrams per day, Americans will reduce their overall risk of heart disease (Hoeg & Brewer 1987). Studies also indicate that soluble fibers, especially those found in cereals and legumes, also help to lower blood cholesterol levels (Lipid Research Clinics Program 1984, Van Horn et al 1986).

Diets for children and adolescents that provide a decreased fat and cholesterol intake and an increased polyunsaturated to saturated fatty acid ratio may be designed to meet all the RDAs (Dwyer 1980). However, it must be remembered that the general health of the population may be improved even without changes in food consumption (AMA 1977). Changes in lifestyle, such as increased physical activity and reduced smoking, have resulted in a decline in blood cholesterol levels and other major risk factors associated with atherosclerotic disease without making changes in nutrition (Wolinsky 1980).

Although the cholesterol-conscious family is already eating less red meat and eggs, more turkey, chicken, and fish, and substituting vegetable oil for animal (saturated) fats, these dietary changes often do not result in improvement of serum cholesterol levels. Moreover, avoiding certain foods without appropriate substitution may be detrimental to the nutritional adequacy of the diet (Lifshitz & Moses 1989). For example, all beef and shellfish have been falsely identified as "bad," cholesterol-laden foods, while veal and prepared cold cuts made from chicken and turkey have been advocated as "good" choices. In Table 24–1, the fat and the cholesterol content of some of children's favorite foods are listed. Contrary to popular ideas, foods that are considered low in cholesterol may actually have as much cholesterol as lean cuts of beef and shellfish such as lobster, clams, and scallops. This may come as as surprise to many families who thought that shellfish, veal, and beef had to be avoided if cholesterol was restricted in the diet.

A key point to remember is that cholesterol comes only from animal products. Fruit, vegetables, or any food that is prepared from plants never had cholesterol and never will. Due to all the attention about cholesterol, many manufacturers have taken this cue to capitalize on the consumer's dread of cholesterol. For foods that are always made without animal products, such as peanut butter, corn oil, and applesauce, adding "no cholesterol" to the label is only stating the obvious.

The kind and the amount of fat in the diet may affect blood cholesterol levels more than the actual amount of cholesterol in the diet (Fig. 24–5 to 24–9). There are two major categories of fats—saturated fats (Fig. 24–6) and unsaturated fats (Fig. 24–7 and 24–8). Saturated fats from animal products, including lard, butter, cheese, and meat, are solid at room temperature. The intake of these types of fats should be limited to 10 percent of the total calories in the diet. In addition, there are vegetable oils, such as coconut and palm kernel oils, that are highly saturated. Unsaturated fats are liquid at room temperature and are either polyunsaturated (safflower oil, sunflower oil, corn oil, and foods such as fish and nuts) (see Fig. 24–7) or monounsaturated (canola oil, olive oil, peanut oil, and foods such as olives and avocado) (see Fig. 24–8).

Consumption of unsaturated fats may help reduce cholesterol levels and does not lower HDL levels ("good cholesterol") as do diets high in saturated fats (Grundy & Bonanome 1987). The intake of polyunsaturated and monounsaturated fats should provide 20 percent of the total calories in the diet (10 percent each). However, just because a food is made with "100 percent vegetable oil" or contains "no animal fat" does not mean it is an appro-

Table 24–1. Fat and Cholesterol Content of Common Foods.*

FOOD	SERVING SIZE	FAT (g)	FAT CALORIES (%)	CHOLESTEROL (mg)
Lamb, loin chop, trimmed	3 oz	8.5	42	80
Milk				
whole	1 cup	8.2	48	30
2% fat	1 cup	4.7	33	18
1% fat	1 cup	2.4	20	10
skim	1 cup	0.6	6	5
Veal				
chop	3 oz	11.4	51	86
cutlet	3 oz	18.0	63	80
Beef				
lean, trimmed	3 oz	5.9	34	56
fatty cut	3 oz	28.2	77	70
Pork				
ham, roasted	3 oz	9.4	45	80
bacon, fried	2 slices (½ oz)	6.2	77	11
Chicken				
light, no skin	3 oz	2.0	13	53
light, skin	3 oz	4.5	29	74
dark, no skin	3 oz	2.2	31	63
dark, skin	3 oz	5.0	43	79
Fish				
flounder, lean	3 oz	1.0	11	59
salmon, red	3 oz	11.2	57	59
tuna, canned, water packed	½ cup	2.5	20	54
shrimp, canned	3 oz	0.9	8	128
lobster, canned	3 oz	1.1	13	71
clams, raw	3 oz	0.8	9	43
Egg	1	5.6	65	274
Organ meats				
beef liver (raw)	3 oz	3.2	25	377
beef kidney	3 oz	10.3	43	600
Oil/fat				
corn oil	1 TB	14.0	100	0
safflower oil	1 TB	14.0	100	0
sunflower oil	1 TB	14.0	100	0
olive oil	1 TB	14.0	100	0
soybean oil	1 TB	14.0	100	0
peanut oil	1 TB	14.0	100	0
cottonseed oil	1 TB	14.0	100	0
vegetable shortening (Crisco)	1 TB	14.0	100	0
bacon fat	1 TB	14.0	100	1
chicken fat	1 TB	14.0	100	9
beef fat	1 TB	11.7	97	14
lard	1 TB	14.0	100	13

Table 24–1. Fat and Cholesterol Content of Common Foods.* *(cont.)*

FOOD	SERVING SIZE	FAT (g)	FAT CALORIES (%)	CHOLESTEROL (mg)
mayonnaise	1 TB	11.2	100	10
butter	1 TB	11.0	99	33
margarine	1 TB	11.0	99	0
Processed luncheon meats				
beef bologna	1 oz	8.1	83	15
turkey ham loaf	1 oz	4.2	54	23
beef frankfurter	1	13.5	86	23
chicken frankfurter	1	8.5	77	23–63
Legumes				
walnuts	1 oz	16.8	88	0
peanuts	1 oz	13.1	73	0
almonds	1 oz	16.2	83	0
cashews	1 oz	12.9	74	0

*The preferred food is the one that provides 30 percent of calories from fat. Note that while the fat and cholesterol content is similar in many products the amounts of saturated fats are quite different (see Table 24–2).

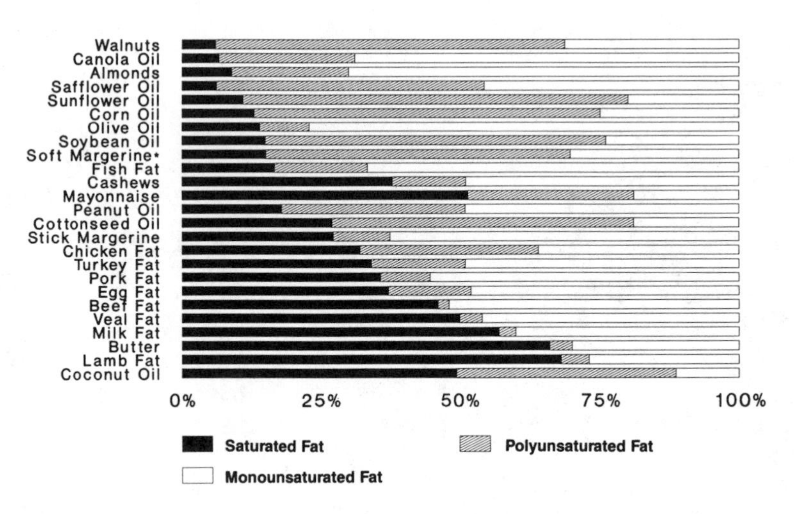

Figure 24–5. Comparison of Dietary Fats in Common Foods.

priate food. For example, potato chips fried in 100 percent natural vegetable oil may contain no cholesterol but are certainly high in total fat and high in hydrogenated fat (Fig. 24–9). Vegetable oils in many prepared products have undergone a process called hydrogenation whereby a liquid oil is hardened to make a more solid fat. During this process, the vegetable oil becomes more

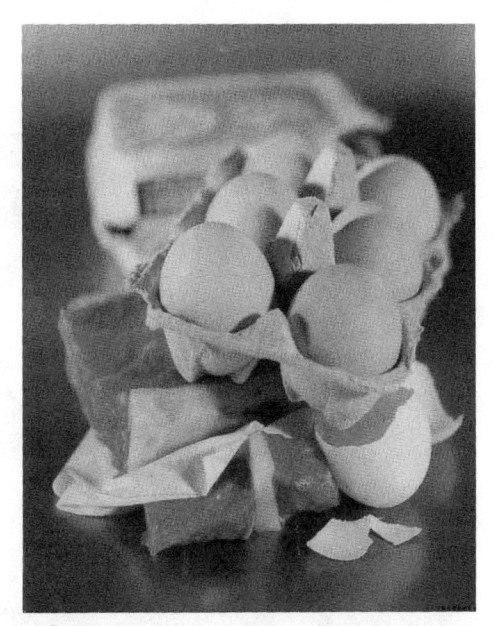

Figure 24–6. Saturated fats. Saturated fats are usually derived from animal products. These include lard, butter, cheese, eggs, and meat. Saturated fats may also come from vegetable sources, including coconut and palm oils, and from the processing and hydrogenation of unsaturated fats (see Fig. 24–9).

saturated and, regardless of the source, saturated fat intake will result in higher cholesterol levels.

Low-fat, low-cholesterol diets are difficult to follow without input from knowledgeable health professionals, as shown below. Mike, an 11-year-old boy, was found to have an elevated serum cholesterol level. The doctor told his parents to modify Mike's diet to be low in fat and cholesterol. They read many articles in newspapers and magazines so they knew what to do . . . or so they thought.

Menu 1 is the low-fat, low-cholesterol menu that Mike was consuming to lower his high cholesterol levels.

MENU 1

Breakfast
1½ cup sugared cereal
1 cup skim milk
½ cup orange juice

Lunch
peanut butter and jelly sandwich
½ cup string beans and carrot sticks

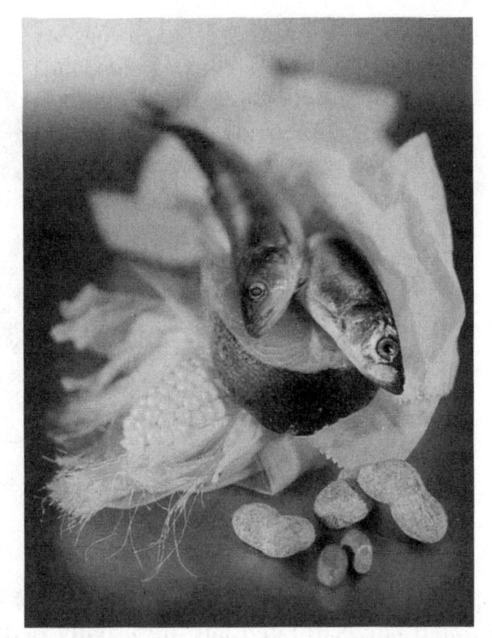

Figure 24–7. Polyunsaturated fats. These fats are usually derived from vegetable sources such as nuts but may also be present in animal food (e.g., fish). The oils derived from safflower, sunflower, and corn are high in this type of fat.

1 cup fruit drink
2 servings pretzel sticks

Snack
1 apple
3 cups unbuttered popcorn
1 cup fruit drink

Dinner
4 ounces breaded chicken without skin
1 baked potato with 1 tsp. margarine
1 cup apple juice

Snack
1 cup skim milk
3 vanilla cookies

Mike was offered only skim milk; other dairy products such as cheese and ice cream were eliminated from his diet because of their high fat and cholesterol content. Red meat and eggs were avoided whereas chicken, fresh fruits,

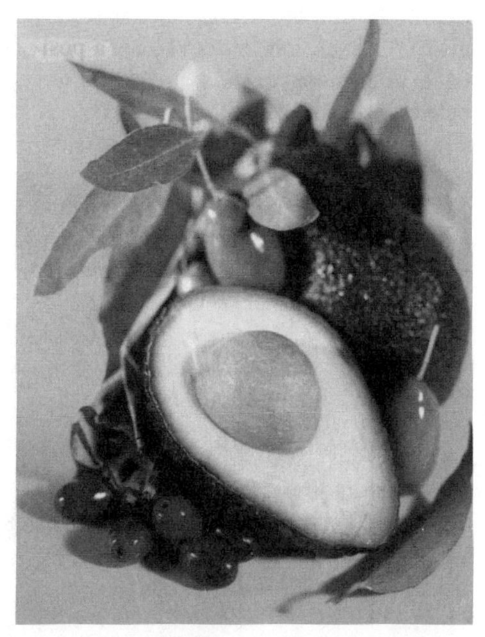

Figure 24–8. Monounsaturated fats. Monounsaturated fats are also found from vegetable sources, including olives and avocado. The oils derived from canola, olives, and peanuts are high in this type of fat.

and vegetables were emphasized. Of course, he did not even get close to shellfish although he really liked it. With this menu, Mike was hungry all the time. This low-cholesterol, low-fat diet was *very* low in calories because Mike was not able to eat enough of the low-fat foods to meet his energy needs. He needed at least 1925 calories per day, more when he played a lot of basketball. However, he ate only a maximum of 1700 calories per day (Fig. 24–10A). Fat contributed only 15 percent of the total calories in the diet, with the carbohydrate content as high as 70 percent. With this low-fat, high-bulk diet, a child not to become satiated before sufficient calories are consumed. The cholesterol intake of 44 milligrams per 1000 calories consumed was also greatly below the generally recommended guidelines of 75 to 100 milligrams per 1000 calories. Many nutrient intakes were also inadequate in this restricted diet. Vitamins D and E, folacin, calcium, zinc, and copper were insufficient to meet Mike's needs (Fig. 24–10B).

Of course, with this dietary intake Mike did not grow; in fact he lost weight during the 6 months he tried to follow the diet. However, his blood cholesterol levels remained high and his doctor referred the child to a medical center. There, Mike's menu was liberalized to include low-fat milk, shellfish, and some of the special desserts that he liked to eat. What a surprise to be

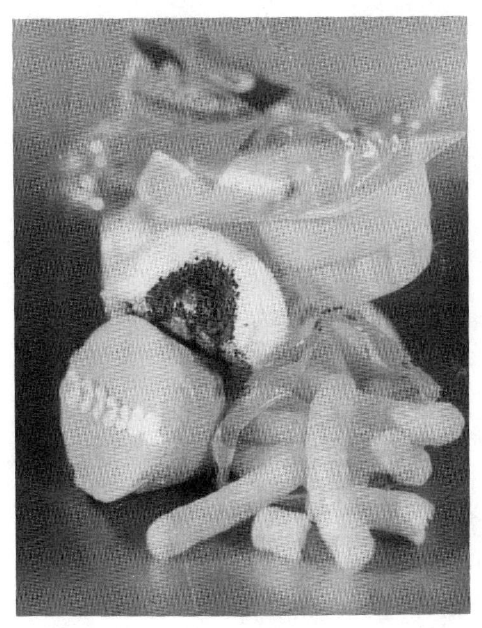

Figure 24–9. Hydrogenated fats. Unsaturated fats from vegetable oils may become hydrogenated when processed. These fats are thereby changed to saturated fats.

able to eat all those goodies and still be on a low-fat, low-cholesterol diet without jeopardizing his health. Menu 2 gives Mike's improved low-fat, low-cholesterol diet.

MENU 2

Breakfast
1½ cup Bran Chex
1 cup 2% milk
¾ cup orange juice

Lunch
peanut butter and jam sandwich on whole-wheat bread
1 cup carrot sticks and green beans
1½ cup apple juice

Snack
2 servings pretzel sticks
chocolate ice milk popsicle

Dinner
10 large shrimp with 1½ tsp. "drawn" margarine
baked potato with 2 tsp. margarine

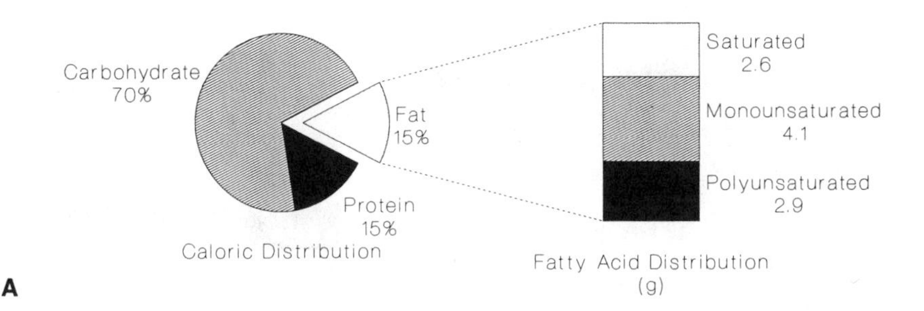

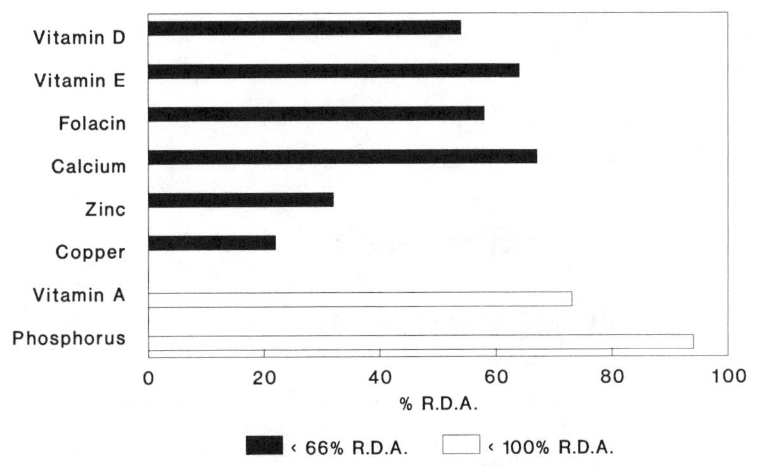

Figure 24–10. **A.** Mike's Low-Fat, Low-Cholesterol Diet (Menu 1). Cholesterol intake is 44 milligrams per 1000 calories. **B.** Inappropriate Nutrient Intakes of Mike's Low-Fat, Low-Cholesterol Diet (Menu 1). Percent of RDAs are for an 11-year-old boy.

salad with 2 tablespoons oil and vinegar dressing
1 cup apple juice

Mike was able to eat enough food to get all the energy he needed for growth and development. The dietary composition of this menu gave him a low-fat diet (30 percent of calories derived from fat) with low cholesterol intake (123 mg). Moreover, the distribution of animal (saturated) versus vegetable (polyunsaturated) fats was ideal (Fig. 24–11A). This diet allowed him to improve the intake of zinc, iron, calcium, and copper. It also provided him with all the vitamin E and folacin he needed (Fig. 24–11B). This menu also has a higher fiber content. The main sources of fiber were high-fiber-containing cereal, whole-wheat bread, fruits, and vegetables. Fiber, particularly soluble fiber from oats, fruits, and vegetables, has been found to be beneficial in helping lower serum cholesterol levels (Van Horn et al 1986).

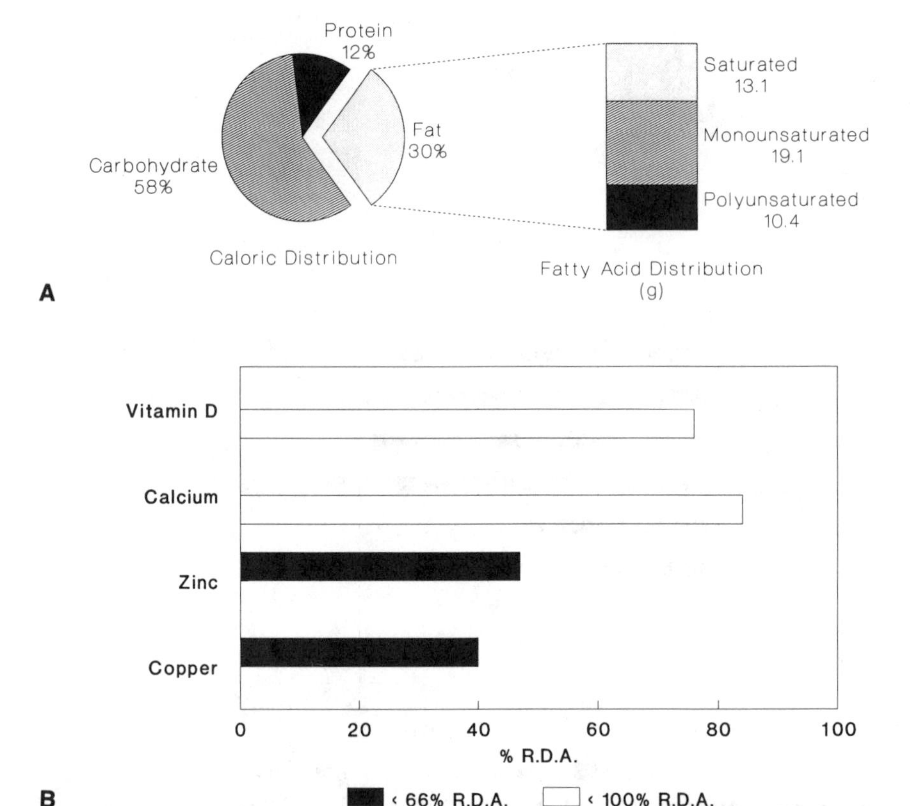

Figure 24–11. **A.** Mike's Improved Low-Fat, Low-Cholesterol Diet (Menu 2). Cholesterol intake is 62 milligrams per 1000 calories. **B.** Inappropriate Nutrient Intakes of Mike's Improved Low-Fat, Low-Cholesterol Diet (Menu 2). Percent of RDAs are for an 11-year-old boy.

CLINICAL INTERVENTION

It is clear that our American diet has traditionally been based on foods that are high in saturated fat and cholesterol. Most authorities agree that fat and cholesterol intakes should be reduced in accordance with the most current nutrition goals (see Chapter 9). A reduction of fat intake to about one third of the calories consumed is easy to aim for, and with minor modifications most adults and children could achieve this level without major dietary changes. A note of caution is important; even the American Heart Association and other organizations do not recommend this reduction in fat and cholesterol in the diet for children less than 2 years of age. The American Academy of Pediatrics has been very vocal in pointing out that infants need fat and cholesterol in their diets for appropriate growth and development. We have recently reported on a number of babies who failed to grow when overzealous mothers decreased the fat content of the diet of infants less than 2 years of age in attempts to avoid atherosclerosis (Pugliese et al 1987).

Human milk, which is the ideal food for all infants, is not low in fat or cholesterol (see Chapter 12), and yet individuals who were breast-fed as babies may have lower blood cholesterol levels in adulthood (Kark et al 1984). Early dietary exposure to cholesterol may modify cholesterol metabolism later in life (Filer 1988). Therefore, humans should not tamper with changing the dietary habits of babies to fit adult ideals.

It should not be forgotten that there are factors other than diet that might be key in the control of high blood cholesterol levels and in reducing the risk of premature atherosclerosis, heart disease, and stroke. Increased exercise and smoking avoidance are essential and of great benefit. Obesity is also a very important risk factor. High fat/calorie intake is usually closely linked to obesity; therefore, children who have a tendency to be overweight may need more attention (Griffin et al 1989) (see Chapter 18).

Children's dietary restrictions require caution and gradual changes to educate their senses, likes, and food preferences while making sure their growth proceeds and their nutritional intake is appropriate. Children with high blood cholesterol levels need to be treated by specific reductions in fat and cholesterol intake in their diets. This should be accomplished only with appropriate supervision and training as it is easy to consume an inadequate diet that may lead to growth failure and/or other complications (Lifshitz & Moses 1989). Moreover, children who are at risk for atherosclerosis and have high blood cholesterol levels may require medical treatment and are best followed by a health care team that includes a physician and a registered dietitian.

When faced with the task of reducing fat and cholesterol intake, parents and children must learn how to make wise food choices. It is at this practical level of selecting meats, preparing foods, eating at restaurants, and dealing with special occasions such as birthday parties that mistakes may be made. In addition, striking a balance between the desire to have the child eat the most ideal diet to lower blood cholesterol levels and the need for the child not to feel alienated or ostracized because he or she eats differently is a very important component in managing a child with hypercholesterolemia. Too much denial of favorite foods will only serve to make those foods even more special and sought after. Again, moderation should be stressed if a healthier style of eating is to be established for a life-time.

Among the variety of meats available, including lamb, veal, beef, pork, poultry, and fish, there are acceptable low-fat, low-cholesterol choices within each category. Of course, all these animal products contribute cholesterol to the diet but depending on the cut of meat, the fat content may vary considerably (see Table 24–1 and Fig. 24–5 to 24–9). For example, a fatty cut of beef such as skirt steak provides over 75 percent of the calories from fat and would not be recommended. However, flank steak, which may provide less than 35 percent of calories from fat, may certainly be an acceptable choice. Therefore, total avoidance of red meat in diets of children with high blood cholesterol is not necessary. In fact, such practices may interfere with the child's ability to ingest adequate amounts of iron and zinc since red meat, including beef and pork, are excellent sources of these nutrients.

The "lower" grades of meat, such as choice or "good," are also lower in fat (Fig. 24–12). The prime cut, highest grade choices, are those with the most fat within the meat (marbling). This increased fat content makes these meats the most tender and therefore they have been the most desirable and expensive choices in America. Using moist methods of cooking such as stewing or using tenderizers may help make the leaner meats more palatable. In light of the efforts to lower fat in the American diet, the meat grading system is also being changed. Choice grades, which have negative connotations as a "lower" grade of meat, are now called "select" in the new grading system established by the USDA.

Fish has received a lot of attention as part of the dietary recommendation to lower blood cholesterol levels and is now a very popular food choice (Kromhout, Bosschieter & Coulander 1985). Fish contains a unique kind of fatty acid, known as omega-3 fatty acid or EPA, which is found in the polyunsaturated part of fish oil. Omega-3 fatty acid has been shown to lower blood cholesterol and triglyceride levels while preserving the level of HDL, or "good," cholesterol (Illingworth, Harris & Conner 1984, Phillipson et al 1985). Fish with a high fat content, such as salmon, mackerel, haddock, trout,

BEEF CUT	NUMBER OF CALORIES	FAT (GRAMS)
Round tip	149	5.0 total 1.8 saturated
Top loin	168	7.1 total 2.7 saturated
Top round	169	4.3 total 1.5 saturated
Eye of round	141	4.0 total 1.5 saturated
Tenderloin	175	8.1 total 3.0 saturated
Top sirloin	162	5.8 total 2.3 saturated

Figure 24–12. The skinniest six. (From the USDA Handbook 8–13 1990 Rev. Figures are for a 3-ounce cooked serving. Beef is trimmed before cooking. Four ounces uncooked meat yield 3 ounces cooked meat. © 1990 Beef Industry Council and Beef Board.)

and herring, contain high amounts of omega-3 fatty acids (Hepburn, Exler & Weihrauch 1986). Therefore, even fatty fish such as salmon, which has 57 percent of calories from fat, may be encouraged in the diet of children with high blood cholesterol levels. The use of fish-oil supplements, however, is not recommended as a component of the nutritional treatment of hypercholesterolemia in children. It should be pointed out that fish is not regulated by the USDA. Most fish is imported and there are no standards to grade the freshness or to determine contamination of the product. Fish might contain bacteria, viruses, parasites, toxins, and other pollutants. Care should be exercised in the selection and preparation of fish before eating it. Shellfish and raw fish need not be avoided because of cholesterol but may need to be avoided because of potential contamination, which could cause infections or other diseases.

Since many of the foods we eat are commercially prepared, reading labels on food products and interpreting their appropriateness is a critical part in modifying children's fat and cholesterol intake. Food labels provide the consumer with product information including the name, manufacturer, and distributor of the product as well as the ingredients, which are listed in descending order of amount. If the product contains fat, the kind must be listed. To avoid products made with saturated fat, products such as bacon, lard, hardened (hydrogenated) fat, coconut, palm, butter, cream, cheese, egg yolk, whole milk, and chocolate should be used sparingly. Do not be fooled by labels that advertise "no cholesterol"; no cholesterol content does not always mean that the product is low in fat or low in saturated fat.

Another advertising trick is to put on the label that a product is 80 percent fat-free. This type of label information is often found on processed luncheon meats and cheeses. Although an 80 percent fat-free turkey bologna may sound like a low-fat product, it really is not! In 1 ounce (28 g) of turkey bologna, 20 percent of the product weight is fat; it would contain 0.2 ounce (5.6 g) of fat. Since each gram of fat has 9 calories, 50.4 calories in this product are from fat. Given the total caloric content (70 kcal) of 1 ounce of turkey bologna, the product has 72 percent of the calories derived from fat, and that fat can add up since most people use at least 3 ounces of meat for a sandwich. Obviously, since the goal is to reduce fat intake to 30 percent of calories from fat, this turkey bologna should not be offered frequently, despite being "80 percent fat free." When faced with a label, an easy thing to do is to estimate the calories from fat. A product that provides more than 30 percent of calories from fat is one that should be used sparingly. Another rule of thumb when trying to select low-fat processed sandwich meats or cheeses is to select products with labels showing 3 grams or less of fat per ounce.

"Fake fat" is now available in local stores. These fat replacements are marketed as a magical cure for obesity and hypercholesterolemia. If history repeats itself, fat substitutes will be as ineffective at altering the fat content of our diets as the advent of sugar substitutes was in reducing sugar consumption and obesity (see Chapters 9 and 18).

Sweets, baked goods, and desserts do not have to be eliminated from a low-fat, low-cholesterol menu, although moderation is generally advised. Most commercially available baked goods incorporate saturated fat such as coconut oil or palm oil and therefore are not acceptable. For the ambitious parent, favorite cookie or cake recipes can be modified to meet the dietary goals of low fat (particularly saturated fat) and low cholesterol. Frozen desserts such as fruit ices, sherbet, sorbet, ice milk, and some low-fat frozen yogurts may be included on a low-fat, low-cholesterol diet without alarm. However, excess intake of refined sugar, even if the fat and cholesterol intakes are reduced, may lead to increased levels of fat (triglyceride) in the bloodstream. As with all diets, a balance must be achieved without excesses or deficiencies in any one food or nutrient.

A low-fat, low-cholesterol diet for the treatment of hypercholesterolemia can best be achieved by making wise substitutions (Table 24–2). No type of food should be eliminated; rather, better choices should be made. With a lot

Table 24–2. Wise Substitutions for the Dietary Treatment of High Blood Cholesterol Levels.

INSTEAD OF	TRY
Whole eggs	Two egg whites or 2 ounces of egg substitute for each whole egg
High fat luncheon meats	Boiled or spiced ham Sliced chicken or turkey breast Wafer-thin meats: lean roast beef, corned beef, pastrami Turkey ham or turkey pastrami
Tuna packed in oil	Tuna packed in water
Hard cheese (cheddar, muenster, Swiss)	Part-skim ricotta and mozzarella cheese; farmer's cheese, hoop cheese; uncreamed pot cheese; dutch cheese; low-fat cheese products
Frying foods in fat	Sauté in nonstick skillet with vegetable cooking spray
Spaghetti sauce containing meat	Meatless spaghetti sauce
Sirloin steak	Flank steak or lean ground beef
Whole milk	Low-fat or skim milk
Sour cream, mayonnaise	Low-fat plain yogurt with added herbs and spices
Butter	Soft tub margarine
Ice cream	Ices; ice milk; sherbet; sorbet; some low-fat frozen yogurts
Puddings made with whole milk	Puddings made with skim milk
Cheesecake	Angel food cake
Corn chips, potato chips	Pretzels; popcorn with no added butter
Croissants, sandwich buns	English muffins; pita bread; water bagels; corn tortilla (not fried); French or Italian bread; whole wheat bread

of knowledge and a little bit of effort, the dietary goals can be achieved and maintained forever.

For children who fail to lower blood cholesterol levels, drug treatment may be indicated. Drugs are expensive, may induce side effects, and do not work efficiently without the necessary dietary treatment. Intensive nutritional intervention combined with drug therapy is urged for individuals at high risk—those whose cholesterol levels remain above 240 milligrams per deciliter despite nutrition intervention, particularly if they have two or more additional cardiac risk factors. A recent scientific discovery has identified a normal body hormone, granulocyte-macrophage colony-stimulating factor, that has been shown to lower serum cholesterol levels. How it works remains unknown but new findings such as this one may lead to new types of treatment and even prevention of atherosclerosis (Nimer et al 1988).

REFERENCES

American Academy of Pediatrics Committee on Nutrition: Prudent life-style for children: Dietary fat and cholesterol. Pediatrics 1986; 78:521–525.

American Academy of Pediatrics Committee on Nutrition: Indications for cholesterol testing in children. Pediatrics 1989; 83:141–142.

American Medical Association Statement. Dietary goals for the US—Supplemental views. Select Committee on Nutrition and Human Needs 1977:670–677.

Bogdanich W. Inaccuracy in testing cholesterol hampers war on heart disease. The Wall Street Journal Vol. CCIX, No. 23, Feb. 3, 1987.

Dwyer J. Diets for children and adolescents that meet the dietary goals. Am J Dis Child 1980; 184:1073–1080.

Dwyer JH, Rieger-Nakorerwa GE, Semmer NK, Fuchs R, Lippert P. Low-level cigarette smoking and longitudinal change in serum cholesterol among adolescents: The Berlin-Bremen Study. JAMA 1988; 259:2857–2862.

Filer LJ. Does diet in infancy influence atherosclerosis in the adult? In Prevention of Adult Atherosclerosis During Childhood. Report of the 95th Ross Conference on Pediatric Research. Columbus, OH: Ross Laboratories, 1988:70–74.

Garcia RE, Moore DS. Routine cholesterol surveillance in childhood. Pediatrics 1989; 89:751–755.

Griffin TC, Christoffel KK, Binns HJ, et al. Family history evaluation as a predictive screen for childhood hypercholesterolemia. Pediatrics 1989; 89:365–374.

Grundy SM, Bonanome A. Workshop on monounsaturated fatty acids. Arteriosclerosis 1987; 7:644–648.

Hepburn FN, Exler J, Weihrauch JL. Provisional tables on the content of omega-3 fatty acids and other fat components of selected foods. J Am Diet Assoc 1986; 86:788–793.

Hoeg JM, Brewer HB. Definition and management of hyperlipoproteinemia. J Am Coll Nutr 1987; 6:157–163.

Illingworth DR, Harris WS, Conner WE. Inhibition of low density lipoprotein synthesis by dietary omega-3 fatty acids in humans. Arteriosclerosis 1984; 4:270–275.

Kark JD, Troya G, Friedlander Y, Slater PE, Stein Y. Validity of maternal reporting of breast feeding history and the association of blood lipids in 17 year olds in Jerusalem. J Epidemiol Community Health 1984; 38:218–225.

Kromhout D, Bosschieter E, Coulander CDL. The inverse relation between fish consumption and 20-year mortality from coronary heart disease. N Engl J Med 1985; 312:1205–1209.

Lauer CM, Lee J, Clarke WR. Factors affecting the relationship between childhood and adult cholesterol levels: The Muscatine Study. Pediatrics 1988; 82:309–318.

Lauer RM, Clarke WR. Use of cholesterol measurements in childhood for the prediction of adult hypercholesterolemia: The Muscatine Study. JAMA 1990; 264:3034–3038.

Lifshitz F, Moses N. Growth failure—A complication of hypercholesterolemia treatment. Am J Dis Child 1989; 83:393–398.

Lipid Research Clinics Program. The Lipid Research Clinics Coronary Primary Prevention Trials results. I. Reduction in the incidence of coronary heart disease. JAMA 1984; 251:351–355.

Nader PR, Taras HL, Sallis JF, Patterson TL. Adult heart disease prevention in childhood: A national survey of pediatricians' practices and attitudes. Pediatrics 1987; 79:843–850.

National Institutes of Health Consensus Conference. Lowering blood cholesterol to prevent heart disease. JAMA 1985; 253:2080–2086.

Newman WP, Freedman DS, Voors AW, et al. Relation of serum lipoprotein levels and systolic blood pressure to early atherosclerosis: The Bogalusa Heart Study. N Engl J Med 1986; 314:138–144.

Newman TB, Browner WS, Hulley SB. The case against childhood cholesterol screening. JAMA 1990; 264:3039–3043.

Nimer SD, Champlin RE, Golde DW. Serum cholesterol-lowering activity of granulocyte-macrophage colony-stimulating factor. JAMA 1988; 260:3297–3300.

Phillipson BE, Rothrock DW, et al. Reduction of plasma lipids, lipoproteins, and apoproteins by dietary fish oils in patients with hypertriglyceridemia. N Engl J Med 1985; 312:1210–1216.

Pugliese MT, Weyman-Daum M, Moses N, Lifshitz F. Parental health beliefs as a cause of non-organic failure to thrive. Pediatrics 1987; 80:175–182.

Roberts L. Measuring cholesterol is as tricky as lowering it. Science 1987; 283:482–483.

Van Horn LV, Liu K, Parker D, et al. Serum lipid response to oat product intake with a modified fat diet. J Am Diet Assoc 1986; 86:759–764.

Weidman W, Kwiterovich P, Jesse MJ, Nugent E. Diet in the healthy child. Task Force Committee of the Nutrition Committee and the Cardiovascular Disease in the Young Council of the American Heart Association. Circulation 1983; 69:1414A.

Wolinsky H. Talking heart. Science (NY) 1980; 21:6–10.

25

Metabolic Disorders

Baby Zachary had frequent feeding problems. He would spit up often and was quite irritable. He was given several different kinds of formulas by his pediatrician but improvement after a formula change only lasted a few days just to be followed by bad days. However, Zachary was thriving well. At 4½ months of age his condition turned worse and his doctor suspected an ear infection as the culprit. Although he was given antibiotics, he became more irritable and sleepy, and none of the formulas that had helped in the past worked this time. Laboratory tests revealed an elevated ammonia level in the blood. Unfortunately, by the time this was uncovered, the baby had lapsed into a coma and was rushed to a specialist in metabolic diseases. When the doctor saw the baby, Zachary's blood ammonia level was 10 times normal and he had brain swelling (cerebral edema). Only with blood filtration (hemodialysis) and special nutritional treatment was the baby able to survive. He had an inborn error of metabolism: partial ornithine transcarboxylase (OCT) deficiency, a rare disorder in which babies cannot metabolize protein.

The study of inborn errors of metabolism began at the turn of the century when Sir Archibald Garrod, Professor of Medicine at Oxford in England, studied patients with diseases that resulted from inherited, life-long defects in the ordered processes of metabolism (Garrod 1908). Since that time, knowledge of inborn errors of metabolism has been slow to develop, but in the past three decades, with the availability of new, sophisticated technologies such as amino acid analysis, our ability to detect and diagnose inborn errors of metabolism has vastly improved. We can now predict the genetic basis and analyze the metabolic consequences of many of these alterations.

In previous decades arrival at a precise diagnosis of a metabolic disease was considered somewhat academic as there was no effective treatment available for most of these conditions. However, that situation has now changed, and increasing numbers of children with these disorders are being successfully treated. Thus, the significance of early diagnosis is often critical to the outcome of the patient.

INBORN ERRORS OF METABOLISM

The inborn errors of metabolism that may occur during infancy are many, each one producing a specific disturbance in the way the body utilizes a particular substance. A partial list of some of the disorders that may lead to metabolic diseases and their principal presenting problem is given in Table 25–1. This list includes a large number of inborn errors of metabolism but it is incomplete. There are many more disorders that are not mentioned in the table; all of them need to be specifically diagnosed to provide appropriate

Table 25–1. Inborn Errors of Metabolism During Infancy.

METABOLIC ACIDOSIS
Glycogen storage diseases
Maple syrup urine disease
Organic acid disorders
Pyruvate catabolic disorders
HYPERAMMONEMIA
Organic acid disorders
Transient hyperammonemia of the newborn (THAN)
Urea cycle defects
HYPOGLYCEMIA
Amino acidopathies
Fatty acid oxidation defect
Fructose 1,6-diphosphatase deficiency
Fructose intolerance
Galactosemia
Glycogen storage diseases
Hormone deficiencies
Maple syrup urine disease
LIVER DYSFUNCTION
α_1-Antitrypsin deficiency
Fructose intolerance
Galactosemia
Glycogen storage diseases
Phenylketonuria
Tyrosinemia
Urea cycle defects

Modified from Slonim AE. Emergencies of inborn errors of metabolism. In Lifshitz F, ed. Pediatric endocrinology. New York: Marcel Dekker, 1990.

therapy (Brusilow, Batshaw & Waber 1982, Wapnir 1985, Muenzer 1986, Goodman 1986, Harkness 1987, Stanley 1987).

Neonatal screening programs are the most effective method of early detection of a number of inborn errors of metabolism. These programs have been operational for more than 20 years in all 50 states and in most other developed countries. In New York the mandate is that all babies be tested for the following seven conditions (Fig. 25–1): phenylketonuria (PKU), maple syrup urine disease, galactosemia, homocystinuria, biotinidase deficiency, hypothyroidism, and sickle-cell disease. However, there are many more potential metabolic problems that are not identified by neonatal screening programs. These need to be recognized by astute physicians for appropriate treatment.

Many inborn errors of metabolism appear during the newborn period with symptoms that typically begin after feedings have been fully initiated. Important signs of incipient problems are breathing difficulties (apnea) or breathing too fast (tachypnea). There may also be severe manifestations of sleepiness (lethargy), weakness (hypotonia), seizures, and coma (Snyderman 1971). Persistent vomiting and failure to thrive (FTT) should always be considered as symptoms indicative of a potential inborn error of metabolism. Abnormal urine or body odor may also be a clue to the diagnosis of a number of these diseases. For example, the urine will smell like maple syrup if the baby has maple syrup urine disease, while a body odor resembling sweaty feet is a clue for isovaleric acidemia (Slonim 1990). Persistent jaundice with liver dysfunction, low blood sugar levels, elevated blood ammonia levels, or metabolic acidosis are strong indicators of inborn errors of metabolism (see Table 25–1). There are many diseases that lead to hyperammonemia and acidosis (Fig. 25–2). A history of an unexplained death in an infant sibling, or the presence of intermarriages within the same family (parental consanguinity) increases the likelihood that a sick infant may be suffering from an inborn error of metabolism.

The clinical manifestations of babies with inborn errors of metabolism are often similar to those that may be seen with infections or with brain injury. Thus, it is important to think of inborn errors of metabolism at the same time as these more common problems are ruled out. However, it should be noted that infants with inborn errors of metabolism may also develop infections or other stresses that may trigger the clinical and biochemical manifestations of the metabolic problem. Infections and stress may disrupt the metabolic equilibrium that existed prior to getting ill. Simple metabolic screening studies of blood and urine may identify the presence of an inborn error of metabolism before permanent damage occurs.

It has been standard teaching that babies with inborn errors of metabolism are normally formed and healthy at birth because the fetus is protected by the exchange of nutrients and metabolites across the placenta, and that only after birth does the disorder become evident. However, this is not always

NEWBORN SCREENING BLOOD COLLECTION FORM
DO NOT USE AFTER JUNE 1989

0 0 6 8 9 1 9 0

Lab I.D. 06891902

☐ *Tests Within Acceptable Limits
☐ SEE ATTACHED REPORT

DOH USE ONLY - - DO NOT WRITE IN SHADED AREA

Infant's Last Name | First Initial | 1 ☐ Male 2 ☐ Female | Multiple Birth A B C OTHER ☐ ☐ ☐ ☐ | Ethnicity/Race 1 ☐ Wht. 3 ☐ Hisp. 2 ☐ Blk. 4 ☐ Asian 5 ☐ Other | ☐ Special Handling

Date of Birth Mo Day Yr | Birth Weight Grams | Date of Specimen Mo. Day Yr. | Specimen Collected 1 ☐ Less than 24 hrs of age 2 ☐ More than 24 hrs of age | 1 ☐ Initial Specimen 2 ☐ Repeat Specimen

Infant's Medical Record No. | ☐ Premature ☐ Transfused. ______ Date | Mother's Social Security No. | Mother's Age

Hospital PFI Code | Hospital of Birth? 1 ☐ Yes 2 ☐ No | ☐ Homebirth | Physician License No | Mother's Name. Last First

Hospital Name: | Physician's Name: | Address:

City | Address | Zip

Zip | Tel ( )

DO NOT USE ADDRESSOGRAPH | Tel ( ) | County of Residence

L-81974

*Tested For Phenylalanine, Leucine, Methionine, Galactose-1-P Uridyl Transferase, Sickle Hemoglobin (SS), Thyroxine

LABORATORY COPY

SATURATE ALL CIRCLES COMPLETELY — See reverse side for instructions

DOH-1514 (1/88) — MCH-3 S&S 903 LOT #WH71

BLOOD COLLECTION FORM
DO NOT USE AFTER JUNE 1989
INSTRUCTIONS

With ballpoint pen, print *all* information requested on form, including current address information.

1. See diagram for puncture site. Avoid previous puncture sites or curvature of the heel.
2. Place infant's limb in a position to increase venous pressure.
3. Warm heel for three minutes.
4. Cleanse puncture site with 70% alcohol.
5. Wipe dry with sterile gauze.
6. Make puncture using sterile lancet with tip not longer than 2.44 mm.
7. Wipe away first drop of blood with dry sterile gauze.
8. Allow second, larger drop of blood to form.
9. Gently apply filter paper to large drop of blood. Allow blood to soak through and completely fill preprinted circle. Apply blood to one side of filter paper only. (Either side may be chosen for procedure.) **Do not use capillary tubes for specimen collection.**
10. Fill circle with **single** application to drop of blood. Do not layer successive drops of blood.
11. Fill all five circles.
12. **Allow blood spots to thoroughly air dry for at least 4 hours** on a flat, nonabsorptive surface, away from direct heat and sunlight. Avoid touching or smearing blood spots. Never superimpose one filter paper on another before thoroughly drying. Do not refrigerate.
13. When placing more than one specimen in an envelope, alternate forms so that blood spots on adjacent forms are not in contact.
14. Mail completed collection forms to the testing laboratory within 24 hours of collection.
15. Specimens identified as **special handling** must be thoroughly dry and then individually sealed in a plastic bag. The outside of the plastic bag **must** be labeled as requiring **special handling.**

Preferred puncture site is indicated by shaded areas on heel.

RIGHT — **ACCEPTABLE** Circle filled and evenly saturated

WRONG — **UNACCEPTABLE** Layering

Insufficient, multiple applications

Serum rings present

Figure 25–1. Five drops of blood are collected from a heel stick and placed on the circles of the newborn screening form. The form is mailed to the state laboratory where the blood drops on the filter paper are titrated for analysis of inborn errors of metabolism.

correct, as inborn errors of metabolism often result in abnormalities detectable at birth (Brown et al 1982, Goodman, Reale & Berlow 1983, Leonard 1986). If an inborn error of metabolism is suspected because of a physical malformation or because of the signs and symptoms mentioned above, the baby needs detailed evaluation to establish an accurate diagnosis. Thus, they should be promptly referred to an Inborn Errors of Metabolism Center,

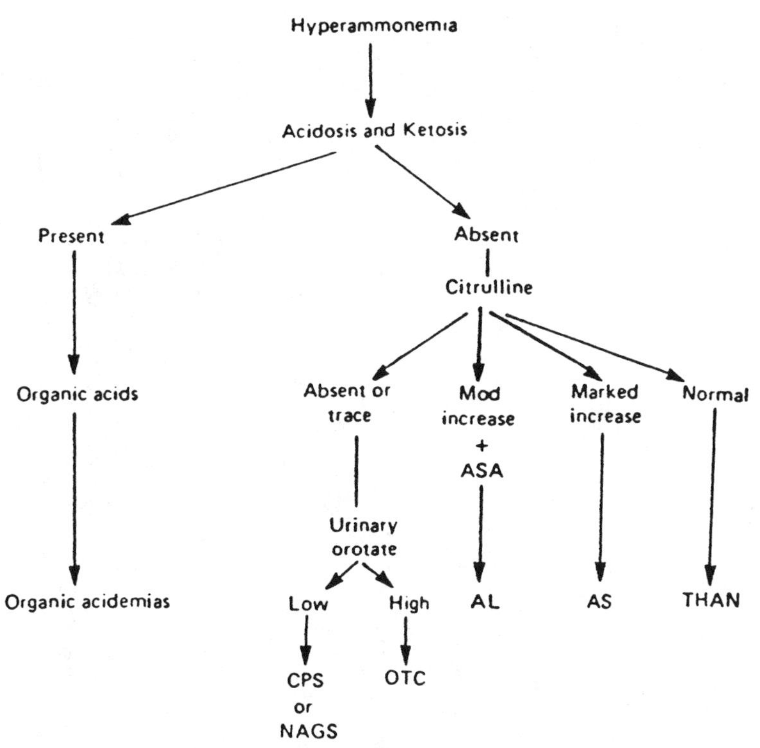

Figure 25–2. Flow chart for diagnosis of hyperammonemia. CPS = carbamoylphosphate synthetase; OTC = ornithine-transcarbamylase; NAGS = acetylglutamate synthetase; AL = argininosuccinate lyase; AS = argininosuccinate synthetase; THAN = transient hyperammonemia of the newborn.

which is a designated center where expertise is available for diagnosis and treatment of these unusual conditions. It should be kept in mind that although individual inborn errors of metabolism are rare, as a group, they are not infrequent. It has been determined that 1 in 5000 live newborn babies have genetic disorders, and many more of the patients who get admitted to tertiary care hospitals might have these types of problems (Cederbaum 1989).

NUTRITIONAL REQUIREMENTS

The nutrient needs and the Recommended Dietary Allowances (RDAs) (Committee on Nutrition 1989) intended for healthy persons are frequently inappropriate for infants and children with specific inherited metabolic disorders. The RDAs may be insufficient or excessive (Table 25–2), or nutrients and other products may become "conditionally" essential or may be needed

Table 25–2. Selected Examples of Disorders and Mechanisms in Which RDAs for Minerals and Vitamins Become Inadequate.

METABOLIC DISORDER		NUTRIENT OF CONCERN		MECHANISM OF DEFICIENCY
Name	**Description**	**Deficiency**	**Excess**	
Abetalipoproteinemia	Lipid disorder associated with low cholesterol levels	Fat-soluble vitamins (A, D, E, K)		Fat malabsorption
Acrodermatitis enteropathica	Gastrointestinal and skin disease with diarrhea and fat malabsorption	Zinc; fat-soluble vitamins (A, D, E, K)		Decreased gastrointestinal absorption
Biotinidase deficiency	Deficiency of enzyme responsible for making biotin available to the body	Biotin		Impaired metabolism of biotin with decreased availability for utilization
Carbohydrate metabolism disorders	Defect in galactose or fructose metabolism	Phosphorus		Trapping of phosphorus by the altered carbohydrate metabolism
Familial hypophosphatemia	Defect in phosphate transport in the kidneys leading to low serum phosphate levels and rickets	Phosphorus; vitamin D		Decreased kidney reabsorption of phosphate Increased requirement for therapy
Hereditary tyrosinemia	Elevated blood and urine tyrosine levels due to deficiency of enzyme responsible for its metabolism; liver damage often occurs	Vitamin D		Impaired synthesis
Homocystinuria	Elevated homocysteine and methionine levels due to deficiency of enzyme responsible for their metabolism	Folate; vitamin B_{12}, vitamin B_6		Excess utilization Increased requirement for potential therapy—cofactor for deficient enzyme
Idiopathic hemochromatosis	Defect in iron metabolism	None	Iron	Excess storage of iron
Maple syrup urine disease	Elevated blood and urine levels of branched-chain amino acids	Thiamin		Increased requirement for potential therapy—cofactor for the deficient enzyme
Menkes' syndrome (steely-hair syndrome)	Defect in copper metabolism	Copper		Decreased gastrointestinal absorption

Organic acid disorders				
Propionic acidemia	Deficiency of biotin-dependent enzyme with accumulation of propionic acid	Biotin		Increased requirement for potential therapy—cofactor for the deficient enzyme
Methylmalonic acidemia	Deficiency of several enzymes with accumulation of methylmalonic acid	Vitamin B_{12} (cobalamin)		Impaired metabolism of vitamin B_{12} to the active form utilized by the body
Phenylketonuria	Elevated blood and urine phenylalanine levels due to deficiency of enzyme responsible for phenylalanine metabolism	Iron		Decreased gastrointestinal absorption
Pyruvate catabolic disorders	Defects in the enzyme systems responsible for production of glucose	Biotin; thiamin		Increased requirement for potential therapy—cofactor for the deficient enzymes
Urea cycle defects	Altered protein metabolism			
	—with phenylacetate therapy	Vitamin B_6		Excess utilization
	—with sodium benzoate therapy	Vitamin B_6; folate; pantothenic acid		Excess utilization
Vitamin B_{12} deficiency disorders				
Intrinsic factor	Deficiency in the intrinsic factor produced in the stomach necessary for vitamin B_{12} absorption	Vitamin B_{12}		Decreased gastrointestinal absorption
Variety of enzyme deficiencies	Deficiency in enzyme systems for vitamin B_{12} metabolism	Vitamin B_{12}		Impaired production of the active form of vitamin B_{12}
Wilson's disease	Defect in copper metabolism with excessive copper accumulation in tissues	Fat-soluble vitamins (A, D, E, K); folate; thiamin; vitamin B_{12}; vitamin B_6; zinc	Copper	Decreased gastrointestinal absorption Decreased metabolism
Williams syndrome	Defect in calcium and vitamin D metabolism	None	Calcium, vitamin D	Increased sensitivity or overproduction of the active form of vitamin D

in larger amounts owing to the metabolic defects that preclude their synthesis (Table 25–3). Consequently, no minimum or recommended daily allowances for nutrients can be established for all patients with inborn errors of metabolism. Each inherited disorder requires a specific recommendation.

Insufficient Nutrients in RDAs

The RDAs are insufficient in many inherited metabolic disorders. Each one of these diseases affects mineral and vitamin utilization through a variety of mechanisms (see Table 25–2). Intestinal malabsorption of zinc is present in acrodermatitis enteropathica (Hambidge & Walravens 1982), in PKU there may be alterations in the absorption of iron (Stephnick-Gropper et al 1988) and in abetalipoproteinemia there may be generalized fat-soluble vitamin malabsorption (Elsas & McCormick 1986).

In other inborn errors of metabolism the body may have an increased requirement for certain nutrients owing to modifications in the way the body

Table 25–3. Examples of "Conditionally" Essential Nutrients with Inborn Errors of Metabolism.

INHERITED METABOLIC DEFECTS OF AMINO ACID METABOLISM	"CONDITIONALLY" ESSENTIAL NUTRIENT
Carbohydrate metabolism disorders	
Galactosemia	Carnitine
Glycogen storage disease	Choline
Hereditary fructose intolerance	
Carnitine biosynthesis disorders	Carnitine
Electron transport disorders	Coenzyme Q_{10}
Homocystinuria	Cystine
Miscellaneous defects	
Wilson's disease	Carnitine
Idiopathic hemochromatosis	Choline
Organic acid disorders	Carnitine
	Choline
Phenylalanine catabolic disorders	
PKU	Tyrosine
Dihydropteridine reductase and biopterin synthetic deficiencies	Tetrahydrobiopterin
Pyruvate catabolic disorders	Lipoic acid
Tyrosinemia	Carnitine
Urea cycle disorders	Arginine
	Glycine
	Hippuric acid
	Citrulline
	Carnitine
	Choline

Adapted from Acosta PB. Mineral and vitamin requirements in patients with selected metabolic disorders. Diet Pediatr Pract 1988; 11(3):1–3.

with a genetic defect disposes of specific substances. In hereditary fructose intolerance and in galactosemia, phosphorus needs are increased because these defects trap phosphate in the cells. In biotinidase deficiency, there is an inability to reuse biotin because it not released from the enzyme compound for further action (Bartlett 1983). In many inborn errors of metabolism that require protein restriction, calorie requirements must be increased to avoid catabolism of protein (Slonim, Coleman & Moses 1984).

Excess utilization of nutrients leading to increased requirements may occur in disorders such as the urea cycle defects (Msall et al 1984), homocystinuria (Bartlett 1983), and propionic acidemia (Petrowski et al 1987). Medications such as sodium benzoate or phenylacetate administered to children with urea cycle defects to help them reduce the toxic levels of ammonia in their blood enhance nitrogen wasting. The loss of protein is also accompanied by increased utilization of specific elements such as glutamate (Newsholme & Leech 1983). In patients with homocystinuria, there may be increased utilization of folate leading to deficiency of this vitamin. In some forms of homocystinuria and maple syrup urine disease, the respective enzyme compounds (holoenzymes) necessary for the appropriate amino acid metabolism may be rapidly degraded in the absence of megadoses of vitamin B_6 or thiamin (Elsas & McCormick 1986). With hereditary deficiencies of transcobalamin II or R binder, not only is vitamin B_{12} poorly absorbed, but the vitamin B_{12} that is absorbed is rapidly lost in the urine (Kapadia & Donaldson 1985).

Several situations exist in which the RDAs for minerals and vitamins are inadequate due to impaired production of active enzyme compounds or active vitamin. Molybdenum (Munich et al 1983), folate (Stanbury et al 1983), vitamin B_{12} (cobalamin) (Cooper & Rosenblatt 1987) and vitamin D (Elsas & McCormick 1986) are nutrients that may not be synthesized to their active products in particular inborn errors of metabolism (see Table 25–1). When this occurs very high doses of the specific vitamin or mineral may correct the problem. For example, some patients with methylmalonic acidemia require megadoses of vitamin B_{12} (cobalamin) for normal enzyme function (Bartlett 1983).

At times there is a lack of action of the vitamin due to target tissue defects. In osteopetrosis, a disorder characterized by fragile (osteosclerotic) bones, defective bone cells (osteoclasts) may fail to respond to vitamin D intakes in the RDA range. Consequently, high doses of the active vitamin D (1,25-dihydroxycholecalciferol) must be given to improve bone formation.

Excessive Nutrients in RDAs

In some metabolic disorders the RDAs for minerals and vitamins are excessive (see Table 25–2). In a condition called Williams syndrome the RDAs for calcium and vitamin D may be toxic due to hypersensitivity to or overproduction of the active form of vitamin D (1,25-dihydroxycholecalciferol) or because of excess storage of this nutrient (Elsas & McCormick 1986). In Wilson's disease and hemochromatosis the RDAs of copper and iron are too high and toxic, respectively.

Conditionally Essential Nutrients

Patients with inborn errors of metabolism often have defects that make them dependent on certain amino acids or other nutrients that are not essential for the normal population. In these situations certain compounds become "conditionally" essential (see Table 25–3). Tyrosine is an essential nutrient in PKU, while cystine is essential in homocystinuria. There may be coenzyme Q_{10} deficiency in patients with cytochrome C oxidase deficiency (Przyrembel 1987). Lipoic acid is of benefit in patients with dihydrolipoyl dehydrogenase deficiency, and tetrahydrobiopterin is of benefit in various genetic defects (Kaufman et al 1982).

Any metabolic disorder that leads to liver-cell dysfunction may cause choline and carnitine to become essential because these compounds may not be synthesized in the liver of these patients (Rudman & Feller 1986). Patients with such diseases may require an exogenous supply of carnitine and choline, for which no RDAs exist. Carnitine becomes essential in other inborn errors of metabolism when there is excess excretion of this element; it occurs in a number of organic acidemias because the carnitine binds with the acyl group of the organic acid and is excreted in the urine (Stanley 1987). Depending on the amount of organic acid synthesized, the liver may or may not be able to keep up with carnitine needs. Also, carnitine is necessary when there is a specific defect in carnitine biosynthesis (Rebouche & Paulson 1986).

NUTRITION INTERVENTION

Nutrition intervention must be individually designed for each inborn error of metabolism. The treatment must aim at either restricting injurious products or supplementing deficient nutrients. The restriction of the injurious products consists of eliminating from the diet the nutrients that are not properly metabolized. For example, in PKU, phenylalanine in the diet must be restricted in amounts sufficient to only meet the requirements. The dietary supplementation of specific nutrients is necessary in certain errors of metabolism because there may be inhibition of the synthesis of essential nutrients and/or other elements (see Tables 25–2 and 25–3).

Patients with inborn errors of metabolism who require specific diets may fail to ingest an adequate diet. For example, because of the restriction of protein intake to limit phenylalanine in the diet of children with PKU there may be a limited consumption of foods rich in iron and other minerals (Stepnick-Gropper et al 1988). In other patients nutrients are utilized to overcome the metabolic alteration; that is, they are given as medication, not as nutrients per se. Vitamins and/or other substances that have the ability to act as "coenzymes" in pharmacologic doses may somehow compensate for the patient's hereditary enzyme defect (see Tables 25–2 and 25–3). Alternatively, the specific enzyme that is lacking in a genetic disease may be able to be replaced through feedings. For example, in lactase-deficient children, the enzyme lactase, which digests the milk sugar lactose, may be added to milk prior to consumption. The patients are then able to drink and enjoy the benefits of milk without ill effects (see Chapter 19).

The nutritional therapies available for patients with inborn errors of metabolism are shown in Table 25–4. Many of the formulas required for treatment of specific disorders are available commercially, but at times special formulas must be individually prepared for the nutritional management of selected patients. An example of the difficulties in the dietary treatment of some inborn errors of metabolism is Zachary, the 4½-month-old baby described above with OTC deficiency. Because he was unable to metabolize protein he developed high blood ammonia levels, which led to seizures, coma, and brain damage. The treatment initially consisted of intravenous nutrition containing a low protein content (0.5 g/kg) but with adequate calories derived from dextrose and intravenous fat emulsion. In addition, he received treatment with sodium benzoate and hemodialysis, which produced a drop in the serum ammonia levels (Batshaw, Thomas & Brusilow 1981). As he began to regain consciousness, continuous nasogastric feedings with a low-protein diet (0.5–1.5 g/kg) were provided until oral feedings could be established. Adequate essential amino acids, calories, and other nutrients for normal growth and development were provided to him with a special formula made from modular feedings, as shown below:

	PROTEIN-FREE DIET POWDER PRODUCT 80056*	COW'S MILK INFANT FORMULA	TOTAL AMOUNT
Amount	53 g	570 mL	1000 mL†
Calories (kcal)	260	380	640
Protein (g)	0	8.55	8.55
Carbohydrate (g)	38.05	41.04	79.09
Fat (g)	11.93	20.5	32.43

*Mead Johnson, Evansville, IN.
†Water added to total volume of 1000 mL.

This combination of infant milk formula and protein-free diet powder provided a 20 calories-per-ounce formula that was low in protein. The caloric distribution was 5 percent protein, 49 percent carbohydrate, and 46 percent

Table 25–4. Nutritional Therapies Available for Patients with Inborn Errors of Metabolism.

I. HISTIDINEMIA

Formula	Manufacturer	Comments
Hist 1	Mead Johnson	For infant feedings; histidine-free L-amino acid powder; incomplete nutritional supplement; high protein (75% calories); fat-free; low carbohydrate; lactose-free; vitamin and mineral fortified.
Hist 2	Mead Johnson	For children; histidine-free L-amino acid powder; incomplete nutritional supplement; high protein (91% protein); fat-free; low carbohydrate; lactose-free; vitamin and mineral fortified; protein to calorie ratio, 22.8 g/100 kcal.

For all formulas listed, histidine from other food sources must be added to meet the child's minimum amino acid requirement for normal growth and development.

II. HOMOCYSTINURIA (VITAMIN B_6–INDEPENDENT FORM) OR HYPERMETHIONINEMIA

Formula	Manufacturer	Comments
Low Methionine Diet Powder	Mead Johnson	For infant feedings; iron-fortified soy protein powder with moderate methionine content (201 mg/100 g); composition similar to standard infant formula; lactose-free; vitamin and mineral fortified.
Hom 1	Mead Johnson	For infant feedings; methionine-free cystine-supplemented L-amino acid powder; incomplete nutritional supplement; high protein (76% calories); fat-free; low carbohydrate; lactose-free; vitamin and mineral fortified; protein to calorie ratio, 19.1 g/100 kcal.
Analog XMET	Ross Laboratories	For infant feedings; methionine-free cystine and glutamine supplemented L-amino acid powder; incomplete nutritional supplement; 11% protein calories, 40% fat calories; lactose free; vitamin, mineral, taurine, carnitine, and trace-element fortified.
Hom 2	Mead Johnson	For children; methionine-free cystine-supplemented L-amino acid powder; incomplete nutritional supplement; high protein (94% calories); fat-free; low carbohydrate; lactose-free; vitamin and mineral fortified; protein to calorie ratio, 23.4 g/100 kcal.
Maxamaid XMET	Ross Laboratories	For children 1–8 years; methionine-free cystine supplemented L-amino acid powder; incomplete nutritional supplement; high protein (28.5% calories); fat-free; high carbohydrate; lactose-free; vitamin and mineral fortified; protein to calorie ratio, 7.14 g/100 kcal.

For all formulas listed, methionine from other food sources must be added to meet the child's minimum amino acid requirement for normal growth and development.

III. HYPERLYSINEMIA OR SACCHAROPINURIA WITH HYPERLYSINEMIA

Formula	Manufacturer	Comments
Lys 1	Mead Johnson	For infant feedings; lysine-free L-amino acid powder; high protein (70% calories); fat-free; low carbohydrate; lactose-free; vitamin and mineral fortified.
Lys 2	Mead Johnson	For children; lysine-free L-amino acid powder; high protein (85% calories); fat-free; low carbohydrate; lactose-free; vitamin and mineral fortified; protein to calorie ratio, 21.25 g/100 kcal.

For all formulas listed, lysine from other food sources must be added to meet the child's minimum amino acid requirements for normal growth and development.

IV. MAPLE SYRUP URINE DISEASE AND OTHER BRANCHED-CHAIN AMINO ACID (BCAA)† METABOLIC DISORDERS‡

Formula	Manufacturer	Comments
MSUD Diet Powder	Mead Johnson	For infants and children; BCAA-free L-amino acid powder; composition similar to standard infant formula; lactose-free; vitamin and mineral fortified.
MSUD 1	Mead Johnson	For infant feeding; BCAA-free L-amino acid powder; incomplete nutritional supplement; high protein (59% calories); fat-free; moderate carbohydrate (41% calories); lactose-free, vitamin and mineral fortified.
Analog MSUD	Ross Laboratories	For infant feeding; BCAA-free glutamine supplemented L-amino acid powder; incomplete nutritional supplement, 11% protein calories, 40% fat calories, lactose-free, vitamin, mineral taurine, carnitine, and trace-element fortified.
MSUD 2	Mead Johnson	For children and adolescents; BCAA-free L-amino acid powder; incomplete nutritional supplement; high protein (71% calories); fat-free; low carbohydrate (29% calories); lactose-free, vitamin and mineral fortified; protein to calorie ratio, 17.8 g/100 kcal.
Maxamaid MSUD	Ross Laboratories	For children 1–8 years; BCAA-free L-amino acid powder; incomplete nutritional supplement; high protein (29% calories); fat-free; high carbohydrate (71% calories); lactose-free; vitamin and mineral fortified; protein to calorie ratio, 7.14 g/100 kcal.
Maxamum MSUD	Ross Laboratories	For children over 8 years and pregnant women; BCAA-free L-amino acid powder; incomplete nutritional supplement; high protein (46% calories); fat-free; moderate carbohydrate; lactose-free; vitamin, mineral, trace-element, taurine and L-carnitine fortified; protein to calorie ratio, 11.5 g/100 kcal.

For all formulas listed, BCAAs from other food sources must be added to meet the child's minimum requirements.

Table 25–4. Nutritional Therapies Available for Patients with Inborn Errors of Metabolism. *(cont.)*

V. PHENYLKETONURIA

Formula	Manufacturer	Comments
Lofenalac	Mead Johnson	For infant feeding; casein hydrolysate powder with low phenylalanine content (80 mg/100 g); composition similar to standard infant formula; lactose-containing; vitamin and mineral fortified.
PKU 1	Mead Johnson	For infant feeding; phenylalanine-free L-amino acid powder; incomplete nutritional supplement; high protein (74% calories); fat-free; low carbohydrate (26% calories): sucrose; vitamin and mineral fortified.
Analog XP	Ross Laboratories	For infant feeding; phenylalanine-free tyrosine and glutamine supplemented L-amino acid powder; 11% protein calories; composition similar to standard infant formula; lactose-free; vitamin, mineral, taurine, carnitine, and trace-element fortified.
Phenyl-Free	Mead Johnson	For children and adolescents; phenylalanine-free L-amino acid powder; incomplete nutritional supplement; 20% protein calories; low fat (15% calories); high carbohydrate (65% calories); lactose-free; vitamin and mineral fortified; protein to calorie ratio, 5 g/100 kcal.
PKU 2	Mead Johnson	For children and adolescents; phenylalanine-free L-amino acid powder; incomplete nutritional supplement; high protein (90.5% calories); fat-free; low carbohydrate (9.5% calories); lactose-free; vitamin and mineral fortified; protein to calorie ratio, 22.64 g/100 kcal.
Maxamaid XP	Ross Laboratories	For children 1–8 years; phenylalanine-free, tyrosine supplemented L-amino acid powder; incomplete nutritional supplement; high protein (28.5% calories); fat-free; high carbohydrate (71.5% calories); lactose-free; vitamin and mineral fortified; protein to calorie ratio, 7.14 g/100 kcal.
PKU 3	Mead Johnson	For pregnant women; phenylalanine-free L-amino acid powder; high protein (97% protein); fat-free; very low carbohydrate; fortified with vitamins, minerals, folic acid, and trace elements; protein to calorie ratio, 24.2 g/100 kcal.
Maxamum XP	Ross Laboratories	For children over 8 years and pregnant women; phenylalanine-free tyrosine supplemented L-amino acid powder; incomplete nutritional supplement; high protein (46% calories); fat-free; moderate carbohydrate (54% calories);

V. PHENYLKETONURIA

Formula	Manufacturer	Comments
		lactose-free; vitamin, mineral, trace-element, taurine, carnitine, and folic-acid fortified; protein to calorie ratio, 11.5 g/100 kcal.

For all formulas listed, phenylalanine from other food sources must be added to meet the child's minimum phenylalanine requirement for normal growth and development.

VI. PROPIONIC OR METHYLMALONIC ACIDEMIAS (VITAMIN B_{12}-INDEPENDENT FORM)

Formula	Manufacturer	Comments
OS 1	Mead Johnson	For infant feedings; isoleucine-, threonine-, methionine- and valine-free L-amino acid powder; incomplete nutritional supplement; high protein (61% calories); fat-free; low carbohydrate; lactose-free; vitamin and mineral fortified.
Analog XMet, Thre, Val, Isoleu	Ross Laboratories	For infant feedings; methionine-, threonine-, and valine-free low isoleucine and glutamine supplemented L-amino acid powder; incomplete nutritional supplement; 11% protein calories, 40% fat calories; lactose-free; vitamin, mineral, taurine, carnitine, and trace-element fortified.
OS 2	Mead Johnson	For children and adolescents; isoleucine-, threonine-, methionine-, valine-free L-amino acid powder; incomplete nutritional supplement; high protein (74% calories); fat-free; lactose-free; vitamin and mineral fortified; protein to calorie ratio, 18.4 g/100 kcal.
Maxamaid XMet, Thre, Val, Isoleu	Ross Laboratories	For children 1–8 years; methionine-, threonine-, valine-, isoleucine-free L-amino acid powder; incomplete nutritional supplement; high protein (28.5% calories); fat-free; high carbohydrate; lactose-free; vitamin and mineral fortified; protein to calorie ratio, 7.14 g/100 kcal.

For all formulas listed, isoleucine, threonine, methionine, and valine from other food sources must be added to meet the child's minimum amino acid requirements for normal growth and development.

VII. TYROSINEMIAS

Formula	Manufacturer	Comments
Low Phe/Tyr Diet Powder (3200AB)	Mead Johnson	For infants and children; casein hydrolysate powder with low phenylalanine (76 mg/100 g) and low tyrosine (38 mg/100 g) content; composition similar to standard infant formula; lactose-free; vitamin and mineral fortified.
Tyr 1	Mead Johnson	For infant feedings; phenylalanine- and tyrosine-free L-amino acid powder; incomplete nutritional supplement; high protein (69%

Table 25–4. Nutritional Therapies Available for Patients with Inborn Errors of Metabolism (*cont.*)

VII. TYROSINEMIAS

Formula	Manufacturer	Comments
		calories); fat-free; low carbohydrate (31% calories); lactose-free; vitamin and mineral fortified.
Analog XPhen, Tyr	Ross Laboratories	For infant feedings; phenylalanine- and tyrosine-free glutamine supplemented L-amino acid powder; incomplete nutritional supplement; 11% protein calories, 40% fat calories; lactose-free; vitamin, mineral, taurine, carnitine, and trace-element fortified.
Analog XPhen, Tyr, Met	Ross Laboratories	For infant feeding of acute tyrosinemia with hypermethioninemia; phenylalanine-, tyrosine-, and methionine-free glutamine supplemented L-amino acid powder; incomplete nutritional supplement; 11% protein, 40% fat calories; lactose-free; vitamin, mineral, taurine, carnitine, and trace-element fortified.
Tyr 2	Mead Johnson	For children and adolescents; phenylalanine- and tyrosine-free L-amino acid powder; incomplete nutritional supplement; high protein (85% calories); fat-free; low carbohydrate; lactose-free; vitamin and mineral fortified; protein to calorie ratio, 21.14 g/100 kcal.

For all formulas listed, phenylalanine and tyrosine from other food sources must be added to meet the child's minimum amino acid requirements for normal growth and development.

VIII. UREA CYCLE DISORDERS: HYPERAMMONEMIA (TYPES I AND II); CITRULLINEMIA; ARGININOSUCCINIC ACIDURIA; HYPERARGININEMIA; HYPERORNITHINEMIA

Formula	Manufacturer	Comments
UCD 1	Mead Johnson	For infant feedings; mixture of essential L-amino acids powder with added cystinine and tyrosine; high protein (92% calories); fat-free; low carbohydrate; lactose-free; vitamin and mineral fortified.
UCD 2	Mead Johnson	For children; mixture of essential L-amino acids powder; high protein (93% calories); fat-free; low carbohydrate; lactose-free; vitamin and mineral fortified; protein to calorie ratio, 23.3 g/100 kcal.

IX. OTHER

Formula	Manufacturer	Comments
Protein-free Diet Powder (Product 80056)	Mead Johnson	For infants and children; protein-free formula base powder; corn oil (41% calories); corn syrup solids (59% calories); other protein sources and adequate sodium, potassium, and chloride must be added in the preparation of the feeding; vitamin and mineral fortified.

IX. OTHER

Formula	Manufacturer	Comments
RCF	Ross Laboratories	For infants and children; carbohydrate-free powder; soy protein isolate (20% calories); soy and coconut oil (80% calories); other carbohydrate sources and iron must be added in the preparation of the feeding; vitamin and mineral fortified.
Caulio XD	Ross Laboratories	Vitamin D–free, low calcium; for patients with hypercalcemia.

†Leucine, isoleucine, valine.
‡Hypervalinemia, methylacetacetic aciduria, leucine-induced hypoglycemia, hyperleucine-isoleucinemia.

fat. Zachary was able to take about 1 liter daily of this diet, with a protein intake of 1.3 grams per kilogram. Additional calories were provided by baby pureed fruits, which are protein-free, and he was able to demonstrate normal weight gain and a slow advancement of his mental development. However, this formula provided somewhat less essential than nonessential amino acids: 3705 milligrams of essential and 4845 milligrams of nonessential amino acids. This imbalance was corrected by adding an essential amino acid powder mixture. The arginine content of the diet was low; therefore, supplementation of arginine or citrulline (100–150 mg/d) is necessary in these patients to drive the urea cycle for maximum nitrogen efficiency (Brusilow 1988).

Although most nutrient intakes based on the above diet exceeded the RDAs for a 4½-month-old baby, babies with OTC deficiency who are treated with sodium benzoate and/or phenylacetate usually require additional supplementation of specific B vitamins such as folic acid, pantothenic acid and/or vitamin B_6 to compensate for excess losses. Therefore, these nutrients were also supplemented in amounts sufficient to prevent deficiency of these vitamins. Although the need for these vitamins may not be very high in patients with OTC deficiency, the requirements for folic acid may be up to 10,000 micrograms per day, and for pantothenic acid and vitamin B_6 up to 1000 milligrams per day in other inborn errors of metabolism that are vitamin-responsive (Acosta 1988).

In other conditions, an inborn error of metabolism will respond to nutritional intervention not so much by the type of feeding given but by the way it is administered. For example, in Type 3 glycogen storage disease low blood sugar levels may be the biggest problem. These patients cannot maintain their blood glucose levels and have protein breakdown owing to their inefficient pathway to make glucose, with resultant malnutrition, growth failure, and muscle weakness (Daeschel et al 1983). However, with continuous nasogastric feedings of a relatively high protein formula (20 to 25 percent of the calories as protein) (Slonim, Coleman & Moses 1984) it is possible to maintain serum glucose levels and to enhance protein utilization, which results in marked clinical improvement (see Fig. 25–3). Thus, continuous feedings, particularly at night, may be necessary for prolonged periods and may be done at home (see Chapters 27 and 29).

Many more inborn errors of metabolism require different treatments (AAP 1985, Wapnir 1985, Caballero 1985). Each one of them varies in respect to nutritional intervention. We cannot cover the details of each disorder and have therefore limited our discussion to the above-mentioned examples to illustrate some of the considerations required for the successful management of patients with inborn errors of metabolism.

CLINICAL INTERVENTION

Inborn errors of metabolism necessitate a precise diagnosis followed by nutrition intervention and careful monitoring. The aim of the treatment of inborn errors of metabolism must be to correct the metabolic alterations and to improve the outcome of the patient. If this objective cannot be accomplished it is hardly worth the effort required in following a difficult treatment. There is general agreement for a restrictive diet for specific disorders such as PKU because of the well-established benefit and improved mental status. However, there is lack of agreement on dietary restriction in other inborn errors of metabolism, such as histidinemia (Tada et al 1982, Levy, Shih & Madigan 1974, Popkin et al 1974). Keeping a child on a low-histidine diet is a very difficult and costly task and since there is no way to assess the effects of dietary restriction this nutritional intervention is generally not recommended. Therefore, the goals of nutritional therapy should be clearly defined, and for that purpose a number of clinical and biochemical parameters should be followed to assess compliance and effectiveness. There is no way to avoid frequent blood tests in children with inborn errors of metabolism.

The nutritional intervention must be specific for the alteration of metabolism being treated. For example, the aim of the dietary treatment of patients with PKU is to keep the blood phenylalanine concentration at a "safe" level; however, there is lack of agreement on what that level should be. Although plasma phenylalanine levels below 8 milligrams per deciliter have been considered acceptable, some scientists have reported higher I.Q. scores in children with PKU whose phenylalanine levels were kept below 5.5 milligrams per deciliter as compared with those having levels between 5.5 and 10 milligrams per deciliter (Dobson et al 1977). However, it is likely that families willing to enforce the stricter, more difficult diet regimen required to maintain lower plasma phenylalanine levels may have a particular psychosocial profile that may bear on their child's intellectual performance independently of the

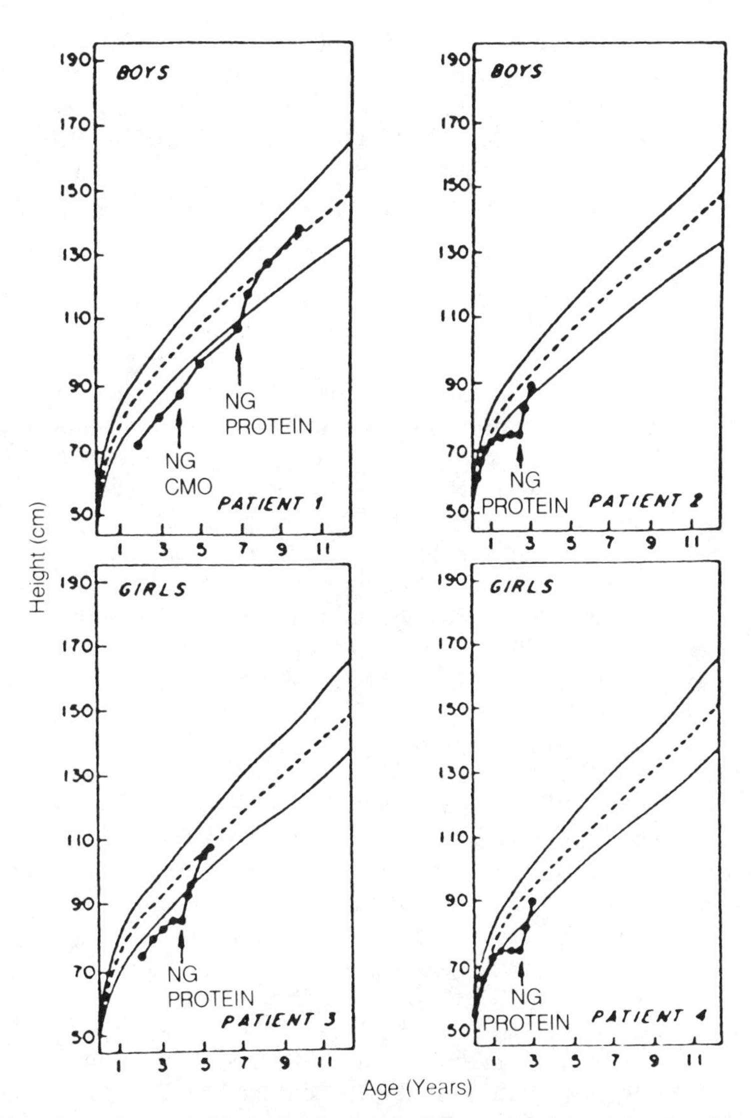

Figure 25–3. These children had growth failure, as shown in the charts, and had severe muscle weakness. After nutritional treatment there was catch-up growth and improved muscle strength, physical activity, and endurance. Also, there was improvement in the anatomic appearance and the EMG tracings of the muscle of these patients.

From Slonim AE, Coleman RA, Moses WS. Myopathy and growth failure in debrancher enzyme deficiency: Improvement with high-protein nocturnal enteral therapy. J Pediatr 1984; 105:906–911.

diet. Beyond 2 years of age the difficulties of keeping the child on a restricted diet increase progressively. Social interaction makes control of actual phenylalanine intake difficult, and there is no precise means of assessing intake other than by measuring blood phenylalanine levels. The commitment and patience of the parents plays a major role at this stage, as the struggle to keep the child on a special diet may place a serious emotional burden on the entire family.

Most experts agree that phenylalanine restriction in classic PKU should continue until at least 10 years of age, but it is less clear when the special diet can be discontinued without risk for the child (Michals et al 1988). Studies have reported a marked fall in I.Q. scores and a higher percentage of electroencephalographic abnormalities and "school problems" after discontinuation of diet therapy (Williamson, Koch & Berlow 1979, Cabalska et al 1977, Smith et al 1978, Holtzman et al 1986), while others found no effect of diet termination (Koff et al 1979, Horner et al 1962). More recently, elevated blood phenylalanine levels were shown to alter neuropsychologic performance, inferring lower learning and social performance (Krause et al 1985, 1986). For each individual patient, careful monitoring and assessment of biochemical, intellectual, and developmental parameters will facilitate individual decisions.

We now have to worry about treatment of mothers-to-be who have specific inborn errors of metabolism. The lack of the enzyme necessary to metabolize phenylalanine (phenylalanine hydroxylase) in the mother-to-be with PKU poses a severe danger to her offspring. In an international survey of pregnant women with PKU and their offspring, a close correlation was reported between maternal plasma phenylalanine levels and the incidence of fetal anomalies such as small head (microcephaly), mental retardation, and heart disease (Lenke & Levy 1980). Because the initiation of diet therapy in the first trimester of pregnancy does not prevent fetal abnormalities, phenylalanine restriction should ideally be started before the time of conception (Rohr et al 1987). Teen-aged female patients with PKU should therefore be informed of the risks of pregnancy and counseled on birth-control methods. Women with PKU who wish to become pregnant should be placed on a phenylalanine-restricted diet and closely monitored prior to the onset of pregnancy.

The considerations for the clinical intervention of patients with PKU discussed above also must be applied for the treatment of patients with other inborn errors of metabolism. However, there may be insufficient data to make appropriate scientific decisions in other conditions in which the experience accumulated is not as extensive as with PKU.

The dramatic positive outcomes that have been accomplished in some patients with inborn errors of metabolism lead to the use and abuse of similar dietary treatments for other inherited metabolic disorders that share some of the abnormalities. For example, the abuse of megavitamins for developmentally impaired children is frequently noted, without any beneficial effects (see Chapter 21). The benefits of such treatments are to be expected only in children afflicted with a specific inherited metabolic condition. Thus, an early, well-documented, and precise diagnosis is required, only to be followed by a specific well-orchestrated treatment. This can be accomplished only with the expertise of a team of sophisticated experts in metabolic disorders, who are often found only in specialized centers devoted to the care of patients with inborn errors of metabolism. Indeed, even in such centers there may be insufficient expertise to diagnose and treat all the various types of inborn errors of metabolism. However, input from other experts at a national and even international level is often available to ensure the best care for patients with inborn errors of metabolism.

REFERENCES

Acosta PB. Mineral and vitamin requirements in patients with selected metabolic disorders. Diet Pediatr Prac 1988; 11:1–3.

American Academy of Pediatrics. Task force on the dietary management of metabolic disorders. Committee on Nutrition, American Academy of Pediatrics, December 1985.

Bartlett K. Vitamin-responsive inborn errors of metabolism. Adv Clin Chem 1983; 23:141–198.

Batshaw ML, Thomas GH, Brusilow SW. New approaches to the diagnosis and treatment of inborn errors of urea synthesis. Pediatrics 1981; 68:290–297.

Brown GK, Hunt SM, Scholen R, et al. B hydroxyisobutyryl coenzyme A deacylase deficiency: A defect in valine metabolism associated with physical malformations. Pediatrics 1982; 70:532–538.

Brusilow SW. Therapy of inborn errors of urea synthesis. In Wapnir RA, ed. Congenital metabolic diseases. New York: Marcel Dekker, 1988:409–418.

Brusilow SW, Batshaw ML, Waber L. Neonatal hyperammonemic coma. Adv Pediatr 1982; 29:69–103.

Caballero B. Dietary management of inborn errors of amino acid metabolism. Clin Nutr 1985; 4:85–94.

Cabalska B, Durynska N, Borzymowska J, et al. Termination of dietary treatment in phenylketonuria. Eur J Pediatr 1977; 126:253–262.

Cederbaum SD. Diagnosing metabolic disease in the neonate. Metabolic Currents, A Timesaver Publication from Ross Laboratories 1989; 2:1–6.

Committee on Dietary Allowances, Food and Nutrition Board, National Research Council. Recommended dietary allowances. 10th ed. Washington, D.C.: National Academy of Sciences, 1989.

Cooper BA, Rosenblatt DS. Inherited defects of vitamin B_{12} metabolism. Ann Rev Nutr 1987; 7:291–320.

Daeschel IE, Janick LS, Kramish MJ, Coleman RA. Diet and growth of children with glycogen storage disease types I and III. J Am Diet Assoc 1983; 83:135–141.

Dobson JC, Williamson ML, Azen C, Kock R. Intellectual assessment of 111 four-year-old children with phenylketonuria. Pediatrics 1977; 60:822–827.

Elsas LJ, McCormick DB. Genetic defects in vitamin utilization. Part I: General aspects and fat soluble vitamins. Vit Horm 1986; 43:103–144.

Garrod AE. Inborn errors of metabolism. Lancet 1908; 2:1–7, 73–79, 142–148, 214–220.

Goodman SI. Inherited metabolic disease in the newborn: Approach to diagnosis and treatment. Adv Pediatr 1986; 33:197–224.

Goodman SI, Reale M, Berlow S. Glutaric aciduria type II: A form with deleterious intrauterine effect. J Pediatr 1983; 102:411–413.

Hambidge KM, Walravens PA. Disorders of mineral metabolism. Clin Gastroenterol 1982; 11:87–118.

Harkness RA. Clinical biochemistry of the neonatal period: Immaturity, hypoxia, and metabolic disease. J Clin Pathol 1987; 40:1128–1144.

Holtzman NA, Kronmal RA, Van Doornick W, Azen C, Koch R. Effect of age at loss of dietary control on intellectual performance and behavior of children with phenylketonuria. N Engl J Med 1986; 314:593–598.

Horner FA, Streamer CW, Alejandring L, Reed LA, Ibott F. Termination of dietary treatment of phenylketonuria. N Engl J Med 1962; 266:79–81.

Kapadia CR, Donaldson RM. Disorders of cobalamin (vitamin B_{12}) absorption and transport. Annu Rev Med 1985; 36:93–110.

Kaufman S, Kapatos G, McInnes RR, et al. Use of tetrahydrobiopterins in the treatment of hyperphenylalaninemia due to defective synthesis of tetrahydrobiopterin: Evidence that peripherally administered tetrahydrobiopterins enter the brain. Pediatrics 1982; 70:376–379.

Koff E, Kammerer B, Boyle P, Pueschel S. Intelligence and phenylketonuria: Effects of diet termination. J Pediatr 1979; 94:534–537.

Krause W, Epstein C, Averbook A, Dembure P, Elsas L. Phenylalanine alters the mean power frequency of electroencephalograms and plasma L-dopa in treated patients with phenylketonuria. Pediatr Res 1986; 20:1112–1116.

Krause W, Halminiski M, McDonald L, et al. Biochemical and neuropsychological effects of elevated plasma phenylalanine in patients with treated phenylketonuria. J Clin Invest 1985; 75:40–48.

Lenke RR, Levy HL. Maternal phenylketonuria and hyperphenylalaninemia. N Engl J Med 1980; 303:1202–1208.

Leonard JV. Teratogenic inborn errors of metabolism. Postgrad Med J 1986; 62:125–129.

Levy HL, Shih VE, Madigan PM. Routine newborn screening for histidinemia. N Engl J Med 1974; 291:1214–1219.

Michals K, Azen C, Acosta P, Koch R, Matalon R. Blood phenylalanine levels and intelligence of 10-year-old children with PKU in the National Collaborative Study. J Am Diet Assoc 1988; 88:1226–1229.

Msall M, Batshaw ML, Suss R, et al. Neurologic outcome in children with inborn errors of urea synthesis. N Engl J Med 1984; 310:1500–1505.

Muenzer J. Mucopolysaccharidoses. Adv Pediatr 1986; 33:269–302.

Munnich A, Saudubray JM, Charpentier C, et al. Multiple olybdoenzyme deficiencies due to an inborn error of molybdenum cofactor metabolism: Two additional cases in a new family. J Inher Metab Dis 1983; 6 Suppl 2:95–96.

Newsholme EA, Leech AR. Biochemistry for the medical sciences. New York: John Wiley & Sons, 1983:421–423.

Petrowski S, Nyhan WL, Reznik V, et al. Pharmacologic amino acid acylation in the acute hyperammonemia of propionic acidemia. J Neurogenet 1987; 4:87–96.

Popkin JS, Clow CL, Scriver CR, Grove J. Is hereditary histidinemia harmful? Lancet 1974; 1:721–722.

Przyrembel H. Therapy of mitochondrial disorders. J Inher Metab Dis 1987; 10 Supp 1:129–146.

Rebouche CJ, Paulson DJ. Carnitine metabolism and function in humans. Annu Rev Nutr 1986; 6:41–66.

Rohr FJ, Doherty LB, Waisbren SE, et al. New England Maternal PKU Project: Prospective study of untreated and treated pregnancies and their outcomes. J Pediatr 1987; 110:391–398.

Rudman D, Feller A. Evidence for deficiencies of conditionally essential nutrients during total parenteral nutrition. J Am Coll Nutr 1986; 5:101–106.

Slonim AE. Approach to diagnosis of inborn errors of metabolism during infancy. In Lifshitz F, ed. Pediatric endocrinology. 2nd ed. New York: Marcel Dekker, 1990:937–951.

Slonim AE. Metabolic myopathies: a consequence of disturbances in energy substrate supply. In Lifshitz F, ed. Common pediatric disorders: Metabolism, heart disease, allergies, substance abuse, and trauma. New York: Marcel Dekker, 1984:55–80.

Slonim AE, Coleman RA, Moses WS. Myopathy and growth failure in debrancher enzyme deficiency: Improvement with high-protein nocturnal enteral therapy. J Pediatr 1984; 105:906–911.

Smith I, Lobascher ME, Stevenson JE, et al. Effect of stopping low-phenylalanine diet on intellectual progress of children with phenylketonuria. Br Med J 1978; 2:723–726.

Snyderman SE. Diagnosis of metabolic disease. Pediatr Clin North Am 1971; 18:199–206.

Stanbury JB, Wyngaarden JB, Fredrickson DS, et al. The metabolic basis of inherited disease. 5th ed. New York: McGraw Hill, 1983: Chapters 5, 6, 7, 24, 58, 59.

Stanley CA. New genetic defects in mitochondrial fatty acid oxidation and carnitine deficiency. Adv Pediatr 1987; 34:59–88.

Stepnick-Gropper SA, Acosta PB, Clarke-Sheehan N, et al. Trace element status of children with PKU and normal children. J Am Diet Assoc 1988; 88:459–465.

Tada K, Tateda H, Arashima S, et al. Intellectual development in patients with untreated histidinemia. J Pediatr 1982; 101:562–563.

Wapnir RA. Congenital metabolic diseases. New York: Marcel Dekker, 1985.

Williamson M, Koch R, Berlow S. Diet discontinuation in phenylketonuria. Pediatrics 1979; 63:823–824.

26

Cancer

"At first it didn't really sink in. I guess it all seemed like a dream. I'd always heard about cancer, of course. But that was always other people. When my doctor told me I had cancer, I started crying. I thought, 'Why did it have to happen to me? Why couldn't it be somebody else?' A lot of other things flashed through my head. I was sure I was going to die. It was a real scary feeling. I worried about myself, and I worried about how my family was going to take it if something happened to me.

"When my doctor tried to tell me more about the cancer, I said, 'Don't go any further, because I don't want to hear any more.' I kept thinking that I wasn't going to live much longer, so it didn't matter how much I knew. Then my doctor said there was a lot they could do for me. I went away and thought about that. And I talked to him again, and I talked with the nurses. They gave me all the hope in the world, and I felt a lot different about having cancer" (United States Department of Health 1987).

Cancer is actually a group of diseases, each one with its own name, its own cause and symptoms, and its own chances for control and cure. Cancer occurs when a particular cell or group of cells in any part of the body gets out of control. These independent cells grow in excess, and crowd out and overcome normal cells. Cancer may take many forms; for example, leukemia, which develops from the white blood cells, or solid tumors, which can form in any tissue of the body.

Despite considerable ongoing research, no one knows why people get cancer, but we do know that cancer may strike one out of every three to four Americans during their lifetime (Simone 1983).

NUTRITION AS A CAUSE OR RISK FOR CANCER

Some authorities believe that up to 90 percent of all cancers are in some way related to diet, environment, and lifestyle (Simone 1983, National Research Council 1982). Of these, up to 40 percent of cancers occurring in men and as many as 60 percent of cancers in women may be related to diet and nutrition alone (Leonard et al 1986). If that is the case, it stands to reason that many cancers may be potentially preventable through modifications of diet and lifestyle habits.

Foods as Cancer Risk Enhancers

Food might be among the most important environmental insults implicated as causes or as factors that increase the risk for cancer. A partial list of potential carcinogens in food is shown in Table 26–1 (Purtilo & Cohen 1985, Guillem,

Table 26–1. Potential Carcinogens in Food.

Natural Sources of Carcinogens in Food
- Mustard
- Horseradish
- Black pepper
- Other spices
- Alcohol
- Mushrooms
- Radishes
- Parsley
- Alfalfa sprouts
- Celery

Naturally Contaminated or Damaged Foods
- Rancid or oxidized fats due to storage
- Molds (aflatoxin) on corn, grains, nuts, peanut butter, breads, cheese, fruit, juices, potatoes

Processing Methods of Foods
- Some food additives
- Frying; charcoal broiling; cooking with extremely high temperatures
- Highly processed foods: beef jerky; some powdered dairy products; processed cheeses; foods with added nitrates and nitrites: pickled or cured items

Pesticides and Chemicals (Examples)
- Daminozide (Alar)
- PCBs

Dietary Habits
- Alcohol
- High fat intake
- Coffee
- Low fiber intake

Adapted from Wallace CL, Watson RR, Watson AA. Reducing cancer risk with vitamins C, E, and selenium. Am J Health Promotion 1988; 3:5-32.

Matsui & O'Brien 1987, Senti 1988). Some of the initiators (carcinogens) are naturally present in fresh foods while others occur only in diseased or contaminated foods or through cooking and preparation, as in charcoal broiling.

Foods may also become contaminated in their natural habitat. For example, molds (aflatoxins) might grow in warm humid climates on corn, grain, and nuts and they may be associated with a variety of undesirable effects including cancer (Wallace, Watson & Watson 1988). Recently, the U.S. corn crop was reported to be contaminated with this toxin because of the summer drought in 1988 (*Newsweek*, March 6, 1989). For Americans, who eat an average of 160 pounds of corn products per year, this potential widespread contamination with aflatoxin is of great concern.

Foods may also contain additives and preservatives that may be the initiators of cancer (Senti 1988). However, the food additives and preservatives are closely regulated by the FDA (Code of Federal Regulations 1985). There are over 500 food ingredients, over 1000 food flavoring agents, 30 color additives, and many artificial sweeteners that have been extensively studied and, to date, they are considered safe for human consumption.

Some preservatives, which are used in processed foods, have been implicated in the genesis of cancer (see Table 26–1). Therefore, food additives such as colorants, which are used strictly for cosmetic reasons, should be minimized as much as possible. In contrast, food preservatives, even when they have been associated with development of cancer, are more acceptable provided they offer a low risk and a high benefit. For example, water in the United States has been considered to be a potential initiator of cancer of the bladder, rectum, and colon (Cantor et al 1987). Water is chlorinated to disinfect it and to limit the growth of potential bacterial pathogens. Thus, no one can deny the benefit of chlorination to humankind in providing clean water. However, this process may be a necessary risk in our world. Further research must be done to establish the safety of many of these substances and the development of "safer" and/or "more effective" preservatives.

Pesticides and chemicals may also play a role in the formation of cancer, but those used for commercial and agricultural purposes in the United States are most often safe (see Chapter 15). The use of pesticides is less controlled in imported products. There are about 50,000 pesticide products in 600 chemical categories used in this country. Nearly 400 of these chemicals were on the market before any regulation was enacted by the Environmental Protection Agency. Although Congress ordered all pesticides to be evaluated by 1997, this agency has developed data on 192 of the older chemicals and it has fully reviewed and registered only two of them. These efforts set tolerance levels for pesticide residues, but monitoring and enforcing those limits is the responsibility of the FDA, which is overburdened and often ineffective in enforcing penalties for violations.

Controversy often arises in regard to specific products. For example, for almost 3 years the Environmental Protection Agency vacillated over daminozide, a chemical that makes apples ripen, redden, and stay fresh. This chemical cannot be cooked or washed off. Daminozide, known by its trade name Alar, has long been a suspected carcinogen. The EPA announced that Alar poses a cancer risk of 1 in 20,000 people when consumed over a 70-year lifetime (*Newsweek*, Feb. 13, 1989). The risk is 50 times greater than the threshold at which EPA is supposed to take action. Despite incomplete and contradictory testing by the FDA and long before the EPA's deadline, public pressure forced American growers to stop using it in 1989.

There are no easy answers to the difficult scientific questions that must be resolved before a product is banned because of possible carcinogenic risks. Large quantities of foods are needed to feed the ever-growing population, and preservatives are needed to protect the food. Sensationalistic reports sporadically hit the media when a product is linked to cancer in laboratory animals and a public outcry is heard regarding the safety of the foods on the market. Recently, the American Council on Science and Health (*New York Times*, April 5, 1989) felt compelled to state that our food supply is safe. As was stated, America's food supply is the safest and most plentiful in the world and pesticides deserve much of the credit. If Americans really want to "go back to nature," they will have to coexist with vermin and insects and the diseases and scarcity of food. Moreover, they state that it is dangerous to focus on unsubstantiated claims regarding safety of the food supply when real problems to our health abound, such as automobile accidents and cigarette smoking. Justifiably, the American Council on Science feels that Americans should count their blessings and reject unproven attacks on the safety of our food supply.

Dietary Habits

It has long been known that certain dietary habits and nutritional deficiencies and excesses may be associated with cancer. Excessive caloric intake leading to obesity and high-fat, low-fiber diets have been shown to be related to the development of cancer (Vaneys 1985, Palmer 1986) (Fig. 26–1). There is also a litany of evidence that supports an association between alcohol or coffee consumption and cancer risk. However, it is often difficult to discern a direct cause and effect given the variety of factors that may influence cancer risk. For example, coffee consumption was implicated as an initiator of pancreatic cancer. However, when coffee consumption was evaluated in light of smoking habits, the effect of drinking coffee on pancreatic cancer was almost entirely limited to cigarette smokers (Gorham et al 1988). Other studies have demonstrated that there may be an additive effect on cancer risk when certain dietary habits are superimposed upon other environmental carcinogens such as smoking. Additionally, individuals who smoke cigarettes and con-

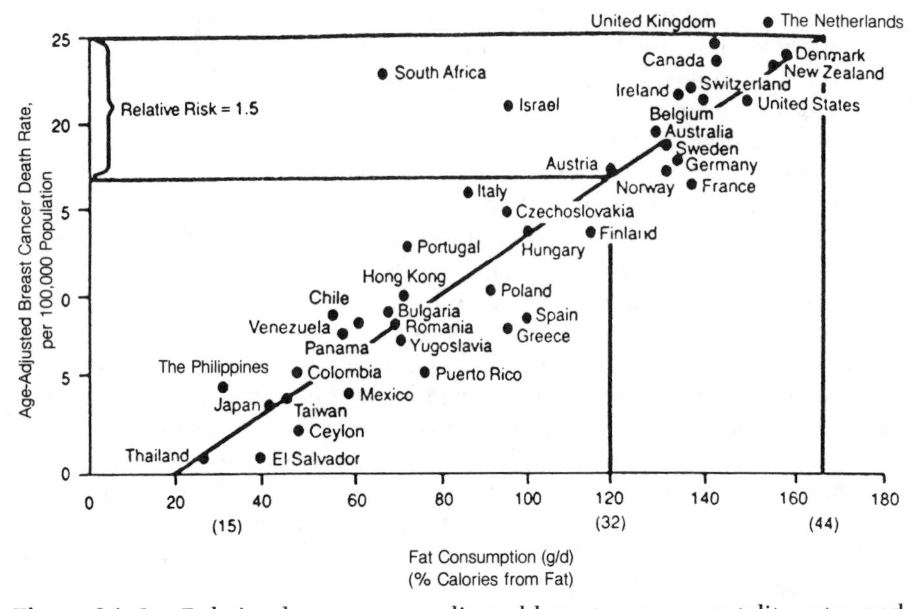

Figure 26–1. Relation between age-adjusted breast cancer mortality rates and per capita fat consumption (adapted from Carroll, Khor, and Willett et al).
From Schatzkin A, Greenwald P, Byar DP, Clifford CK. The dietary fat-breast cancer hypothesis is alive. JAMA 1989; 261:3283-3287.

sume diets high in fat and cholesterol may have an even greater risk of lung cancer than those who smoke but consume less fat and cholesterol (Goodman et al 1988). Alcohol ingestion and nutritionally inadequate diets associated with very poor living conditions have also been related to esophageal cancer (Segal, Reinach & de Beer 1988). Thus, it appears that environmental factors such as smoking and poor living conditions may be a necessary, fertile setting for dietary factors to initiate these dreaded diseases.

NUTRITION IN CANCER PREVENTION

Food is not only a potential cancer threat, it may also have protective effects. A great variety of dietary substances might be natural protectors that inhibit rather than enhance cancer production. Vitamins C and E and the mineral selenium (Wallace, Watson & Watson 1988) are antioxidants—that is, they compete against free radicals, natural initiators of malignancies. Antioxidants decrease the exposure of cells to toxic forms of oxygen. Without antioxidants, free radicals would enhance the process of oxidation and trigger the formation of cancer initiators. This mutagenic process is comparable to the oxidation that produces spoilage and rancidity of foods (Simone 1983). A certain amount of free-radical damage is a normal event that occurs continuously in the human body. However, the body contains complex protective systems to destroy these toxic substances. Only when the body is weakened or exposed to continuous free-radical insult does the cancer occur.

Other vitamins, minerals, and substances in food may inhibit carcinogenesis by a variety of mechanisms. Vitamin A, vitamin D, retinoid, carotenoids, zinc, magnesium, iron, molybdenum, and certain amino acids have been shown to alter tumor formation (Shils 1988). Certain carotenoids, which are the compounds necessary for formation of retinol (vitamin A), can neutralize or "quench" the reactivity of oxygen by dissipating the energy throughout the carotenoid molecule (Fig. 26–2). This process defuses the singlet oxygen (oxidant) to "normal" oxygen, which is much less likely to generate potentially damaging free radicals. A large amount of literature suggests that carotenoids decrease the risk of cancer (Ziegler 1989). A group of fatty acids known as CLA also may inhibit cancer formation. It is believed that CLA can establish a permanent defense against cancer by becoming incorporated into cells. These CLAs have been detected in beef, milk, and cheeses such as Cheez Whiz and parmesan cheese (*Newsweek*, March 9, 1989). However, the effect of preventing or reducing the risk of cancer through these dietary constituents has been primarily demonstrated in experimental animals, not in human beings. Therefore, at present, supplementation with any of the abovementioned nutrients to alter cancer incidence or to reduce cancer growth is not indicated.

STEP 1:	$^1O_2$ + Beta Carotene singlet oxygen energized	→→→	O_2 + Beta Carotene energized
STEP 2:	Beta Carotene energized	→→→	Beta Carotene + Heat

Figure 26–2. Beta carotene picks up a singlet oxygen (oxidant). The energized carotene molecule dissipates the potentially harmful oxygen by releasing a small amount of heat, converting it to "normal" oxygen, which is less likely to generate free radicals. They occur without loss of the beta carotene molecules.

From Krinsky WI. Antioxidant functions of beta carotene. In Vitamin nutrition information source. Vol. 1. No. 5, 1990.

Diets for Cancer Risk Reduction

To date, no magic nutrition bullet exists that will prevent or cure cancer. Thus, a well-balanced varied diet is still the best approach for maintaining health and preventing cancer. However, certain guidelines have been recommended to reduce cancer risk (Table 26–2) (Palmer 1986). These recommendations must be followed with caution and in moderation, especially for children. They have not been proven either effective or safe, and they may result in adverse consequences. For example, lowering saturated fat intake to prevent heart disease has been associated with an increased risk of colon cancer in males (National Research Council 1982). Also, low-fat, low-cholesterol diets may result in FTT in infants and children (Pugliese et al 1987, Lifshitz et al 1987, Lifshitz & Moses 1989). High-fiber diets may reduce the chances of developing colon cancer and other diseases, but these diets may induce gastrointestinal problems such as abdominal pain, gas, and bowel irregularity and may cause the child to become satiated before adequate intake is consumed. High-fiber diets also have been associated with vitamin and mineral deficiencies when consumed over prolonged periods (Kelsay 1978).

Although the dietary recommendations for reducing cancer risk are well-publicized (Fig. 26–3), only a small proportion of the population is modifying their diet (Patterson & Block 1988). Since much of the research regarding diet and cancer remains controversial, it is reasonable that the adoption of and

Table 26–2. Dietary Guidelines to Lower Cancer Risk.*

1. Eat a variety of foods.
2. Avoid obesity and maintain normal weight and growth.
3. Emphasize complex carbohydrate intake.
4. Increase consumption of fruits and vegetables, especially citrus fruits (vitamin C), green/yellow vegetables (vitamins C and A), and cruciferous vegetables (provitamin A).
5. Increase fiber intake.
6. Decrease fat intake to 30–35% of total energy intake.
7. Avoid highly processed food, cooking/frying at high temperatures, and charcoal broiling.
8. Reduce exposure to contaminated and/or damaged foods.
9. Avoid excess alcohol ingestion and spices.

*These recommendations must be modified in accordance with the needs of children at various stages of development (see Chapter 9).

Adapted from recommendations established by the following scientific and health organizations in the United States: National Research Council, Commission on Life Sciences. Diet, nutrition, and cancer. Washington, D.C.: National Academy of Sciences, 1982; American Cancer Society. Nutrition and cancer: Cause and prevention. New York: American Cancer Society, 1984; National Cancer Institute. Cancer prevention: Good news, better news, best news. NCI Publication No. 84-2671. Washington, D.C.: U.S. Government Printing Office, 1984; National Cancer Institute. Diet, nutrition and cancer prevention: A guide to food choices. NIH Publication No. 85-2711. Washington, D.C.: U.S. Government Printing Office, 1984; U.S. Department of Agriculture and Department of Health and Human Services. Nutrition and your health: Dietary guidelines for Americans. Washington, D.C.: U.S. Department of Agriculture and Department of Health and Human Services, 1985.

Great American Food Fight Against Cancer
Tips For
Dining Out And Traveling

- Select a restaurant that will offer a variety of foods and variety of choices. If a restaurant is unfamiliar to you, call in advance and inquire about menu options and methods of cooking.
- Try to pick a restaurant with a salad bar which offers many low-fat, high-fiber choices. Steer clear of high-fat toppings such as cheese, bacon bits, croutons, and regular dressings. Soup and salad make a great combination, but be sure to choose clear broth soups instead of creamy ones.
- Read the menu carefully. Avoid items that are buttered, fried, breaded, creamed, and browned. If you're not sure about a recipe, don't be shy about asking your server. And don't be afraid to ask if items can be prepared in a different manner or substituted. You can also ask that an item, such as high-fat french fries or chips or bread, not be brought with the meal.
- Always be clear about what you order. Don't assume your server knows exactly what you want.
- Always ask for sauces and salad dressing to be delivered on the side. Order breads and toast without butter or margarine.
- Lean meats, poultry, and fish are healthiest baked or broiled. Look for menu items that are roasted, steamed, poached, and stir-fried. Ask to have these items prepared without added fat.
- Cut down on portion sizes by ordering appetizers as the main course, ordering a la carte, sharing food with a companion, or taking home part of your meal in a doggie bag.
- Order desserts with less fat and sugar, such as fresh fruit, sherbert, sorbets, frozen yogurt, and angel food cake.
- Even at fast food restaurants you can make a difference by looking for a salad bar, skipping the cheese and mayonnaise on sandwiches, eating smaller portions, and choosing low-fat milk, juice, or tea instead of shakes and malts.
- Airlines offer special meals, such as low-fat ones. Check with the airline or your travel agent before you fly.
- Keep low-fat, high-fiber snacks at work and in your car. That way you always have a smart snack on hand and can avoid vending machines. Most snack items found in vending machines are high in fat and calories.
- Contact your local American Cancer Society for more tips.

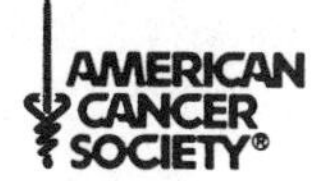

Figure 26–3. Advertisement by the American Cancer Society encouraging diet for cancer risk reduction.

compliance with these dietary recommendations are slow to take hold. Attempts to reduce the risk of cancer must take into account a person's entire lifestyle, not just one factor, such as dietary habits or specific nutrient supplementation.

MALNUTRITION IN THE CANCER PATIENT

Cancer itself often causes malnutrition (cancer cachexia) (Fig. 26–4). Involuntary weight loss is often the first sign of disease, and anyone who loses weight without an apparent cause should visit a physician. Long before the development of sophisticated chemotherapeutic treatment modalities, as many as 23 percent of patients with cancer were dying from protein-calorie malnutrition (marasmus), not from their underlying disease (Warren 1932). Today, malnutrition is still a problem among patients with cancer. Up to 50 percent of cancer patients are malnourished (Nixon et al 1980), and when the disease affects the gastrointestinal tract, malnutrition occurs in even higher propor-

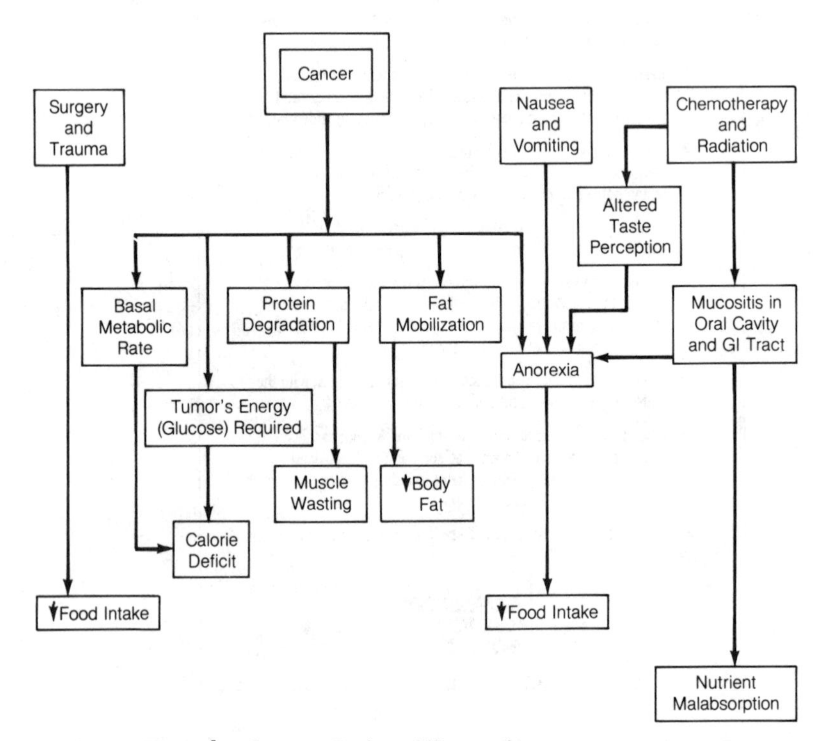

Figure 26–4. How the Cancer Patient Wastes Away.

tions. For example, up to 65 percent of patients with pancreatic and abdominal cancer were malnourished (Meguid et al 1983). Children with solid tumors such as stage IV neuroblastoma and Ewing's sarcoma are often malnourished at diagnosis (Carter et al 1983, Rickard et al 1985), and malnutrition appears to be a poor prognostic sign for the child with cancer (Donaldson et al 1981, Van Eys 1984).

The precise cause of malnutrition in cancer patients is not completely understood (Van Eys 1985). Malnutrition in patients with GI cancers who are unable to eat or absorb nutrients is understandable. Cachexia in patients with cancers in locations other than the GI tract is a common problem, which could be due to an altered metabolism. The tumor itself may produce substances that interfere with normal metabolic processes (Costa 1977) and induce increased breakdown of protein (Blackburn et al 1977) and increased glucose production (Meguid et al 1981). These abnormalities in carbohydrate and protein metabolism would lead to continued mobilization and ineffective repletion of host tissue even with improved nutritional intake.

In addition, the cancer victim usually becomes anorexic, perhaps owing to factors produced by the cancer itself (Kern & Norton 1988) or to depression and anxiety that may follow diagnosis of the disease. The treatment of cancer with chemotherapy and radiation therapy may also induce severe anorexia and an inability to eat due to nausea, vomiting, diarrhea, constipation, and ulcerations of the intestinal tract (mucositis) and mouth (stomatitis). These adverse side effects may vary depending on the drug, dose, duration of treatment, and individual tolerance (Kokal 1985). In addition, the drugs used in the treatment of cancer may have negative effects on specific nutrients. Listings of commonly used drugs in the treatment of cancer are available to identify potential drug–nutrient interactions that may alter the patient's nutritional status (Lenssen & Aker 1985).

Altered food preferences may occur in children with cancer, especially if the ingestion of "favorite" foods is associated with nausea and vomiting because of chemotherapy (Dickerson 1984). Also, there may be an altered taste threshold in these children that affects their food preferences and desire to eat (Barale, Aker & Martinsen 1982). Patients with cancer often report that meat has a "funny," metallic taste, or that sweets are harder to taste and the bitterness of foods is more pronounced.

Malnutrition in the cancer patient may be part of a vicious cycle. It will further aggravate the patient's anorexia, worsen the nutritional status, compromise immune function with lower resistance to infections, and produce weakness and a general decrease in stamina and feelings of well-being. In addition, a malnourished patient may not be able to tolerate the stress of cancer therapy, especially surgical intervention, as well as a well-nourished patient could (Meguid & Meguid 1988).

BOGUS NUTRITION CURES FOR CANCER

Despite the advances made in the medical treatment of cancer, unconventional cancer treatments continue to hold the interest of the media and engender hope in patients with cancer. More than 70 unproven cancer cures are on file at the American Cancer Society (ACS) (ACS 1982, Ross 1985). Up to 30 percent of cancer patients have tried some type of unorthodox treatment for their disease. Many of these bogus cures involved dietary modification, including vitamin and mineral supplementation.

Patients with cancer or parents of children with cancer search for a cure; often, they assume that anything is worth a try. Typically those who seek unorthodox treatments are well-off and have a high educational level (Cassileth et al 1984). Bogus nutrition cures are attractive because they appear "natural" or "nontoxic" as compared with conventional chemotherapy or radiation, and these cures give control to the patients at a time when they feel that their lives are out of their control.

The most frequent nutrition cures attempt to "detoxify the body" by using coffee or castor-oil enemas, special diets, megavitamin supplements, minerals, pancreatic enzymes, or Laetrile. Dietary treatments may eliminate animal protein, including meat and milk products (Shils & Hermann 1982) or other foods, as with the Zen macrobiotic diet that at its most "potent" level includes only grains (see Chapter 15).

These bogus nutritional treatments are of concern because the patient may forego appropriate medical treatment. When nutritional therapies are employed they may receive inadequate diets and/or excess vitamins, minerals, or other factors with potential toxicity (see Chapter 9). In fact, toxicity with vitamins A and B_{12} in cancer patients has been described (Shils & Hermann 1982).

CLINICAL INTERVENTION

It is important for everybody to eat a well-balanced, varied diet throughout life (see Chapter 9), and this is especially true for children with cancer. Unfortunately, eating is often the last thing on the minds of these children. They usually experience eating problems that interfere with the dietary intake and may lead to malnutrition (cancer cachexia). The eating problems fall into five general categories: loss of appetite, tired feeling, nausea and vomiting, mouth soreness and dryness, and intestinal upset. These complaints are real and difficult to deal with, but they need to be overcome to maintain or improve the patient's nutritional status and improve the quality of his or her life. However, there is no evidence at this time that changes in dietary intake will prevent a recurrence of the cancer.

The nutritional status of a child with cancer requires immediate assessment at the time of diagnosis and prompt intervention. Special attention must be given to specific conditions of the cancer, such as the location of the tumor and the nutritional impact of the therapies used for treatment of the disease. The nutritional recommendations must change with the progression of the disease and treatment regimens.

The nutritional requirements of patients with cancer have recently been reviewed (Dempsey & Mullen 1985, Hoffman 1985). These children have greater nutrition needs, but their ability to meet these demands is reduced. An exception to increasing requirements is the necessity to limit folic-acid intake when the chemotherapeutic agent methotrexate is administered. This drug exerts its action by interfering with folic-acid metabolism, and increased ingestion of folic acid would limit this drug's effectiveness.

Energy needs of children with cancer vary depending on the stage of the disease and other factors. For example, the activity of the patient while in the hospital for treatment may be curtailed while the amount of stress he or she experiences is increased. In addition, other complications associated with the disease process and/or its treatment will serve to increase the requirements of children with cancer. As with any other child, a good index of sufficient energy intake is continued growth along normal patterns (see Chapter 10).

Protein and other specific nutrient needs might be increased during the process of nutritional rehabilitation in the malnourished child with cancer. However, the presence of compromised renal function, which may occur particularly with certain chemotherapies, may contraindicate higher protein intake. Children with cancer have increased requirements due to chemotherapy, fever, diarrhea, and vomiting, all of which enhance water losses. On the other hand, impaired liver and kidney function might decrease the child's ability to handle fluid, and controlling fluid intake may be necessary (see Chapter 23).

Meal times should be separated from the times that treatment or medical intervention is given. The meals should be offered in a relaxed setting and the child can view this time as separate from the unpleasantness of being sick. Friends and family may make meals more fun; soft music can help enhance the atmosphere, and food should be presented in an attractive manner (e.g., favorite dishes, tablecloth, flowers, etc.). Ideally, positive reinforcement without negative pressure to eat is recommended for encouraging children who refuse to eat (Handen, Mandell & Russo 1986).

The best way to feed children with cancer is to ask them how they feel and find out what foods they like and don't like. Not all children have the same response to their illness or to the variety of treatments that may be employed. They need to be offered food they like in a manner that promotes maximum intake. In general, children with cancer will say that they are just not hungry and thus may not eat enough to maintain their nutrition. Loss of appetite, not being hungry, bad taste of food, bitter metal taste in the mouth or tongue, or feeling full too soon are real problems to be dealt with in the nutritional rehabilitation of cancer victims.

The complaint of early satiety can be addressed by offering small, frequent meals of nutritious, preferred foods such as cheese, muffins, yogurt, and peanut butter. Low-calorie, nutrient-poor liquids should be limited before and during meals, whereas nutritious drinks such as juices, milk, and milkshakes may be offered. Often, fatty and greasy foods cause delayed gastric emptying. This will aggravate and extend the feeling of fullness. These items may need to be limited in the child's diet.

The recommendations to limit fluids during meals, avoid high-fat foods, and eat small portions may also be beneficial for the child with nausea and vomiting. In addition, salty rather than sweet foods may be better tolerated as well as dry toast or crackers and cool clear drinks such as ginger ale, ice chips, popsicles, and juices. Sometimes the smell of food can dissuade a child from eating. If this is the case, offer the child foods that do not require cooking or entertain the child in another room where kitchen odors are limited. The child will be able to tell you which smells make him or her nauseated and these items should be avoided.

In general, it is important to listen to the child and be responsive to his or her feelings when it comes to food. Patience is the key. Quite often, a food that is well-liked one day will be hated the next; therefore, other options should be readily available. Care must be taken that meal time and food do not become the battleground for the family to express their anxieties and fears about having a child with cancer.

Physicians should not wait until the child is malnourished to establish a nutrition support program. High-calorie supplements are recommended from the beginning of treatment. The amount of supplement might vary, and they should be offered only after the child has tried to eat food. If the patient will not or cannot eat enough, nasogastric or intravenous feedings may be necessary (see Chapters 27 and 28). In patients with normal function of the gastrointestinal tract the use of enteral nutrition is preferred. Although enteral feedings have been shown to be less psychologically stressful, parenteral nutrition may be needed if enteral feedings are not tolerated (Padilla & Grant 1985).

The diagnosis of cancer will affect not only the patient but also the parents, siblings, and extended family. Acknowledging sad feelings and crying are healthy outlets for emotions. During this period, a child with cancer may challenge the "limits" that had previously been set. Although a normal feeling might be to let sick children have their way, "giving in" may serve only to increase the anxiety since the patient may perceive that things are really worse than they actually are. As with all children, children with cancer should be permitted to exert some control, but not to the extent that it would jeopardize their health.

REFERENCES

American Cancer Society. Unproven methods of cancer management. New York: American Cancer Society, 1982.

Barale K, Aker SN, Martinsen CS. Primary taste thresholds in children with leukemia undergoing marrow transplantation. JPEN 1982; 6(4):287–290.

Blackburn GL, Maini BS, Bistrian BR, et al. The effect of cancer on nitrogen, electrolyte, and mineral metabolism. Cancer Res 1977; 37:2348–2353.

Cantor KP, et al. Bladder cancer, drinking water source, and tap water consumption: A case-control study. J Natl Cancer Inst 1987; 79:1269–1279.

Carter P, Carr D, van Eys J, et al. Nutritional parameters in children with cancer. J Am Diet Assoc 1983; 82(6):616–622.

Cassileth BR, Lusk EJ, Strouse TB, et al. Contemporary unorthodox treatments in cancer medicine. Ann Intern Med 1984; 101:105–112.

Code of Federal Regulations. Title 21: Food and Drugs, Parts 170–199 rev. Washington, D.C.: U.S. Government Printing Office, 1985.

Costa G. Cachexia, the metabolic component of neoplastic diseases. Cancer Res 1977; 37:2327–2335.

Dempsey DT, Mullen JL. Macronutrient requirements in the malnourished cancer patient. How much of what and why? Cancer 1985; 55:290–294.

Dickerson JWT. Nutrition in the cancer patient: A review. J Roy Soc Med 1984; 77:309–315.

Donaldson SS, Wesley MN, DeWys WD, et al. A study of the nutritional status of pediatric cancer patients. Am J Dis Child 1981; 135:1107–1112.

Goodman MT, Kolonel LN, Yoshizawa CN, Hankin JH. The effect of dietary cholesterol and fat on the risk of lung cancer in Hawaii. Am J Epidemiol 1988; 128:1241–1255.

Gorham ED, Garland CF, Garland FC, Benenson AS, Cottrell L. Coffee and pancreatic cancer in a rural California county. West J Med 1988; 148:48–53.

Guillem J, Matsui M, O'Brien C. Nutrition in the prevention of neoplastic disease in the elderly. Clin Geriatr Med 1987; 3:373–387.

Handen BL, Mandell F, Russo DC. Feeding induction in children who refuse to eat. Am J Dis Child 1986; 140:52–54.

Hoffman FA. Micronutrient requirements of cancer patients. Cancer 1985; 55:295–300.

Kelsay JA. A review of research on the effects of fiber intake in man. Am J Clin Nutr 1978; 31:142–159.

Kern KA, Norton JA. Cancer cachexia. JPEN 1988; 12:286–298.

Kokal WA. The impact of antitumor therapy on nutrition. Cancer 1985; 55:273–278.

Lenssen P, Aker SN, eds. Nutritional assessment and management during marrow transplant: A resource manual. Seattle, WA: Fred Hutchinson Cancer Research Center, 1985.

Leonard T, Mohs M, Ho E, Watson R. Nutrient intake, cancer causation and prevention. Prog Food Nutr Sci 1986; 10:237–277.

Lifshitz F, Moses N. Growth failure—A complication of hypercholesterolemia treatment. Am J Dis Child 1989; 83:393–398.

Lifshitz F, Moses N, Cervantes C, Ginsberg L. Nutritional dwarfing in adolescents.

Semin Adolesc Med 1987; 3:255–266.
Meguid MM, Aun F, Soeldner JS, et al. Insulin half-life in man after trauma. Surgery 1981; 89:650–653.
Meguid MM, Debonis D, Mequid V, et al. Nutritional support in cancer. Lancet 1983; 2:320–323.
Meguid MM, Meguid V. Nutrition—A useful adjunct to cancer therapy. Nutrition 1988; 4:320–323.
National Research Council, Commission on Life Sciences. Diet, nutrition and cancer. Washington, D.C.: National Academy of Sciences, 1982.
Nixon DW, Heymsfield SB, Cohen AE, et al. Protein-calorie undernutrition in hospitalized cancer patients. Am J Med 1980; 68:683–690.
Padilla GV, Grant MM. Psychosocial aspects of artificial feeding. Cancer 1985; 55:301–307.
Palmer S. Dietary considerations for risk reduction. Cancer 1986; 58:1949–1953.
Patterson BH, Block G. Food choices and the cancer guidelines. Am J Pub Health 1988; 78:282–286.
Pugliese M, Weyman-Daum M, Moses N, Lifshitz F. Parental health beliefs as a cause of non-organic failure to thrive. Pediatrics 1987; 80:175–182.
Purtilo D, Cohen S. Diet, nutrition and cancer. An update on a controversial relationship. Postgrad Med 1985; 78:192–194, 199–203.
Rickard KA, Loghmani ES, Grosfeld JL, et al. Short- and long-term effectiveness of enteral and parenteral nutrition in reversing or preventing protein-energy malnutrition in advanced neuroblastoma. Cancer 1985; 56:2881–2897.
Ross WE. Unconventional cancer therapy. Compr Ther 1985; 11:37–43.
Segal I, Reinach SG, de Beer M. Factors associated with oesophageal cancer in Soweto, South Africa. Br J Cancer 1988; 58:681–686.
Senti FR. Food additives and contaminants. In Shils ME, Young VR, eds. Modern nutrition in health and disease. New York: Lea & Febiger, 1988:698–711.
Shils ME. Nutrition and diet in cancer. In Shils ME, Young VR, eds. Modern nutrition in health and disease. New York: Lea & Febiger 1988:1380–1422.
Shils ME, Hermann MG. Unproved dietary claims in the treatment of patients with cancer. Bull NY Acad Med 1982; 58:323–340.
Simone C. Cancer and nutrition. New York: McGraw-Hill, 1983.
Van Eys J. Nutrition in the treatment of cancer in children. J Am Coll Nutr 1984; 3:159–168.
Van Eys J. Nutrition and cancer: Physiological interrelationships. Ann Rev Nutr 1985; 5:435–461.
Wallace CL, Watson RR, Watson AA. Reducing cancer risk with vitamins C, E, and selenium. Am J Health Promotion 1988; 3:5–16, 32.
Warren S. The immediate causes of death in cancer. Am J Med Sci 1932; 184:610–615.
Ziegler R. A review of epidemiologic evidence that carotenoids reduce the risk of cancer. J Nutr 1989; 119:116–122.

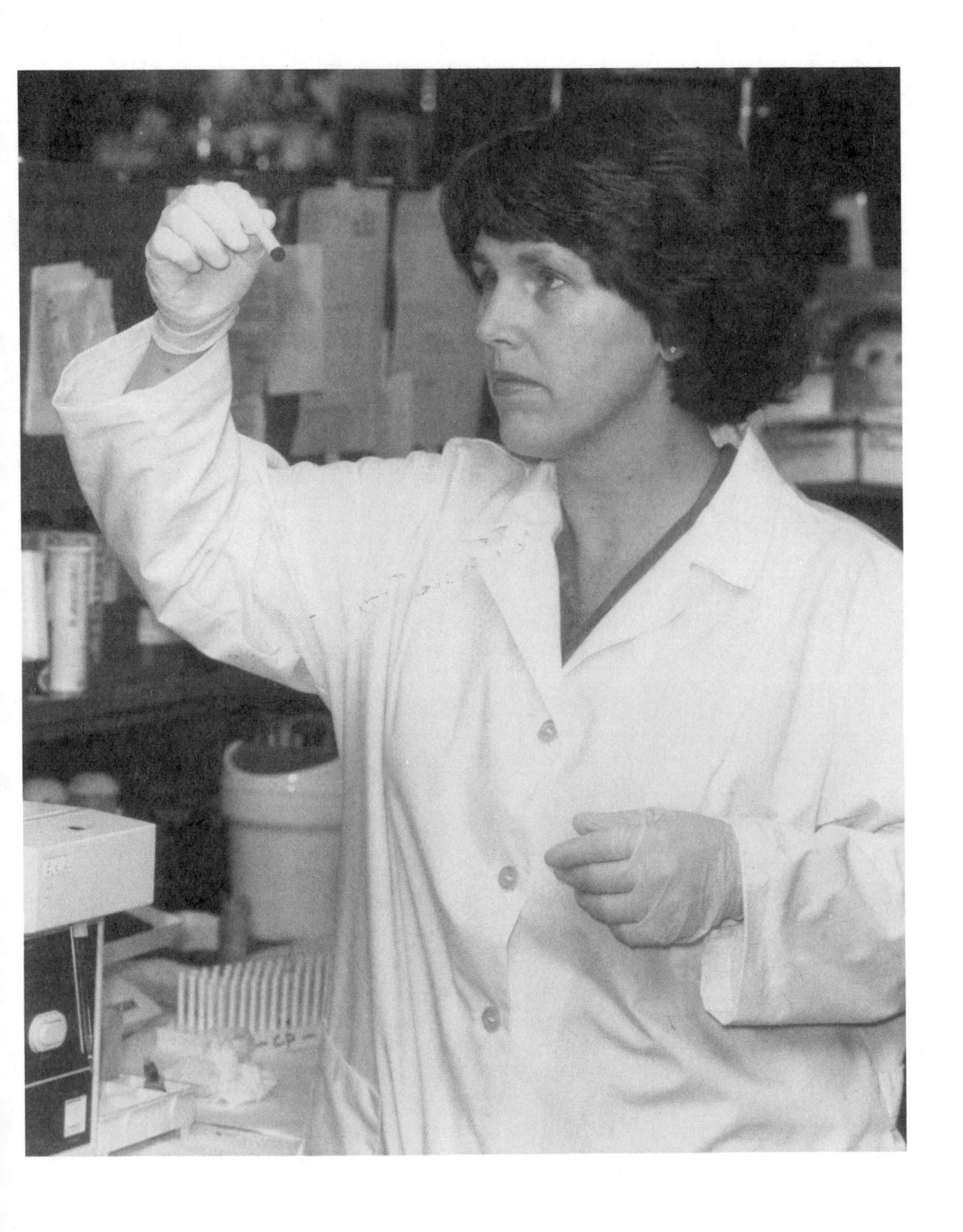

PART IV

High-Tech Nutrition

27

Enteral Nutrition

Charlie, a 14-year-old boy, had had chronic inflammatory bowel disease, or Crohn's disease, since age 8 years. The doctors told him that his poor growth and lack of sexual development were due to poor nutrition. Because of his Crohn's disease, he could not eat as much as the doctors advised. He was not hungry and, if he forced himself to eat, he would have stomach pain and have to run to the toilet because of cramps and diarrhea. He tried to eat more because he was not happy being short and looking like a 10-year-old while his friends were all blooming. When tube feedings were recommended to improve his nutritional status he was shocked, saddened, and afraid. His parents were very upset too; but what a difference the tube feedings made. Soon after they were started, he began feeling better, gaining weight, and growing for the first time in years.

WHO SHOULD GET ENTERAL NUTRITION

Those who are unable to eat, cannot eat enough, will not eat, or should not eat are candidates for enteral nutrition as long as there is a functional gastrointestinal system. Enteral nutrition is more nutritionally complete, less expensive, safer, and less time consuming than intravenous (parenteral) nutrition (see Chapter 28). Enteral alimentation may be given alone as a complete diet, or in addition to other oral feedings. It may also be given in conjunction with parenteral alimentation, particularly for transitional purposes when weaning a patient off intravenous feeding. The use of the GI tract for feeding provides advantages beyond nutritional repletion (Green 1985). Studies have demonstrated that enteral feedings enhance the return of GI function and structural integrity of the GI mucosa. For these reasons, if the alimentary canal is functional, it should be used.

TUBE FEEDINGS

If a patient is unable to consume adequate nutrition with oral enteral nutritional supplements and/or other foods, tube feeding should be considered. The clinical disorders that warrant the use of enteral tube feedings are listed in Table 27–1.

SELECTION OF FEEDING TUBES

Nasogastric and Nasoduodenal Tubes

The most commonly used feeding tubes are nasogastric and nasoduodenal (Fig. 27–1). Small-bore, soft, and flexible feeding tubes are those most beneficial for enteral feedings. A nasogastric feeding tube is easily inserted and can be left in place for several weeks or reinserted with each feeding depending on the patient's preference. The nasoduodenal feeding tubes are usually more difficult to place in the correct position, so frequent reinsertions are not done

Table 27–1. Clinical Disorders in Which Enteral Tube Feeding Has Been of Value.

Weight loss associated with chronic illness
Cancer
Eating disorders or psychiatric problems
Surgery
Neurologic disease with inability to swallow; mental retardation
Inborn errors or metabolism, such as glycogen storage disease
Increased metabolic rate, e.g., burns and postsurgery
Prematurity or low birth weight
Failure to thrive
Chronic diarrhea
Inflammatory bowel disease
Short-bowel syndrome
Pancreatic insufficiency
Swallowing problems, gastroesophageal reflux, delayed gastric emptying
Radiation enteritis
Cystic Fibrosis with malnutrition
Upper gastrointestinal obstruction or surgery
Heart failure—limited cardiac reserve in congenital heart disease

Modified from Greene HL. Use of continuous nasogastric feedings in malabsorption syndromes of infancy. In Lifshitz F, ed. Nutrition for special needs in infancy, protein hydrolysate. New York: Marcel Dekker, 1985:202.

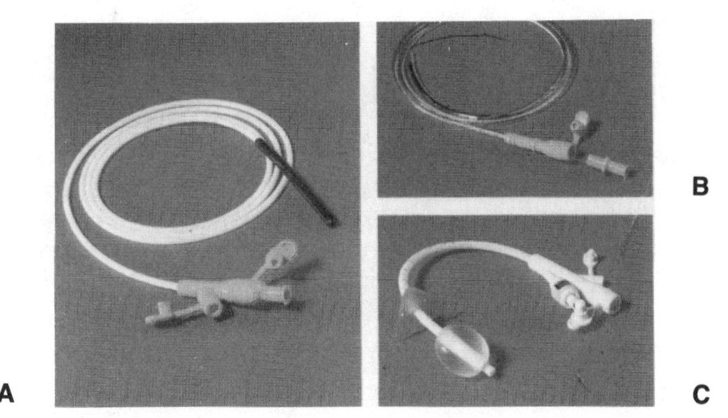

Figure 27–1. Various enteral feeding tubes: nasogastric (A), nasoduodenal (B), and gastrostomy (C). (Courtesy of Ross Laboratories, Columbus, OH.)

easily. Many nasogastric and nasoduodenal tubes are weighted at the proximal tip, which may facilitate placement and increase the likelihood that the tube will remain in the proper position. Nonweighted tubes may become more easily displaced with coughing or vomiting. Many tubes come with a stylet, which eases intubation in some patients. A stylet should never be inserted into a tube that is already placed in a patient. This can cause perforation of the gastrointestinal tract.

Nasogastric and nasoduodenal feeding tubes are available in various sizes, from very small infant tubes to larger adult-size tubes. The smallest lumen tube in which the feeding and medications flow easily is the safest tube to use. Larger lumen tubes may allow for an easier flow of a thicker formula and/or a larger volume but they have potential complications such as irritation or trauma to the upper GI tract or partial airway obstruction. The incidence of the complications outweighs any potential benefits. The tube should be of sufficient length to be properly positioned in the stomach or small intestine. Tubes that have a Y or double-exit port can facilitate verifying placement, flushing, and injecting medications. Care must be taken with feeding-tube insertion. Nasally inserted tubes should never be forced. If a tube cannot be easily passed through one side of the nose, the other side should be tried. If both sides are obstructed, the physician should be contacted. Infants and children may need to be restrained during feeding-tube insertion. After the tube is in place, the patient should be held, cuddled, and comforted (Paine 1986).

Nasogastric tubes deliver the feeding directly into the stomach and are thus considered more physiologic. However, when patients have delayed gastric emptying or gastroesophageal reflux, it may be necessary to use a nasoduodenal tube. Infusion beyond the pyloric sphincter often prevents regurgitation and aspiration, although reflux of the formula into the stomach may not be totally eliminated. The rate of the feeding will also affect the degree of reflux (Rombeau & Caldwell 1984).

Feeding Gastrostomy and Jejunostomy Tubes

When the need for enteral tube feedings is anticipated to be long-term, gastrostomy tubes can be either surgically or percutaneously inserted in the patient (Patterson & Andrassy 1983). These types of feeding tubes allow the patient increased mobility, while they are easily concealed, are very stable, and save the need for repeated nasoduodenal intubations (Fig. 27–2). Children with chronic neurologic, craniofacial, and esophageal disorders who cannot use nasogastric or nasoduodenal tubes may need gastrostomy or jejunostomy tubes for enteral feedings. Patients with mental illness and/or mental retardation who have an inadequate caloric intake may also require a feeding gastrostomy tube to facilitate their care.

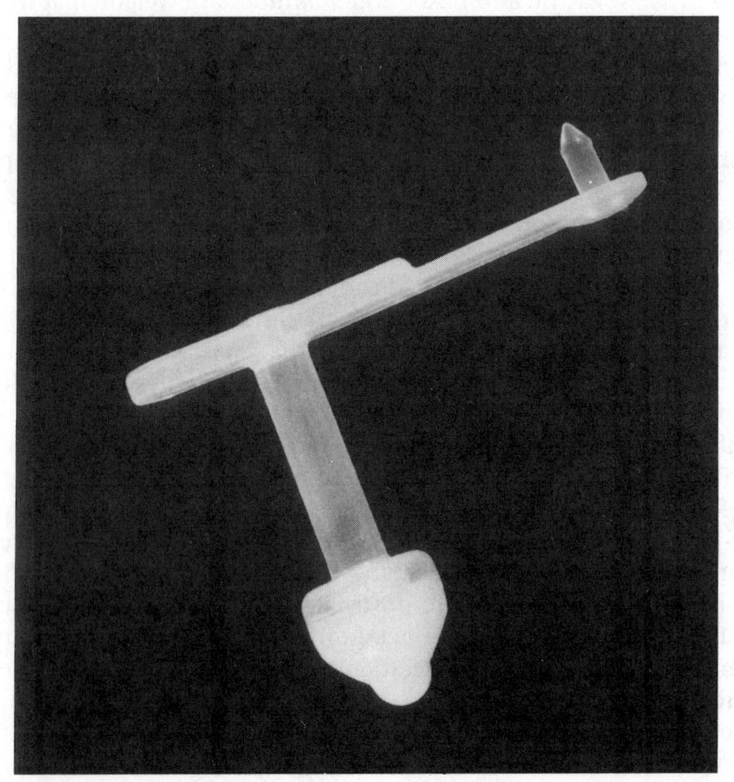

Figure 27–2. Button replacement gastrostomy device (BRGD). (Courtesy of C.R. Bard, Tewksbury, MA.)

Surgical gastrostomies can be performed under local anesthesia via a stab wound. Most surgeons prefer the construction of a feeding gastrostomy by laparatomy (surgery of the abdomen) with a serous- or mucous-lined tube, which avoids major reconstruction of the stomach. However, since the late 1970s, percutaneous gastrostomy feeding-tube placement has also been utilized (Sacks & Glotzer 1979). This procedure allows the tube to be placed into the stomach via endoscopic placement, without general anesthesia and without surgery of the abdomen (Ponsky, Gauderer & Stellato 1983).

Many patients need additional surgical procedures to ensure that gastrostomy feedings will work appropriately. Patients with feeding problems who require gastrostomy feeding might also have abnormalities of the esophagus (GI reflux) and/or delayed gastric emptying. Indeed, GI reflux is particularly prevalent in patients who have psychomotor retardation and developmental delay. These patients are at risk of developing severe complications of GI reflux, including esophageal ulceration, strictures, and narrowing. For this reason, some physicians recommend that a fundoplication (tightening of the entrance to the stomach) and pyloroplasty (loosening of the outlet of the stomach) be performed concurrently with gastrostomy placement to ensure successful feedings (Jolley, Smith & Tunell 1985). However, performance of these procedures increases the surgical risk and may cause future complications with dumping syndrome (Hirsig et al 1984).

The most common disadvantage of a feeding gastrostomy or jejunostomy tube is that they are invasive surgical procedures. Also, there may be skin irritation or infection at the exit site of the tube (Starkey, Jefferson & Kirby 1988), peritonitis, and risk of dislodgement of the tube and/or intra-abdominal leaks (Wasiljew, Ujiki & Beal 1982). These complications can often be prevented with good skin care at the tube exit site (Picco, Baranuski, Polyak 1985) and by frequent verification of the tube placement.

It should be kept in mind that a gastrostomy or jejunostomy is often performed on chronically ill, malnourished, and debilitated patients who are otherwise poor operative risks because of malnutrition. While considered a technically simple procedure, problems may occur in this patient population (Torosian & Rombeau 1980). For example, the sutures may fail to heal, especially if there is gastric distention. Wound infection may also result at times, and may lead to more severe systemic infections. The mouth of the gastrostomy or jejunostomy may retract or become narrow, or the stomach may stick out through the wound. The feeding tube may break or become obstructed, be accidentally removed, or even migrate into the esophagus or jejunum. These and other complications lead to surgical revision of the gastrostomy in about 2 percent of cases (Cataldi-Betcher et al 1982). However, despite the risks, when this procedure is indicated and appropriately done, it may be life-saving and allow for long-term enteral feedings, with recovery of the patient.

CONTINUOUS-DRIP FEEDINGS

Tube feedings are administered by either continuous drip or by bolus. The method of administration depends on the type and location of the feeding tube, the type of formula, and the patient's degree of GI function. Continuous-drip feedings provide enteral nutrition by a slow constant drip during the entire day, best delivered by an enteral pump. This delivery method is often the best way to initiate enteral nutrition, especially in children and infants. The younger and the sicker the patient, the more likely that he or she will tolerate continuous-drip feedings better than any other feeding method. Indeed, continuous-drip feedings are often the only route for enteral nutritional rehabilitation of premature infants or acutely ill patients.

The constant, slow rate of continuous feedings may diminish the GI reflux often associated with bolus feedings. For infants or children with limited stomach capacity, a large volume of formula may be given continuously throughout the day and be well tolerated. This may allow the patient to receive a higher caloric and nutritional load than would be possible with bolus feedings. Also, better intestinal absorption of the formula occurs when continuous feedings are given as compared with other feedings (Greene 1985). There is greater energy, protein, fat, and mineral absorption because there is more time for the digestive process to take place; thus, continuous feedings are associated with a greater body weight gain, decreased stool sugars, and less water and mineral losses than bolus feedings. In addition, there is diminished stomach and intestinal distention and less mass propulsion of enteric contents. Therefore, continuous-drip feedings may be useful even in patients whose GI tract function is markedly impaired (Walker & Hendrick 1985).

Continuous-drip feedings can be used with all types of feeding tubes and all defined formula diets. However, pureed table food should not be used for this type of infusion. Problems associated with a fluctuating infusion rate are best avoided when the feedings are regulated with an enteral pump (Orvieto, Kirsch & Goldberger 1983). The ability of a pump to run at a low, accurate rate and to have small incremental changes is important for pediatric patients whose nutritional requirements may be quite precise. Infants and children need pumps with much lower delivery rates than adolescent or adult patients. Factors to consider when choosing an enteral pump include operating pressure, accuracy, rate, weight, size, duration of battery before recharging, alarms, ancillary supplies, and cost (Table 27–2).

The initiation of continuous feedings in a patient whose GI tract has not been used for a while may be best accomplished by starting with a dilute, hypotonic formula given at a slow continuous infusion rate. Once this initial type and amount of formula has been tolerated for 24 hours, the rate and concentration of the feedings may be slowly increased (generally, the formula is advanced every 1 or 2 days). When giving enteral-tube feedings, it is advis-

Table 27–2. Questions to Ask When Selecting an Enteral Pump.

1. What is its size and weight?
2. Is it easily attached to a portable pole?
3. Can the patient wear the pump and easily ambulate?
4. What is the usual length of operation for the pump battery?
5. Is the battery rechargeable? If yes, how long does it take?
6. What are the pump's minimum and maximum infusion rates?
7. What are the increments of infusion rate?
8. Is the pump easy to operate?
9. Is the pump accurate, reliable, and durable?
10. Does the pump have alarms? If so, for what and are they easily heard?
11. Does the pump require special tubing or containers? If so, what is the cost and can they be reused?
12. Are additional supplies necessary? If so, what are their costs?
13. What is the average breakdown record of the pump?
14. Can the pump be easily repaired?
15. Can it be easily cleaned?
16. How long does the pump last? Is it guaranteed?
17. What is the price?

able that the type, quantity, and rate of infusion of the formula not be changed all at once. If there are undesirable effects of enteral feedings, the culprit can more easily be detected and quickly corrected if only one change is made at a time.

At times it is advantageous to administer continuous enteral drips for only part of the day. This is referred to as cyclic drip feedings. Cyclic drip feedings are frequently administered at night, while the patient sleeps, over a 10- to 12-hour cycle. This method of feeding frees the patient from the pump and tube during part or all of the daytime hours. However, cyclic drips can be used only when the patient tolerates a high enough rate of infusion and volume of formula to meet all nutrient requirements in a shorter time period and can adjust to many hours without any feeding.

The transition from continuous-drip to cyclic-drip feedings should be done by slowly increasing the rate of the enteral tube feeding and by decreasing the infusion time of the formula needed during a day in accordance with the patient's tolerance. This may be a slow adjustment process, and may take days or weeks to accomplish. Similarly, it is prudent to gradually taper the rate of infusion in patients receiving cyclic infusions throughout the night. Tapering cyclic-drip feedings can be accomplished by decreasing the infusion rate by 50 percent 1 hour before its completion. If further tapering is needed, the rate of the infusion can then be decreased again by another 50 percent after 30 minutes. The formula is then stopped after 30 minutes of this slower rate with safety and without problems such as reactive low blood sugar (hypoglycemia). When a transition from continuous tube feedings to oral feedings is initiated, the tube feedings should be discontinued at least 1 hour prior to meal time to encourage oral intake.

BOLUS FEEDINGS

Bolus feedings are also referred to as intermittent feedings. The major advantage of bolus feeding is its similarity to a normal pattern of eating, which includes three or more meals per day. Bolus feedings are often indicated for children who have good digestive function but have chronic neurologic or esophageal disorders, feeding problems, or eating disorders, and for children who need supplementation to their regular diets and cannot drink supplements. Bolus tube feedings are also preferable because of the shortened time the patient is connected to a feeding system and the lower cost for supplies. Bolus feedings are only given for brief periods four or more times a day, and do not require special equipment. However, infants, acutely ill children, and children with vomiting, reflux, delayed gastric emptying, malabsorption, and diminished GI function are not candidates for bolus feedings.

Each bolus feeding is delivered over 20 to 30 minutes or longer. The length of time of the feeding depends on the patient's tolerance to the volume and to the formula used. A large volume or a rapidly administered bolus feeding can lead to gastric distention and regurgitation. To decrease the chances of these complications, each feeding should be dripped more slowly than it would take to eat an equivalent meal. This can be accomplished by dripping the feedings by gravity. Feedings should never be pushed or forced with a syringe; this can lead to aspiration. The patient should sit up or be propped up to avoid reflux, vomiting, and aspiration while the feeding is being given. Bolus feedings may be given directly into the stomach via a nasogastric tube or via gastrostomy. Bolus feedings should not be used with nasoduodenal tubes or jejunostomy because the stomach's regulating mechanism for the emptying of its contents into the small intestine is bypassed.

TYPES OF ENTERAL FORMULAS

An ever-expanding array of enteral formulas is available in the market (see Tables 27–3 to 27–7). These formulas often compensate for specific physiologic GI deficits, and they are especially prepared by professionals, thereby decreasing the chance of error and contamination. However, the composition, cost, and medical indications of each formula vary considerably. Thus, health care professionals should be familiar with the benefits of various products in order to select the most appropriate enteral supplement for the treatment of a specific problem (Wilson 1987).

Children and adolescents with minimal or no digestive dysfunction frequently do well with either pureed table foods or with blenderized enteral feedings, but patients with marked GI dysfunction need more processed, refined, elemental, or specialized formulas. When selecting an enteral feeding, the amount and the type of carbohydrate, protein, fat, and osmolality must be considered. Patients who have specific food allergies, such as egg or milk, may not tolerate enteral products made with these proteins. Also, lactose, the milk sugar present in some enteral formulas, is not absorbed by the majority of individuals and may lead to diarrhea if given to lactose-intolerant patients. In addition, it should be remembered that the prices of these products vary widely. Generally, the less refined the nutrients, the lower the cost; elemental and specialized formulas are usually the most expensive. Special packaging (ready to use, with tubing, etc.) also increases the price; however, these products may be cost-effective when time factors are taken into consideration and may diminish complications such as bacterial contamination or incorrectly prepared formula.

Most of the commercially prepared enteral formulas are listed in various books, which contain tables and charts of the composition and specific indications for use of each formula (Moses 1985). However, it should be remembered that new products are always being developed and that the composition of the formulas change; thus, tables and charts in books become outdated. Therefore, it is best to check the composition listed on the formula container prior to initiating enteral feedings. It must be remembered that the formula should provide complete RDAs for all nutrients and it should meet the patient's specific needs (Lifshitz, Moses & Carrera 1988).

The volume of enteral formula given to a patient is not equivalent to the amount of water required by patients given enteral feedings. The total water content of each formula or blenderized diet varies. One can assume that isocaloric formulas, which provide 1 calorie per milliliter, are the formulas that contain sufficient water content to meet the needs of the patient. When hypercaloric formulas are fed, the amount of water is insufficient. For example, if a 1.5 calories per milliliter formula is used, there is only about 80 percent free water, and for those with caloric density of 2.0 calories per milliliter there will only be 60 percent of its volume as water. In patients who are getting formulas with increased calories and those unable to relate thirst and drink water voluntarily, water can be added by flushing it through the feeding tube. Water intake is a very important consideration in providing tube feedings.

Most enteral formulas are appropriate for nasogastric or nasoduodenal tube feedings. However, an intact protein formula should not be used as jejunal feedings; a protein hydrolysate formula must be selected because the feeding infuses directly into the jejunum and bypasses gastric and duodenal digestion, which breaks down protein.

Infant formulas can be classified as milk-based, soy-based, protein hydrolysate, and special infant formulas (see Chapter 13). Infants who need enteral feedings may be given milk-based formulas, which are well tolerated by patients with no GI abnormalities and should be considered as the first choice, second only to human-milk feedings. For an infant who does not tolerate the milk-based formula and/or for the one with specific metabolic problems or intolerances such as galactosemia or lactose intolerance, there are a great number of specific formulas that may be utilized (see Chapters 13, 25, and 29). These specialized formulas should not be used for any purpose other than those specified, as they may not meet the RDAs for all nutrients to support normal growth.

Blenderized formulas are meal-replacement feedings for children who can tolerate a normal diet and do not have increased metabolic needs (Table 27–3). These formulas usually contain beef puree, vitamins, and minerals. Blenderized formulas are available with and without lactose and can be successfully used for bolus feedings. These types of feedings may be advantageous for children with gastrostomy tubes who have chronic feeding problems such as esophageal, neurologic, and swallowing disorders with an otherwise intact, functional digestive tract.

Home-prepared blenderized feedings may be used instead of purchasing commercially available formulas, but these should be designed by a dietitian to ensure that the nutritional needs of the patient are met. A variety of foods from each food group should be selected for the formula; including meat, cereal, vegetables, fruits, fats, and milk. Substitutions, additions, or exclusions should not be undertaken without first consulting a dietitian. In making blenderized feedings at home, foods that contain nuts, seeds, whole grains, or coconut should not be used. Fruits and vegetables should be well-cooked or canned, and all seeds and tough skin removed before blenderizing. For easy puree of meats, tender cuts cooked by a moist heat method should be selected. Strained baby meats may be used, but combination dinners should be avoided because they contain less protein. Raw eggs are not acceptable; they contain a substance, avidin, that binds with the nutrient biotin, making it unavailable for absorption. Biotin deficiency may result from long-term ingestion of uncooked eggs. To prevent spoilage, formula should be

Table 27–3. Blenderized Formulas.

FORMULA	MANUFACTURER	COMMENTS
Vitaneed	Sherwood Medical	Tube feeding; isotonic lactose-free; low sodium content; 1.0 kcal/mL
Compleat Regular	Sandoz Nutrition	Tube feeding; with lactose; hypertonic; 1.0 kcal/mL
Compleat Modified	Sandoz Nutrition	Tube feeding; isotonic lactose-free; low sodium content; 1.0 kcal/mL

made fresh every day and refrigerated in a covered container until it is used. The decreased cost is a major benefit of homemade pureed and blenderized diets. However, the potential for the patient to receive an inadequate, incomplete, or contaminated diet and the additional time needed to prepare the pureed feedings at home are disadvantages.

Whole protein supplemental formulas are quite numerous, and may differ in their composition, characteristics, and indications (Table 27–4). The protein sources of these formulas are derived from either caseinate or soy protein isolate. The standard whole protein formulas usually contain 30 to 40 grams of protein per liter. There are also high-nitrogen formulas that may contain as much as 70 grams of protein per liter. The caloric density (kcal/mL) of standard formulas is usually 1.00 to 1.06 calories per milliliter, but there are also high-calorie formulas that provide 1.50 to 2.00 calories per milliliter. Some formulas are isotonic (300 mOsm/kg water), while others are hypertonic (as high as 750 mOsm/kg water). Isotonic formulas are usually better tolerated in patients with compromised GI function, whereas hypertonic formulas may result in diarrhea and abdominal cramping. Whole protein supplemental formulas are nutritionally complete and contain vitamins, minerals, and electrolytes to meet all the RDAs when given in sufficient quantity to meet the patient's calorie and nitrogen needs.

Protein hydrolysates, semi-elemental or *elemental formulas*, are comprised of peptides, small peptides, and amino acids and thus are more processed or predigested than other formulas (Lifshitz 1985) and may be better absorbed (Meredith et al 1990). Some of these products are available only in powder form and must be reconstituted (mixed) specifically for each patient's needs (Table 27–5). The protein content varies from 21 to 45 grams of protein per liter, with the high-nitrogen formulas providing 38 to 45 grams of protein per liter. The caloric densities range from 1.00 to 1.06 calories per milliliter. The osmolality of these formulas is usually high, ranging from 400 to 810 milliosmol per kilogram of water, with most formulas between 450 and 650 milliosmol per kilogram of water.

Semi-elemental and elemental formulas are used for patients with either (1) severe malabsorption; (2) failure to tolerate other formulas; and/or (3) jejunal feedings. Short-gut syndrome, inflammatory bowel disease with fistulas, cystic fibrosis, burns, and AIDS are conditions that often require the use of protein hydrolysate feedings.

Modular supplements provide specific nutrients but are not complete enteral feedings when given alone (Table 27–6). Modular supplements are very concentrated forms of protein, carbohydrate, or fat that can be diluted and combined with other nutrients to customize a formula to meet a patient's special needs. It is important to keep in mind that the addition of these modular supplements to a nutritionally complete formula will make an unbalanced

Table 27–4. Whole Protein Supplements and Formulas.

FORMULA		
LACTOSE-CONTAINING	**MANUFACTURER**	**COMMENTS**
Carnation Instant Breakfast Powder	Carnation	Oral feeding; milk to be added; hypertonic; high protein; 1.1 kcal/mL
Sustacal Powder	Mead Johnson	Predominantly for oral feeding with added flavorings; milk to be added; hypertonic; high protein and calories; 1.85 kcal/mL
Sustagen Powder	Mead Johnson	Predominantly for oral feeding with added flavorings; milk to be added; hypertonic; high protein and calories; 1.85 kcal/mL
Meritine Liquid/ Powder	Sandoz Nutrition	Predominantly for oral feeding with added flavorings; hypertonic; high protein; 1 kcal/mL
Forta Shake	Ross Laboratories	Oral feedings; milk to be added; hypertonic; high protein; low fat; 1.2 kcal/mL
Nutrament	Dracket Products	For oral supplements; 1 kcal/mL; high protein; readily available in supermarkets; slightly cheaper than other products
LACTOSE-FREE		
Pre-Attain	Sherwood Medical	Tube feeding; low osmolality (150 mOsm/kg); low carbohydrate; available in ready-to-use closed-system feeding; 0.5 kcal/mL
Attain L.S.	Sherwood Medical	Tube feeding; low carbohydrate; low sodium; 1.0 kcal/mL
Attain	Sherwood Medical	Tube feedings; isotonic; available in ready-to-use closed-system feeding; 1.0 kcal/mL
Magnacal	Sherwood Medical	Predominantly for tube feedings; hypertonic; high fat (36%); 2.0 kcal/mL
Sustacal Liquid	Mead Johnson	Predominantly for oral feeding with added flavorings; hypertonic; high protein; low fat (21%); 1.0 kcal/mL
Sustacal HC	Mead Johnson	Similar to Sustacal Liquid with 34% corn oil; 1.5 kcal/mL
Isocal	Mead Johnson	Tube/oral feedings; isotonic; low electrolyte content; MCT oil 20% of fat; 1.06 kcal/mL
Isocal HCN	Mead Johnson	Predominantly for tube feedings; hypertonic; high fat, MCT oil 30% of fat; 2 kcal/mL
Isocal HN	Mead Johnson	Predominantly for tube feedings; isotonic; high nitrogen; 1.0 kcal/mL
Ensure Liquid	Ross Laboratories	Predominantly for oral feedings with added flavorings; hypertonic; low residue; 1.06 kcal/mL
Ensure Plus	Ross Laboratories	Similar to Ensure Liquid; with 1.5 kcal/mL and greater osmolality
Ensure HN	Ross Laboratories	Similar to Ensure Liquid; high nitrogen with 1.06 kcal/mL and greater osmolality
Ensure Plus HN	Ross Laboratories	Similar to Ensure Liquid; high nitrogen with 1.5 kcal/mL and greater osmolality
Osmolite	Ross Laboratories	Predominantly for tube feeding; isotonic; low

Table 27–4. Whole Protein Supplements and Formulas. *(cont.)*

FORMULA	MANUFACTURER	COMMENTS
		electrolyte content; MCT oil 50% of fat; 1.0 kcal/mL
Osmolite HN	Ross Laboratories	Similar to Osmolite; high nitrogen with 1.06 kcal/mL
Two Cal HN	Ross Laboratories	Tube/oral feedings; hypertonic; high fat; MCT oil; 2.0 kcal/mL
Forta Drink	Ross Laboratories	Oral feedings; hypertonic; high protein and carbohydrate; low fat; 0.56 kcal/mL
Pediasure	Ross Laboratories	Oral feeding for children; hypertonic; high fat; low carbohydrate; 1.0 kcal/mL
Travasorb MCT	Baxter Health Care	Predominantly for tube feeding; isotonic; high protein; MCT oil for fat malabsorption; 1.0 kcal/mL
Travasorb Liquid	Baxter Health Care	Tube/oral feedings; hypertonic; 1.06 kcal/mL
Citrotein	Sandoz Nutrition	Predominantly oral feeding with added flavorings; hypertonic; high protein and carbohydrate; low fat; clear liquid; 0.66 kcal/mL
Precision Isotonic	Sandoz Nutrition	Predominantly for tube feedings; isotonic; low electrolyte content; 1.0 kcal/mL
Isotein HN	Sandoz Nutrition	Predominantly for tube feedings; isotonic; high protein; low fat; MCT oil; 1.2 kcal/mL
IsoSource	Sandoz Nutrition	Predominantly for tube feedings; isotonic; 1.25 kcal/mL
Resource	Sandoz Nutrition	Predominantly for oral feedings with added flavors; hypertonic; 1.06 kcal/mL; ready-to-use box packaging
Resource Plus	Sandoz Nutrition	Predominantly for oral feeding with added flavors; hypertonic; 1.5 kcal/mL; ready-to-use box packaging
Newtrition Vanilla, Chocolate	Knight Medical	Predominantly oral feedings with added flavorings; hypertonic; 1.06 kcal/mL
Newtrition Isotonic	Knight Medical	Tube/oral feedings; isotonic; MCT oil 19% of fat; ready-to-use box packaging; 1.06 kcal/mL
Newtrition High Nitrogen	Knight Medical	Tube/oral feedings; isotonic; high protein; MCT oil 50% of fat; ready-to-use box packaging; 1.24 kcal/mL
Newtrition	Knight Medical	Ready-to-use closed enteral nutrition delivery system for tube feedings; isotonic; 1.06 kcal/mL

Table 27–5. Protein Hydrolysates (Elemental and Semi-elemental Formulas).

FORMULA	MANUFACTURER	COMMENTS
Criticare HN	Mead Johnson	Tube feedings; hypertonic; low fat; high carbohydrate; moderate protein (14% of calories); small peptide formulation; lactose-free; 1.06 kcal/mL
Vital HN	Ross Laboratories	Tube feedings; hypertonic; high carbohydrate; low fat; 45% of fat from MCT oil; lactose-free; 1.0 kcal/mL
Tolerex	Norwich Eaton	Tube/oral feedings; hypertonic; low protein (8% of calories) and fat; high carbohydrate; lactose- and sucrose-free; 1.0 kcal/mL
Vivonex HN	Norwich Eaton	Tube feeding; hypertonic; low fat; high protein (18% of calories); high carbohydrate; lactose and sucrose-free; 1.0 kcal/mL
Vivonex T.E.N.	Norwich Eaton	Tube feeding; hypertonic; low fat; high carbohydrate; moderate protein (15% of calories); lactose- and sucrose-free; 1.0 kcal/mL
Travasorb STD	Baxter Health Care	Tube feeding; hypertonic; low fat; high carbohydrate; 60% of fat from MCT oil; lactose-free; 1.0 kcal/mL
Travasorb HN	Baxter Health Care	Tube feeding; hypertonic; low fat; high nitrogen and carbohydrate; moderate protein; 60% of fat from MCT oil; lactose- and sucrose-free; 1.0 kcal/mL
Peptamen	Baxter Health Care	Tube feeding; isotonic; 70% of fat from MCT oil; small peptide formulation; lactose-free
Reabilan	O'Brien	Tube feeding; isotonic; 40% of fat from MCT oil; small peptide formulation; lactose- and sucrose-free; 1.0 kcal/mL
Reabilan HN	O'Brien	Tube feeding; high protein (17% of calories); 38% of fat from MCT oil; small peptide formulation; lactose- and sucrose-free; 1.3 kcal/mL
Pepti 2000	Sherwood Medical	Tube feeding; hypertonic; low fat; high carbohydrate; small peptide formulation; 1.0 kcal/mL

feeding and, therefore, should be used only to compensate for specific problems (see Chapters 11 and 21).

Specialized (disease-specific) formulas are manufactured and recommended for specific clinical disorders (Table 27–7). There are formulas specifically intended for patients with hepatic, pulmonary, and renal diseases, as well as for patients with increased metabolic needs such as occurs in trauma. There are also specialized formulas designed for the treatment of specific inborn errors of metabolism (see Chapter 25). These formulas vary dramatically and should not be compared with each other because they are indicated for quite different disorders. They should be used only for the purposes for which they are clearly specified.

Table 27–6. Modular Formulas.

FORMULA	MANUFACTURER	COMMENTS
Protein Supplements		
Casec	Mead Johnson	Calcium caseinate; 88 g protein/100 g powder; 4.0 kcal/g
Propac	Sherwood Medical	Whey; 77 g protein/100 g powder; 4.0 kcal/g
Promod	Ross Laboratories	Whey and soy lecithin; 75 g protein/100 g powder; 5.6 kcal/g
Nutrisource Protein	Sandoz Nutrition	Lactalbumin and egg white solids; 76 g amino acids/100 g powder; 4 kcal/g
Nutrisource Amino Acids—High Branched Chain	Sandoz Nutrition	Balances of essential and nonessential L-amino acids; 97 g amino acids/100 g powder; 3.9 kcal/g
Carbohydrate Supplements		
Moducal	Mead Johnson	Maltodextrin 95 g carbohydrate/100 g powder; 3.8 kcal
Sumacal	Sherwood Medical	Maltodextrin 95 g carbohydrate/100 g powder; 3.8 kcal/g
Polycose	Ross Laboratories	Glucose polymers from hydrolyzed corn starch; 94 g carbohydrate/100 g powder; 80 g carbohydrate/100 mL liquids, 3.8 kcal/g and 2.0 kcal/mL
Nutrisource Carbohydrate	Sandoz Nutrition	Corn syrup solids; 80 g carbohydrate/100 mL liquid; 3.2 kcal/mL
Fat Supplements		
MCT Oil	Mead Johnson	Coconut oil; 93 g oil/100 mL; 7.7 kcal/mL
Microlipid	Sherwood Medical	Safflower oil; polyglycerol; 50 g fat/100 mL; 4.5 kcal/mL
Lipomil	Upjohn	Corn oil; 66 g fat/100 mL; 6.0 kcal/mL
Nutrisource Lipid—Long Chain	Sandoz Nutrition	Soybean oil; polyglycerol; 24 g fat/100 mL; 2.2 kcal/mL
Nutrisource Lipid—Medium Chain	Sandoz Nutrition	Medium-chain triglyceride; polyglycerol, lecithin; 22 g MCT/100 mL; 2.0 kcal/mL

DISADVANTAGES, SIDE EFFECTS, AND COMPLICATIONS OF ENTERAL FEEDING

The disadvantages of enteral feedings include the potential for bacterial contamination owing to formula handling and preparation (Mandel et al 1985), difficulty in regulating flow rate of delivery, particularly when no enteral pump is used, limited mobility of the patient when connected to the feeding system, and the cost of formula and equipment for enteral nutrition.

The most frequent side effects encountered with enteral feedings are adverse GI symptoms (see Table 27–8). Poorly tolerated enteral feedings produce a number of problems, including diarrhea, nausea, vomiting,

Table 27–7. Special Formulas.

FORMULA	MANUFACTURER	COMMENTS
Traumacal	Mead Johnson	Tube feeding; hypertonic; high protein with 22% from branched-chain amino acids; MCT oil; for hypermetabolic patients (e.g., trauma); 1.5 kcal/mL
Sustacal with Fiber	Mead Johnson	Predominantly oral feeding; hypertonic; lactose-free; high-fiber liquid supplement for constipation; 1.0 kcal/mL
Stresstein	Sandoz Nutrition	Tube feedings; hypertonic; high protein with 40% from branched-chain amino acids; low fat with MCT oil; for hypermetabolic patients under stress; 1.2 kcal/mL
Traum-Aid HBC	American McGaw	Tube/oral feeding; hypertonic; high protein with 36% branched-chain amino acids; low fat with MCT oil; for trauma patients; 1.0 kcal/mL
Enrich	Ross Laboratories	Predominantly oral feedings; hypertonic; lactose-free; high-fiber liquid supplement; for constipation; 1.1 kcal/mL
Jevity	Ross Laboratories	Tube feeding; isotonic; lactose- and gluten-free; 50% of fat from MCT oil; for constipation, intolerances to long-chain fat; 1.06 kcal/mL
Pulmocare	Ross Laboratories	Tube/oral feeding; hypertonic; lactose-free; high fat; low carbohydrate; for patients with respiratory problems; 1.5 kcal/mL
Ross SLD	Ross Laboratories	Tube/oral feeding; clear liquid; high protein and carbohydrate; low fat; for patients following surgery; 0.7 kcal/mL
Travasorb Renal	Baxter Health Care	Tube/oral feeding; hypertonic; low protein with essential amino acids for patients with renal disease; not a complete nutritional supplement; 1.4 kcal/mL
Amin-Aid	American McGaw	Tube/oral feeding; hypertonic; low protein with essential amino acids for patients with renal disease; low electrolytes; not a complete nutritional supplement; 1.9 kcal/mL
Travasorb Hepatic	Baxter Health Care	Tube feeding; hypertonic; high branched-chain amino acids for patients with liver disease; 1.1 kcal/mL
Hepatic Aid II	American McGaw	Tube feeding; hypertonic; high branched-chain amino acids; low electrolytes for patients with liver disease; 1.2 kcal/mL

cramping, and distention (Konstantinides & Shronts 1983). These adverse effects are usually related to feedings that are too rapidly infused or to formula intolerance, such as a formula with too high an osmolality for the patient to tolerate (Keohane et al 1981, Niemier et al 1983). The patient's degree of intestinal-function deficit is often the main factor determining the tolerance of a given product. Also, the use of antibiotic therapy may lead to diarrhea

Table 27–8. Complications of Enteral Feedings.

SYMPTOM	CONTRIBUTING FACTORS	TREATMENT OR PREVENTION
Gastrointestinal		
Diarrhea Nausea Vomiting Cramping Distention Hyperactive bowel	Too rapid infusion High osmolality Formula intolerance/sensitivity Lactose intolerance Intestinal function deficits Contamination of formula	Decrease rate and/or volume of infusion Decrease concentration/osmolality Use continuous drip Use lactose-free formula Pay attention to clean technique
Gastric	Delayed gastric emptying Inactivity Cold formula	Slow or stop feeding Reduce rate, concentration, and volume of feeding Use formula at room temperature Position patient with head of bed elevated 30 degrees Medicate to increase gastric motility Use nasoduodenal tube
Constipation	Inadequate water intake Inadequate bulk Impaction Decreased GI motility Medications (narcotics)	Increase free water Give prune juice Use stool softener Increase patient's activity and ambulation Increase bulk of formula
Mechanical		
Aspiration	Decreased gag reflux Displaced feeding tube Deflated tracheostomy cuff Coma Decreased gastric motility Clogged tube	Stop feeding and suction trachea Use jejunal feeding tube Inflate cuff before feeding and keep inflated 1 hour after feeding completed Medicate to increase gastric motility Elevate head of bed 30 degrees or more Hold feedings when gastric residuals high Flush tube and check placement every 4–8 hours
Nasal or pharyngeal irritation	Large lumen, nonflexible tube Pulling of tube Belligerent and uncooperative patients	Use small lumen, flexible, soft tube Position tube without pressure Provide mouth and nares care every 4 hours while awake Retape tube every day Mittens to be worn on hands
Metabolic		
Hyperglycemia Glycosuria Hyperosmolar dehydration	Stress response High rate/high carbohydrate formula Inadequate fluid coverage Diabetes mellitus Drug therapy (steroids)	Stop formula, hydrate patient Treat with insulin and electrolytes Reduce rate of formula when resumed

Table 27–8. Complications of Enteral Feedings. *(cont.)*

SYMPTOM	CONTRIBUTING FACTORS	TREATMENT OR PREVENTION
Overhydration	Intravenous fluid Parenteral nutrition	Decrease volume and intake of IV fluids or nutritional supplements Use more concentrated formulas
Mineral and electrolyte losses	Diarrhea Vomiting	Replace losses
Failure to gain weight	Inadequate nitrogen to calorie ratio Insufficient feedings Vitamin and mineral deficits	Change formula Increase amount of feeding Provide all RDAs of all nutrients Perform frequent nutritional assessment

Adapted from Konstantinides NN, Shronts E. Tube feeding, managing the basics. Am J Nutr 1983; 83:1312–1319

independently of the formula selection or to the method of administration (Keohane et al 1983). Antibiotics may produce alterations in bowel flora or allow the development of *Clostridium difficile* toxin, which may lead to severe enterocolitis. In all cases the treatment of these GI complaints must be specifically aimed at eliminating the source of the problem. To avoid most of these problems it is best to advance the enteral nutrition by first increasing the daily volume until an adequate quantity is provided and then slowly increasing the concentration of the formula.

Incorrect placement of enteral feeding tubes can bring potentially life-threatening complications. The likelihood of aspiration can be decreased by verifying tube placement prior to each bolus feeding or every 4 hours for continuous drips, placing patients in an upright position or elevating the head at least 30 degrees during and for at least 30 minutes after feedings, and using a nasoduodenal or jejunostomy tube rather than a nasogastric tube. In addition, monitoring of gastric residuals in patients with nasogastric tubes or gastrostomy tubes will help detect patients with delayed gastric emptying and those at risk for aspiration. To avoid aspiration, bolus tube feedings are contraindicated for children and adolescents with GI reflux, delayed gastric emptying, and vomiting. If aspiration is suspected, as described below, tube feedings must be stopped immediately and the trachea suctioned.

The most serious metabolic complication of enteral tube feeding is hyperosmolar dehydration and coma. When administered in a large volume, high-caloric density, undiluted formula may lead to high blood sugar and glycosuria. If this progresses untreated, osmotic diuresis (increased urine output), dehydration, and coma ensue. Hyperosmolar coma is a rare and life-threatening complication to enteral tube feedings. Factors other than enteral feedings that can contribute to a high blood sugar are diabetes mellitus, stress response, and steroid therapy. Hyperosmolar dehydration without hyperglyemia can also be precipitated by the hyperosmolality of the enteral tube feedings. Hyperosmolar dehydration and coma are virtually always preventable by (1) monitoring urine output, sugar, and acetone; (2) balancing fluid intake and output; and (3) making appropriate changes in formula type, volume, concentration, and rate of feeding as needed. When hyperosmolar dehydration and/or coma occur, treatment must be immediate; it consists of hydration, insulin, and electrolyte replacement as indicated by a physician.

Infants who solely receive enteral tube feedings for an extended time may be at risk for later acquiring eating disorders if they do not have any oral intake. For example, infants who are not given oral feedings for the first few months of life may develop a rumination disorder, failure to chew, refusal of solids, and vomiting (Kennedy-Caldwell & Caldwell 1984). To diminish these problems with high-risk infants, pacifiers and other forms of oral stimulation are often used so the infants experience sucking and develop oral motor skills during tube feedings. In addition, oral stimulation may shorten the time from weaning off enteral feedings onto bottle feedings and may subsequently increase weight gain.

CLINICAL INTERVENTION

Prevention of complications is an important aspect of caring for patients who receive enteral tube feedings. Aspiration, one of the most serious complications, may sometimes be prevented with astute verification of nasogastric or nasoduodenal tube placement. The initial placement of these tubes is verified by x-ray study when first inserted, and thereafter the tube location should be checked before each bolus feedings or at least every 4 to 8 hours if the patient is receiving continuous feedings.

There are two clinical methods to verify the presence of a nasogastric or nasoduodenal tube in the stomach or small bowel. The first method is to rapidly instill air (1–10 mL, depending on the size of the patient) into the feeding tube while listening with a stethoscope for the sound of the injected air slightly below the xiphoid process for nasogastric tubes or the midabdomen (below the pylorus) for nasoduodenal tubes. The second method for checking placement of these tubes is to attempt to aspirate a small quantity of fluids. Gastric secretions may be easily aspirated and verified by pH measurements. However, feeding tubes may collapse very easily and not permit aspiration of fluid. Thus, the lack of aspirant indicates either a poor test of placement or an improperly placed feeding tube. If there is ever any doubt about the placement of a feeding tube, the enteral feeding should be withheld until placement can be verified by x-ray studies.

Some nutrition services add dye such as methylene blue or add grape juice to enteral feedings. This makes the feeding an easily recognizable bright blue color, which distinguishes it from bronchopulmonary secretions. If suction of the patient's respiratory tract yields blue aspirate, it is clearly evident that the patient has aspirated. A nasogastric or nasoduodenal tube may have a mark where it exits the nose. By checking the level of the marking prior to administering feedings, it may determine if the feeding tube has moved. The location of the tube should be verified prior to resuming the feedings.

Feeding tubes should be carefully and securely taped to either the nose or the cheek without pressure to the nares (Fig. 27–3). A minimal amount of hypoallergenic tape is used and changed daily to keep the nose clean and dry. The external nares should be cleaned to remove mucus crust formation and checked at least every 4–8 hours for signs of pressure or erosion. Infants and children may need to wear mittens to prevent them from pulling out the tube. Frequent mouth care is also important since nasally placed tubes cause patients to mouth breathe, which, combined with lack of chewing or salivation, causes a dry mouth. Frequent mouth rinses, lip moisturizer, and ice chips or sour candy to suck may stimulate salivation and alleviate some of

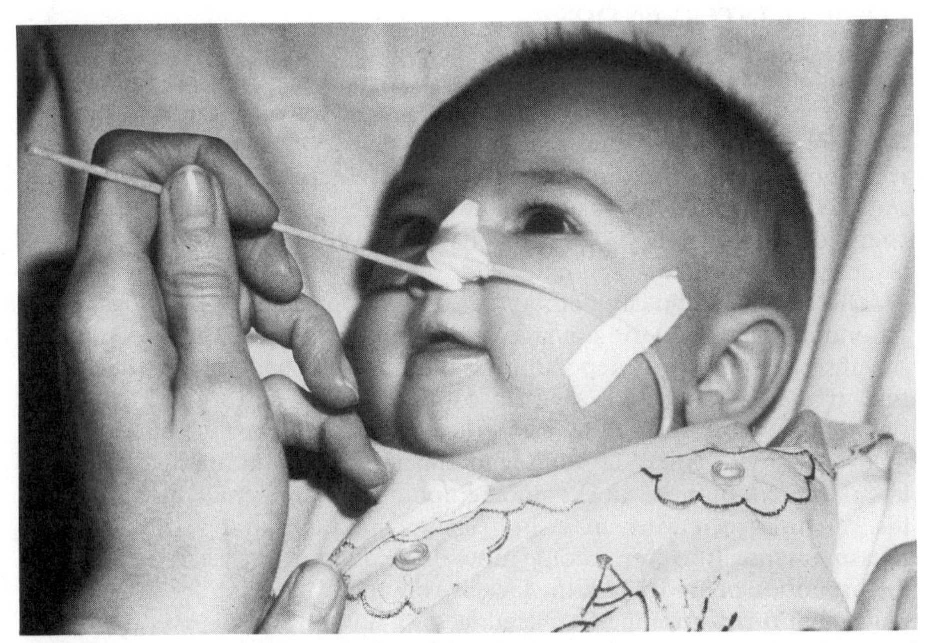

Figure 27–3. Care of nares and nasoduodenal tube. (Used with permission of Home Nutritional Services, Parsippany, NJ.)

this discomfort. If the patient complains of a sore throat, anesthetic lozenges or spray may be helpful. It is also important for the patient to brush his or her teeth twice daily; even if there is no oral intake, bacteria still form on the teeth and gums.

Some patients prefer to insert their feeding tube prior to each feeding, rather than continuously leaving it in place. This procedure can usually easily be taught to children and adolescents. A simple technique is to have the patient suck on small ice chips or sip water while swallowing the small flexible feeding tube. This facilitates intubation, and many children learn to do this quite rapidly with relative ease. The ability to remove the feeding tube after each feeding may increase their acceptance of the enteral feedings and improve their body image.

Countless feeding systems are available to deliver the formula to the patient; these comprise the feeding container and the administration tubing. When choosing an enteral feeding system, an often overlooked but important consideration is the system's similarity to the intravenous system. If the enteral feeding system is not easily distinguished from the intravenous system, enteral nutrition may be mistakenly instilled into a vein instead of the digestive tract (Ament 1987). The enteral tubing should not be the same size as the intravenous tubing; the end of the enteral tubing should not fit into the intravenous tubing and thereby the enteral tubing will not be inadvertently attached to an intravenous tubing.

Other variations and considerations include durability, ease of filling, accurate markings for determining volume, ease of rinsing and cleaning, ability to reuse the system, ease of making additions to the solution, and ability to flush tubing or add medication without disconnecting the system. When evaluating the cost of the system, time factors for dietary, nursing, or pharmacy staff should be included. A system that initially appears expensive may be cost-effective when waste and cost of personnel are factored into the evaluation (Pemberton et al 1985). Young children may see an infusion pump as a new toy. To avoid problems, extra extension tubing can be attached to the administration set and the pump kept a distance from the patient (Paine 1986). Covering the pump or its controls is also helpful to prevent children from gaining access to the pump.

Gastrostomy and jejunostomy tubes require frequent meticulous skin care to prevent irritation or erosion and infection at the tube's exit site. There should be no pressure on the tube or skin, and the tube should be securely anchored. This helps prevent accidental dislodgement of the feeding tube while maintaining skin integrity. Some manufacturers recommend dressing changes, while others do not. If a dressing is necessary, the skin is inspected daily and with each dressing change to note leakage around the tube, which rapidly leads to skin excoriation. Leakage around the gastrostomy or jejunostomy may indicate a peritoneal leak into the abdominal cavity, which is a serious complication. The surgeon should be notified whenever this problem is noted. Skin protectors or barriers, such as those used around wounds and ostomies, may be useful in preventing skin breakdown. These barriers are placed on the skin around the tube before gauze is applied as a dressing.

When patients are given their enteral feedings, the head of the bed should be raised at least 30 degrees during the feeding and for 30 minutes after the feeding is stopped to decrease the incidence of regurgitation and aspiration. Patients receiving bolus feedings are often able to sit in an upright position to facilitate feedings. Patients receiving nasogastric or gastrostomy feeding should have gastric residuals checked often, and feedings should be withheld until residuals decrease. Since the aspirated content of the stomach is rich in electrolytes, all residuals should always be given back to the patient through the feeding tube to prevent problems caused by fluid and electrolyte losses via discarded gastric content.

Occlusion of small-bore feeding tubes may occur in 6 to 10 percent of patients. All feeding tubes should be flushed with a small quantity of warm water or saline before and after each feeding to maintain patency of the tube and to avoid problems with water deficits. Patients who receive continuous feedings should have their tubes flushed once every 4 to 8 hours. Other types of irrigants such as cranberry or other juices (Wilson & Haynes-Johnson 1987) are not recommended because they increase the incidence of tube occlusion and necessitate more frequent tube replacement when obstruction of the tube occurs. Carbonated beverages, pancreatic enzymes (Viokase) and the proteolytic enzyme papain (Meat Tenderizer) have been used to unclog tubes; the best result has been obtained with a pancreatic enzyme solution (Marcuard, Stegall & Trogdon 1989). Viokase solution is flushed through the tube after attempts are made to drain any residual fluid from the clogged tube. Viokase powder is mixed with 5 milliliters of water and used immediately. The solution is clamped in the tube for 3 minutes. After that, the tube is unclamped and an attempt is made to flush it with sterile water. If the tube is still obstructed, the above procedure can be repeated once; if unsuccessful, the tube must be removed.

Since diarrhea is a frequent consequence of tube feedings, the amount of stool losses should be measured to determine how much fluid replacement is needed. Because most tube feedings have little bulk, constipation may also be a side effect. There are several formulas available with added fiber to minimize this problem. Constipated patients may require either stool softeners, laxatives, or bulk-forming agents. Stool softeners and laxatives in liquid form can be administered through the feeding tube. However, bulk-forming agents (such as Metamucil) clog feeding tubes, and therefore, if needed, they must be taken orally.

Patients often require numerous medications via their feeding tube. Pills and the contents of capsules that can be crushed to a fine powder and dissolved in warm water can be injected into feeding tubes. Elixirs and liquid medications can usually be directly instilled or diluted and then injected into the feeding tube and flushed with water or saline. Enteric-coated pills, time-released capsules, and those that cannot be crushed to a fine powder should not be pushed through feeding tubes because they will clog them. Hypertonic or irritating medications should always be diluted in at least as much water as when taken orally to avoid GI ulceration or even necrotizing enterocolitis. Also, any medication that is recommended to be given with meals needs to be diluted with water and administered during a feeding. Medications should not be mixed together but always administered separately with a flush between medication (Burns, McCall & Wirsching 1988).

Few medications are compatible with enteral formulas. Most medications cause precipitation or a reaction, and thus they should not be added to the formula (Wright & Robinson 1986). Some medications may affect nutrient absorption or be associated with GI tract problems (Paine 1986). The reader is referred elsewhere for more details regarding physical compatibility of commonly used medications with different types of enteral formulas (Burns, McCall & Wirsching 1988).

Improper handling of enteral formulas allows organisms to grow in the formula or for toxins to form (Mandel et al 1985, Freedland et al 1989). Formulas should always be checked to determine whether they have expired. The tops of cans should be cleaned before opening; the can should be refrigerated after opening and discarded if open for more than 24 hours. Feedings that require mixing or diluting, such as powders or concentrated formulas, are more likely to become contaminated than canned, undiluted liquid feedings (Freedland et al 1989). Most continuous feedings should not be hung for longer than 4 hours as they may spoil, and the administration bags and tubing should be washed and rinsed every 4 hours to enhance patency and diminish bacterial growth. These bags and tubing should not be re-used beyond 2 or 3 days. All feedings should be taken from the refrigerator 30 to 60 minutes prior to administering. Feedings should not be given cold, nor should feedings be hung with an ice pouch to keep them cold. Cold feedings are poorly tolerated and cause cramping (Kagawa-Busby et al 1980).

Daily weights, intake and output measurements every 8 to 12 hours, urine sugar and acetone every 4 to 8 hours, daily stool count, and weekly blood chemistry and nutritional assessments are monitored in stable patients receiving enteral feedings. Acutely ill patients require more extensive monitoring. Conversely, once patients have been stable on tube feedings without side effects and without changes in formula, they may no longer need urine sugar and acetone monitored. However, all hospitalized patients on tube feedings should continue to have daily monitoring of weight and intake and output of fluids. The intake of enteral feedings can then be modified appropriately. One final consideration is to give enteral feedings only to patients who have active bowel sounds. Absence of bowel sounds, or decreased intestinal propulsion activity, can lead to obstruction if the patient is tube fed.

When initiating tube feedings, the rationale and goals of therapy should be clearly explained to the parents and the patient so they can accept the treatment and not have misconceptions. Their participation in the tube-feeding process should be encouraged. All procedures should be simply explained and demonstrated when possible. Having a child handle a feeding tube and perhaps insert it into a doll may be helpful (Paine 1986).

To prevent developmental or psychosocial problems in patients receiving tube feedings, attention must be given to the specific developmental and emotional needs of each age group. Infants should be held and comforted during feedings. Normal feeding times may need to be simulated and normal activities maintained. Patients should be encouraged to interact normally with other children. Meals are a social experience for children. They can be taught to play without dislodging their tube. Adolescents may be particularly sensitive to alterations in body image at a time when the need for acceptance by peers is very strong. Encouragement to participate in daily activities, non-judgmental acceptance of their behavior, and allowing teenagers as much control as is realistic may alleviate problems with tube feedings in this group (Paine 1986).

REFERENCES

Ament ME. Parenteral nutrition of the pediatric patient at home. In Lifshitz JZ, ed. Home nutritional therapy. Clinical nutrition supplement. St. Louis: C.V. Mosby, 1987:17–25.

Burns PE, McCall L, Wirsching R. Physical compatibility of enteral formulas with various common medications. J Am Diet Assoc 1988; 88:1094–1096.

Cataldi-Betcher E, Seltzer M, Slocum B, et al. Complications occurring during enteral nutrition support: A prospective study. JPEN 1982; 7:546–552.

Freedland CP, Roller RD, Wolfe BM, Flynn NM. Microbial contamination of continuous drip feedings. JPEN 1989; 13:18–22.

Greene HL. Use of continuous nasogastric feedings in malabsorption syndromes of infancy. In Lifshitz F, ed. Nutrition for special needs in infancy—Protein hydrolysates. New York: Marcel Dekker, 1985:201–211.

Hirsig J, Baals H, Tuchschmid P, et al. Dumping syndrome following Nisien fundoplication: A cause of refusal to feed. J Pediat Surg 1984; 19:155–157.

Jolley SG, Smith EI, Tunell WP. Protective antireflux operation with feeding gastrostomy: Experience with children. Ann Surg 1985; 201:736–740.

Kagawa-Busby K, Heitkemper M, Hansen B, et al. Effects of diet temperature on tolerance of enteral feedings. Nurs Res 1980; 29:276–280.

Kennedy-Caldwell C, Caldwell M. Pediatric enteral nutrition in enteral and tube feeding. In Rombeau JL, Caldwell M, eds. Enteral and tube feeding. Philadelphia: W.B. Saunders, 1984:434–474.

Keohane P, Attrill H, Jones B, et al. The role of lactose and *Clostridium difficile* in the pathogenesis of enteral feeding associated diarrhea. Clin Nutr 1983; 1:259–264.

Keohane P, Attrill H, Love M, et al. Relation between osmolality of diet and gastrointestinal side effects in enteral nutrition. Br Med J 1981; 288:678–680.

Konstantinides NN, Shronts E. Tube feeding, managing the basics. Am J Nutr 1983; 83:1312–1319.

Lifshitz F, Moses N, Carrera E. Normal and abnormal nutrition in children. In Silverberg M, Daum F, eds. Pediatric gastroenterology. New York: Yearbook, 1988:146–233.

Lifshitz F, ed. Nutrition for special needs in infancy—Protein hydrolysates. New York: Marcel Dekker, 1985.

Mandel J, Hamilton B, Hamilton T, et al. A study of microbial contamination of enteral nutrient solutions. Nutr Support Serv 1985; 5:58–60.

Marcuard SP, Stegall KL, Trogdon S. Clearing obstructed feeding tubes. JPEN 1989; 13:81–83.

Meredith J, et al. Visceral protein levels in trauma patients are greater with small peptide diet taken with intact protein diet. J Trauma 1990; 30:825–829.

Moses N. Infant formula and enteral products to meet nutritional needs. In Lifshitz F, ed. Nutrition for special needs in infancy—Protein hydrolysates. New York: Marcel Dekker, 1985:267–296.

Niemier P, Vanderveen T, Morrison J, et al. Gastrointestinal disorders caused by medication and electrolyte solution osmolality during enteral nutrition. JPEN 1983; 7:387–389.

Orvieto A, Kirsch J, Goldberger J. Evaluation of enteral delivery systems. Nutr Support Serv 1983; 3:44–49.

Paine JS. Practical aspects of nasogastric feeding in pediatric patients from a ward nursing perspective. Nutr Support Serv 1986; 6:11–14.

Patterson RS, Andrassy RJ. Needle-catheter jejunostomy. Am J Nutr 1983; 83:1325–1326.

Pemberton LB, Lyman B, Covinstey J, et al. An evaluation of a closed enteral feeding system. Nutr Support Serv 1985; 5:36–42.

Picco C, Baranoski S, Polyak E. Skin care and the gastrostomy tube site. Nutr Support Serv 1985; 5:49–50.

Ponsky JL, Gauderer MWL, Stellato TA. Percutaneous endoscopic gastrostomy. Review of 150 cases. Arch Surg 1983; 118:913–914.

Rombeau JL, Caldwell MD. Enteral and tube feeding. Philadelphia: W.B. Saunders, 1984.

Sacks BA, Glotzer DJ. Percutaneous reestablishment of feeding gastrostomies. Surgery 1979; 85:575–576.

Starkey JF, Jefferson PA, Kirby DF. Taking care of percutaneous endoscopic gastrostomy. Am J Nutr 1988; 88:42–46.

Torosian MH, Rombeau JL. Feeding by tube enterostomy. Surg Gynecol Obstet 1980; 150:918–924.

Walker A, Hendrick S. Manual of pediatric nutrition. Enteral nutrition: Support of the pediatric patient. Philadelphia: W.B. Saunders, 1985:63–68.

Wasiljew BK, Ujiki GT, Beal JM. Feeding gastrostomy: Complications and mortality. Am J Surg 1982; 143:194–195.

Wilson MF, Haynes-Johnson V. Cranberry juice or water? A comparison of feeding tube irrigants. Nutr Support Serv 1987; 7:23–24.

Wilson SE. Pediatric enteral feedings. In Grand RJ, Sutphen JL, Dietz WH, Butterworth S, eds. Pediatric nutrition. Theory and practice. Boston: Butterworth, 1987:771–786.

Wright B, Robinson L. Enteral feeding tubes as drug delivery systems. Nutr Support Serv 1986; 6:33–48.

28

Total Parenteral Nutrition

Sammy, a 3-year-old boy, had a neuroblastoma, a tumor of the adrenal glands. A year ago he underwent surgery to have it removed, but the tumor recurred. The cancer did not respond to chemotherapy and radiation therapy so the doctors planned to give him a huge radiation dose to eliminate the tumor. This would also destroy his bone marrow. Therefore, he needed a bone-marrow transplant to survive. Furthermore, the radiation treatment would injure the lining of his entire gastrointestinal tract. He wouldn't be able to eat or absorb food because of ulcers in his mouth and damage to his intestines. Thus, Sammy would need intravenous nutrition.

Sammy would have to be in a special bone-marrow transplantation unit for 1 to 2 months, requiring strict protective isolation while recovering from the severe irradiation. The newly transplanted bone marrow would begin functioning to give him new sources of red and white blood cells to protect him against infections. Additionally, the total parenteral nutrition (TPN) would provide him with all of his nutrition while his intestines recovered. These treatments were expected to cure Sammy of his neuroblastoma.

HISTORY OF INTRAVENOUS NUTRITION

Intravenous nutrition as it is known today has been used since the late 1960s. However, the concept on which this treatment is based is not new. Long ago, when it was suspected that ingested food was absorbed from the intestine into the bloodstream, physicians reasoned that intravenous administration of nutrients would prevent starvation of patients who could not eat. In the late 1600s, initial attempts to feed by vein were made by infusion of substances such as wine, honey, milk, and oils, with disastrous results (Rhoads, Dudrick & Vars 1986).

One of the earliest reports of successful intravenous nutrition in children was published by Helfrick and Abelson in 1944. A 5-month-old male with severe malnutrition received alternate infusions by peripheral vein of a mixture of casein hydrolysate as a protein source and an olive oil–lecithin homogenate as a fat source. This regimen, which delivered 130 calories per kilogram per day, was given for 5 days. By the end of this period, "the fat pads of the cheek had returned, the ribs were less prominent, and the general nutritional status of the body was much improved." However, the use of a central venous catheter inserted into the large blood vessel of the heart (vena cava) (Rhoads, Dudrick & Vars 1986) is the event that made long-term administration of concentrated nutrient infusates possible. The high blood flow of the central vein allowed immediate dilution of the highly concentrated solutions, thereby preventing damage to the vein. Central venous administration of glucose, protein hydrolysate, electrolytes, minerals, and vitamins produced normal growth and development in an infant who was born without a small intestine (Wilmore & Dudrick 1968). This dramatic demonstration was the beginning of TPN.

TPN is often referred to as hyperalimentation because of the extra calories given to prevent negative nitrogen balance. TPN can provide the essential nutrients to maintain a positive nitrogen balance and achieve weight stability or weight gain. TPN can also allow normal growth and development in infants and children with complex medical problems. However, intravenous nutrition should be used only when oral diets or enteral feedings are unsuccessful or impossible.

TPN is relatively safe when performed in medical centers where specialized care is available. There, the benefits outweigh potential risks and the common complications of TPN can usually be prevented or rapidly treated. It is common to find most infants in tertiary care neonatal ICUs receiving TPN.

WHO SHOULD GET TPN

The best route for satisfying nutritional requirements for patients with a functional GI tract is through oral nutrition. When oral or enteral feedings become inadequate or impossible, however, intravenous nutrition is indicated. Specific conditions that may require TPN include mechanical obstruction, postoperative illness, short-gut syndrome, fistula, inflammatory and malabsorptive processes, very severe diarrhea, chronic inflammatory bowel disease, or in some patients with renal failure or hepatic dysfunction. TPN may also be indicated when the alimentary tract is partially functional but enteral nutrition is improbable, such as low-birth-weight infants and patients with cancer undergoing chemotherapy or irradiation. TPN can also be of value for restoring the nutritional status of patients in whom the use of the GI tract is avoided for psychologic reasons, as in patients with anorexia nervosa. Finally, there are conditions in which TPN may be considered because oral intake is hazardous owing to a high risk of aspiration pneumonia. These include patients with cerebrovascular accidents, coma, tetanus, laryngeal incompetence, and tracheoesphageal fistulas. However, enteral feedings via gastrostomy or jejunostomy are often successful and should be used whenever possible (see Chapter 27).

NUTRITIONAL ASPECTS OF TPN

A patient requiring TPN usually is suffering from acute or chronic malnutrition and other medical complications. TPN should provide nutrients in amounts sufficient to achieve anabolism (tissue build-up) and to correct the malnutrition. The energy requirements of these patients go beyond the needs for resting metabolism, growth, physical activity, and specific dynamic action of food. TPN provides additional energy to account for the increased energy expenditure of the patient in a particular disease state and to allow for nutritional recovery. The daily recommendations for infants and children receiving intravenous nutrition are listed in Table 28–1. Intravenous nutrition must

Table 28–1. Daily Recommendations for Infants and Children Receiving Intravenous Nutrition.

AGE (yr)	FLUID* (mL/kg)	ENERGY† (kcal/kg)	CARBOHYDRATE‡ (g/kg)	PROTEIN§ (g/kg)	FAT‖ (g/kg)
0–1	125–150	100–120	13	3.0–3.5	4
1–3	100	90–110	10	2.6–3.0	4
3–6	90	75–100	8	2.0	4
7–12	70	60–80	8	2.0	4
Adults	35	35–60	2	1.2	2

*If greater volumes are required to achieve appropriate nutritional support, fluid intakes may gradually be increased in infants by increments of 10 mL/kg/d to total volume of 200 mL/kg/d (Kerner 1983); fluid requirements increase 12 percent for each degree of fever and to replace excessive losses.

†Energy requirements increase as follows: 12 percent for each degree of fever above 37°C; 20–30 percent with major surgery; 40–50 percent with severe sepsis; 40–100 percent with long-term growth failure.

‡Dextrose infusion should not exceed 1 g/kg/hr. In very small babies, or babies who are sick at birth, lower glucose intakes should be given (3.5–5.0 mg/kg/min) to avoid hyperglycemia and osmotic diuresis.

§To promote efficient protein utilization for tissue synthesis, recommend 24 to 40 calories from nonprotein sources for each gram of protein given. If insufficient nonprotein calories are given, protein is used for energy, not anabolism (150 to 250 nonprotein calories: 1 g nitrogen ratio). The protein needs for premature babies are 4 g/kg; for pregnant women 3 g/kg; for renal insufficiency 0.8 g/kg.

‖Fat infusion should not exceed 40 to 50 percent of total calories.

Adapted from Khalidi N, Coran AG, Wesley JR. Guidelines for parenteral nutrition in children. Nutr Support Serv 1984; 4:27–28.

provide fluid, energy, protein, carbohydrate, and fat in accordance with the age and size of the patient. Most traditional methods of delivery of the nutrients is a two-plus-one method, where lipid emulsions are given separately from the dextrose–amino acid mixture. However, three-in-one (total nutrient admixture) parenteral nutrition methods, in which all three solutions are given simultaneously, have been proven to be safe and economical for the nutritional support of infants (Rollins et al 1990).

Carbohydrate Source

Hypertonic glucose solutions have been the major energy source of intravenous nutrition solutions in the United States. A minimum of 100 grams of carbohydrate per day will prevent ketosis and decrease protein catabolism in adults. A proportionately smaller amount will suffice for children. However, glucose must not be the only source of calories in intravenous solutions. Protein and fat sources must be included since intravenous glucose infusions alone or TPN with high glucose concentration may cause fatty infiltration of the liver, increased water retention, and excessive carbon monoxide production. The latter would be particularly detrimental to a ventilator-dependent patient or to one with compromised respiratory function. Initially, more calories than could be provided by glucose alone are needed to spare the protein for tissue synthesis. As the patient improves and gains weight, the amount of nonprotein calories from glucose and fat sources should be adjusted downward.

Protein Source

Several mixtures of crystalline amino acids are available, including special pediatric formulations (Table 28–2). The manufacturers and compositions often change and therefore the reader is referred directly to the product information. The quantities of nitrogen to be given vary in accordance with the needs of the growing child. Ideally, the patient should receive all 20 amino acids necessary to build protein. The indispensable or essential amino acids should be maintained at about equal amounts with the nonessential amino acids to promote tissue build-up in infants, children, and malnourished adults. Amino acid solutions usually contain all the essential amino acids that the body cannot manufacture. However, these solutions do not necessarily provide ideal amino acid composition. Many amino acid solutions are not designed for children and contain both insufficient amounts of some amino acids and excessive amounts of others (Table 28–3). For example, phenylalanine is present at a threefold greater level than that needed by a normal child. This is important since this amino acid could potentially be toxic, as seen in patients with hyperphenylalaninemia. In contrast, other amino acids usually considered nonessential are excluded. In the immature infant, tyrosine, cystine, and taurine are considered essential amino acids. Therefore, pediatric amino acid mixtures are now supplemented with cysteine hydrochloride and may contain tyrosine derivatives (e.g., N-acetyl-tyrosine) (Helms et al 1988). Further research is needed to determine whether these are efficacious in meeting cystine and tyrosine requirements. Taurine has also been added to some amino acid solutions for special cases such as low-birth-weight infants and renal insufficiency. Other nonessential amino acids may be needed to promote tissue build-up in patients and young babies who cannot manufacture these amino acids because of their immaturity or their disease. In some formulations, amino acids are present in unbalanced amounts; that is, they are present in quantities that may differ from the usual amino acid composition found in blood. To date, the consequences of these imbalances have not been determined, although these solutions do induce a positive effect on nitrogen balance and growth. It should also be remembered that for optimal utilization of parenteral amino acids, energy requirements must be simultaneously met by infusion of glucose and fat (see Table 28–1). Without the nonprotein source of energy, protein will be used inefficiently for energy, and anabolism or tissue growth will not occur.

Recent research has proposed that glutamine, a nonessential amino acid, may become temporarily essential in some critically ill patients. Some animal studies have suggested that the addition of glutamine to TPN may enhance skeletal muscle protein synthesis, improve nitrogen retention, and decrease hepatic steatosis (Hammerqvist et al 1989, Grant & Snyder 1990). Other studies have demonstrated no difference in glutamine-enriched TPN as compared with standard TPN (Shulman et al 1990). Further work is needed before additional glutamine is considered.

Fat Source

The intravenous fat emulsions available in the United States are soybean oil and safflower oil emulsion with egg yolk, phospholipids, and glycerol (Table 28–4). Infusions of fat provide a large amount of energy (9 kcal/g fat) and are available in small volumes of isotonic fluid, which can be administered via peripheral veins or admixed to the TPN solution. This contrasts with the irritating hypertonic glucose solutions used for TPN that must be administered through central venous catheters. Fat emulsions prevent and correct the essential fatty acid deficiency that occurs when no fat is given. Low-birth-weight infants or those who are malnourished with depleted fat stores may be especially prone to essential fatty acid deficiency. In addition, L-carnitine, the cofactor needed to shunt fatty acids into the cell mitochondria, must be given to babies receiving fat emulsions. Although blood L-carnitine levels do not fall below normal in adults before 20 to 30 days of unsupplemented TPN solutions, this cofactor is needed and should be given, especially to newborn

Table 28–2. Available Amino Acid Infusates for Intravenous Nutrition.*

PRODUCT NAME (Manufacturer)	PERCENT AMINO ACID	NITROGEN (g/100 mL)	OSMOLALITY (mOsm/L)	HOW SUPPLIED (mL)	COMMENTS
Special Pediatric Formulations†					
Aminosyn PF (Abbott)	7	1.07	586	250	Indicated for low-birth-weight infants; when administered with L-cysteine hydrochloride, results in plasma amino acid patterns similar to breast-fed infants; complete amino acid formula with high concentrations of histidine and taurine; low phenylalanine, methionine, and glycine; low pH; minimizes liver problems associated with TPN.
	10	1.56	834	100	
TrophAmine (Kendall McGaw)	6	0.93	525	500	
Standard Formulations					
Aminosyn (Abbott)	3.5	0.55	357	1000	
	5.0	0.786	500	250, 500, 1000	
	7.0	1.1	700	5000	
	8.5	1.34	850	500, 1000	
	10.0	1.57	1000	500, 1000	
Aminosyn with Electrolytes (Abbott)	3.5	0.55	477	1000	With added electrolytes.
	7.0	1.1	1013	500	With added electrolytes.
	8.5	1.34	1160	500	With added electrolytes.
Freamine III (Kendall McGaw)	8.5	1.3	810	500, 1000	
	10.0	1.53	950	1000	
FreAmine III with Electrolytes (Kendall McGaw)	3.0	0.46	405	1000	With added electrolytes.
Novamine (Baxter)	8.5	1.35	785	500, 1000	
	11.4	1.8	1049	250, 500, 1000	
ProcalAmine (Kendall McGaw)	3.0	0.46	735	1000	Ready-to-use pre-mixed TPN solution with protein and carbohydrate

					(glycerol); 130 nonprotein calories per liter
Travasol (Baxter)	5.5	0.924	575	500	
	8.5	1.42	890	500	
	10.0	1.65	1000	250, 500, 1000	
Travasol with Electrolytes (Baxter)	3.5	0.59	450	500, 1000	With added electrolytes.
	5.5	0.924	850	500	With added electrolytes.
	8.5	1.42	1160	500	With added electrolytes.
VeinAmine (Cutter Medical)	8.0	1.33	950	500	With added electrolytes.
Disease-Specific Formulations					
Amines with Histidine (Baxter)	5.2	0.660	416	400	Three special formulations for renal failure; provides 8 essential amino acids including histidine; use with caution in pediatric patients, especially low-birth-weight patients. The absence of arginine in Amines with Histidine may accentuate the risk of hyperammonemia in infants.
Aminosyn-RF (Abbott)	5.2	0.787	475	300	
RenAmin (Baxter)	6.5	1.0	600	250, 500	
Branchamin (Baxter)	4.0	0.44	316	500	Two special formulations for hepatic failure/hepatic encephalopathy; mixture of essential and nonessential amino acids with a high concentration of branched-chain amino acids (BCAAs): isoleucine, leucine, valine; contraindicated with certain inborn errors of metabolism; use with caution in pediatric patients.
HepatAmine (Kendall McGaw)	8.0	1.2	785	500	
Freamine HBC (Kendall McGaw)	6.9	0.973	670	750	Special formulation for hypermetabolic states, stress, and trauma; provides a mixture of amino acids with high concentrations of BCAAs.

*Not a complete listing of all types of amino acid infusates available for intravenous nutrition.
†Need to add L-cysteine.

Table 28–3. Amino Acid Composition of TPN Solution Compared with the Requirements of a Child.

	AMINO ACID SOLUTION* (mg)	AMINO ACID REQUIREMENTS† (mg)
Essential Amino Acids		
Leucine	1700	750–1000
Phenylalanine	1700	250–500
Lysine	1590	1200–1600
Methionine	1590	400–800
Isoleucine	1315	500–750
Valine	1260	400–600
Threonine	1150	800–1000
Tryptophan	495	60–120
Nonessential Amino Acids		
Alanine	5700	N/A‡
Glycine	5700	N/A‡
Arginine	2850	N/A‡
Proline	1150	N/A‡
Tyrosine	110	N/A‡
Histidine§	1205	N/A‡
Serine	—	N/A‡
Glutamic acid	—	N/A‡
Aspartic acid	—	N/A‡
Asparagine	—	N/A‡
Glutamine	—	N/A‡
Taurine	—	N/A‡
Cysteine	—	N/A‡

*Composition based on Travasol (Baxter Health Care, Inc.) crystalline amino acid infusion.
†From the American Academy of Pediatrics Committee on Nutrition. Special diets for infants with inborn errors of amino acid metabolism. Pediatrics 1976; 57:786.
‡N/A = information not available.
§Histidine is considered an essential amino acid in infants and in patients with renal failure; 16–34 mg/kg.

children and those who have limited nutrient stores. Unlike adults, babies are unable to synthesize carnitine from the dietary amino acids lysine and methionine (Novak et al 1981). Therefore, L-carnitine supplementation during TPN in newborns is recommended (Orzali et al 1983, 1984). In cases of L-carnitine deficiency, fat cannot be utilized by the cells of the body. This cofactor is needed at a dose of 10 milligrams per kilogram per day to prevent deficiency due to limited stores of L-carnitine at birth. Furthermore, 2 grams of L-carnitine is beneficial in sick adults by reducing the amount of acid formation in the blood (lactate and pyruvate) even before L-carnitine levels in the blood are deficient (Gibault et al 1988).

Vitamins and Minerals

Intravenous nutrition solutions must also contain vitamins and minerals (Tables 28–5 to 28–7). These nutrients must be present in sufficient quantities

Table 28–4. Composition of Available Intravenous Fat Emulsions.*

	INTRALIPID (KABI-VITRUM) SOYBEAN		LIPOSYN II (ABBOTT) SAFFLOWER/ SOYBEAN		SOYACAL (ALPHA) SOYBEAN		TRAVAMULSION (BAXTER) SOYBEAN	
Oil (%)	10	20	10	20	10	20	10	20
Fatty acid pattern (% of total)								
Linoleic	54	50	65.8	65.8	49–60		56	56
Oleic	26	26	17.7	17.7	21–26		23	23
Linolenic	8	9	4.2	4.2	6–9		6	6
Caloric content (cal/mL)	1.1	2.0	1.1	2.0	1.1	2.0	1.1	2.0
Osmolality (mOsm/L)	230	330	276	258	315		270	300
Egg yolk								
Phospholipids (%)	1.2		1.2		1.2		1.2	
Glycerol (%)	2.25		2.5		2.2		2.5	
Fat particle size (u)	0.5		0.4		0.83		0.5	
How supplied (mL)	50, 100, 500		50, 100, 200, 500		50, 100, 250, 500		500	

Note: Infants require 10 mg/kg/d of L-carnitine supplementation.
Adults may also need 2 g/d of L-carnitine when fat emulsions are given for long periods of time or sooner if the patient has an infection.

*Not a complete listing of all available intravenous fat emulsions.

Table 28–5. Daily Requirements of Minerals and Electrolytes and Composition of Intravenous Preparations.*

	RECOMMENDED DIETARY ALLOWANCES AND ESTIMATED SAFE AND ADEQUATE INTAKE OF NUTRIENTS			RECOMMENDATIONS FOR PARENTERAL NUTRITION	PREPARATION	
	Infants <1 year	Children 1–10 years	Children >11 years		Type	Concentration
MINERALS						
Calcium, mg	360–540	800	1200	10–60 mg/kg	Calcium gluconate	8.0 mg/mL
(mEq)	(18–27)	(40)	(60)	(0.5–3.0 mEq/kg)		(0.4 mEq/mL)
Phosphorus, mg	240–360	800	1200	15.5–31 mg/kg	Potassium phosphate	93 mg/mL
(mmol)	(7.7–11.6)	(25.8)	(38.7)	(0.5–1.0 mM/kg)		(3 mmol/mL)
Magnesium, mg	50–70	150–250	300–400	6–12 mg/kg	Magnesium sulfate	12.0–48 mg/mL
(mEq)	(4.2–5.8)	(12.5–20.8)	(25–33.3)	(0.5–1.0 mEq/kg)		0.8–4.0 mEq/mL
Electrolytes						
Sodium, mg	115–750	325–1800	900–2700	46–92 mg/kg	Sodium chloride	57.5–92 mg/mL
(mEq)	(5–32.60)	(14.1–78.3)	(39.1–117.4)	(2.0–4.0 mEq/kg)	Sodium acetate	(2.5–4.0 mEq/mL)
						46–92 mg/mL
						(2–4 mEq/mL)
Potassium, mg	350–1275	550–3000	1525–4575	78–156 mg/kg	Potassium acetate	78–156 mg/mL
(mEq)	(9.0–32.7)	(14.1–76.9)	(39.1–117.3)	(2.0–4.0 mEq/kg)		(2–4 mEq/mL)
Chloride, mg	275–1200	500–2775	1400–4200	—	Potassium chloride	71 mg/mL
(mEq)	(7.7–33.8)	(14.1–78.2)	(39.4–118.3)			(2 mEq/mL)

*Not a complete listing of all the types of additives commercially available.

Adapted from the Food and Nutrition Board, National Research Council. Recommended dietary allowances. 9th ed. Washington, D.C.: National Academy of Sciences 1980; and Khalidi N, Coran AG, Wesley JR. Guidelines for parenteral nutrition in children. Nutr Support Serv 1984; 4:27–28.

Table 28–6. Daily Intravenous Requirements for Trace Metals for Infants and Children and Commercial Formulations for Intravenous Use.*

	DAILY INTRAVENOUS REQUIREMENTS			TYPE OF SALT	FORMULATION'S‖ CONCENTRATION (mg/mL)	
TRACE METAL	Preterm Infants (μg/kg)	Term Infants (μg/kg)	Children (μg/kg) [maximum μg/d]		Single Item	Multiple
Zinc	400	250 (<3 mo) 100 (>3 mo)	50 [5000]	Chloride; sulfate	1.0, 4.0, 5.0	1.0–5.0
Copper†	20	20	20 [300]	Chloride; sulfate	0.4	0.1–1.0
Chromium‡	0.20	0.20	0.20 [5.0]	Chloride	0.004	0.001–0.01
Manganese†	1.0	1.0	1.0 [50]	Chloride; sulfate	0.1	0.025–0.5
Selenium‡	2.0	2.0	2.0 [30]	Selenione acid	0.04	0
Iron	NK§	NK§	NA‖	NA§	—	0
Molybdenum‡	0.25	0.25	0.25 [5.0]	Ammonium molybdate	0.025	0
Iodide	1.0	1.0	1.0 [1.0]			

*When intravenous nutrition only partially provides infants nutrition or is limited to <4 weeks, only zinc is necessary. Otherwise, complete supplementation of trace elements is recommended. Not a complete listing of all types of additives commercially available.
†Omit in patients with obstructive jaundice.
‡Omit in patients with renal dysfunction.
§Not known.
‖Iron dextran preparations are frequently used for TPN, usually for the treatment of iron deficiency.
NA Information not available.

Adapted from Greene HL, Hambidge KM, Schanler R, Tsang RC. Guidelines for the use of vitamins, trace elements, calcium, magnesium, and phosphorus in infants and children receiving total parenteral nutrition: Report of the Subcommittee on Pediatric Parenteral Nutrient Requirements from the Committee on Clinical Practice Issues of the American Society for Clinical Nutrition. Am J Clin Nutr 1988; 48:1324–1342.

Table 28–7. Daily Requirements for Vitamins and the Nutritional Composition of Recommended Intravenous Multivitamin Preparations.

	RECOMMENDED DAILY DIETARY ALLOWANCES AND ESTIMATED SAFE AND ADEQUATE INTAKES OF NUTRIENTS			RECOMMENDED MULTIVITAMIN FOR IV USE (mg/kg/d)	
VITAMINS	**Infants <1 year**	**Children 1–10 years**	**Children >11 years**	**Preterm Infants**	**Infants and Children**
A (IU)	1332–1400	1332–2331	2664–3330	0.5	1.0
D (IU)	400	400	400	160*	400*
E (IU)	4.5–6.0	7.5–10.5	12–15	2.8	7
K (μg)	10–20	15–60	50–100	80	200
C (mg)	35	45	50–60	25	80
Thiamin (mg)	0.3–0.5	0.7–1.2	1.1–1.4	0.35	1.2
Riboflavin (mg)	0.4–0.6	0.8–1.4	1.3–1.7	0.15	1.4
Niacin (mg)	6–8	9–16	14–18	6.8	17
B_6 (mg)	0.3–0.6	0.9–1.6	1.8–2.0	0.18	1.0
Folacin (μg)	30–45	100–300	400	56	140
B_{12} (μg)	0.5–1.5	2.0–3.0	3.6	0.3	1.01.0
Biotin (μg)	35–50	65–120	100–200	6	20
Pantothenic acid (mg)	2–3	3–5	4–7	2	5

Adapted from the Food and Nutrition Board, National Research Council. Recommended dietary allowances. 9th ed. Washington, D.C.: National Academy of Sciences, 1980; Multivitamin preparations for parenteral use. A statement by the Nutrition Advisory Group. JPEN 1979; 3:258–262; and Greene HL, Hambidge KM, Schanler R, Tsang RC. Guidelines for the use of vitamins, trace elements, calcium, magnesium, and phosphorus in infants and children receiving total parenteral nutrition: Report of the Subcommittee on Pediatric Parenteral Nutrient Requirements from the Committee on Clinical Practice Issues of the American Society for Clinical Nutrition. Am J Clin Nutr 1988; 48:1324–1342.

*Units per day per patient.

to reverse prior deficiencies as well as to meet the increased metabolic demands associated with the disease, to allow tissue growth, and to compensate for excessive urinary losses, particularly of water-soluble vitamins.

Notice that most major minerals and trace elements in the commercial formulation provide sufficient quantities to avoid deficiencies (see Table 28–5). However, there are some inadequacies that may be of importance (Hack, Merritt & Cheng 1988). For example, iron is not contained in the intravenous nutrition solutions and it is not routinely administered. Iron deficits could ensue if TPN is given for prolonged periods and/or if there are ongoing losses. In babies, the average loss of iron is up to 2 milligrams per kilogram per day, and in adults it is more than 1 milligram per kilogram per day (Fairbanks & Besitler 1988). Thus, it may take up to 6 months to deplete the stores of this element. However, increased iron losses are usually ongoing in patients who are receiving TPN, who get frequent, repeated blood drawings for monitoring that could lead to more rapid iron loss. Also, the increased growth and weight gain that occurs with recovery from malnutrition increases the demand for iron and other minerals. The use of intravenous iron is a controversial issue, and further studies are needed to evaluate its use in children and infants.

Calcium and phosphorus requirements for intravenous fluids can often only be met when given through a central vein. These minerals might precipitate in TPN if present in high concentrations. If fluid restriction is warranted, the child may not be able to be given all the necessary calcium and phosphorus (Greene et al 1988). In premature infants or newborn babies who need intravenous nutrition the concentration of calcium and phosphorus may be increased to 600 milligrams per liter and 450 milligrams per liter, respectively (see Chapter 11).

Other essential trace elements such as selenium and molybdenum are not routinely included in intravenous nutrition solutions since their roles in body functioning have not been clearly defined. Selenium deficiency has been documented to be a problem in long-term TPN and thus it should be supplemented. Molybdenum has been found to be deficient in a patient receiving TPN for 1 year (Abumrad et al 1981). This deficiency caused headaches, night blindness, nausea, vomiting, disorientation, and coma, and when molybdenum was supplemented symptoms improved. However, no studies on the requirements and the possible toxic effects of this element have been carried out. Therefore, we do not recommend molybdenum supplementation to TPN for general use.

On the other hand, the presence of excess trace elements such as aluminum could also cause trouble in TPN administration. Although this mineral is not added to intravenous nutrition solutions and is not mentioned in any table of contents of these formulations, it is a contaminant that was shown to be an important factor in the development of metabolic bone disease, neurologic symptoms, and abnormal blood formation in patients on TPN treatment for 6 months or longer (Klein et al 1982, 1984). Aluminum toxicity in infants receiving intravenous nutrition has also been recognized (Koo & Kaplan 1988). Aluminum in TPN solutions may be highly toxic because it bypasses the major protective barrier of aluminum absorption—the GI tract. Calcium gluconate for intravenous use is heavily contaminated with aluminum and accounts for 90 percent of the aluminum content in intravenous solutions. The aluminum concentration of the TPN solutions should be below 11 micrograms per liter to avoid toxicity, but most solutions do not meet this standard.

Given the recommended dose of pediatric multivitamin preparation for intravenous use, most vitamin needs are met (see Table 28–7). However, it should be mentioned that vitamin needs and requirements are primarily based on oral nutrition studies (Greene et al 1986). Requirements for intravenous nutrition might not be the same. For example, riboflavin blood levels in babies receiving TPN increase over 100-fold with the current recommended dose of this vitamin (Moore et al 1986). In contrast, the addition of vitamins to the TPN solutions, which contain fat emulsions, results in insufficient levels of vitamin A but not vitamins D and E. In addition, losses of vitamins, such as retinol, into the TPN bag and tubing may cause vitamin deficiencies. Alternative methods of delivery may need consideration. Biotin requirements are also greater than those provided by the standard multivitamin preparation for IV use, and biotin deficiency has been reported in patients on long-term TPN. Folacin requirements are met for children under 10 years of age, but additional supplementation should be added for adolescents as their needs are increased up to 200 micrograms per day. Administration of parenteral vitamins, especially the water-soluble type, are often given in excess of established dietary recommendations. This increased intake is provided to overcome the potential higher losses through the kidney with intravenous nutrition compared with oral feedings. However, care must be taken in giving parenteral doses of water-soluble vitamins to infants and children with compromised renal function. Toxicity of these nutrients, although rare, may occur in sick or very small babies. Therefore, further studies are needed to determine optimal requirements of vitamins with TPN.

The total volume of TPN administered is also very important (see Table 28–1). Many factors influence fluid requirements during intravenous nutrition. Metabolic water formed by the conversion of protein, carbohydrate, and fat must be considered when calculating fluid balance. Care must be taken to avoid excessive fluid and electrolytes in patients who are very young, critically ill, or in kidney or liver failure. However, sufficient water must be provided to allow for the metabolic utilization of all the energy that is being administered and to prevent dehydration and/or other problems.

An example of the intravenous nutrition solutions required by a 2-year-old patient who weighs 10 kilograms is shown below. This patient's need for water and all major nutrients can easily be met by using standard formulations available for intravenous nutrition therapy as shown below.

	DAILY REQUIREMENTS	SOLUTIONS TO BE USED TO MEET REQUIREMENTS			FINAL TPN COMPOSITION
		Type	Concentration	Amount	
Fluid	1000 mL	—	—	1100 mL	1000 mL
Calories	900–1100 kcal	—	—	—	1004 kcal
Dextrose	100 ≤240 g	Dextrose	40%	500 mL	200 g
Protein	26–30 g	Amino acid	5.5%	500 mL	27.5 g
Fat	≤40 g	Fat emulsion	10%	100 mL	10.0 g
Vitamins		MVI			
Minerals		MTE			

Notice that all the above considerations for TPN are appropriate for a child weighing 10 kg who starts this therapy in a good nutritional state (Dempsey et al 1987). However, this patient is severely malnourished. He has the weight of a 1-year-old child and may have multiple nutrient deficits that have not been addressed by this TPN formulation. Therefore, the TPN for this child should be modified and adjusted as he begins to gain weight, and treatment for previous nutritional deficiencies must be given for full nutritional recovery. The calories and nutrients provided by the TPN, which induce growth, enhance the need for some of the minerals and vitamins; consequently, the patient may require higher quantities than those provided by the standard intravenous nutrition formulations. Also, other conditions may increase the specific needs for some nutrients; for example, in burn patients the need for copper, zinc, and manganese are greatly exaggerated.

TECHNIQUES OF INTRAVENOUS NUTRITION THERAPY

Intravenous Nutrition by Central Vein Infusion

TPN consists of infusing a concentrated nutrient solution through a catheter at a constant rate into a large vessel with a rapid blood flow (Fig. 28–1). There are at least eight sites that can be used for catheter placement: the large veins in the neck area (the two external jugulars and the two internal jugulars), the veins in the chest area (the two subclavian veins), and the large veins leading from the legs (the two femoral veins). In infants, TPN is usually accomplished by placing an in-dwelling venous catheter through either the internal or ex-

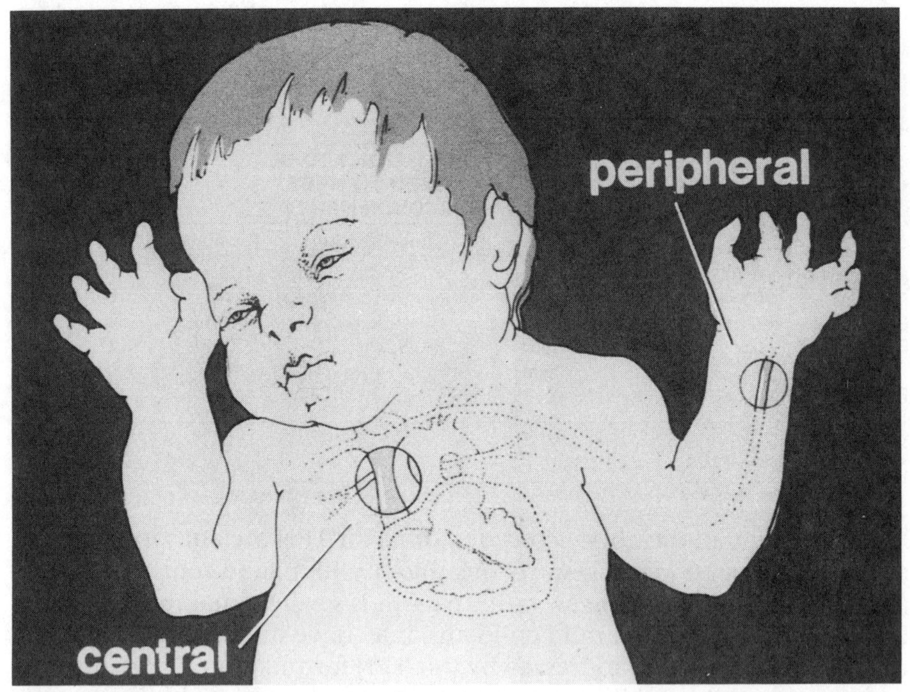

Figure 28–1. Intravenous nutrition by central or peripheral vein infusion. (Used with permission of Home Nutritional Service, Parsippany, NJ.)

ternal jugular vein, inserting it until the distal tip of the catheter is in the superior vena cava just above the right atrium of the heart (Fig. 28–2). In older children and adolescents, the catheter can be placed directly through the subclavian vein into the superior vena cava. With either route of placement, the distal portion of the catheter is usually tunneled under the skin to exit either through the scalp or the chest. The channeling of the catheter to a point distant from the cut-down site protects the catheter from the infants' wandering hands, makes maintenance and care of the catheter site easier, and may diminish infection rates.

There are several theoretical disadvantages to placing catheters in the groin area. The primary one is that introduction of the catheter through a cutdown in the groin area increases the risk of infection. Nonetheless, it appears that such catheters, if tunneled subcutaneously to an exit site on the abdominal wall or the thigh, represent no greater risk with respect to infection than the usual superior vena cava catheters. Catheter exit sites adjacent to ileostomies, colostomies, or jejunostomies have a potentially greater risk of becoming infected from stool cross-contamination. However, meticulous attention

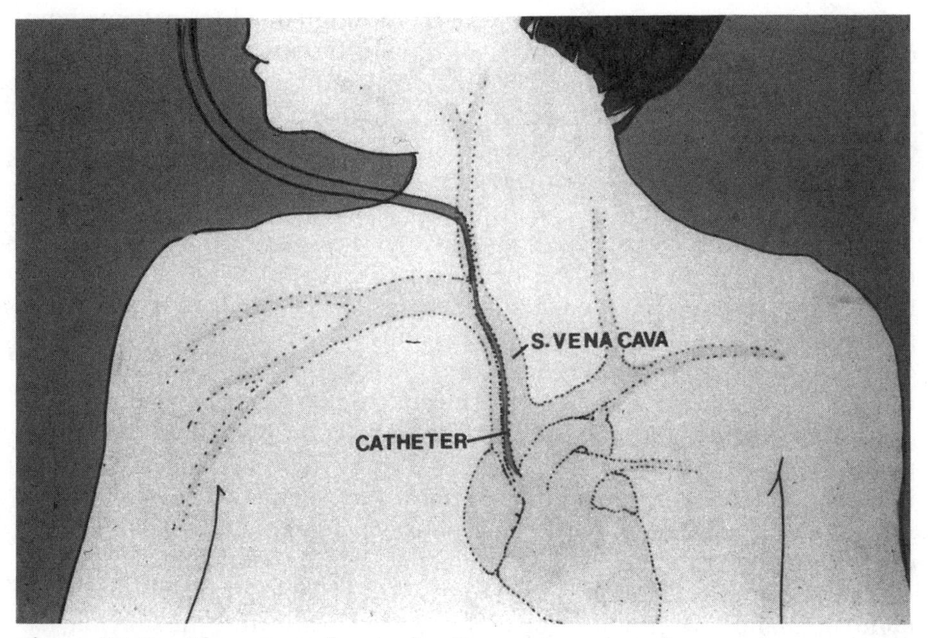

Figure 28–2. Placement of an in-dwelling catheter into the superior vena cava. (Used with permission of Home Nutritional Service, Parsippany, NJ.)

to hand-washing in between caring for the ostomy and the catheter may materially reduce the risk. Placement of the catheter also depends, in part, on cosmetic appearance. Teenagers, especially, may object to catheter placement in the jugular or subclavian veins because the exit site on the chest wall is easily seen and may impose limitations on the type of clothing that can be worn.

Silastic, polyethylene, and hydrophilic rather than polyvinyl catheters are preferable and are generally used. The latter catheters have a tendency to become very rigid once they have been in place for even a short period of time and a fibrin sheath often develops around the catheter inside the vein. The other types of catheters remain soft and flexible for many years. Double- and triple-lumen catheters are beneficial when patients require various simultaneous infusions such as TPN, antibiotics, chemotherapy, and blood products, or frequent blood drawing. However, each additional lumen increases the risk of complications, especially infection, and should be used only when needed for long-term use.

The most commonly known catheters, the Broviac and the Hickman, have been available for many years. The Hickman catheter, having the larger internal diameter and the thickest wall, is recommended for patients who may require blood products in addition to intravenous nutrition, and who may require frequent blood samples. However, because of its long length and large bore size, it cannot be used in young children. An infant-size Broviac catheter is available that is satisfactory for placement in patients less than 1 year of age; the standard Broviac catheter is recommended for use in children after the first year of life.

There are other central venous access devices—ports—that are inserted entirely beneath the skin in a subcutaneous pocket and are usually threaded into the subclavian vein. The major advantage of a port is its lack of external parts; thus, it is very useful for long-term infusion, particularly at home (see Chapter 29). However, these devices require more meticulous and complicated skin preparation, special noncoring needles pre-bent at a 90-degree angle, and puncture of the skin to access the catheter or infuse any solution. A port may be preferable for some patients because it allows increased freedom, is cosmetically preferable, and may decrease the potential for complications such as catheter breakage or site infections. The diaphragms of these ports can withstand approximately 2000 punctures without problems developing at the puncture site. Multiple lumen ports are available for patients who require simultaneous infusions. However, the need to puncture the skin may be undesirable to some patients.

All TPN should be infused with a pump to ensure the patient's safety during the administration of the solution. Infusion pumps using ready-to-use cassettes are the safest, most-accurate method. Thus, in smaller children or in those who cannot afford extra fluid or errors, a pump that utilizes a cassette and has a greater degree of accuracy is preferable. Children older than 10 years may use intravenous infusion pumps that do not involve cassettes. These pumps, however, require care and monitoring, may have a 6 to 10 percent error rate, and often extra solution is infused.

Intravenous Nutrition by Peripheral Vein Infusion

Intravenous nutrition by peripheral vein infusion is also known by the term peripheral parenteral nutrition (PPN) (see Fig. 28–1). Since intravenous fat emulsions were introduced in 1977, PPN has become an increasingly popular method of nutritional support because of its apparent simplicity and safety (Blackburn et al 1973). PPN may help with maintenance and/or restoration of nutritional status, thereby reducing morbidity and mortality (Mullen et al 1980).

Healthy infants and children (excluding premature infants) can tolerate 5 to 7 days of fasting without incurring significant nutritional deficits, provided they are not hypermetabolic and are given hydration with intravenous solutions containing 5 to 10 percent glucose (Seashore & Hoffman 1983). Since it is easier to maintain lean body mass than to restore it, every effort should be made to identify those children who will be without food intake for more than 5 to 7 days and begin PPN as soon as possible. There may also be some children in whom a few days of PPN is indicated during transition to enteral feedings or TPN. These exceptions, however, should be infrequent if careful thought is given to patient selection. Inevitably, there will be errors of judgment and some children will resume oral feedings sooner than expected.

The major problem of PPN is that it often provides insufficient nutrition (Seashore & Hoffman 1983). PPN can provide the total nutritional requirements of patients only if fluid intake is 25 to 50 percent higher than the usual maintenance volumes and if fat emulsion is included at appropriate doses. Under ordinary circumstances in babies, when the fluid intake is limited to the usual total volume of fluid (150 mL/kg/d) and the intravenous lipid intake is limited to ordinary amounts (3 g/kg/d), the maximum energy intake that can be delivered via peripheral vein is approximately 80 calories per kilogram per day. Obviously, this is less than what can be achieved with conventional TPN (usually more than 100 kcal/kg/d). While PPN treatment clearly slows the rate of nitrogen loss, the patients may remain in negative nitrogen balance despite this type of nutrition. Even the staunchest advocates of PPN agree that it is not appropriate for long periods, and that in order to achieve nitrogen equilibrium the total protein and energy requirements of the patient must be provided at all times. Hypocaloric PPN provides no clinical advantage over glucose alone. However, the difference in cost is striking: 1 liter of 5 percent glucose usually costs 30 times less than 1 liter of intravenous nutrition.

Despite PPN's inability to deliver many calories there are a number of patients for whom this route of delivery may suffice. The efficacy of such a regimen in low-birth-weight infants was demonstrated in a controlled study (Anderson et al 1979). Infants on PPN should receive progressively increasing amounts of glucose, amino acids, and lipids (see Chapter 11). Once the maximum levels are achieved they should be maintained for the duration of the treatment, although these levels must be recalculated and the amounts increased as body weight increases. Even when sufficient PPN is ordered to cover all the needs, the child may actually receive less. Difficulties maintaining high flow rates through small, fragile veins, infiltrated IVs that are not replaced promptly, and interruptions of the flow of nutrients to administer medications are all very real problems in infants and children. When oral feedings are initiated the PPN should be progressively and proportionately reduced in relation to the increase in oral caloric intake.

The standard intravenous solutions used for PPN usually provide appropriate quantities of electrolytes, magnesium, phosphorus, trace minerals, and vitamins, and are similar to TPN solutions. However, the amount of calcium that can be given by peripheral-vein infusion is usually less than would be necessary for positive calcium balance, but this has not been a problem since PPN is not usually given for long periods.

Choice of Peripheral versus Central Vein Intravenous Nutrition

The idea that PPN is easier and less time-consuming than successful TPN is fallacious. The supervision required for successful PPN certainly is equal to, and may even be greater than, that required for successful TPN, because a single PPN site rarely lasts more than 24 hours. Furthermore, the complications of therapy associated with TPN and PPN are similar. Thus, it seems reasonable to base the choice of delivery route for parenteral nutrition on an individual patient's clinical condition and nutritional needs rather than on the perceived ease or difficulty of a particular technique.

Currently, it is generally agreed that intravenous nutrition, administered either by central vein or by peripheral vein, is indicated for any patient who is unable to tolerate sufficient enteral feedings for a significant period of time. There is less agreement, however, concerning the definition of a "significant period of time." A reasonable guideline is to use intravenous nutrients to prevent depletion of the patient's body stores. For example, the well-nourished patient who must forego enteral feedings for only 2 or 3 days is unlikely to require TPN. On the other hand, small infants as well as patients with preexisting malnutrition are likely to experience significant depletion of their limited nutrient stores with even this short a period of fasting.

PPN regimens almost certainly maintain existing body composition; thus, this route of delivery is a reasonable choice for the normally nourished infant who is not likely to tolerate an adequate enteral regimen within a short period of time, for example, less than 2 weeks. On the other hand, TPN is a more reasonable choice for infants and older children, regardless of initial nutritional status, who will be intolerant of enteral feedings for longer than 2 weeks who require normal growth rather than simple maintenance of existing body composition.

COMPLICATIONS OF INTRAVENOUS NUTRITION

Metabolic Complications

Glucose intolerance is the most common metabolic complication of intravenous nutrition. Two opposite and extreme manifestations of this complication may occur: (1) very high blood glucose levels leading to hyperosmolar nonketotic hyperglycemia owing to an inability to utilize the high concentration of glucose in TPN solutions; and (2) very low blood sugar levels leading to severe hypoglycemia that results from sudden cessation of the concentrated glucose infusion.

Complications relative to amino acid metabolism alterations may occur. For example, hyperchloremic metabolic acidosis occurs due to excessive chloride content in the crystalline amino acid solution. High ammonia levels are observed especially in premature infants and in patients with hepatic disorders who cannot handle the protein load, as is prerenal azotemia, when excessive total dose or rate of protein is given without sufficient fluids. The major concern with respect to the metabolic consequences of currently available amino acid mixtures used for TPN is that none of the solutions result in a completely normal plasma amino acid pattern. Abnormalities in serum amino acids have long been recognized to be associated with mental retardation in patients with various inborn errors of metabolism (e.g., phenylketonuria). Also, there is a concern that some of the currently available amino acid mixtures do not contain appreciable amounts of cystine and tyrosine, which are thought to be essential for newborns. The lack of other amino acids may decrease the efficacy of protein synthesis; work is on-going to determine whether the addition of glutamine to intravenous feedings will make any difference to the patient (Hammerqvist et al 1989, Grant & Snyder 1990, Shulman et al 1990).

Even less well understood are the metabolic abnormalities related to either of the lipid emulsions, which usually induce a difference in fatty acid patterns of serum and tissue lipids. With soybean oil emulsion, the percentage of arachidonic acid decreases, while safflower oil emulsion decreases the percentage of linolenic acid. High cholesterol and high phospholipid blood levels are also common findings in both adult and pediatric patients who receive the soybean oil emulsion. Hyperphospholipidemia may result from accumulation of the egg yolk phospholipid used as the emulsifying agent, but the cholesterol content of the emulsion is not sufficient to explain the hypercholesterolemia. Essential fatty acid metabolism may also be impaired by inadequate essential fatty acid feedings, by vitamin E administration, or by L-carnitine deficiency (Orzali et al 1983, 1984, Gibault et al 1988). Additionally, there are concerns with the use of parenteral lipids in patients with pulmonary disease (Kerner 1983) and/or high bilirubin levels (Thiessen, Jacobsen & Broderson 1972). Fat emulsions have also been thought to induce liver injury, coagulation disturbances, and allergies.

Mineral and vitamin deficiencies are known to occur with TPN. Low serum phosphorus, calcium, and magnesium levels are often found in such patients, although other more unusual deficiencies, such as selenium, chromium, or molybdenum, have also been reported (Abumrad et al 1981). Metabolic bone disease may also be the result of long-term TPN due to hypercalciuria (Lipkin et al 1988) and/or to aluminum overload (Sedman et al 1985).

TPN may result in jaundice owing to elevation of conjugated bilirubin in blood (Hughes et al 1983). The reason is unclear, but many factors have been suggested to have a role in the pathophysiology of this complication. There may be an inflammatory response and liver-cell injury or there may be a failure of bile secretion resembling mechanical bile-duct obstruction rather than a primary liver injury. The damage to the liver cells could be the result of backflow of bile from the bile ducts into the liver, which follows introduction of enteral nutrition. Another complication may be fatty liver, particularly when excess carbohydrate is being administered.

Mechanical Complications

The infusion of concentrated solutions (800–1000 mOsm/kg) may lead to local injury if they infiltrate into the surrounding tissues. Also, they may induce vein inflammation (thrombophlebitis) and clogging (phlebothrombosis). Blockage of great veins may occur, but may not become a clinical problem until they prevent catheterization, cause emboli, or become septic (see below). When these conditions develop, thrombosis can become a major threat to survival. Mechanical complications are less common with PPN than with TPN, but PPN may also cause significant morbidity, particularly if the intravenous site is not changed every 2 days or if the infusate contains high calcium concentrations.

Mechanical malfunction of catheters has posed potential hazards to intravenous nutrition recipients. Air emboli may occur during the process of central venous catheter insertion, when the syringe is removed, or if the intravenous line becomes inadvertently detached from the intravenous catheter. Other complications related to central catheters include malposition, pneumothorax, dislodgment, and leaks.

Septic Complications

Septic complications are frequent because of the deficient immune mechanisms of patients who are recipients of intravenous nutrition. Although intravenous nutrition solutions are able to sustain growth of many pathogens, solution contamination is rare as a cause of sepsis. The frequent cause of sepsis is growth of organisms at the catheter hub and along the course of the catheter resulting from contamination of the sterile closed system. These infections occur less frequently when meticulous attention to aseptic technique occurs and with implementation of procedures and techniques that are aimed at reducing the incidence of sepsis. Utmost care with aseptic techniques and maintenance of a closed system are essential whenever intravenous nutrition by central vein infusion is used.

Other Complications

Allergic reactions may be seen in patients with specific hypersensitivity or allergy to the amino acid preparations or fat emulsion, for example, if the patient is sensitive to egg proteins found in the emulsion. Other idiosyncratic reactions can occur with lipids and for this reason a test dose should be given to determine if a sensitivity exists.

Finally, death resulting from overzealous nutritional support has been reported (Weinsier & Krumdieck 1980). This is of particular importance, as it may occur whenever there is an overzealous refeeding of a malnourished patient. Cachectic patients are relatively well adapted to their calorically deprived state, and thus they are prone to acute metabolic imbalances and other incompatibilities when given TPN. Developmental delays in infants on long-term TPN have also been identified (Allen & Harper 1983) as well as feeding difficulties later on when oral intake is started (Handen et al 1986).

CLINICAL INTERVENTION

Safe, effective, and efficient use of intravenous nutrition can best be accomplished with standardized procedures within each institution. Strict adherence to aseptic techniques is necessary to maintain an acceptable infection rate of less than 1 percent. The central venous catheter used for TPN should always be inserted under sterile conditions in an operating or treatment room—not at the patient's bedside. In addition, to reduce the risk of infections a central catheter that has been used for other infusions without strict adherence to aseptic technique should not be used for TPN. The TPN administration system should always be a closed system, used only for TPN. Therefore, the TPN system and catheter should not be used for central venous pressure readings, medication administration, piggyback of additional solution, withdrawing blood, or flushing. If the TPN catheter is used for other purposes in an emergency situation, the catheter should be changed before TPN is resumed.

After catheter insertion, its placement must be confirmed by x-ray study or fluoroscopy before the TPN is initiated. TPN solution should be administered at a maximum of one third the desired rate and volume for the first 24 hours. If no complications ensue, it can be increased to two thirds the optimal rate and volume for the following 24 hours. Thereafter a full rate and volume can be given unless the patient develops metabolic problems. A reverse tapering schedule occurs when discontinuing TPN; it is decreased by one third each day until the patient is able to be weaned off the parenteral nutritional support. It is advisable to use intravenous nutrition equipment that has tubing, pump set, and filter all in one; if this is not available, the system should have as few connectors and junctions as possible. There should *never* be a Y connector or stoplock added to the system. If Y injection sites are part of the tubing and cannot be eliminated, they should never be used.

A sudden unexplained spike in the temperature of the patient can be caused by a contaminated intravenous nutrition solution. The solution should be immediately changed. Cultures should be obtained from the suspect intravenous nutrition solution, with fluid samples obtained both distal and proximal to the filter. Blood cultures should be obtained peripherally and from the catheter. Other causes of sudden unexplained high fever include inflammation, infection, and septic embolus. When a patient has acute sepsis or septic shock the catheter should be immediately pulled, rather than waiting for results of cultures.

If a catheter infection is suspected a physician should evaluate the patient to rule out other causes of fever. If another source of infection cannot be found and catheter infection is suspected, intravenous antibiotics may be tried prior to discontinuing TPN. If a fungal infection such as *Candida* is present and the catheter is suspected of being infected, the catheter should be pulled and intravenous antifungal medications started. Better yet, patients should be carefully observed for symptoms of *Candida* such as thrush or a rash; when these are detected antifungals should be started immediately before it infects the TPN catheter.

The intravenous nutrition solution should always be prepared under aseptic conditions in a pharmacy clean room under a laminar flow hood or class 100 clean room. Similarly, any additions to the intravenous nutrition solution are made under the same safeguards. The intravenous nutrition solution should be prepared daily and then refrigerated. It should be removed from the refrigerator 1 hour before infusing into the patient, and it should never be hung for more than 24 hours. The intravenous nutrition administration set, including pump set and filter, should be changed daily. If an extension tube is used, this should be changed with each dressing change.

The catheter exit site must be meticulously dressed and observed for signs of infection. Sterile dressing changes are performed every 48 to 72 hours, often on Monday, Wednesday, and Friday, and as needed when the dressing becomes soiled or loose. The nurse performing the procedure should wear a mask and sterile gloves and use standard cleansing techniques. If the patient can tolerate it, he or she should also wear a mask or turn his or her head in the opposite direction of the catheter site. Cleaning and changing the dressing on a catheter exit site should be performed efficiently and quickly. It may be necessary to have someone hold the infant's or child's hands as the procedure is being performed.

The connection between the catheter hub and the administration tubing should be visible so it can easily be managed and changed. This connection and all connections should be taped together to prevent accidental loosening or disconnection. Connections that screw together also decrease the chance of loose connections. It is important to keep the tubing away from the reach of the infant or child. If a jugular line is in place, it can be taped behind the ear and a cap placed on the child to hold the tubing in place and keep it out of reach. Subclavian lines may require close-fitting undershirts to keep the catheter and tubing out of reach of grabbing hands. Catheters that are tunneled through subcutaneous tissue may be more secure and stable and more difficult to accidentally pull. In addition to bacterial contamination, a loose connection within the tubing can cause problems such as an air embolus, excessive bleeding, or a clotted catheter.

An infusion pump should always be used to administer intravenous nutrition to provide an accurate, constant, prescribed rate with alarms to notify the health care practitioner of problems within the system. Particular attention should be paid to the quantity of pressure (psi) that a pump delivers prior to sounding an alarm. Some infusion pumps deliver very high pressures, which may be undesirable with infants and children. The infusion rate should be constant and accurate and not fluctuate to compensate for errors. For example, when the infusion is behind schedule, the rate should not be increased to make up the difference. Changes in rate could cause alterations in blood sugar or lead to fluid imbalance. A filter is also used in the system to prevent particles, bacteria, viruses, and air from reaching the patient. A 0.22-micron filter is used on TPN, unless total nutrient admixture is used with the lipids mixed into the TPN, in which case a larger bore 1.2-micron filter, which permits passage of lipids, is used.

A patient suspected of having an air embolus should immediately be placed on the left side, with the head down and the feet up, and a physician immediately contacted. An air embolus can be fatal, but most air emboli are absorbed, and symptoms such as difficulty breathing, shortness of breath, cyanosis, and lightheadedness subside within 20 minutes. An air embolus can also occur when the tubing at the catheter hub is changed. To diminish the chances of this occurring, the patient should be positioned flat in bed and asked to perform the Valsalva maneuver (hold breath and bear down) during the connection change. If a silicone catheter is used, the tubing can be changed easily by clamping the catheter with a smooth edge (never a rough) clamp, and thus preventing air embolus or catheter breakage. The use of a Groshong catheter or port, which has an internal valve that prevents air from entering or blood from exiting, may prevent these complications.

Patients receiving lipids must be monitored for signs and symptoms such as difficulty breathing, fever, flushing, alterations in heart rate, or other allergic reactions. If these occur, the rate of administration should be slowed or discontinued. Lipids are contraindicated in patients with liver disease or lipemia, and are used with caution in patients with active pancreatitis. Before lipids are started, patients should have their serum cholesterol and triglyceride levels measured. The serum should also be checked for lipemia each time lipids are administered. If the blood remains turbid (lipimec) 4 hours after the lipid infusion, administration should be discontinued.

Lipids are more easily administered when mixed into the intravenous solution. This is referred to as total nutrient admixture, or 3-in-1 solution. The

Table 28–8. TPN Worksheet and Nutritional Requirements for Children Ages 3 to 6.

Patient: ____________________ Physician: ____________________

Primary Nurse: ____________________ Nutritionist: ____________________

Diagnosis: ____________________

initial wt ________ (kg) ideal wt ________ (kg) birth date ______

current wt ________ (kg) height ________ (cm)

Date
weight (kg)
Total Volume, mL
hr infusion
rate of infusion
taper rate
sterile water
multivitamins
trace minerals
Dextrose, %
mL
g
kcal CHO
Amino Acids, %
mL
g
g N
kcal PRO
Lipids, %
mL
g
kcal FAT

Nutritional aspects of prescribed TPN/day [estimated needs of patient/kg/day]:
fluid (mL) [90]
kcal/kg [75–110]
CHO/kg (g) [8]
PRO/kg (g) [2]
FAT/kg (g) [2]
Nonprotein kcal
Total kcal
NonPROkcal/g Nitrogen

Percentage total TPN kcal from carbohydrate, protein, fat:
CHO [40–70%]
PRO [8–18%]
FAT [0–35%]

Composition of prescribed TPN/day [estimated parenteral requirements of patient/kg/day]:
Calcium (mEq) [0.5–3.0]
Phosphorus (mM) [0.5–1.0]
Magnesium (mEq) [0.5–1.0]
Sodium (mEq) [2.0–4.0]
Potassium (mEq) [2.0–4.0]
Chloride (mEq) [2.0–4.0]

Other fluid patient is receiving [] oral _____ mL qd, [] IV _____ mL qd, [] enteral _____ mL qd

rate must be calculated so the TPN part of the lipid solution infuses at the same rate as the TPN solution without lipids. If lipids are given separately, they should be given peripherally or through another lumen of the catheter, via an infusion pump, and should not be piggybacked into the TPN.

Careful monitoring of patients will often prevent or diminish complications (Tables 28–8 and 28–9). Freshly double-voided urine is monitored for sugar and acetone at least every 6 hours, around the clock, the entire time a patient receives TPN. If a patient spills 2+ or more sugar, the physician should be notified. Intravenous nutrition, oral or enteral feeding intake, and all output including stool, ostomy, drainage tubes, urine, and enuresis are monitored every 8 hours during TPN administration. The patient should be weighed and the fluid balance be calculated every 24 hours. The schedule for monitoring the TPN patient varies, but a minimum of a weekly lipid clearance test and blood for routine chemistries are needed. Other assessments including measurements of serum and urine minerals should be performed.

Despite the overall efficiency of intravenous nutrition, this procedure is not without problems. The complications that arise from the lack of optimal components in the intravenous nutrition solution culminated in great advances in human nutrition knowledge. Definition of the intravenous nutrition requirements and the availability of new and better products continues to improve and facilitate the use of this method of nutritional rehabilitation. Research in this area will no doubt continue to yield very important informa-

Table 28–9. Monitoring of Patients Receiving TPN.

Daily
Oral and IV intake and output (precise food balance)
Weight
Urine for sugar and acetone every 6 hours
Serum turbidity 4–6 hours after fat emulsion infusion
Serum electrolytes and glucose, BUN, creatinine
Weekly
Lipid clearance test
Hemoglobin, hematocrit, white blood cell count, differential
Serum mineral levels: calcium, magnesium, phosphorus
Serum proteins: total protein, albumin, transferrin (pre-albumin, retinal binding protein)*
Liver function tests: SGOT, LDH, alkaline phosphatase, bilirubin
Biweekly
Height
24-hour urine for urea nitrogen, calcium, creatinine
Serum zinc, copper, with simultaneous 24-hour urine collection for same minerals
Serum trace elements and vitamins
Amino acid levels
Monthly
Anthropometric assessment of arm circumference and tricep skinfold
Serum iron, total iron-binding capacity, ferritin

*More adult nutritional variations are considered.

tion, which will lead to reformulations of available products or to new products, and as in the past some of the abnormalities associated with TPN may no longer occur.

REFERENCES

Abumrad NN, Schneider AJ, Steel D, Rogers LS. Amino acid intolerance during prolonged total parenteral nutrition reversed by molybdate therapy. Am J Clin Nutr 1981; 34:2551–2559.

Allen SS, Harper KL. Developmental delay in infants on long-term TPN. Nutr Supp Serv 1983; 3:42–43.

Anderson TL, Muttart CK, Bieber MA, et al. A controlled trial of glucose versus glucose and amino acids in premature infants. J Pediatr 1979; 94:947–951.

Blackburn GL, Flatt JP, Clowes GHA, et al. Peripheral intravenous feeding with isotonic amino acid solutions. Am J Surg 1973; 125:447–454.

Dempsey DT, Mullen JL, Rombeau JL, et al. Treatment effects of parenteral vitamins in total parenteral nutrition patients. JPEN 1987; 11:229–237.

Fairbanks VF, Besitler E. Iron. In Shils ME, Young VR, eds. Modern nutrition in health and disease. 7th ed. Philadelphia: Lea & Febiger, 1988: 193–226.

Gibault JP, Frey A, Guiraud M, Scirardin H, Bouletreau P, Bach AC. Effects of L-carnitine infusion in intralipid clearance and utilization. Study carried out in septic patients of an intensive care unit. JPEN 1988; 12:29–34.

Grant JP, Snyder BA. Effect of glutamion on total fat content of the liver. ASPEN Jan. 1990 (abstract).

Greene HL, Moore ME, Phillips B, et al. Evaluation of a multiple vitamin preparation for total parenteral nutrition II. Blood levels of Vitamin A, D, and E. Pediatrics 1986; 77:539–547.

Greene HL, Hambidge KM, Schanler R, Tsang RC. Guidelines for the use of vitamins, trace elements, calcium, magnesium, and phosphorus in infants and children receiving total parenteral nutrition: Report of the Subcommittee on Pediatric Parenteral Nutrient Requirements from the Committee on Clinical Practice Issues of the American Society for Clinical Nutrition. Am J Clin Nutr 1988; 48:1324–1342.

Hack S, Merritt RJ, Cheng M. Trace element status in pediatric patients receiving parenteral nutrition. JPEN 1988; 12:105.

Hammerqvist F, Wernerman J, Ali R, et al. Addition of glutamine to total parenteral nutrition after elective surgery spares free glutamine in muscle, counteracts the fall in muscle protein synthesis, and improves nitrogen balance. Ann Surg 1989; 209:455–461.

Handen BL, Mandell F, Russo DC. Feeding induction in children who refuse to eat. Am J Dis Child 1986; 140:52–54.

Helfrick FW, Abelson NW. Intravenous feeding of a complete diet in a child: Report of a case. J Pediatr 1944; 25:400–403.

Helms RA, Johnson MR, Christensen ML, Lazar LF. Evaluation of two pediatric amino acid formulations. JPEN 1988; 12:45 (abstract).

Hughes CA, Talbot IC, Ducker DA, Hzrran MJ. Total parenteral nutrition in in-

fancy: Effect on the liver and suggested pathogenesis. Gut 1983; 24:241–248.
Kerner JA. Fat requirements. In Kerner JA, ed. Manual of pediatric parenteral nutrition. New York: John Wiley, 1983: 103.
Klein GL, Alfrey AC, Miller NL, et al. Aluminum loading during total parenteral nutrition. Am J Clin Nutr 1982; 35:1425–1429.
Klein GL, Berquest WE, Ament ME, et al. Hepatic aluminum accumulation in children on total parenteral nutrition. J Pediatr Gastroenterol Nutr 1984; 3:740–743.
Koo WWK, Kaplan LA. Aluminum and bone disorders: With specific reference to aluminum contamination of infant nutrients. J Am Coll Nutr 1988; 7:199–214.
Lipkin EW, Oh SM, Chestnut CH, Chait A. Mineral loss in the parenteral nutrition patient. Am J Clin Nutr 1988; 47:515–523.
Moore MC, Greene HL, Phillips B, et al. Evaluation of a pediatric multiple vitamin preparation for total parenteral nutrition in infants and children. I. Blood levels of water soluble vitamins. Pediatrics 1986; 77:530–538.
Mullen JL, Buzby GP, Matthews DC, et al. Reduction of operative morbidity and mortality by combined preoperative and postoperative nutritional support. Ann Surg 1980; 192:604–613.
Novak M, Monkus EF, Chung D, et al. Carnitine in the perinatal metabolism of lipids. I. Relationship between maternal and fetal plasma levels of carnitine and acylcarnitines. Pediatrics 1981; 67:95–100.
Orzali A, Donzelli F, Enzi G, Rubaltelli FF. Effect of carnitine on lipid metabolism in the newborn. I. Carnitine supplementation during total parenteral nutrition in the first 48 hours of life. Biol Neonate 1983; 43:186–190.
Orzali A, Maetzke G, Donzelli F, Rubaltelli FF. Effect of carnitine on lipid metabolism in the neonate. II. Carnitine addition to lipid infusion during prolonged total parenteral nutrition. J Pediatr 1984; 104:436–440.
Rhoads JE, Dudrick SJ, Vars HM. History of intravenous nutrition. In Rombeau JL, Caldwell MD, eds. Parenteral nutrition. Vol. 2. Philadelphia: W.B. Saunders, 1986: 1–8.
Rollins SJ, Elsberry VA, Pollack KA, et al. Three-in-one parenteral nutrition: A safe and economical method of nutritional supplement for methods. JPEN 1990; 14:290–294.
Seashore JH, Hoffman M. Use and abuse of peripheral parenteral nutrition in children. Nutr Supp Serv 1983; 3:8–13.
Sedman AB, Klein GL, Merritt RJ, et al. Evidence of aluminum loading in infants receiving intravenous therapy. N Engl J Med 1985; 312:1337–1343.
Shulman RJ, Burrin DC, Reeds PJ, et al. Effect of glutamine and glutamic acid on small intestinal growth and differentiation in the newborn miniature pig. ASPEN Jan. 1990, abstract.
Thiessen H, Jacobsen J, Broderson R. Displacement of albumin-bound bilirubin by fatty acids. Acta Paediatr Scand 1972; 61:285–288.
Weinsier RL, Krumdieck CL. Death resulting from overzealous total parenteral nutrition: The refeeding syndrome revisited. Am J Clin Nutr 1980; 34:393–399.
Wilmore DM, Dudrick SJ. Growth and development of an infant receiving all nutrients by vein. JAMA 1968; 203:860–864.

29

Home Nutritional Therapy

Jeffrey, a very active 7-year-old, was swimming with his friends on a hot summer day. The swimming pool looked so nice and clear after his parents installed a new automatic pool cleaner. While they were playing in the pool, the automatic pool cleaner suddenly attached to Jeffrey's rear end . . . they could not do a thing before the vacuum's pressure pulled out his bowel through his rectum! Jeffrey's life was saved, but he was left with almost no small bowel and no colon. He slowly recovered, but since he was left without intestines and thus could not absorb any food, he needed intravenous nutrition. The doctors and nurses taught Jeffrey and his parents the techniques of intravenous nutrition so they could do it at home. This was the only way Jeffrey could go home and resume as close to normal a life as possible (modified from a case study by Tims 1989).

HOME PARENTERAL NUTRITION

Home parenteral nutrition (HPN) for adolescents and adults evolved in the early 1970s and became more commonly used in the 1980s. HPN is now a reality and can be quite successful when all factors that influence its outcome are considered (Fig. 29–1). Home nutritional therapy requires the availability of a nutritional support team involved in the long-term care of the patients (Fig. 29-2). HPN became a reality even for the very young only after small pediatric catheters for infants became available and enough experience was gathered to decrease the fears of complications of intravenous nutrition (Cannon et al 1980).

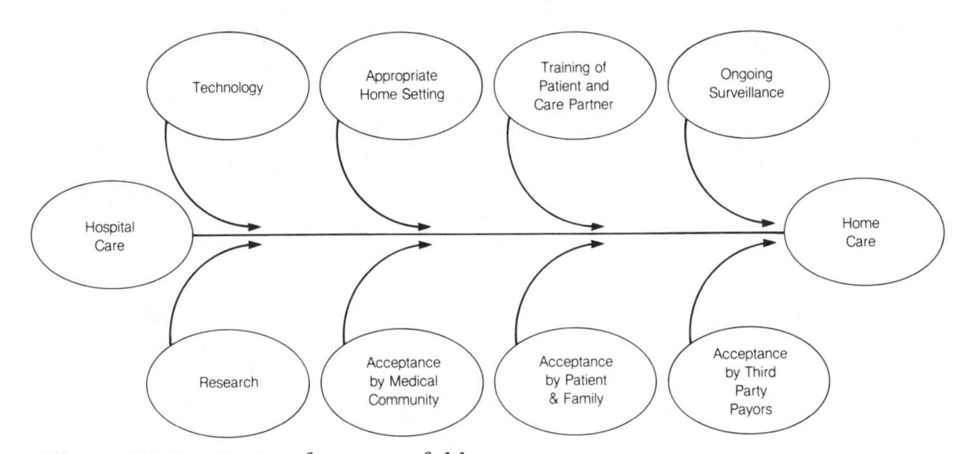

Figure 29–1. Factors for successful home care.

Adapted from Lifshitz JZ. Home parenteral nutrition. In Lifshitz JZ, ed. Home nutritional therapy. St. Louis: C.V. Mosby, 1987:7–16.

HPN is a means by which all or part of the body's nutritional requirements for weight maintenance and growth can be provided intravenously through a central venous catheter for prolonged periods. HPN is now the treatment of choice for chronically ill patients who have long-term intravenous nutrition requirements. This form of high-tech nutrition is the only one available for patients with little hope of restoring or maintaining nutrition by oral or enteral means.

HPN evolved from hospital-based intravenous nutrition treatment when it became apparent that patients needed prolonged hospitalization solely for long-term nutritional support. If these patients were discharged and parenteral nutrition discontinued, their nutritional status would seriously deteriorate and the patient would die. HPN has radically altered attitudes and treatment toward patients with intestinal catastrophes, massive small-bowel resection, or other abnormalities that in the past resulted in death. These patients may now maintain excellent nutrition at home and may resume a nearly normal life.

HPN is an example of how medical care, once restricted to the hospital, can be provided at home effectively, conveniently, and inexpensively. As the expense of health care is close to 12 percent of our gross national product, less expensive means of delivering health care attain even greater significance (Schneider 1986). Specialized support systems have been developed to help

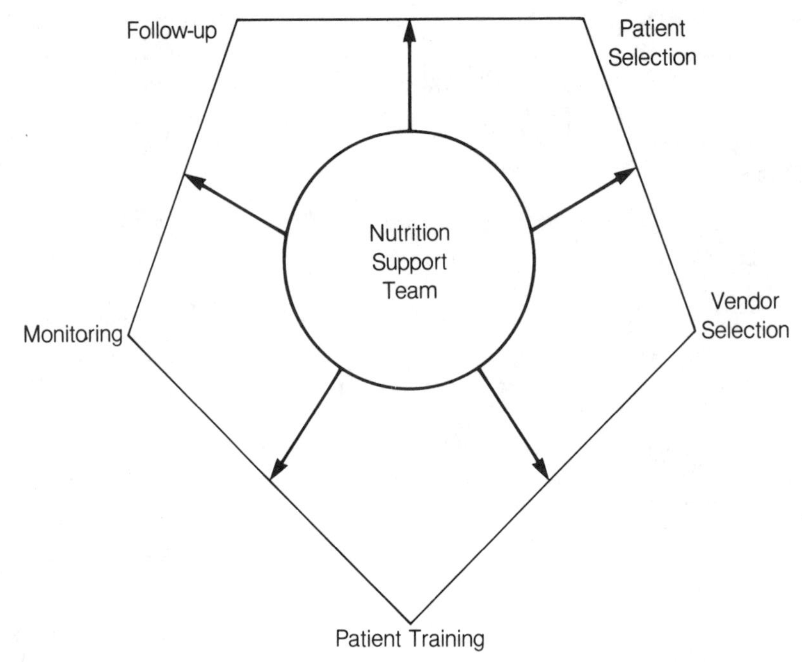

Figure 29–2. Requirements for successful home nutritional therapy.

the patient and the physician ensure the success of HPN. This contributes to the reduced cost of health care and allows the patient to integrate into a life at home as normal as possible.

CANDIDATES FOR HPN

HPN should be considered for any infant, child, or adolescent whose only reason for remaining in the hospital is to receive intravenous nutritional support. HPN is a valuable mode of therapy for children who are unable to tolerate oral diets or whose medical problems prevent use of the GI tract for prolonged periods. Sometimes, these concerns are recognized immediately, as, for example, after the resection of a considerable length of intestine. At other times it may not be evident until after enteral feeding has been attempted without success.

Major indications for HPN include the following conditions: (1) intestinal catastrophes; (2) short-bowel syndrome; (3) chronic malabsorption states; (4) motility disorders; (5) inflammatory bowel disease with complications or failure of ordinary treatment; (6) enterocutaneous or other enteral fistulas; (7) some instances of chronic diarrhea; (8) malignancy (with or without antineoplastic therapy); (9) radiation enteritis; (10) obstruction; (11) graft-versus-host disease after bone-marrow transplantation; (12) rehabilitation after surgery for abdominal congenital anomalies; and (13) AIDS with malnutrition and failure of oral or enteral feedings.

In all these conditions, the major problem is that the digestive tract either in whole or in part is not functional. Thus, the only way to sustain life is through intravenous nutrition, which will be necessary for prolonged periods.

METHOD OF HPN

The techniques, infusion devices, and formulation of parenteral nutrition solutions for HPN are similar to those used for intravenous nutrition in patients in a hospital setting (Broviac & Scribner 1974, Jeejeebhoy et al 1976). These are discussed in detail in Chapter 28 and therefore will not be addressed here. However, the addition of certain trace elements, such as selenium (1.4 mEq) and chromium (0.14–0.20 μg), makes solutions typically used for HPN unique (Nicholas, Meng & Caldwell 1977, Jeejeebhoy et al 1977, Freund, Atamian & Fischer 1979, Lane et al 1982, Howard et al 1983). These elements are not necessary when intravenous nutrition is given for less than 1 month (Fleming et al 1982). Although patients receiving long-term HPN have been shown to become deficient in other trace elements such as nickel, rubidium, and cobalt, no supplementation is provided since their biologic function is unknown.

Since one of the goals for patients on HPN is to assume as normal a life as possible, it seems only appropriate that the patient be disconnected from the infusion system for as long as possible. Thus, most patients who receive HPN are candidates for cyclic parenteral nutrition—that is, nocturnal infusions for 10 to 12 hours (Table 29–1).

However, HPN can also be successful when continuous intravenous nutrition is provided throughout an entire 24-hour period. HPN has proven to be a remarkable technique that has allowed patients to live who, heretofore, would have died or become nutrition cripples (Wretlind 1981). This high-tech nutrition technique will be needed by patients who require intravenous nutrition because of inappropriate intestinal function until bowel transplantation becomes a reality (Starzl et al 1989). The latter is still many years away, and for patients who do not have functional intestines, the indefinite use of parenteral long-term nutrition is the only means presently available to sustain their life.

Table 29–1. Typical Schedule of a Patient Receiving HPN Each Night.

TIME	EVENT
8:00 PM	Remove nutrition solutions from refrigerator
	Make any necessary additions to solution
8:45 PM	Set up the infusion pump
9:00 PM	Start infusion with pump set at 50 mL/hr for 1 hour
10:00 PM	Increase rate to 100 mL/hr for 9 hours
7:00 AM	Decrease infusion to 50 mL/hr for 30 minutes
7:30 AM	Decrease infusion to 25 mL/hr for 30 minutes
8:00 AM	Stop infusion and heparin-lock catheter
	Change dressing if necessary; inspect exit site
	Monitor weight, temperature, intake, and output
8:30 AM	Test urine for sugar and acetone

CLINICAL EXPERIENCE

In 1986 there were approximately 3000 patients being treated with HPN, and over 20,000 had received the benefits of this treatment since its inception (Ament 1987). Almost 30,000 patients are projected to receive HPN in 1991 (Biomedical 1989). One patient who has been treated with home HPN owing to a short bowel syndrome for over 17 years recently gave birth to twins (Lifshitz 1989). Another patient who had small-bowel bypass surgery for obesity treatment 14 years earlier received HPN from the 27th week of her pregnancy when twin gestation was diagnosed. She gained weight and delivered healthy twins of appropriate weight for gestational age (Karamatsu et al 1987).

The longest and the largest clinical experience with HPN in children is from a group at UCLA (Ament 1987). They reviewed their experience with 102 pediatric patients who received HPN for prolonged periods, their youngest patient being 1 month old and the oldest being 17 years. The duration of therapy for the 102 children reported by the UCLA group was 75,000 patient-days of HPN; the average length for each patient was 735 days. They utilized 234 catheters for intravenous nutrition, and the average duration of use was 380 days per catheter. The longest time a single catheter was used was 1962 days!

Patients with short-bowel syndrome comprised the largest group of children the UCLA group treated with HPN. Ninety percent of these patients had congenital problems such as intestinal atresia (being born without part of the intestine) or alterations in the development of the abdomen (omphalocele or gastroschisis). However, many patients were born intact but in the first month of life or later had a subsequent loss of their intestine due to intestinal torsion (volvulus), necrotizing enterocolitis, or trauma (Dorney et al 1985). Unfortunately, a delay in diagnosis was often the cause for infarction of the small intestine, thereby necessitating its surgical removal.

Long-term HPN allowed for the survival of patients with short-bowel syndrome. Eventual adaptation to enteral feedings from HPN was possible for patients who had as little as 11 cm (4 in.) of small bowel if the valve that separates the small intestine from the large intestine (the ileocecal valve) was intact. Survival and adaptation also occurred in patients who had 25 cm (10 in.) of small intestine without the ileocecal valve.

Chronic intestinal pseudo-obstruction syndrome is another indication for long-term HPN (Schuffler et al 1981). This was the problem in 10 percent of the patients treated by the UCLA group (Ament 1987). Twenty percent of the patients treated with long-term HPN by the UCLA group had inflammatory bowel disease (Ostro, Greenberg & Jeejeebhoy 1985). The indications for HPN in these patients were complications of the disease such as short-bowel syndrome, failure to gain weight and grow despite medical therapy, enterocutaneous fistula, and intractable disease with failure to respond to medications.

Other clinical conditions necessitating long-term HPN include severe chronic diarrhea owing to congenital alterations such as hypoplastic villus syndrome, immunodeficiency/graft-versus-host disease following bone-marrow transplantation, cystic fibrosis, and intestinal lymphoangiectasia. In these patients, HPN improved nutritional status, and kept the patients alive, but their primary problem did not necessarily improve. Also, patients with malignant tumors who had complications as a result of radiation therapy required HPN to keep them alive independently of the evolution of their cancer (Ament 1987).

COMPLICATIONS OF HPN

HPN patients have had remarkably few complications related to this treatment despite great fears that this type of long-term feeding could not be accomplished at home. Indeed, the number of complications of HPN patients treated by experienced teams is no worse than when TPN is given in hospital centers (Ament 1987). These patients have had few complications related to therapy, including rehospitalization for infection-related processes, malfunction of the catheter, and fluid and electrolyte imbalances.

In the series at UCLA (Ament 1987), 42 catheters were changed because they became clogged, 9 were broken, and 3 were pulled out by the patient. Sixty of the 102 patients (58 percent) did not have any catheter-related infection; however, there were 97 episodes of confirmed catheter-related infections in 42 patients. Significant abnormalities in fluid and electrolyte balance requiring hospitalization virtually never occurred. Macrocytosis (large red blood cells) developed in three patients, along with lightening of hair and skin color and abnormalities in liver enzyme levels (Vinton, Dahlstrom & Ament 1986). All these patients had abnormally low levels of selenium in blood, and all abnormalities reversed toward normal when selenium was added to the intravenous solution. Clinically apparent biotin deficiency developed in one patient before biotin was added to the intravenous solutions (Kien et al 1981).

Metabolic bone disease manifested by bone pain, spontaneous fractures, hypercalcemia, and intermittent hyperphosphatemia has been a problem with long-term HPN (Shike et al 1980, Klein et al 1980). Aberrations in vitamin D and calcium metabolism, and aluminum overload, have been implicated in the above-mentioned problems (Sedman et al 1985). Cholelithiasis, cholecystitis, and chronic liver disease may also occur in HPN patients. At times, removal of the gallbladder was needed because of recurrent right-upper-quadrant and midepigastric abdominal pain, with or without jaundice and/or vomiting (Ament 1987).

HOME ENTERAL NUTRITION

Home enteral nutrition (HEN) through feeding tubes is based on similar principles and techniques to those used for enteral nutrition in the hospital (McArdle et al 1981) (see Chapter 27). Therefore, it is important to identify patients who, because of their underlying disorders, may be subject to progressive malnutrition and debility. When this is the case and nutritional therapy is needed for prolonged periods, enteral tube feeding at home may sustain or improve proper energy–protein balance and weight in patients with an accessible and functioning GI tract.

Enteral tube feeding at home is not a new concept or practice, but it has been underutilized because its potential benefits have not been appreciated, and/or because of fears regarding insertion of enteral tubes. Also, it has been misdirected because in the past only the terminally ill or the institutionalized patient were committed to such an endeavor. The practice of HEN needs to be expanded so that patients with a variety of disorders can be successfully treated with this technique. Positive nitrogen balance, progressive weight gain, and restoration of lean body tissue can be achieved with HEN while the medical or surgical disease is being corrected or controlled (Newmark et al 1981, Chrysomilides & Kaminski 1981). HEN may also result in improvement in the primary disease. This may occur directly or indirectly from nutritional therapy. Examples of diseases improved by HEN include inborn errors of metabolism and Crohn's disease (Goode et al 1976, Greene et al 1980).

Often, children with failure to thrive due to organic or nonorganic causes are managed by usual means for long periods without appropriate weight gain and growth. The use of HEN may be a rapid and efficient way to reverse the malnutrition and the anorexia of these children. An example of a baby who benefitted from HEN is discussed below.

Seth had a severe congenital heart disease. He was born with a reversal of the large blood vessels that circulate the blood from the heart (transposition of the great vessels). He needed a partial cardiac repair at birth with cardiac surgery, and required heart medications to keep him alive, but he failed to thrive. The doctors wanted him to gain weight so he could receive an operation to complete the repair of the heart defect. How could this be done if he had no strength to eat?

With feedings, Seth would sweat profusely and tire easily. In fact, he could consume only 3 ounces over a 4-hour period of feeding. Therefore, Seth was only able to take 15 to 17 ounces of a 20-calorie-per-ounce infant formula a day. This level of intake (300–340 kcal/d) did not meet his caloric requirements, especially given his increased needs due to the heart condition and great energy expenditure with feeding. At his present weight of 9.9 pounds (4.5 kg), Seth required at least 120 calories per kilogram or 540 calories a day to maintain normal growth. Even when the doctors increased the caloric density of the formula to 27 calories per ounce, he could not take the 20 ounces a day plus additional free water that he needed to be able to grow. This was not unexpected since this sick baby struggled taking just 17 ounces a day!

The addition of modular supplements of carbohydrate or fat to the formula would increase the caloric supply but would result in an unbalanced dietary intake (Table 29–2). For example, adding carbohydrate or fat results in a drop in the proportion of calories derived from protein below the requirements for this child. Also, multiple vitamins and minerals would be deficient even though sufficient calories were attained. In addition, high sugar feedings may lead to more accumulation of fat in the liver, increased water retention, and excessive carbon monoxide production, which could be harmful to a baby with compromised cardiac function. With a high-fat formula, gastric emptying, which is already compromised in patients with heart disease, would be delayed further, not withstanding poor digestibility and absorption of some fat modular supplements in malnourished children. Also, bolus feedings may be detrimental to a patient with insufficient cardiac reserve.

In contrast, continuous infusion of nutrients makes feedings more efficient and easier to induce a positive nitrogen balance (see Chapter 27). This patient, with insufficient cardiac function, needed all the help of continuous feedings to faciliate the intake and assimilation of nutrients to allow him to grow. Therefore, nasogastric tube feedings were recommended as an excellent alternative to oral feedings for this baby. A continuous feeding of regular infant formula (20 kcal/oz) could be administered at a rate of 35 milliliters per hour. With these continuous nasogastric tube feedings all the patients' nutri-

Table 29–2. Various Methods for Nutritional Management of a Baby with Congenital Heart Disease and Failure to Thrive.

	DAILY REQUIREMENTS*	DAILY ORAL FEEDINGS†	ORAL FEEDINGS PLUS CARBOHYDRATE MODULAR SUPPLEMENT‡	ORAL FEEDINGS PLUS FAT MODULAR SUPPLEMENT§	CONTINUOUS TUBE FEEDINGS‖
Fluid	100–150 mL/kg	510 mL (17 oz)	510 mL (17 oz)	494 mL (16.5 oz)	840 mL (28 oz)
Calories	120–150 kcal/kg; 540–675 kcal/d	76 kcal/kg; 340 kcal	102 kcal/kg; 460 kcal/d	127 kcal/kg; 570 kcal/d	124 kcal/kg; 560 kcal/d
Protein	2.2 g/kg; 9.9 g	1.7 g/kg; 7.6 g	1.4 g/kg; 6.2 g/d	1.5 g/kg; 6.6 g/d	2.8 g/kg; 12.6 g/d
Vitamin A (IU)	1399	1062	868	930	1750
Vitamin D (IU)	400	212	174	186	350
Vitamin E (IU)	4.5	10.6	8.7	9.3	17.5
Vitamin K (IU)	12.0	29.2	24.1	25.8	48.1
Thiamin (mg)	0.3	0.27	0.22	0.25	0.44
Riboflavin (mg)	0.4	0.53	0.44	0.47	0.88
Vitamin B_6 (mg)	0.3	0.21	0.17	0.19	0.35
Vitamin B_{12} (mg)	0.5	0.8	0.6	0.7	1.3
Niacin (mg)	6.0	4.2	3.5	3.8	7.0
Folacin (μg)	30	53.1	43.7	46.8	87.5
Vitamin C (mg)	35	27.6	22.7	24.3	45.5
Calcium (mg)	360	234	193	207	385
Phosphorus (mg)	240	160	132	141	263
Magnesium (mg)	50	26.6	21.8	23.4	43.8
Zinc (mg)	3	2.7	2.2	2.3	4.4
Iron (mg)	10	0.5	0.4	0.5	0.9

*Requirements based on a 10-pound (4.5 kg) baby with heart defects and failure to thrive.
†Enfamil 20-calories-per-ounce formula (Mead Johnson Nutritional Division, Evansville, IN 47721).
‡14-ounces Enfamil, 20 calories per ounce plus 3 ounces glucose polymers, which provides an additional 180 calories (Polycose, Ross Laboratories, Columbus, OH 43216).
§15-ounces Enfamil, 20 calories per ounce plus 3 tablespoons Lipomul, which provides an additional 270 calories (UpJohn Company, Kalamazoo, MI 49001).
‖Continuous nasogastric tube feedings with Enfamil 20-calories-per-ounce formula at a rate of 35 milliliters per hour.

tional needs were met, with the exception of iron, which can be given as needed to avoid deficiency.

NUTRITION SUPPORT TEAM

Pediatric patients needing home nutritional therapy usually have multiple problems that require an interdisciplinary expertise to meet their needs. Therefore, a team approach to HPN and HEN generally works best (Fig. 29–3). The team should include a physician coordinator, whose primary responsibility is nutritional care of patients; a nurse; a nutritionist; a pharmacist; a social worker; a home-care nurse and social worker; an infectious disease representative; a consultant psychiatrist; and a consultant surgeon (Lifshitz 1987). It is the responsibility of the nutrition support team to decide on the suitability of patients for HPN or HEN and to manage the care of these patients.

Once a patient is identified as a candidate for HPN or HEN, a meeting

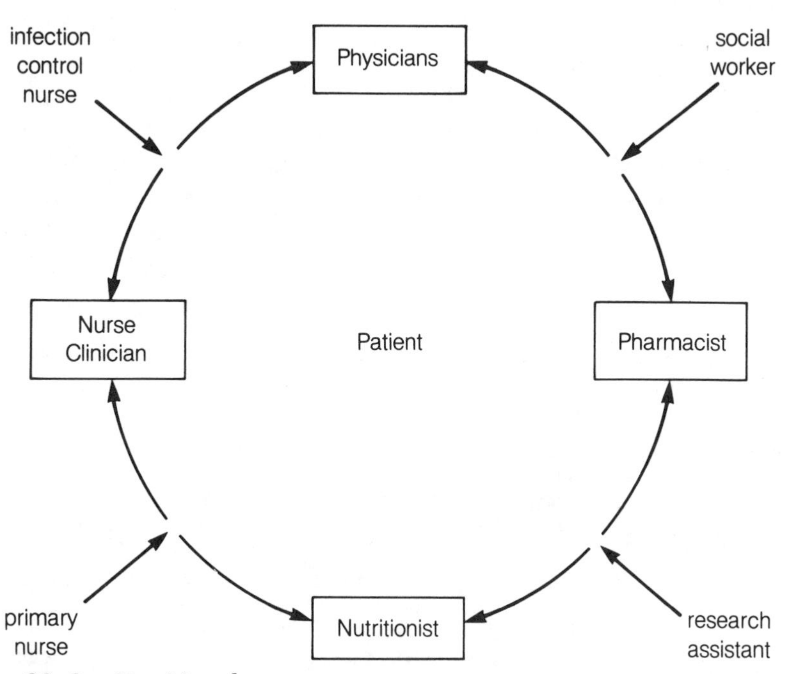

Figure 29–3. Nutritional support team.

Adapted from Lifshitz JZ. Home parenteral nutrition. In Lifshitz JZ, ed. Home nutritional therapy. St. Louis: C.V. Mosby, 1987:7–16.

should be held by the nutrition support team, with the primary care physician and the primary nurse. Medical criteria should include evidence that the patient cannot meet nutritional requirements by oral intake, will require parenteral and/or enteral nutrition beyond the allocated hospital stay, and will benefit from home nutrition support. Special needs of the patients or family are also identified at this meeting, such as the psychosocial status of the family and the needs for home health assistance, home nursing care, psychiatric counseling, and/or medical assistance program to pay for the high cost of HPN or HEN. Appropriate arrangements must be made to fulfill those needs prior to the patient's discharge from the hospital.

A family conference is held to explain the rationale for HPN or HEN, the goals of therapy, the role of each team member, the estimated course and length of therapy, the time commitment, and financial considerations. A primary issue to address is the willingness of the family to provide or assist with home nutritional therapy and to comply thoroughly with all procedures. It is important to address all the questions the family may have (Table 29–3). These cannot be addressed in one session and may require several hours of reassurance to alleviate all the fears and concerns. Often, simple questions denote great fears that need to be answered for a home nutrition therapy to be successful.

For home nutritional therapy to be feasible and effective, the patient must have a competent, supportive caregiver. A stable home situation to support reliable and consistent care is very important. Infants and children require complete parental/caregiver assistance. Older children and adolescents may be capable of providing much of their own care. Under careful supervision, responsible siblings may also assist the patient. It is important for the person assuming the primary care responsibility to have a backup caregiver. Counseling and emotional support may be necessary for the parents to avoid their

Table 29–3. The Ten Most Frequently Asked Questions When Starting HPN or HEN.

1. How long will my child require such care?
2. How many hours per day will it require?
3. How dangerous is it?
4. Can my child bathe or shower with the HPN catheter in place?
5. What do we do if there is a fire in our house or apartment when the child is receiving HPN?
6. What do we do if the power fails?
7. How expensive is it?
8. Who will pay for it?
9. Who will do the HPN or HEN care if I am sick and cannot do it?
10. What if I need to be away from my child for a week and there is no one available to help do the HPN or HEN?

Adapted from Ament M. Parenteral nutrition of the pediatric patient at home. In Lifshitz JZ, ed. Home nutritional therapy. St. Louis: C.V. Mosby, 1987:17–27.

being overwhelmed with the burden of responsibility. Parents often state the need for an occasional vacation from the administration of HPN and HEN. Nurses from HPN and HEN vendors or parents of other HPN or HEN children may be able to serve as backup caregivers so the parents can have a break from the home nutritional therapy routine.

CLINICAL INTERVENTION

Training the patient and family is one of the most important factors in preparing for hospital discharge and HPN or HEN (Lifshitz 1987). The patient and the caregiver must be trainable in all procedures required for successful HPN or HEN (Tables 29–4 and 29–5). Educational status is not the only criterion for determining trainability. It is time-consuming but possible to teach HPN to an adult who can neither read nor write. The patient's and caregiver's motivation, ability to follow directions, and desire to perform all tasks correctly and precisely are the most important considerations.

Teaching the parent and additional members of the household HPN techniques and total independence usually requires 1 to 2 weeks, although the time varies with the level of medical sophistication of the family. Extra days may be necessary for metabolic adjustments and psychologic adaptation, and to allow sufficient practice for the patient and caregiver to feel comfortable with HPN, HEN, or both.

The team nurse coordinates a teaching plan to meet the needs of the fam-

Table 29–4. Teaching Requirements for HPN.

A. General Principles
   1. Disease process
   2. Intravenous nutrition
   3. Aseptic and clean technique
   4. Intravenous catheter
B. Specific Feeding Techniques
   1. Catheter care
   2. Pump operation
   3. Starting, monitoring, and stopping the infusion
   4. Flushing the catheter
   5. Making additions to nutrition solutions
C. Problem-Solving, Monitoring, and Complications
   1. Pump, administration set, filter
   2. Catheter occlusion, kink, position, infection, repair
   3. Hypoglycemia, hyperglycemia, urine testing
   4. Fluid balance, intake and output, weight
   5. Signs and symptoms of infection
   6. When to call nurse and/or physician

Table 29–5. Teaching Requirements for HEN.

A. General Principles
   1. Disease process and why HEN is needed
   2. Formula type and feeding schedule
   3. Clean technique, hand-washing, cleaning utensils
   4. Preparation and storage of formula
      a. Measuring formula and additives
      b. Mixing formula
B. Specific Feeding Techniques
   1. Preparation of each feeding
      a. Setting up and filling feeding set
      b. Checking tube placement and gastric residuals
   2. Operation of pump
   3. Administration of feeding
      a. Patient position
      b. Flushing the tube
      c. Care of tube and equipment
      d. Skin care
C. Problem-Solving, Monitoring, and Complications
   1. Pump, alarms, feeding set
   2. Gastrointestinal symptoms
   3. Clogged tube
   4. Displaced tube, aspiration, peritonitis
   5. Nutritional status
   6. Blood sugar increase or decrease
   7. Fluid balance, intake and output, weight
   8. Assessment of skin at tube site
   9. When to call nurse, nutritionist, and/or physician

Adapted from Mueller KJ. Home tube feeding instruction packet. The American Diabetes Association, 1986.

ily. The goals of the instruction are threefold: (1) to teach the administration of parenteral or enteral nutrition so that it can be performed safely; (2) to educate the family regarding potential complications and appropriate responses; and (3) to facilitate the family and the patient to return to as normal a lifestyle as possible.

Many different types of instruction manuals are available from home nutrition therapy teams and companies. They are written for either patient–family teaching or as procedures and guidelines for health care personnel to use to establish teaching protocols. Each procedure requires written step-by-step instructions that are simple and easy to follow. Repeated demonstrations are the primary teaching methods. The patient and the caregiver practice with all equipment for HPN, and a catheter or port and chest mold should be used until the caregiver is competent enough to practice with the actual patient catheter. Multiple short teaching sessions facilitate instruction and are more easily followed than lengthy detailed sessions. All supplies are to be taken out and prepared for use before each procedure. Every step is to be followed exactly. The procedure manual is used to ensure that a step has not been forgotten. After the nurse has certified the patient and the caregiver competent in all procedures, they should perform the entire HPN or HEN procedure in the hospital without assistance, but with supervision for a few days. The above teaching schedule is ideal for total independence, but is not always possible with the reimbursement environment which promotes short hospital stays.

SELECTION OF VENDOR

Numerous hospital home-care departments or nutritional support services provide all the personnel, support, supplies, and solutions necessary for their HPN or HEN patients (Table 29–6). This requires adequate coordination of services, space, centralized distribution, and billing management to ensure prompt and easy patient services. Under such a system, the patients can see their physicians or other team members when picking up solutions. The advantages of the system vary with each hospital and are generally dependent

Table 29–6. Services Provided by HPN/HEN Vendors.

A. Nursing
   1. Predischarge home and social situation assessment
   2. In-hospital teaching by HPN specialist
   3. Primary nursing with home follow-up visits
   4. Frequent consultation with patient's physician
   5. 24-hour availability with on-call staff
B. Pharmacy
   1. Pre-mixed nutrition solutions
   2. All solutions available
   3. Other therapies available
   4. Specialized mixing facility
C. Operations
   1. All ancillary supplies and pumps available
   2. Non–product specific
   3. One-stop shopping for all supplies
   4. Frequent deliveries by vendor
   5. Home inventory
D. Insurance
   1. Predischarge qualification
   2. Accept Medicare, Medicaid, and private insurance
   3. Seek alternative sources of coverage
   4. Assignment of benefits
   5. Direct billing to carrier
   6. Complete insurance management

Adapted from Lifshitz JZ. Home parenteral nutrition. In Lifshitz JZ, ed. Home nutritional therapy. St. Louis: C.V. Mosby, 1987:7–16.

on the number of personnel dedicated to providing these services. Decreased cost and increased accountability are the major benefits. The disadvantages of hospital-based vendors for HPN or HEN include the need for patients to travel to obtain their solutions and supplies and the need to coordinate home nursing visits.

Most hospitals are not able to provide HPN or HEN services and seek outside vendors to provide these services along with other aspects of home care to their patients (Lifshitz 1987). There are commercial companies that can deliver all necessary materials to patients in need of home nutritional therapy. The equipment comes from a single source and is delivered to patients at predetermined intervals. In addition, the commercial vendors employ nurses who visit the family regularly and can draw blood in the home should the need arise. The disadvantage of this approach is that the home nutrition therapy team transfers direct control to the vendor, and the vendor may have poor quality control and/or subcontract crucial services, such as nursing.

Several factors must be considered when choosing a vendor. The first is the total number of patients and the experience and time commitment of the personnel who will be providing these patient services. To provide a high-quality HPN or HEN program, the personnel involved must be specialists in nutritional support and must devote the majority of their time to this endeavor. It is important to consider vendors with experience in the care of children.

Cost is another crucial consideration. Vendors often misrepresent the high cost of their products and services. Chronically ill children on home nutritional support can quickly consume the entire family's life-time insurance coverage. Vendors should provide the referring physician with written guaranteed charges and be held accountable for maintaining these rates.

REFERENCES

Ament ME. Parenteral nutrition of the pediatric patient at home. In Lifshitz JZ, ed. Home nutritional therapy. St. Louis: C.V. Mosby, 1987:17–25.

Biomedical Business International Home Infusion Therapy Markets. Reprint 2821, Oct. 1989, Maxwell/MacMillan Corporation.

Broviac JW, Scribner BH. Prolonged parenteral nutrition in the home. Surg Gynecol Obstet 1974; 139:24–28.

Cannon RA, Byrne WJ, Ament ME, Gates B, O'Connor M, Fonkalsrud EW. Home parenteral nutrition in infants. J Pediatr 1980; 96:1098–1104.

Chrysomilides SA, Kaminski MV Jr. Home enteral and parenteral nutrition support. Am J Clin Nutr 1981; 34:2271–2275.

Dorney S, Ament ME, Vargas J, et al. Improved survival in very short small bowel of infancy with use of long-term parenteral nutrition. J Pediatr 1985; 107:521–525.

Fleming CR, Lie JY, McCall JT, O'Brien JF, Baille EE, Thistle JT. Selenium deficiency and fatal cardiomyopathy in a patient on home parenteral nutrition. Gastroenterology 1982; 83:689–693.

Freund H, Atamian S, Fischer JE. Chromium deficiency during total parenteral nutrition. JAMA 1979; 241:496–498.

Goode A, Feggetter JG, Hawkins T, Johnston IDA. Use of an elemental diet for long-term nutritional support in Crohn's disease. Lancet 1976; 1:122–124.

Greene HL, Slonim AE, Burr IM, Moran JR. Type I glycogen storage disease: Five years of management with nocturnal intragastric feeding. J Pediatr 1980; 96:590–595.

Howard L, Bigaouette J, Chub R, Krenzer BE, Smith D, Tenny C. Water soluble vitamin requirements in home parenteral nutrition. Am J Clin Nutr 1983; 37:421–428.

Jeejeebhoy KN, Chu RC, Marliss EB, Greenberg GR, Bruce-Robertson A. Chromium deficiency, glucose intolerance, and neuropathy reversed by chromium supplementation in a patient receiving long term parenteral nutrition. Am J Clin Nutr 1977; 30:531–538.

Jeejeebhoy KN, Langer B, Tsallas G, Chu RC, Kukis A, Anderson GH. Total parenteral nutrition at home: Studies in patients surviving 4 months to 5 years. Gastroenterology 1976; 71:943–953.

Karamatsu JT, Boyd AT, Cooke J, Vinall PS, McMahon MJ. Intravenous nutrition during a twin pregnancy. JPEN 1987; 11:499–501.

Kien CL, Kohler E, Goodman SJ, et al. Biotin responsive in vivo carboxylase deficiency in two siblings with secretory diarrhea receiving total parenteral nutrition. J Pediatr 1981; 99:546–550.

Klein GL, Targoff CM, Ament ME, Sherman DJ, Bluestone R, Young JW. Bone disease associated with total parenteral nutrition. Lancet 1980; 2:1041–1044.

Lane HW, Barroso AO, Englert D, Dudrick SJ, MacFayden BS Jr. Selenium status of seven chronic intravenous hyperalimentation patients. JPEN 1982; 6:426–431.

Lifshitz JZ. Home parenteral nutrition. In Lifshitz JZ, ed. Home nutritional therapy. St. Louis: C.V. Mosby, 1987:7–16.

Lifshitz JZ. Personal communication, 1989.

McArdle AH, Palmason C, Morency I, Brown RA. A rationale for enteral feeding as the preferable route for hyperalimentation. Surgery 1981; 90:616–623.

Newmark SR, Simpson S, Beskitt P, et al. Home tube feeding for long term nutritional support. JPEN 1981; 5:76–79.

Nicholas GE, Meng HC, Caldwell WD. Vitamin requirements in patients receiving total parenteral nutrition. Arch Surg 1977; 112:1061–1065.

Ostro MJ, Greenberg GR, Jeejeebhoy KN. Total parenteral nutrition and complete bowel rest in the management of Crohn's disease. JPEN 1985; 9:280–287.

Schneider PJ. The home health care revolution. Nutr Clin Prac 1986; 1:177,–178.

Schuffler MD, Rohrmann CA, Chaffee RG, et al. Chronic intestinal pseudo-obstruction. A report of 27 cases and a review of the literature. Medicine 1981; 60:173–196.

Sedman AB, Klein GL, Merrit RJ, et al. Evidence of aluminum loading in infants receiving intravenous therapy. N Engl J Med 1985; 312:1337–1343.

Shike M, Harrison JE, Sturtridge WC, et al. Metabolic bone disease in patients receiving long-term total parenteral nutrition. Ann Intern Med 1980; 92:343–350.

Starzl TE, Rowe MI, Todo S, et al. Transplantation of multiple abdominal viscera. JAMA 1989; 261:1449–1457.

Tims R. One child's experience with total parenteral nutrition. ASPEN Miami, Jan. 1989.

Vinton NE, Dahlstrom KA, Ament ME. Macrocytosis and pseudo-albinism—New manifestations of selenium deficiency. Clin Res 1986; 34:139A.

Wretlind A. Parenteral nutrition. Nutr Rev 1981; 39:257–265.

30

Medical Ethics of Nutrition Support

Over twenty years ago the medical profession and the public at large were openly confronted with the ethics of using extraordinary means to sustain life in the Karen Ann Quinlan case in New Jersey. Since then, newspapers and courts often debate similar dramas, and many more unresolved cases linger on in hospitals, long-term-care facilities, and homes.

The medical ethics of high-tech nutrition need to be considered by everybody involved with patients in need of such treatment (Hitz & Fenster 1986). Medical science now possesses the capability of sustaining life with nutritional support in cases where, only decades ago, death would have been a certainty. This capability is accompanied by numerous ethical considerations. Modern medicine has realized very definite benefits from high-tech nutrition. However, from the solution may arise a new problem; it is a tragedy that the quality of the life preserved may be less than desirable (Green 1986).

Feeding is an expression of faithfulness to the patient, a symbol of caring and compassion (Miles 1985). Survival is impossible without food and fluids. Withholding such basic and essential needs is sometimes difficult for health care professionals to accept, as they are taught to preserve and nurture life. One of the dilemmas facing the medical profession is in the area of providing nutritional support to the terminally ill, hopeless patient (Boisaubin 1984). It is difficult when faced with such a situation not to do everything technologically possible to provide the nutrition needed.

Courts have generally agreed that there is no legal difference between artificial feeding via gastrostomy, nasogastric tube, or venous routes and any other medical treatment such as intravenous hydration, mechanical respiration, or hemodialysis (Schneidereman & Spragg 1985). Also, there is a clear precedent that allows competent adult patients the right to refuse any treatment, including artificial feeding. Moreover, under appropriate circumstances, a surrogate, often a family member or guardian, may order the termination of artificial feeding on the behalf of an incompetent patient (Annas 1985).

However, there are exceptions to those rules, as in the case of Elizabeth Bouvia, a young woman with cerebral palsy who sought a court injunction to prevent the hospital staff from force-feeding her. She asserted that her paralytic condition prevented her from committing suicide by any other method. The courts did not allow it, as they felt especially responsible for protecting the rights of individuals who are unable to do so themselves.

When dealing with the ethics question, the first decision the physician must make regarding nutrition support or any other method of treatment is whether it is medically indicated; that is, whether it will contribute to preserving the patient's life or alleviate his or her suffering. If it will not, then the indication for such treatment is unjustified. Therefore, it is important that everyone involved understand the type of patient under consideration for treatment.

A brain dead patient is one who has irreversible cessation of all brain functions. By accepted medical standards, to be brain dead is to be considered medically and legally dead. No further treatment is required because the possibility of effective treatment is nonexistent (Wanzer et al 1984).

A persistent vegetative state patient is one in whom the thinking part of the brain as well as most other cerebral functions are largely and irreversibly destroyed. However, some brainstem functions may persist, such as respiration or circulation. When such a state has been documented in a patient, it is morally and legally justifiable to withhold antibiotics, artificial nutrition and hydration, and other life-sustaining treatment, thus permitting death (Dresser 1985).

In all other types of patients, the ethical dilemmas are more complicated. Even in patients who are severely and irreversibly demented, or who have a permanent impairment of competence, the decisions are never easy. This is particularly true in children, where the state of the patient and the chances for recovery are more difficult to ascertain.

It is important to remember that a comatose patient who fails to respond within a couple of weeks after injury has an increasingly slim chance of ever recovering. When a person becomes unconscious, the part that makes that person unique and special is lost; only the biological functions remain. These patients should receive care according to their prior wishes, if known, or if not known, according to their families' wishes. However, the focal point of the decision should be the prospect of a reasonable possibility to return to cognitive and sapient life, as distinguished from forced continuance of a biologic vegetative existence. Prolongation of life should not mean a mere suspension of the act of dying, but it should contemplate, at the very least, a return toward a normally functioning, integrated existence (Wanzer et al 1984).

The terminal patient must also be considered in this discussion. We usually associate terminal with the dying process. It has been defined as "the time in the course of irreversible illness when treatment will no longer influence it" (Miles 1985). If the purpose of nutritional support is to maintain or restore health, it would seem that we have no responsibility in providing support to the terminal patient unless it is requested by the patient or family or if the patient is able to benefit from it in some way (Boisaubin 1984). Once the irreversibility of the illness is imminently certain, the focus changes from prolonging life to postponing death and improving the quality of life.

One main concern in withholding nutrition and fluids is that the caregivers could be seen as directly responsible for the patient's death, which would be comparable to murder in some people's eyes. For someone who is terminally or irreversibly ill and for whom death is unquestionable, it is a matter of allowing that person to die, which in some cases may be more humane (Green 1986). If the decision is made to end the use of extraordinary means of treatment—that is, mechanical ventilation or artificial feedings—all participants in the decision should realize that the patient's death will follow. We believe it is important to medicate such patients before these treatments are withdrawn in order to eliminate the discomfort of agonal efforts on the part of the patient as death ensues. As an unavoidable side effect of the medication, this distress may be shortened to minutes instead of days (Schneiderman & Spragg 1985). The administration of narcotics is morally obligatory and is necessary to keep the patient comfortable. Other medications, such as substances to support blood pressure or cardiac function, are superfluous. Above all, sensitive reactions to the patient's needs for pain relief, communication, and human touch are of utmost importance.

It is often helpful to differentiate between ordinary/extraordinary treatment or benefit/burden when considering what treatment should be given (Lynn & Childress 1983, Curran 1985). This may seem to be a relatively simple procedure, but decisions in these situations are based on more than objective considerations. Personal values, fear of legal liability, monetary burden, and the use of increasingly scarce health care resources can complicate the dilemma. Added to these factors is the expectation that once a treatment is initiated, it will be continued indefinitely. Even conservative, ethical standards state that extraordinary care is not morally obligatory when it is medically futile or when it provides no benefits only prolonging the process of dying without or alleviating suffering.

As these issues evolve, physicians should encourage their patients to have living wills, or should talk with patients and their families to determine their wishes. In the absence of these documents, hospitals, health care providers, and nursing homes may establish an ethics committee to whom these cases may be presented, and a decision can be made that will be in the patient's best interest.

The decision not to nourish and hydrate patients will continue to be a difficult one for patients, family, caregivers, and the courts. Many interests are hanging in the balance, such as the fear of abandonment, decreased levels of care, and the threat of financial hardship. The acceptance of euthanasia is also a problem for all those involved with life-and-death matters. A number of institutions in the Netherlands have developed procedures and policies to enable physicians and health care providers to participate in active euthanasia in an acceptable and controllable manner, however uncomfortable the practice is (Wachter 1989). Only open and ongoing discussion will facilitate greater understanding and, it is hoped, guide us in providing the most humane treatment.

REFERENCES

Annas GJ. Fashion and freedom: When artificial feeding should be withdrawn. Am J Public Health 1985; 75:685–688.

Boisaubin EV. Ethical issues in the nutritional support of the terminal patient. J Am Diet Assoc 1984; 84:529–531.

Curran WJ. Defining appropriate medical care: Providing nutrients and hydration for the dying. N Engl J Med 1985; 313:940–942.

Dresser RS. Discontinuing nutrition support: A review of the case law. J Am Diet Assoc 1985; 85:1289–1292.

Green WP. Nutrition and ethics: A moral dilemma. Am Health Care Assoc 1986; 2:19–21.

Hitz MJ, Fenster K. Medical ethics and nutrition support: The dichotomy of a decision. Nutr Supp Serv 1986; 11:19–21.

Lynn J, Childress JF. Must patients always be given food and water? The Hastings Center Rep 1983; 13:17–21.

Miles SH. The terminally ill elderly: Dealing with the ethics of feeding. Geriatrics 1985; 40:112–120.

Schneiderman LJ, Spragg RG. Ethical decisions in discontinuing mechanical ventilation. N Engl J Med 1985; 318:984–988.

Wachter MAM. Active euthanasia in the Netherlands. JAMA 1989; 262:3316–3319.

Wanzer SH, Adelstein J, Cranford RE, et al. The physician's responsibility toward hopelessly ill patients. N Engl J Med 1984; 310:955–959.

Guide to Tables and Figures

Index